HEPATOBILIARY CANCER

EDITORS

Yuman Fong, MD, FACS
Murray F. Brennan Chair in Surgery
Co-Director, Center for Image-guided Interventions
Member, Departments of Surgery and Radiology
Memorial Sloan-Kettering Cancer Center
Professor of Surgery, Weill Cornell Medical College
New York

Jia-Hong Dong, MD, FACS
Professor and Chairman
Hospital & Institute of Hepatobiliary Surgery
Chinese PLA General Hospital
Chinese PLA Medical Postgraduate School
Beijing, China

SECTION EDITORS

Ghassan K. Abou-Alfa, MD
Associate Member
Memorial Sloan-Kettering Cancer Center
Associate Professor, Weill Cornell Medical College
New York

Gary E. Deng, MD, PhD
Associate Member, Attending Physician
Integrative Medicine Service
Memorial Sloan-Kettering Cancer Center
New York

Damian E. Dupuy, MD, FACR
Director of Tumor Ablation at Rhode Island Hospital
Professor of Diagnostic Imaging
The Warren Alpert Medical School of Brown University
Providence, Rhode Island

2014
People's Medical Publishing House - USA
Shelton, Connecticut

People's Medical Publishing House-USA
2 Enterprise Drive, Suite 509
Shelton, CT 06484
Tel: 203-402-0646
Fax: 203-402-0854
E-mail: info@pmph-usa.com

© 2014 PMPH-USA, LTD

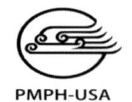

All rights reserved. Without limiting the rights under copyright reserved above, no part of this publication may be reproduced, stored in or introduced into a retrieval system, or transmitted, in any form or by any means (electronic, mechanical, photocopying, recording, or otherwise), without the prior written permission of the publisher.

14 15 16 17/Sheridan/9 8 7 6 5 4 3 2 1

ISBN-13	978-1-60795-016-5
ISBN-10	1-60795-016-2
eISBN-13	978-1-60795-222-0

Printed in the United States of America by Sheridan Books, Inc.
Editor: Carole Wonsiewicz; Copyeditor/Typesetter: diacriTech; Cover designer: Mary McKeon

Library of Congress Cataloging-in-Publication Data
Hepatobiliary cancer (Fong)
  Hepatobiliary cancer / [edited by] Yuman Fong, Jia-Hong Dong ; section editors, Ghassan K. Abou-Alfa, Gary Deng, Damian E. Dupuy.
    p. ; cm.
  Includes bibliographical references.
  ISBN-13: 978-1-60795-016-5
  ISBN-10: 1-60795-016-2
  ISBN-13: 978-1-60795-222-0 (eISBN)
  I. Fong, Yuman, editor of compilation. II. Dong, Jia-Hong, editor of compilation. III. Abou-Alfa, Ghassan K., editor. IV. Deng, Gary, editor. V. Dupuy, Damian E., editor. VI. Title.
  [DNLM: 1. Liver Neoplasms—diagnosis. 2. Biliary Tract Neoplasms—diagnosis. 3. Biliary Tract Neoplasms—therapy. 4. Liver Neoplasms—therapy. WI 735]
  RC280.L5
  616.99'436—dc23
                                           2013035047

Sales and Distribution

Canada
Login Canada
300 Saulteaux Cr., Winnipeg, MB
R3J 3T2
Phone: 1.800.665.1148
Fax: 1.800.665.0103
www.lb.ca

Foreign Rights
John Scott & Company
International Publisher's Agency
P.O. Box 878
Kimberton, PA 19442
USA
Tel: 610-827-1640
Fax: 610-827-1671

Japan
United Publishers Services Limited
1-32-5 Higashi-Shinagawa
Shinagawa-ku, Tokyo 140-0002
Japan
Tel: 03-5479-7251
Fax: 03-5479-7307
Email: kakimoto@ups.co.jp

United Kingdom, Europe, Middle East, Africa
Eurospan Limited
3, Henrietta Street, Covent
Garden,
London WC2E 8LU, UK
Within the UK: 0800 526830
Outside the UK: +44 (0)20 7845 0868
http://www.eurospanbookstore.com

Singapore, Thailand, Philippines, Indonesia, Vietnam, Pacific Rim, Korea
McGraw-Hill Education
60 Tuas Basin Link
Singapore 638775
Tel: 65-6863-1580
Fax: 65-6862-3354
www.mcgraw-hill.com.sg

Australia, New Zealand
Elsevier Australia
Locked Bag 7500
Chatswood DC NSW 2067
Australia
Tel: 161 (2) 9422-8500
Fax: 161 (2) 9422-8562
www.elsevier.com.au

Brazil
SuperPedido Tecmedd
Beatriz Alves, Foreign Trade Department
R. Sansao Alves dos Santos, 102 | 7th floor
Brooklin Novo
Sao Paolo 04571-090
Brazil
Tel: 55-16-3512-5539
www.superpedidotecmedd.com.br

India, Bangladesh, Pakistan, Sri Lanka, Malaysia
CBS Publishers
4819/X1 Prahlad Street 24
Ansari Road, Darya Ganj, New Delhi-110002
India
Tel: 91-11-23266861/67
Fax: 91-11-23266818
Email:cbspubs@vsnl.com

People's Republic of China
People's Medical Publishing House
International Trade Department
No. 19, Pan Jia Yuan Nan Li
Chaoyang District
Beijing 100021
P.R. China
Tel: 8610-67653342
Fax: 8610-67691034
www.pmph.com/en/

Notice: The authors and publisher have made every effort to ensure that the patient care recommended herein, including choice of drugs and drug dosages, is in accord with the accepted standard and practice at the time of publication. However, since research and regulation constantly change clinical standards, the reader is urged to check the product information sheet included in the package of each drug, which includes recommended doses, warnings, and contraindications. This is particularly important with new or infrequently used drugs. Any treatment regimen, particularly one involving medication, involves inherent risk that must be weighed on a case-by-case basis against the benefits anticipated. The reader is cautioned that the purpose of this book is to inform and enlighten; the information contained herein is not intended as, and should not be employed as, a substitute for individual diagnosis and treatment.

DEDICATION

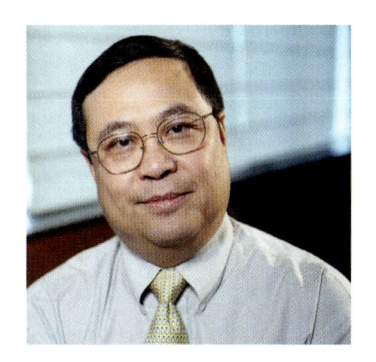

This book is dedicated to Stephen Lowry who passed away suddenly and tragically in 2011. He was past Chairman of Surgery at the University of Medicine and Dentistry of New Jersey and one of the major figures in surgical oncology. His contributions to surgical oncology, to the understanding of infection and sepsis, and to education are too numerous to list. He was the best educator, researcher, teacher, role model, and friend. He is sorely missed.

YUMAN FONG

Stephen F. Lowry, MD, MBA, FACS, FRCS (Ed.) (Hon)
November 1, 1947 – June 4, 2011

A pre-eminent surgeon-scientist and expert in inflammation and inflammatory disorders, he served as Richard Harvey Professor and Chair of the Department of Surgery and Senior Associate Dean for Education at the University of Medicine and Dentistry of New Jersey-Robert Wood Johnson Medical School in New Brunswick. He was instrumental in creating and leading the Division of Surgical Sciences which focuses on core research issues of inflammation and developmental biology and the interfaces among science, technology, and clinical medicine.

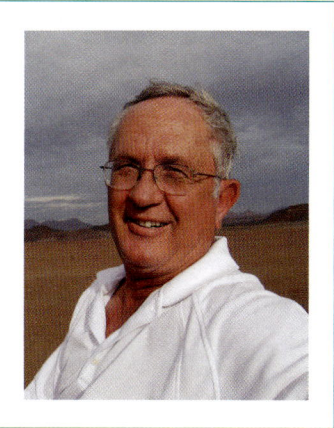

CONTENTS

Preface ix

Author listing xi

Section I: Biliary Tumors (Yuman Fong) — 1

1. Hilar Cholangiocarcinoma — 3
Aram Demirjian, Steven C. Cunningham & Timothy M. Pawlik

2. Peripheral Cholangiocarcinoma — 23
Sachin Patil & Ronald S. Chamberlain

3. Gallbladder Cancer — 61
Anu Behari & Vinay K. Kapoor

Section II: Liver Tumors (Jia-Hong Dong) — 89

4. Benign Liver Lesions — 91
Daniel E. Abbott & David Bentrem

5. Primary Hepatic Malignancies — 111
Jia-Hong Dong

6. Colorectal Cancer Liver Metastases — 137
T. Peter Kingham & Yuman Fong

7. Metastatic Neuroendocrine Tumors to the Liver — 157
Saboor Khan, David M. Nagorney & Florencia G. Que

8. The Role of Liver-Directed Therapy for Noncolorectal, Non-neuroendocrine Liver Metastasis — 177
Junaid Haroon & Ronald S. Chamberlain

9. Surgical Resection for Non-colorectal, Non-neuroendocrine Liver Metastases — 211
Christoph Kahlert & Jergen Weitz

Section III: Diagnosis (Yuman Fong) — 221

10. Imaging of Hepatobiliary Cancer: Ultrasonography, CT, PET-CT, and MRI — 223
Thorsten Persigehl & Lawrence H. Schwartz

v

11. Diagnostic and Therapeutic Approaches for Patients With Liver Tumors 247
Kimberly Moore Dalal

Section IV: Surgical Therapies (Yuman Fong) 267

12. Techniques for Hepatic Resection 269
Clifford S. Cho

13. Liver Transplantation for Malignant Tumors 293
Vatche G. Agopian & Henrik Petrowsky

Section V: Ablative Therapies (Damian E. Dupuy) 317

14. Ablation Therapy for Hepatocellular Carcinoma 319
Jason D. Iannuccilli & Damian E. Dupuy

15. Transcatheter Ablative Therapy for Liver Tumors 355
Karen T. Brown & Anne M. Covey

16. High Intensity Focused Ultrasound for Liver Tumors 369
Kelvin K. Ng

17. Radiotherapy for Liver Cancers 377
Guo-Liang Jiang & Jian-Dong Zhao

18. Yttrium-90 Microsphere Radiomicrosphere Therapy of Hepatic Malignancies 391
Seza A. Gulec, Tushar C. Barot & Yuman Fong

Section VI: Systemic and Regional Chemotherapies and Biologic Therapies (Ghassan K. Abou-Alfa) 411

19. Systemic Chemotherapy for Hepatocellular Carcinoma 413
Syed A. Hussain & Daniel H. Palmer

20. Intraarterial Chemotherapy for Liver Tumors 425
Maeve A. Lowery & Nancy E. Kemeny

21. Novel Therapeutics for Liver Tumors 437
Ghassan K. Abou-Alfa, Celina Ang & Eileen M. O'Reilly

22. Immunotherapies for Liver Tumors 453
Tetsuya Nakatsura & Yusuke Nakamura

Section VII: Complementary Therapies and Supportive Care (Gary E. Deng) — 475

23. Integrative Oncology: Complementary Therapies in Cancer Care — 477
Gary E. Deng & Barrie R. Cassileth

24. Natural Medicine and Complementary and Alternative Therapy in Primary Liver Cancer: Scientific Research and Clinical Applications — 493
Hao Chen & Zhiqiang Meng

Index — 503

PREFACE

Liver and biliary malignancies remain common causes of cancer deaths worldwide. The associated liver parenchymal injury from viral hepatitis and other diseases make such malignancies particularly difficult to manage. Until recently, most cases of liver or biliary malignancies resulted in fatality. Over the last two decades great strides have been made in the treatment of these cancers. These improvements have come not only in surgery, radiation therapy and chemotherapy, but also from advances in interventional oncology and integrative medicine. The modern approach for treatment of these malignancies is truly a successful multidisciplinary collaboration with a resultant improvement in prolongation of life, relief of symptoms, and cure.

The current textbook reflects the multi-disciplinary nature of the field of hepatobiliary cancer. It represents a collaboration of world authorities in surgery, chemotherapy, radiation therapy, medical oncology, and integrative medicine. The book begins with a concise discussion of the major tumor types of hepatobiliary cancers before moving on to diagnosis and detailed discussions of individual therapies. These chapters summarize not only the state-of-the-art in the field but also potential directions for future evolution. Algorithms of care combining the various treatment modalities are presented throughout.

Three decades ago a diagnosis of liver or biliary cancer was most often a hopeless diagnosis with few treatment options, but today there are an abundance of effective therapies. These range from potentially curative surgery by resection or transplantation, to life-prolonging, minimally invasive therapies used by interventional oncologists, to palliative procedures in integrative medicine, radiation oncology, and medical oncology. The sum of these therapies provides significant prolongation of quality of life. As a concise summary of the present state-of-the art, our book is designed to be sufficiently comprehensive for expert practitioners, but also useful for students and educators.

We thank each world-recognized authority who authored a chapter, and our three section editors: Ghassan Abou-Alfa, Damian Dupuy, and Gary Deng. Their valuable contributions to the field and the book are gratefully appreciated. We also thank Carole and Martin Wonsiewicz from Peoples Medical Publishing for their tireless efforts in organizing and producing this book. We are especially indebted to our brave patients who have educated us daily on these disease processes, and allowed us to study treatments and outcomes by their data. Our sincere hope is that this valuable information will contribute to the improvement of care for the next generation of patients. Finally, we thank our families for giving us support and allowing us the time not only to participate in clinical care but to engage in these academic efforts that will continue to educate the next generation of caregivers of the infirmed.

Yuman Fong
Jia-Hong Dong

AUTHOR LISTING

Daniel E. Abbott, MD
Assistant Professor of Surgery
Division of Surgical Oncology
Department of Surgery, University of Cincinnati
Cincinnati, Ohio
Chapter 4: Benign Liver Lesions

Ghassan K. Abou-Alfa, MD
Associate Member
Gastrointestinal Oncology Service
Memorial Sloan-Kettering Cancer Center
Associate Professor, Weill Cornell Medical College
New York, NY
Chapter 21: Novel Therapeutics for Liver Tumors

Vatche G. Agopian, MD
Assistant Professor of Surgery
Division of Liver and Pancreas Transplantation
Department of Surgery
David Geffen School of Medicine
University of California
Los Angeles, California
Chapter 13: Liver Transplantation for Malignant Tumors

Celina Ang, MD
Fellow, Medical Oncology
Memorial Sloan-Kettering Cancer Center
New York, NY
Chapter 21: Novel Therapeutics for Liver Tumors

Tushar C. Barot, MD
Research Fellow
Department of Surgical Oncology and Radiology/Nuclear Medicine
Florida International University College of Medicine
Miami, Florida
Chapter 18: Yttrium-90 Microsphere Radiomicrosphere Therapy of Hepatic Malignancies

Anu Behari, MS
Assistant Professor
Department of Surgical Gastroenterology
Sanjay Gandhi Post-Graduate Institute of Medical Sciences
Lucknow, INDIA
Chapter 3: Gallbladder Cancer

David Bentrem, MD, MSCI
Associate Professor
Department of Surgery
Feinberg School of Medicine
Northwestern University
Chicago, Illinois
Chapter 4: Benign Liver Lesions

Karen T. Brown, MD, FSIR
Professor of Clinical Radiology
Weill Medical College of Cornell University
Memorial Sloan-Kettering Cancer Center
New York, NY
Chapter 15: Transcatheter Ablative Therapy for Liver Tumors

Barrie R. Cassileth, PhD
Laurance S. Rockefeller Chair in Integrative Medicine
Chief, Integrative Medicine Service
Memorial Sloan-Kettering Cancer Center
New York, NY
Chapter 23: Integrative Oncology: Complementary Therapies in Cancer Care

Ronald S. Chamberlain, MD, MPA, FACS
Chairman and Surgeon-in-Chief
Department of Surgery
Saint Barnabas Medical Center
Livingston, New Jersey
Professor of Surgery
University of Medicine and Dentistry of New Jersey
Newark, New Jersey
Chapter 2: Peripheral Cholangiocarcinoma
Chapter 8: The Role of Liver-Directed Therapy for Non-colorectal, Non-neuroendocrine Liver Metastasis

Hao Chen, MD
International Center of Integrative Oncology
Fudan University Cancer Hospital
Shanghai, China
Chapter 24: Natural Medicine and Complementary and Alternative Therapy in Primary Liver Cancer: Scientific Research and Clinical Applications

Clifford S. Cho, MD, FACS
Associate Professor, Department of Surgery
Section of Surgical Oncology
University of Wisconsin School of Medicine and Public Health
Madison, Wisconsin
Chapter 12: Techniques for Hepatic Resection

Anne M. Covey MD, FSIR
Associate Professor of Radiology
Memorial Sloan-Kettering Cancer Center
New York, NY
Chapter 15: Transcatheter Ablative Therapy for Liver Tumors

Steven C. Cunningham, MD, FACS
Co-Director of Pancreatic and Hepatobiliary Surgery
Saint Agnes Hospital Center
Baltimore, Maryland
Chapter 1: Hilar Cholangiocarcinoma

Kimberly Moore Dalal, MD
Medical Director, Surgical Oncology
Palo Alto Medical Foundation
Mills-Peninsula Division, Department of Surgery
Burlingame, California
Chapter 11: Diagnostic and Therapeutic Approaches for Patients With Liver Tumors

Aram Demirjian, MD
Assistant Professor, Department of Surgery
Division of Hepatobiliary and Pancreatic Surgery
University of California
Irvine, California
Chapter 1: Hilar Cholangiocarcinoma

Gary E. Deng, MD, PhD
Associate Member/Attending Physician
Integrative Medicine Service
Memorial Sloan-Kettering Cancer Center
New York, NY
Chapter 23: Integrative Oncology: Complementary Therapies in Cancer Care

Jia-Hong Dong, MD, FACS
Professor and Chairman
Hospital and Institute of Hepatobiliary Surgery
Chinese PLA General Hospital
Chinese PLA Medical Postgraduate School
Beijing, CHINA
Chapter 5: Primary Hepatic Malignancies

Damian E. Dupuy, MD, FACR
Director of Tumor Ablation
Rhode Island Hospital
Professor of Diagnostic Imaging
The Warren Alpert Medical School of Brown University
Providence, Rhode Island
Chapter 14: Ablation Therapy for Hepatocellular Carcinoma

Yuman Fong, MD, FACS
Murray F. Brennan Chair in Surgery
Co-Director, Center for Image-guided Interventions
Member, Departments of Surgery and Radiology
Memorial Sloan-Kettering Cancer Center
Professor of Surgery
Weill Cornell Medical College
New York, NY
Chapter 6: Colorectal Cancer Liver Metastases
Chapter 18: Yttrium-90 Microsphere Radiomicrosphere Therapy of Hepatic Malignancies

Seza A. Gulec, MD, FACS
Professor of Surgery
Department of Surgical Oncology and Radiology/Nuclear Medicine
Florida International University College of Medicine
Miami, Florida
Chapter 18: Yttrium-90 Microsphere Radiomicrosphere Therapy of Hepatic Malignancies

Junaid Haroon, MD
Department of Surgery
Saint Barnabas Medical Center
Livingston, New Jersey
Chapter 8: The Role of Liver-Directed Therapy for Non-colorectal, Non-neuroendocrine Liver Metastasis

Syed A. Hussain, MD
Clinical Senior Lecturer and Consultant in Medical Oncology
Department of Molecular and Clinical Cancer Medicine
University of Liverpool
Liverpool, UNITED KINGDOM
Chapter 19: Systemic Chemotherapy for Hepatocellular Carcinoma

Jason D. Iannuccilli, MD
Assistant Professor Diagnostic and Interventional Radiology
The Alpert Medical School of Brown University
Providence, Rhode Island
Chapter 14: Ablation Therapy for Hepatocellular Carcinoma

Guo-Liang Jiang, MD, FACR (Hon)
Department of Radiation Oncology
Fudan University Shanghai Cancer Center
Shanghia, CHINA
Chapter 17: Radiotherapy for Liver Cancers

Christoph Kahlert, MD
Surgical Fellow
Department of General, Visceral and Thoracic Surgery
University of Dresden
Dresden, GERMANY
Chapter 9: Surgical Resection for Non-colorectal, Non-neuroendocrine Liver Metastases

Vinay K. Kapoor, MS, FRCS, FACS, FACG
Professor of Surgical Gastroenterology
Sanjay Gandhi Post-Graduate Institute of Medical Sciences (SGPGIMS)
Lucknow UP, INDIA
Chapter 3: Gallbladder Cancer

Nancy E. Kemeny, MD
Attending, Department of Medicine
Gastrointestinal Oncology Service
Memorial Sloan Kettering Cancer Center
Professor of Medicine
Weill Cornell Medical College
New York, NY
Chapter 20: Intraarterial Chemotherapy for Liver Tumors

Saboor Khan, PhD, FRCS, FACS
Consultant Hepatobiliary Pancreatic and General Surgeon
University Hospitals Coventry and Warwickshire
Coventry, UNITED KINGDOM
Formerly HPB Scholar, Mayo Clinic
Rochester, Minnesota
Chapter 7: Metastatic Neuroendocrine Tumors to the Liver

T. Peter Kingham, MD
Assistant Professor, Division of Hepatopancreatobiliary Surgery
Department of Surgery
Memorial Sloan-Kettering Cancer Center,
New York, NY
Chapter 6: Colorectal Cancer Liver Metastases

Maeve A. Lowery, MD
Department of Medicine,
Gastrointestinal Oncology Service
Memorial Sloan-Kettering Cancer Center
New York, NY
Chapter 20: Intraarterial Chemotherapy for Liver Tumors

Zhiqiang Meng, MD, PhD
Associate Professor and Director,
Department of Integrative Oncology
International Center of Integrative Oncology
Fudan University Cancer Hospital
Shanghai, CHINA
Chapter 24: Natural Medicine and Complementary and Alternative Therapy in Primary Liver Cancer: Scientific Research and Clinical Applications

David M. Nagorney, MD
Professor of Surgery
Division of General Surgery
Mayo Clinic College of Medicine
Rochester, Minnesota
Chapter 7: Metastatic Neuroendocrine Tumors to the Liver

Yusuke Nakamura, MD, PhD
Professor of Department of Medicine
Section of Hematology/Oncology
Professor of Department of Surgery
Deputy Director, Center for Personalized Therapeutics
Knapp Center for Biomedical Discovery
Pritzker School of Medicine
University of Chicago
Chicago, Illinois
Chapter 22: Immunotherapies for Liver Tumors

Tetsuya Nakatsura, MD, PhD
Chief, Division of Cancer Immunotherapy
Research Center for Innovative Oncology
National Cancer Center Hospital East
Kashiwa, JAPAN
Chapter 22: Immunotherapies for Liver Tumors

Kelvin K. Ng, MS, PhD, FRCS Ed (Gen)
Honorary Clinical Associate Professor
Department of Surgery
The University of Hong Kong
Hong Kong, CHINA
Chapter 16: High Intensity Focused Ultrasound for Liver Tumors

Eileen M. O'Reilly, MD
Associate Attending Physician
Gastrointestinal Oncology Service
Memorial Sloan-Kettering Cancer Center
Associate Professor
Weill Cornell Medical College
New York, NY
Chapter 21: Novel Therapeutics for Liver Tumors

Daniel H. Palmer, MD
Professor of Medical Oncology
University of Liverpool
Liverpool, UNITED KINGDOM
Chapter 19: Systemic Chemotherapy for Hepatocellular Carcinoma

Sachin Patil, MD
Surgical Research Fellow
Saint Barnabas Medical Center
Livingston, New Jersey
Chapter 2: Peripheral Cholangiocarcinoma

Timothy M. Pawlik, MD, MPH, PhD, FACS
Professor of Surgery and Oncology
Chief, Division of Surgical Oncology
John L. Cameron M.D. Professor of Alimentary Tract Diseases
Director, Johns Hopkins Medicine Liver Tumor Center Multi-Disciplinary Clinic
Johns Hopkins Hospital
Baltimore, Maryland
Chapter 1: Hilar Cholangiocarcinoma

Thorsten Persigehl, MD
Department of Radiology
Columbia University Medicine Center
New York
Department of Radiology
University Hospital Cologne
Cologne, GERMANY
Chapter 10: Imaging of Hepatobiliary Cancer: Ultrasonography, CT, PET-CT, and MRI

Henrik Petrowsky, MD
Professor of Surgery and Vice Chair
Section Head of Hepato-Pancreato-Biliary Surgery
Swiss HPB and Transplant Center
Department of Surgery University Hospital
Zurich, SWITZERLAND
Chapter 13: Liver Transplantation for Malignant Tumors

Florencia G. Que, MD, FACS
Associate Professor of Surgery
Mayo Clinic College of Medicine
Rochester, Minnesota
Chapter 7: Metastatic Neuroendocrine Tumors to the Liver

Lawrence H. Schwartz, MD
Chairman, Department of Radiology
Columbia University Medical Center (CUMC)
New York
Chapter 10: Imaging of Hepatobiliary Cancer: Ultrasonography, CT, PET-CT, and MRI

Jergen Weitz, MD
Chairman Department of Visceral, Thoracic and Vascular Surgery
University Hospital Carl Gustav Carus of the Technical University
Dresden, GERMANY
Chapter 9: Surgical Resection for Non-colorectal, Non-neuroendocrine Liver Metastases

Jian-Dong Zhao, MD
Department of Radiation Oncology
Fudan University Shanghai Cancer Center
Shanghia, CHINA
Chapter 17: Radiotherapy for Liver Cancers

SECTION I

Biliary Tumors

Yuman Fong

CHAPTER 1

Hilar Cholangiocarcinoma

Aram Demirjian, Steven C. Cunningham & Timothy M. Pawlik

Cholangiocarcinoma is a primary tumor that arises from the ductal epithelium of the biliary tree. Cholangiocarcinoma, first reported by Durand-Fardel[1] in 1840, remains a relatively uncommon cancer that accounts for approximately 3% of all gastrointestinal cancers worldwide.[2,3] The vast majority (~90%) of cholangiocarcinoma lesions are adenocarcinomas,[4] with <5% being of squamous cell origin. Although cholangiocarcinoma can arise from anywhere in the biliary tree, most cholangiocarcinomas arise in the extrahepatic tree. Specifically, although 5%–15% of cholangiocarcinomas are intrahepatic in location, 20%–30% can be found in the distal common bile duct and 60%–70% arise at the bifurcation of the right and left hepatic ducts.[4–6] The subset of cholangiocarcinoma lesions that involve the confluence of the right and left hepatic ducts are known as "hilar" or "Klatskin" tumors, named after the Yale physician who brought wider attention to this tumor in 1965.[7] We herein review the epidemiology, preoperative workup, as well as surgical management and outcome of patients with hilar cholangiocarcinoma. Adjuvant therapy including systemic and radiotherapy is reviewed, as well as palliative approaches to the patient with unresectable hilar cholangiocarcinoma.

Epidemiology and Risk Factors

Although most cholangiocarcinoma lesions arise in the extrahepatic biliary tree, the worldwide incidence of extrahepatic cholangiocarcinoma is decreasing in contrast with the incidence of intrahepatic cholangiocarcinoma that is on the rise (Figure 1-1).[4,8] For example, in the United States, the age-adjusted incidence of extrahepatic cholangiocarcinoma has decreased from 1.08 per 100,000 to 0.82 per 100,000 individuals over a 20-year period.[9,10] A similar decrease in the incidence of extrahepatic cholangiocarcinoma has also been reported in other countries worldwide.[3,9,10] Epidemiologic data on the incidence of hilar cholangiocarcinoma are complicated by the fact that some registry–based studies either have not traditionally included hilar cholangiocarcinoma or have classified Klatskin tumors as intrahepatic.[9] In addition, in some instances, data for extrahepatic cholangiocarcinoma have been combined with gallbladder cancer for the purposes of ICD coding.[3,9] Despite these shortcomings, the decreasing incidence of extrahepatic cholangiocarcinoma appears genuine, although the reasons for this remain unclear.

A number of risk factors can predispose an individual to hilar cholangiocarcinoma. Hilar cholangiocarcinoma is more common in men with a reported age-adjusted incidence in the United States of 1.2 per 100,000 for men versus 0.8 per 100,000 per women.[11] The risk of hilar cholangiocarcinoma also increases with age as most patients are diagnosed in the seventh decade of life. Additional risk factors include history of sclerosing cholangitis, hepatolithiasis, choledochal cysts, thorotrast exposure, parasitic infection (e.g., *Opisthorcosis viverrini*), viral hepatitis, and cirrhosis. Primary

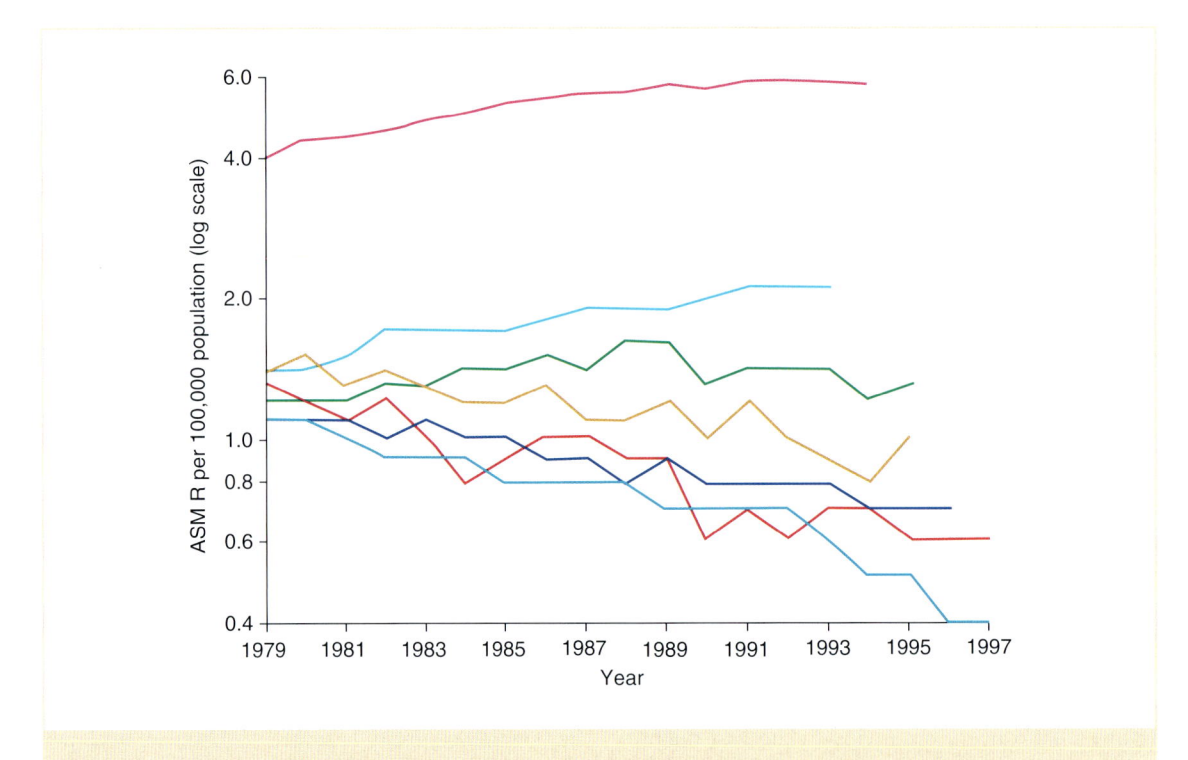

Figure 1-1: International age-standardized mortality for extrahepatic cholangiocarcinoma. Reprinted from Khan SA, Thomas HC, Davidson BR, Taylor- Robinson SD.*Lancet*. 2005;366:1303–1314 with permission from Elsevier Inc © 2005.[4]

sclerosing cholangitis (PSC) is one of the most well-established and strongest factors is associated with hilar cholangiocarcinoma. Patients with PSC are at risk for developing hilar cholangiocarcinoma at an earlier age with a median diagnosis in the fifth decade of life.[12,13] In fact, the lifetime risk of cholangiocarcinoma may be as high as 10%–20% among patients with PSC.[14,15] Although PSC may play a larger role in risk of hilar cholangiocarcinoma in Western countries, parasitic infections and choledochal cysts may be a more important risk factor in Eastern countries where these conditions are more common. In one study from Thailand, patients with a past or present infection with *O. viverrini* were noted to have a nearly fivefold (odds ratio = 4.8) increased risk of cholangiocarcinoma.[16] Choledochal cysts, in which there is congenital cystic dilation of the bile duct, has been reported to have a 5%–30% lifetime risk of cholangiocarcinoma,[17,18] probably secondary to bile stasis and long-standing inflammation inducing carcinogenesis within the bile duct epithelium.[19]

Overall, data on trends in extrahepatic cholangiocarcinoma-associated mortality have shown a decrease in age-adjusted mortality rates. Over a 20-year period from 1979 to 1998, the age-adjusted mortality rate for extrahepatic cholangiocarcinoma in the United States was reported to decrease from 0.6 per 100,000 to 0.3 per 100,000.[3,10] Utilizing the Surveillance Epidemiology and End Results database, Nathan et al. reported on 2107 patients with extrahepatic cholangiocarcinoma who had undergone resection from 1973 to 2002.[20] In this study, multivariate modeling of survival after surgery for extrahepatic cholangiocarcinoma revealed a 23.3% increase in adjusted survival in each decade studied, resulting in a cumulative 53.7% improvement from 1973 through 2002. Similar trends in improved mortality related to extrahepatic cholangiocarcinoma have been note in other countries worldwide including Australia, France, and England. For unclear reasons, however, the age-adjusted mortality associated with extrahepatic cholangiocarcinoma was noted to increase over the same period in other countries such as Japan.[3]

Preoperative Evaluation

Clinical Presentation and Diagnostic Workup

Although intrahepatic cholangiocarcinoma often presents with no or minimal signs or symptoms, hilar cholangiocarcinoma usually presents in a jaundiced patient. Other symptoms may include weight loss, pale stools, dark urine, and pruritus.[21] Cholangitis is an uncommon presentation. Although most patients with a hilar strictures and jaundice have cholangiocarcinoma,[22] up to 20% of patients with this clinical presentation will have either another malignancy causing obstruction of the hepatic confluence or a benign biliary stricture.[23,24] Definitive diagnosis of a hilar cholangiocarcinoma can be difficult, especially in patients with a history of PSC-associated strictures. Other possible diagnoses in the differential include choledocholithiasis, iatrogenic bile duct strictures, and gallbladder cancer, among others. Because of the notorious difficulty in definitively diagnosing hilar cholangiocarcinoma, the clinician must maintain a high index of suspicion and have a low threshold to initiate further investigative studies.

In addition to ascertaining any possible risk factors for hilar cholangiocarcinoma in the patient's medical history, laboratory examinations including liver panel and tumor markers such as carbohydrate antigen (CA) 19-9 and carcinoembryonic antigen (CEA) should be obtained. Patients with hilar cholangiocarcinoma and obstruction of the hepatic duct confluence generally have an elevation in serum bilirubin and alkaline phosphatase. The overall accuracy of tumor markers for diagnosing hilar cholangiocarcinoma remains somewhat poor. The sensitivity and specificity of CA 19-9 have been reported to be 76% and 92%, respectively, in differentiating nonmalignant versus malignant bile duct strictures.[25] In one study, patients with higher CA 19-9 levels were more likely to have unresectable cholangiocarcinoma at the time of staging. CA 19-9, however, can also be elevated in the setting of other malignancies such as pancreatic cancer, and less commonly, colorectal or gastric cancer. In addition, CA 19-9 levels may be affected by serum bilirubin levels. As most patients with a hilar stricture present with elevated serum bilirubin levels, CA 19-9 should be reassessed after biliary drainage. Although CEA is primarily a tumor marker of colorectal cancer, some reports have suggested that an increase in both CEA and CA 19-9 may increase the detection rate of cholangiocarcinoma.[26]

Cross-Sectional Imaging

Transabdominal ultrasound is often the first imaging test employed for patients presenting with jaundice due to its low cost, low risk, and ready availability.[27] Ultrasound can evaluate hepatic blood flow when combined with Doppler (duplex) imaging and can help identify intrahepatic biliary dilation in the absence of a dilated common bile duct, which may suggest a hilar biliary obstruction.[27] Ultrasound alone, however, is inadequate, and cross-sectional imaging should always be obtained when a patient presents with jaundice and any suspicion of a hilar lesion.

Cross-sectional imaging includes multiphase, contrast-enhanced computed tomography (CT) or magnetic resonance imaging with cholangiopancreatography (MRI/MRCP). High-quality cross-sectional imaging is critical for both diagnosis and planning of treatment. If possible, it is best to obtain cross-sectional imaging before placement of a biliary stent to facilitate better assessment of the biliary stricture in the absence of a foreign body. In this way, imaging can better evaluate the biliary ductal system, level of obstruction, and extent of tumor involvement. Hilar vascular structures such as the hepatic artery and portal vein must be carefully inspected to determine anatomic variants and associated tumor involvement. Vascular encasement, as well as long-standing biliary obstruction, can cause an "atrophy-hypertrophy" complex resulting in segmental or hemi-liver atrophy and compensatory contralateral hepatic hypertrophy. In fact, up to 30% of patients undergoing operative exploration for hilar cholangiocarcinoma demonstrate some degree of lobar atrophy.[28] On cross-sectional imaging, evidence of locoregional adenopathy can sometimes be detected.[29]

High-quality multiphase (liver/pancreas-protocol) CT allows for rapid high-resolution scanning with fewer motion artifacts compared with MRI. For patients being elevated for a hilar stricture/mass, CT should include the use of thin collimation in the arterial, portal venous, and equilibrium or delayed phases.[29] CT data should be reconstructed with 1–5 mm slice thickness for axial images, and coronal images should also be routinely included, as this may more optimally display the imaging findings and delineate anatomic relationships for surgical planning.[30] CT characteristics of hilar cholangiocarcinoma can be variable with hilar cholangiocarcinoma appearing as either an ill-defined or a focal mass. In general, hilar cholangiocarcinoma often appears initially hypovascular with more heterogeneous hypervascular enhancement on the delayed images.[29] The accuracy of CT to detect cholangiocarcinoma varies between 75% and 100%.[29,31] Unno and colleagues reported that the accuracy of CT to define the extent of tumor spread along the axis of the bile duct was 80%, whereas the accuracy for diagnosing extension into the hepatic parenchyma and vascular structures was 100%.[32] Other studies have reported an accuracy of 86% and 93%, respectively, for CT to predict portal venous and hepatic artery invasion.[33] In a study by Aloia et al., the authors reported that high-resolution CT could predict resectability with a sensitivity and specificity of 94% and 79%, respectively, and a negative and positive predictive value of 92% and 85%, respectively.[34] This study, however, suffered from a small sample size ($n = 32$) making definitive conclusions difficult.

In recent years, MRI and MRCP have gained increasing use in diagnosing and determining resectability of hilar cholangiocarcinoma.[35,36] MRI can help identify the site of biliary ductal narrowing and evaluate for choledocho- and hepatolithiasis, as well as the extent of vascular involvement. On cross-sectional MR images, hilar cholangiocarcinoma often appears as hypointense to the liver on T1-weighted images and moderately intense with a high signal on T2-weighted images.[37] The majority of lesions are hypovascular compared with the adjacent liver parenchyma with a heterogeneous enhancement that increases on delayed images.[36,37] MRCP can accurately reflect the anatomic changes of the bile duct. The acquired cholangiographic images obtained at MRCP have been reported to be comparable to more invasive procedures such as endoscopic retrograde cholangiopancreatography (ERCP) or percutaneous transhepatic cholangiography (PTC).[38,39] In fact, MRCP may be preferable to ERCP or PTC because of its noninvasive nature and because it allows visualization of both the obstructed and nonobstructed ducts (Figure 1-2). In addition, MRI provides information about lobar atrophy, locoregional extension of disease, and distant metastasis. The overall accuracy of MRI/MRCP to detect cholangiocarcinoma ranges from 80% to 95%,[31,40,41] with the sensitivity of MRCP to detect radial extension ranging from 71% to 96%.[37,42,43] Although MRI/MRCP may be considered to be the imaging technique of choice for bile duct cancers, some data have suggested that MRCP and CT are equally accurate in evaluating the biliary ductal extension of hilar cholangiocarcinoma. Cho and colleagues reported that among operated patients, the diagnostic accuracy of MRCP was 71% versus 64% for CT ($P = 0.93$).[42] Although the authors concluded that MRCP and CT were equivalent, the small number of patients in the study ($n = 33$) may have contributed to a type II statistical error, making

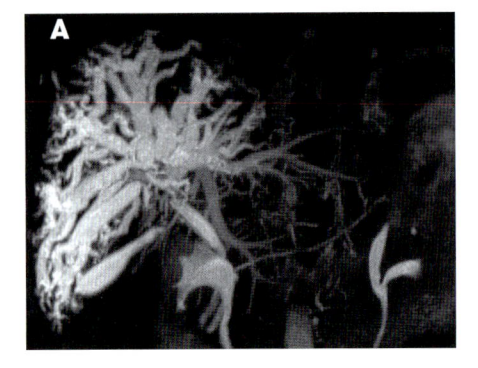

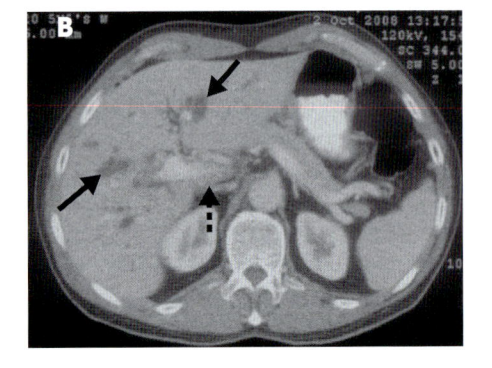

Figure 1-2: (A) MR cholangiopancreatography demonstrating hilar obstruction secondary to tumor with associated biliary dilatation. (B) Axial computed tomography image demonstrating bilateral biliary ductal dilatation (solid arrows) and a hilar soft tissue mass encasing the right portal vein (dashed arrow).

interpretation of the data difficult. Regardless, MRCP has been reported to be accurate for treatment planning in up to 75% of patients,[31,40] and MRI/MRCP can accurately predict resectability in 70%–80% of patients. Underestimation of the extent of ductal involvement is more common than overestimation,[44] and therefore, patients who may appear resectable on cross-sectional imaging can still be found to be unresectable at the time of surgery.

The role of 18-fluorodeoxyglucose (FDG)–positron emission tomography (PET) in the management of hilar cholangiocarcinoma remains unclear. The usefulness of FDG-PET may depend, in part, on the morphologic subtype of cholangiocarcinoma. For example, PET seems to be more helpful in detecting nodular cholangiocarcinoma as compared to infiltrating tumors.[45] In a study by Kato and colleagues, patients with extrahepatic cholangiocarcinoma were evaluated with CT and FDG-PET. In this series, 80% of patients were correctly interpreted as having a malignant lesion by CT scan compared with only 60% by PET scan.[46] Although PET may not be helpful to evaluate the primary lesion, some data have suggested that PET did change the surgical management in up to 30% of patients due to the detection of previously occult metastasis.[46] These data, however, are limited, and many experienced hepatobiliary surgeons do not routinely obtain PET scans before surgery. When a PET scan is obtained, it does need to be interpreted with caution as in-dwelling biliary stents, and a history of sclerosing cholangitis can lead to false-positive results.[45]

Direct Cholangiography and Cholangioscopy

Direct cholangiography includes both ERCP and PTC. The main benefits of this modality include direct imaging of the biliary tree and the ability to proceed with therapeutic interventions such as biliary drainage.[27] Traditionally, ERCP or PTC was a standard method for the evaluation of hilar strictures with biopsy of the suspicious lesion at the time of surgery. Unfortunately, the accuracy and usefulness of biopsy remains somewhat poor with only a reported sensitivity of 40%–80%.[47] In addition, although certain cholangiographic features may be more suspicious for a malignant process, cholangiographic findings are rarely specific enough to diagnose the lesion definitively. Given that tissue diagnosis is often not feasible and therefore is not requisite for surgical resection, as well as the availability of MRCP, it is not necessarily mandatory to obtain either an ERCP or a PTC before surgery. ERCP or PTC, however, is still commonly performed to help elucidate the degree of tumor extension/stricture.

Direct cholangiography with ERCP or PTC may also be warranted when biliary drainage is required before surgery. In general, preoperative biliary drainage should be aggressively pursued in patients with a bilirubin level >7 mg/dL. At the time of resection, most patients with hilar cholangiocarcinoma will require either an extended right hepatectomy or a left hemi-hepatectomy. In the setting of a planned major hepatectomy, preoperative normalization of the bilirubin level (e.g., <7 mg/dL) may be beneficial as severe cholestasis has been shown to compromise hepatocyte function and regeneration.[48,49] Some surgeons have argued that PTC is highly preferable to ERCP in patients requiring preoperative biliary drainage.[2] PTC has been advocated over ERCP, because some surgeons believe not only that it allows better evaluation of the intrahepatic biliary tree but also that in-dwelling PTC catheters may facilitate the biliary-enteric anastomosis at the time of surgery. However, neither of these claims are universally accepted. MRCP can now effectively evaluate the intrahepatic ductal system just as effectively as PTC. Furthermore, some surgeons find the presence of the PTC catheter at the time of surgery can hinder the formation of enteric anastomoses to small, segmental bile ducts. As such, whether to utilize PTC or ERCP to drain preoperatively, the biliary tree should be individualized and be based on not only surgeon preference but also biliary anatomy and location of the obstructing lesion.

Another more recent advance in the evaluation of the biliary tree has been the introduction of direct cholangioscopy. Although first described in a more rudimentary form in the late 1970s,[50] with modern fiber optics and improved image quality, cholangioscopy has been gaining increasing utility.[51] Unlike direct cholangiography that can only identify areas of stricture and filling defects, direct cholangioscopy can more directly evaluate the underlying bile duct anomaly. With direct cholangioscopy, a cholangioscope is advanced inside the bile duct while sterile saline solution is continuously flushed through the channel of the miniscope to facilitate visualization.[51] Certain visual characteristics such as polyps, nodules, irregular vascular or mucosal patterns, and ulcerations are suggestive of a malignant process.[52] In a study by Chen and colleagues, direct cholangioscopy was shown to be clinically feasible, provide adequate samples for histologic diagnosis, and successfully guide therapeutic interventions.[52] In another study that assessed 97 patients, ERCP with tissue sampling was compared with ERCP plus cholangioscopy.[51] In this study, the addition of direct cholangioscopy was associated with a 15% increase in diagnostic accuracy (78%–93%) and a 42% increase in diagnostic sensitivity (58%–100%).

Portal Vein Embolization

In a subset of patients, planned resection of the liver may result in an inadequate size of the future liver remnant (FLR). As noted, many patients with hilar cholangiocarcinoma will require a major hepatectomy leaving only a remnant liver volume of 20%–25%. If an inadequate FLR is anticipated, formal volumetric calculations should be performed to assess the exact volume of the FLR. Patients with an FLR < 20%–25% have been found to have an increase in major complications, postoperative liver insufficiency/failure, and mortality.[53,54] As such, patients who have an anticipated FLR of <20% (or 30%–40% in the setting of underlying liver steatosis, fibrosis, etc.) should be considered for portal vein embolization (PVE) to induce hypertrophy of the contralateral hemiliver. PVE involves selective cannulation of either the right or the left portal vein using fluoroscopic guidance and the subsequent embolization of the selected vessel with embolic materials such as cyanoacrylate, tris-acryl gelatin microspheres, polyvinyl alcohol, or coils. PVE has been demonstrated to be safe and effective with complications in 5%–8% of cases[55] and can increase the FLR[56] by 8%–16% depending on the degree of preoperative underlying hepatic dysfunction. In general, PVE should be considered only in patients who are undergoing an extended right hepatic resection; patients undergoing extended left hepatic resections rarely need PVE, because the remaining segments commonly represent an FLR of ≥30%. PVE can be used in a safe and effective manner to help induce hypertrophy in the FLR thereby making major liver resection for hilar cholangiocarcinoma safer by reducing the risk of postoperative liver insufficiency.

Classification and Staging of Hilar Cholangiocarcinoma

Classification and staging of hilar cholangiocarcinoma has three goals: define the extent of biliary involvement, assist in providing information on the potential for resectability, and stratify patients into risk groups regarding risk of recurrence and survival. Although the Bismuth–Corlette classification is an anatomic description of the lesion that defines extent of biliary tumor involvement, the Memorial Sloan Kettering Cancer Center (MSKCC) staging system provides a composite score that helps predict resectability. In contrast, the American Joint Committee on Cancer (AJCC) staging system utilizes the standard tumor node metastasis (TNM) system derived from pathologic data.

The Bismuth–Corlette classification (Figure 1-3) describes the anatomic location and extent of tumor within the biliary tree. In this classification scheme, type I tumors arise below the confluence of the right and left hepatic ducts; type II lesions reach the confluence of the ducts, but not beyond; type IIIa tumors occlude the common hepatic duct and extend into the main right hepatic duct, whereas type IIIb tumors occlude the common hepatic duct but extend into the left hepatic duct; type IV tumors block the confluence and extend into both the right and the left hepatic ducts.[57] Of note, the Bismuth–Corlette classification only includes longitudinal extension of the tumor and does not incorporate radial tumor extension. In contrast, the group from MSKCC has proposed a clinical T-staging system that includes both longitudinal and radial extension of hilar cholangiocarcinoma. In a study of 225 patients with hilar cholangiocarcinoma, patients were assigned a clinical "T score" based on preoperative MRCP and duplex ultrasound.[58] The "T score" was determined using three factors: location and extent of biliary involvement, presence or absence of portal vein involvement, and signs of hepatic lobar atrophy (Table 1-1). Both resectability and overall survival were associated with the T score, with a higher T score being correlated with an increased risk of unresectability. In fact, none of the patients with T3 lesions were resectable at the time of surgery.[58] The MSKCC hilar cholangiocarcinoma scoring system has subsequently been independently validated.[59]

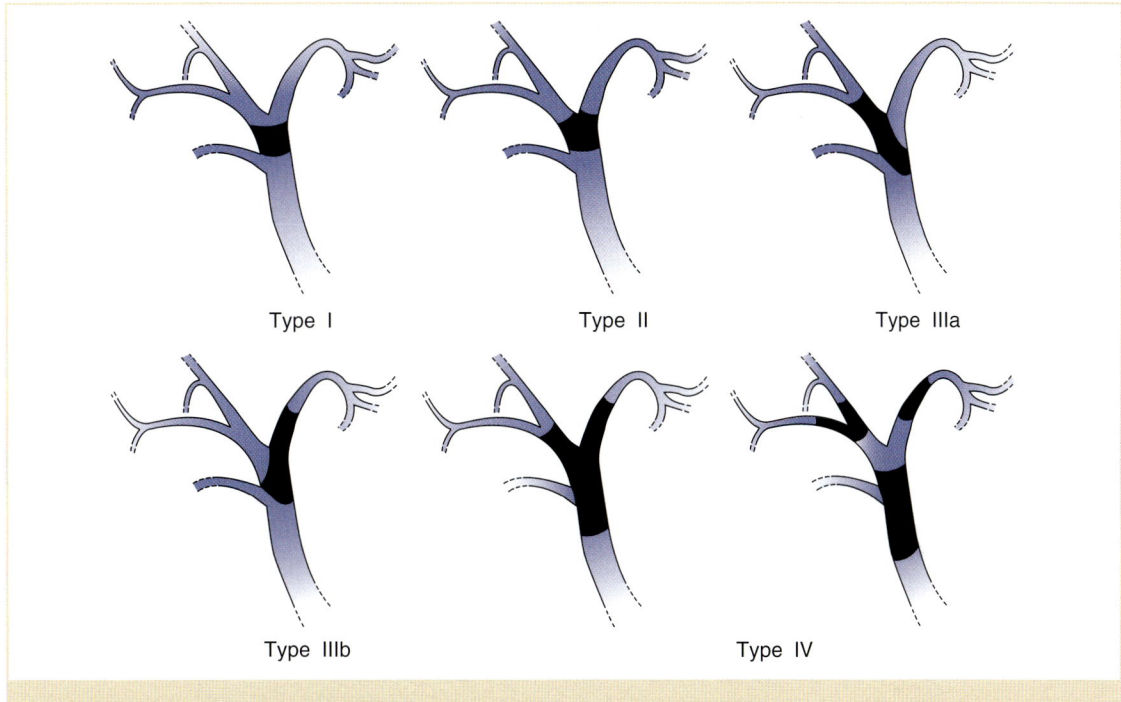

Figure 1-3: Bismuth–Corlette classification of hilar cholangiocarcinoma.

TABLE 1-1: Jarnagin–Blumgart T-stage Criteria[58]

Stage	Histology
T1	Tumor involving biliary confluence ± unilateral extension to second-order biliary radicles
T2	Tumor involving biliary confluence ± unilateral extension to second-order biliary radicles and *ipsilateral* portal vein involvement ± *ipsilateral* hepatic lobar atrophy
T3	Tumor involving biliary confluence ± unilateral extension to second-order biliary radicles; *or* unilateral extension to second-order biliary radicles with *contralateral* portal vein involvement; *or* unilateral extension to second-order biliary radicles with *contralateral* hepatic lobar atrophy; *or* main or bilateral portal vein involvement

From Jarnagin WR, Fong Y, DeMatteo RP, et al. Staging, resectability, and outcome in 225 patients with hilar cholangiocarcinoma. *Ann Surg.* 2001;234:507–519 with permission from Lippincott Williams & Wilkins.

The most commonly used staging system for hilar cholangiocarcinoma is the AJCC or TNM staging system (Table 1-2).[60] The AJCC staging system is based on histopathologic analysis of the specimen and therefore cannot assist in preoperative decision making. Of note, the staging of cholangiocarcinoma has undergone important changes in the latest seventh edition of AJCC staging manual.[60] For the first time, extrahepatic bile duct tumors have been separated into perihilar (proximal/Klatskin) and distal groups with separate staging classifications defined for each. As a result of this, the T-stage classifications have also undergone some important revisions that make the T-stage definitions more specific and relevant to hilar tumors. In addition, lymph node metastasis has been reclassified as stage III (upstaged from stage II), and the stage IV grouping defines unresectability based on local invasion (IVA) or distant disease (IVB).

TABLE 1-2: Tumor Node Metastases Staging System for Perihilar Cholangiocarcinoma

Primary tumor (T)	
TX	Primary tumor cannot be assessed
T0	No evidence of primary tumor
Tis	Carcinoma in situ
T1	Tumor confined to the bile duct, with extension up to the muscle layer or fibrous tissue
T2a	Tumor invades beyond the wall of the bile duct to surroundings adipose tissue
T2b	Tumor invades adjacent hepatic parenchyma
T3	Tumor invades unilateral branches of the portal vein or hepatic artery
T4	Tumor invades main portal vein or its branches bilaterally; or the common hepatic artery; or the second-order biliary radicals bilaterally; or unilateral second-order biliary radicals with contralateral portal vein or hepatic artery involvement
Regional lymph nodes (N)	
NX	Regional lymph nodes cannot be assessed
N0	No regional lymph node metastasis
N1	Regional lymph node metastasis (including nodes along the cystic duct, common bile duct, hepatic artery, and portal vein)
N2	Metastasis to periaortic, pericaval, superior mesenteric artery, and/or celiac artery lymph nodes
Distant metastasis (M)	
M0	No distant metastasis
M1	Distant metastasis

Anatomic stage/prognostic groups			
0	Tis	N0	M0
I	T1	N0	M0
II	T2a–b	N0	M0
IIIA	T3	N0	M0
IIIB	T1–3	N1	M0
IVA	T4	N0–1	M0
IVB	Any T	N2	M0
	Any T	Any N	M1

Note: cTNM is the clinical classification, pTNM is the pathologic classification.
Source: Used with the permission of the American Joint Committee on Cancer (AJCC), Chicago, Illinois. The original source for this material is the *AJCC Cancer Staging Manual*, Seventh Edition (2010) published by Springer Science and Business Media LLC, www.springer.com.[60]

Surgery for Hilar Cholangiocarcinoma

Surgical resection of hilar cholangiocarcinoma is the only potentially curative therapeutic option. Resection should therefore be undertaken in those patients who are appropriate surgical candidates and who have potentially resectable disease. Unfortunately, the resectability rate for cholangiocarcinoma is highly variable ranging from 28% to 95% at different centers.[58,61-64] There are several accepted criteria for unresectability for hilar cholangiocarcinoma (Table 1-3). In addition to standard factors such as excessive patient comorbidity and the presence of distant metastases, there are a

TABLE 1-3: Criteria for Unresectability[58]

Tumor-Related Criteria of Unresectability
1. Biliary duct involvement to secondary radicles bilaterally
2. Main portal vein encasement or occlusion[a]
3. Hepatic lobe atrophy with contralateral encasement or occlusion of portal vein
4. Hepatic lobe atrophy with contralateral involvement of secondary biliary radicles
5. Secondary biliary radicle involvement with contralateral portal vein branch encasement or occlusion

[a]Relative criterion. Portal vein resection and reconstruction may be possible. de Jong MC, Marques H, Clary BM, et al: The impact of portal vein resection on outcomes for hilar cholangiocarcinoma: a multi-institutional analysis of 305 cases. Cancer. 2012 Oct 1; 118(19):4737–47.

number of local factors that may preclude curative resection of hilar cholangiocarcinoma.[58] These local factors include bilateral segmental ductal extension, unilateral segmental ductal extension with contralateral vascular encasement, unilateral lobar hypertrophy with contralateral segmental ductal or vascular involvement, and encasement of the main portal vein or hepatic artery.

Resection of hilar cholangiocarcinoma can be technically challenging due to its proximity to the hilum and the adjacency of major vascular structures. The goal of surgical resection is to extirpate all disease with negative surgical (R0) margins while preserving an adequate liver remnant. Whereas in the past the surgical approach for hilar cholangiocarcinoma often consisted solely of an extrahepatic bile duct resection, over the past 20 years there has been an increase in the routine use of hepatic resection in patients with hilar cholangiocarcinoma.[2,28] In fact, among series with low rates of liver resection, the rate of obtaining a negative surgical margin has been reported to range from only 10% to 30%.[65–67] In contrast, in those centers that have routinely adopted hepatic resection as a component of the surgical strategy for hilar cholangiocarcinoma, the reported higher rates of negative surgical margins are much higher ranging from 68% to 95%.[28,68–70] As such, most experienced liver surgeons advocate for the routine incorporation of hepatic resection for hilar cholangiocarcinoma (Figure 1-4).

In general, the type of major hepatic resection required is dictated by the longitudinal extent of disease and the Bismuth–Corlette classification (Figure 1-5). After dividing the common bile duct just cephalad to the pancreas, a frozen section margin should be obtained. In unusual cases where this margin is positive for cancer, a pancreaticoduodenectomy will be required, and only in highly selected cases, should this be done in addition to a hilar and hepatic resection to achieve an R0 resection. If the distal margin is negative, then the common bile duct is reflected cephalad to aid in the exposure and dissection of the structures within the hepatoduodenal ligament. The ligamentum teres is reflected anterior and cephalad to expose the base of segment 4b, where the hepatoduodenal ligament and Glisson's capsule fuse. An incision is made at the base of segment 4b to lower the hilar plate (Figure 1-6). Sometimes division of the bridging tissue between segments 3 and 4 will assist in hilar exposure. If the tumor does not invade the portal vein, then with the common bile duct reflected cephalad, the plane between the posterior wall of the duct and the anterior surface of the portal vein may be dissected. Typically, the left hepatic duct is divided first in the umbilical fissure proximal to the tumor and if this margin is negative on frozen section, then an extended right hepatectomy may be performed. If the left hepatic duct margin is involved by tumor, and a negative right hepatic duct tumor margin can be obtained proximal to the tumor, then a left/extended left hepatectomy may be performed to achieve a complete resection. The role of routine major hepatic resection for a Bismuth–Corlette type I lesions is somewhat more debated due to the location of the lesion below the confluence below the right and left hepatic ducts. There are data, however, to support the use of hepatic resection even in this subset of patients as Ikeyama et al. demonstrated a survival benefit from right hepatectomy in patients with type I lesions.[71]

In addition to either a right or a left hemihepatectomy, strong consideration should be given to resection of the caudate lobe (segment 1). The caudate lobe bile ducts can enter both the right and the left hepatic ducts, but the primary drainage of the caudate lobe is into the left hepatic duct.[69,72]

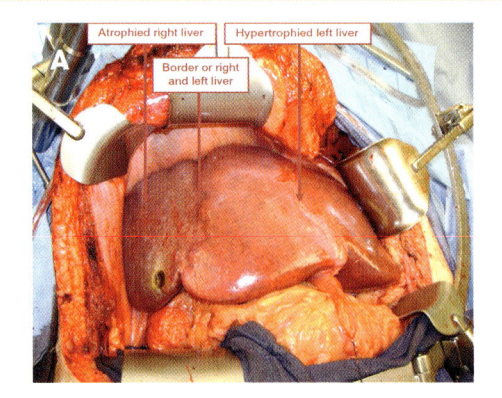

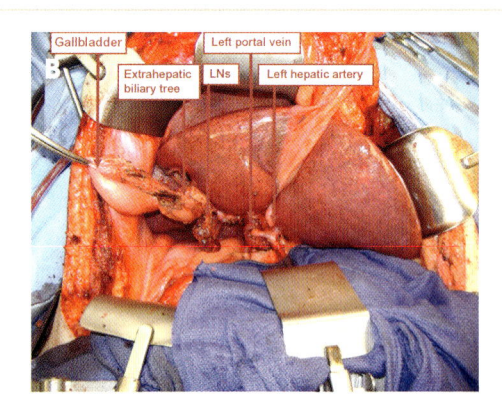

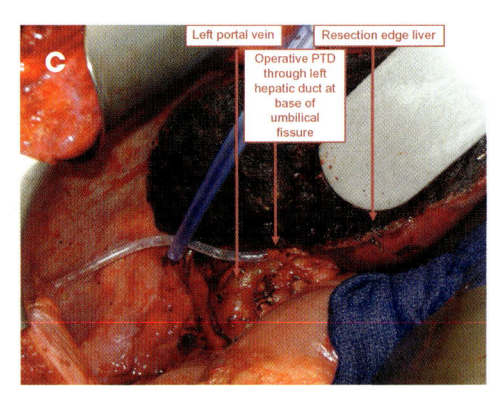

Figure 1-4: (A) Intraoperative photo of patient with right hilar cholangiocarcinoma. Note the atrophy of the right hemi-liver with the compensatory hypertrophy of the left liver. (B) Intraoperative photo illustrating hilar dissection with transection of the extrahepatic biliary tree, right portal vein and right hepatic artery. (C) Intraoperative photo following extended right hemi-hepatectomy illustrating operative percutaneous transhepatic drain (PTD) that was placed through left hepatic duct at the time of surgery.

Some studies have shown a decrease in local recurrence and an improvement in long-term survival among patients who have undergone concomitant caudate lobe resection.[73,74] As such, most surgeons advocate for routine resection of the caudate lobe. Resection of the caudate should be complete or at a minimum involve the caudate process and paracaval process portions of the caudate lobe in all cases, whereas the Spiegel lobe portion of caudate should be resected for Bismuth–Corlette IIIb cases.

At the time of surgery, removal of clinically suspicious nodal disease is mandatory. The surgeon should, however, routinely perform a hilar and pericholedochal lymphadenectomy even when no clinical disease is detected. Lymph node metastases from hilar cholangiocarcinoma are found in up to 30%–50% of cases, and therefore, a full lymphadenectomy should be performed in all surgical cases.[75,76]

In some cases, the hilar tumor will invade or involve major vascular structures such as the main portal vein or the hepatic artery. Portal vein resection and reconstruction can be performed safely, although with some increase in perioperative morbidity and mortality. Most surgeons advocate resection of the portal vein in select circumstances where the vein needs to be resected due to local tumor involvement. Neuhaus and colleagues, however, have advocated for routine portal vein resection as part of a "no touch" technique, claiming that resection "en bloc" of the bile duct and portal vein adheres more to oncological principles.[62] Although Neuhaus and colleagues have reported improved survival with

Hilar Cholangiocarcinoma

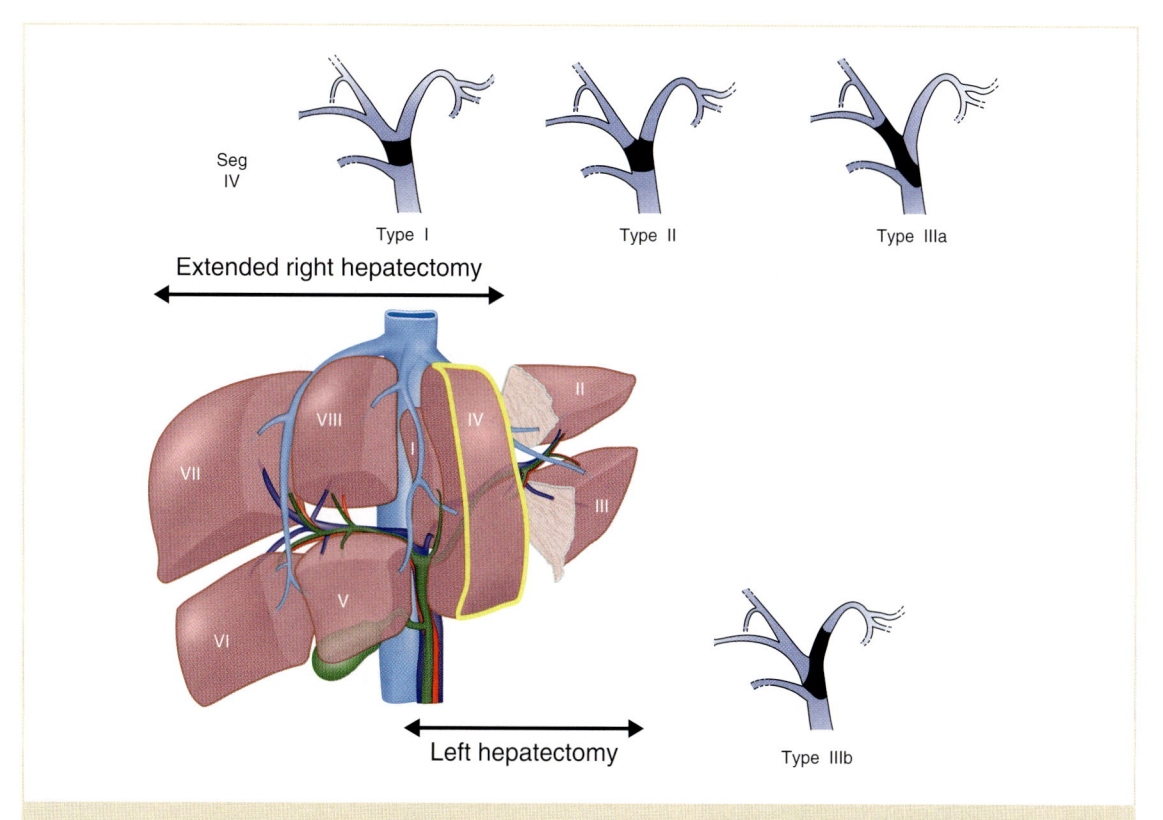

Figure 1-5: Schematic demonstrating the indications for extended right or left hemi-hepatectomy depending on the location of the lesion.

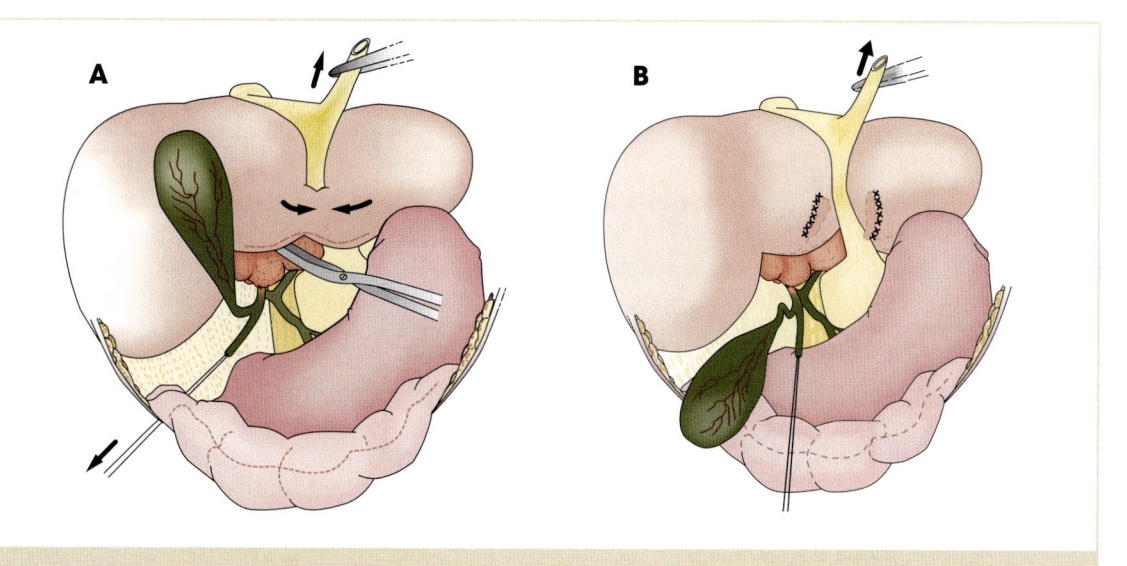

Figure 1-6: Dissection of the hilus of the liver. (A) With firm upward traction on the ligamentum teres, dissection at the base of the quadrate lobe (scissors) lowers the hilar plate. (B) The bridge of tissue at the base of the umbilical fissure (arrows in [A]) is divided, further exposing the hilar structures.

the "no touch" technique, mortality rates were high (17%), and other studies have failed to show similar improvements with routine resection of the portal vein.[77,78] Although portal vein resection may be considered at the time of surgery because of the acceptable perioperative risk and possible association with improved survival, resection of the hepatic artery is usually not justified.[79,80]

Following surgery for hilar cholangiocarcinoma, perioperative mortality ranges from 0% to 15%. Overall, most centers have reported five-year survival rates that range from 20% to 45% (Table 1-4).[81] Factors that have been most commonly associated with a worse long-term survival include lymph node metastasis, poor tumor differentiation, and perineural invasion.[58,73,82–84] Another modifiable factor that has been shown to impact survival significantly is resection margin status. As previously noted, obtaining a margin-negative (R0) resection has been repeatedly shown to improve both local recurrence rates and long-term survival.[2,28] As such, the primary goal of surgical resection should be a margin-negative resection, which most commonly requires a major hepatic resection.

Transplantation

Given the difficulties in resecting hilar cholangiocarcinoma, orthotopic liver transplant (OLT) has been proposed as an alternative treatment option. Unfortunately, initial results with transplantation for cholangiocarcinoma were dismal, with five-year survival rates ranging from 0% to 23% with prohibitively high recurrence rates.[85,86] As such, OLT was largely abandoned as a treatment option for patients with hilar cholangiocarcinoma. More recently, however, over the last decade, there has been a renewed interest in hilar cholangiocarcinoma as an indication for OLT.[87] On the basis of the known palliative efficacy of radiotherapy, the transplant team at the University of Nebraska established a strategy using high-dose neoadjuvant brachytherapy and 5-fluorouracil (5-FU) followed by liver transplantation.[88] The Mayo Clinic has subsequently adopted and championed

TABLE 1-4: Results of Surgical Resection[3]

Author (Year)[ref]	Resected (N)	Liver Rx (%)	5-y Survival, R0 (%)	5-y Survival, all (%)	Mortality (%)
Suigura (1994)[69]	83	100	33	20	8
Su (1996)[70]	49	50	34	15	10
Nagino (1998)[71]	138	90	26	NR	10
Miyazaki (2007)[79]	76	86	40	26	15
Madariaga (1998)[73]	28	100	25	9	14
Kosuge (1999)[61]	65	80	52	35	9
Neuhaus (1999)[62]	95[b]	85	37	22	6
Jarnagin (2001)[58]	80	78	30	NR	10
Kondo (2004)[70]	40	78	NR[a]	NR	0
Rea (2004)[73]	46	100	30	26	9
Nishio (2005)[77]	301	95	27	22	8
Dianant (2006)	99	38	33	27	15
Wahab (2006)[78]	73	100	NR	13	11
DeOliveira (2006)[6]	173	20	30	10	5

Abbreviations: NR, not reported; Rx, resection.
[a]Three-year survival = 44%.
[b]Includes 15 hepatectomies with liver transplantation.
[c]Three-year survival = 62%.

this neoadjuvant/transplantation approach for select patients with hilar cholangiocarcinoma. Patients are carefully screened and then treated with external beam radiation therapy (45 Gy) with continuous 5-FU followed by intrabiliary brachytherapy and capecitabine administered until the time of transplantation. Patients must then undergo an abdominal exploration close to the time of OLT. Although many patients fail to reach OLT due to the strict inclusion criteria and rigid neoadjuvant schedule, results among the select group of individuals who do receive OLT have been encouraging. Specifically, the reported five-year survival for all patients who begin neoadjuvant therapy is 54% (61% for patients with underlying PSC and 42% for those with de novo cholangiocarcinoma). Data from the Mayo Clinic have noted a five-year survival after transplantation of 73% (79% for patients with underlying PSC and 63% for those with de novo cholangiocarcinoma).[87] Transplantation for hilar cholangiocarcinoma remains controversial, however, and the data have been questioned due to the very strict patient selection and the absence of pathologic confirmation of disease on some ex-plant specimens.

Adjuvant Therapy for Hilar Cholangiocarcinoma

Systemic Chemotherapy

A subset of patients with hilar cholangiocarcinoma will be unresectable, and even among patients with resected disease, relapse rates can be high.[89,90] There is therefore a need for effective systemic chemotherapy to treat patients with hilar cholangiocarcinoma. Randomized phase III studies to examine systemic chemotherapy for cholangiocarcinoma have been very limited due to the heterogeneity of this patient cohort (i.e., intrahepatic, extrahepatic, and gallbladder), as well as the small number of patients. Several studies have evaluated various regimens in patients with advanced disease, including oxaliplatin and 5-FU gemcitabine alone, and gemcitabine plus capecitabine.[91–93] Response rates have largely ranged from 20% to 30%. Wagner et al. reported on 37 patients with histologically proven, advanced, or metastatic bile duct cancer who were treated with gemcitabine, oxaliplatin, and 5-FU as part of a phase II trial.[94] The response rates were 19%, and the median overall survival was 10 months. In a separate phase II trial examining combined gemcitabine plus capecitabine in patients with advanced biliary malignancies, Knox and colleagues reported an overall objective response rate of 31%, with an additional 42% of patients having stable disease, for a disease control rate of 73%.[93] Among treated patients with advanced disease, the median overall survival time was 14 months and the median progression-free survival time was seven months. Patients included in this study, however, had various biliary tract cancers with only 53% having cholangiocarcinoma. In a study that included only patients with pathologically proven cholangiocarcinoma, Charoentum et al. reported on their experience with gemcitabine and cisplatin in 42 patients with inoperable or metastatic disease. The overall response rate was 21% with a median survival of 11 months.[95] In another study also examining gemcitabine plus cisplatin, Meyerhardt and colleagues reported a partial response rate of 21% and a 36% incidence of stable disease using this combined chemotherapy regimen.[96] In a separate retrospective study, Murakami et al.[97] reported on 42 patients with hilar cholangiocarcinoma and noted an association between gemcitabine-based adjuvant chemotherapy and prolonged survival. In fact, the five-year survival among those patients receiving adjuvant gemcitabine-based chemotherapy was 57% compared with 23% for those patient who did not receive adjuvant therapy. Although the role of adjuvant therapy for patients with resected hilar cholangiocarcinoma remains not established, adjuvant chemotherapy utilizing the agents highlighted above should be strongly considered in those patients with lymph node metastasis given their worse prognosis.

Loco-Regional Therapies

The use of radiotherapy in the adjuvant setting for hilar cholangiocarcinoma also remains poorly defined. Although some retrospective studies have suggested no survival benefit for radiation therapy in the adjuvant setting,[98–100] other studies have noted an improvement in long-term outcome with the addition of radiotherapy following resection of hilar cholangiocarcinoma.[101,102] Specifically, Cheng et al. analyzed data from 75 patients undergoing surgical resection of hilar cholangiocarcinoma.[101] In this study, the authors noted that adjuvant radiotherapy was among the most significant independent predictors of survival (HR 4.3, 95% CI 3.6–4.9) with nearly a 10% increase in five-year survival compared to surgery alone.[101] Although the role of routine adjuvant radiation therapy for hilar cholangiocarcinoma in patients who undergo an R0 resection remains unclear, the use of adjuvant radiation therapy in patients undergoing an R1 resection should be strongly considered.

The role of radiation therapy for inoperable hilar cholangiocarcinoma is more defined. In those patients with inoperable disease, nonoperative biliary drainage in conjunction with external beam radiation therapy is a reasonable approach. The group from MSKCC has reported that biliary drainage with external beam radiation is a safe and effective method to palliate unresectable hilar cholangiocarcinoma.[103] The authors also noted that radiotherapy was associated with maintaining a reasonable quality of life. Biliary drainage and chemoradiotherapy are, therefore, probably the most common palliative therapeutic approaches in patients with inoperable hilar cholangiocarcinoma.

Another loco-regional treatment for hilar cholangiocarcinoma includes photodynamic therapy (PDT). PDT is a form of ablative therapy in which a photosensitizing drug is administered systemically and allowed to accumulate in the tumor of interest. The lesion is then exposed to a certain wavelength of laser light causing a photodynamic reaction that liberates oxygen cytotoxic radicals to cause local cell death. PDT has been used with some success in cancers of the lung, bladder, and esophagus, with tumor regression observed.[104–107] Several studies have specifically examined the role of PDT in treating patients with inoperable hilar cholangiocarcinoma and have noted an improvement in symptoms and survival.[108–110] Recently, the use of PDT has also been examined in the neoadjuvant setting in a phase II pilot study.[111] In a small number of patients (*n* = 7), PDT was administered in the area of tumor infiltration and 2 cm beyond, followed by curative-intent resection six weeks later. A margin-negative resection (OLT in one patient) was performed in all cases, and postoperative complications were minor. Two patients had a recurrence (6 and 19 months postoperatively) and the one-year recurrence-free survival rate[111] was 83%. These results, although difficult to interpret due to the small sample size, may suggest a future role of PDT in the treatment of patients with hilar cholangiocarcinoma.

Palliative Therapy for Hilar Cholangiocarcinoma

The majority of patients with hilar cholangiocarcinoma are unresectable at the time of presentation, and for this reason, palliation is a key component in the management of this disease. A recent publication by the British Association for the Study of Liver suggested that the primary goal of palliation should be to maximize patient quality of life, with survival being the secondary consideration.[21] There are various methods of palliation, all of which have as their goal adequate and durable relief of biliary obstruction and thereby improved quality of life.[112]

Surgical Palliation

Generally, a minimum of two segments or sectors of the liver (approximately 25%–50% of the total liver volume) must be drained in order to effectively alleviate symptoms such as jaundice and pruritis.[113] For maximum efficiency, atrophic segments should be avoided. Surgical palliation is achieved through a biliary–enteric bypass procedure. Given its relatively longer extrahepatic course, the left main hepatic duct is a good candidate for anastomosis to a Roux-en-Y jejunal limb.[113] Alternatively, if the degree of hilar involvement precludes this, a segment III Roux-en-Y cholangiojejunostomy can be fashioned (Figure 1-7).[114] If the left hemi-liver is atrophic, then a right-sided hepaticojejunostomy is required. With hilar involvement, a bypass may be created using the anterior sectoral ducts V and VI, which can be exposed just under the liver parenchyma in the gallbladder fossa.[113,115]

Surgical palliation should be considered in cases where the patient is found to be unresectable at the time of laparotomy. Biliary bypass procedures can be performed in this setting with acceptable rates of perioperative morbidity and mortality and provide effective and durable relief of biliary obstruction.[116] In addition, surgical bypass likely decreases the number of future procedures and has lower long-term morbidity than noninvasive techniques.[115] It should

Hilar Cholangiocarcinoma

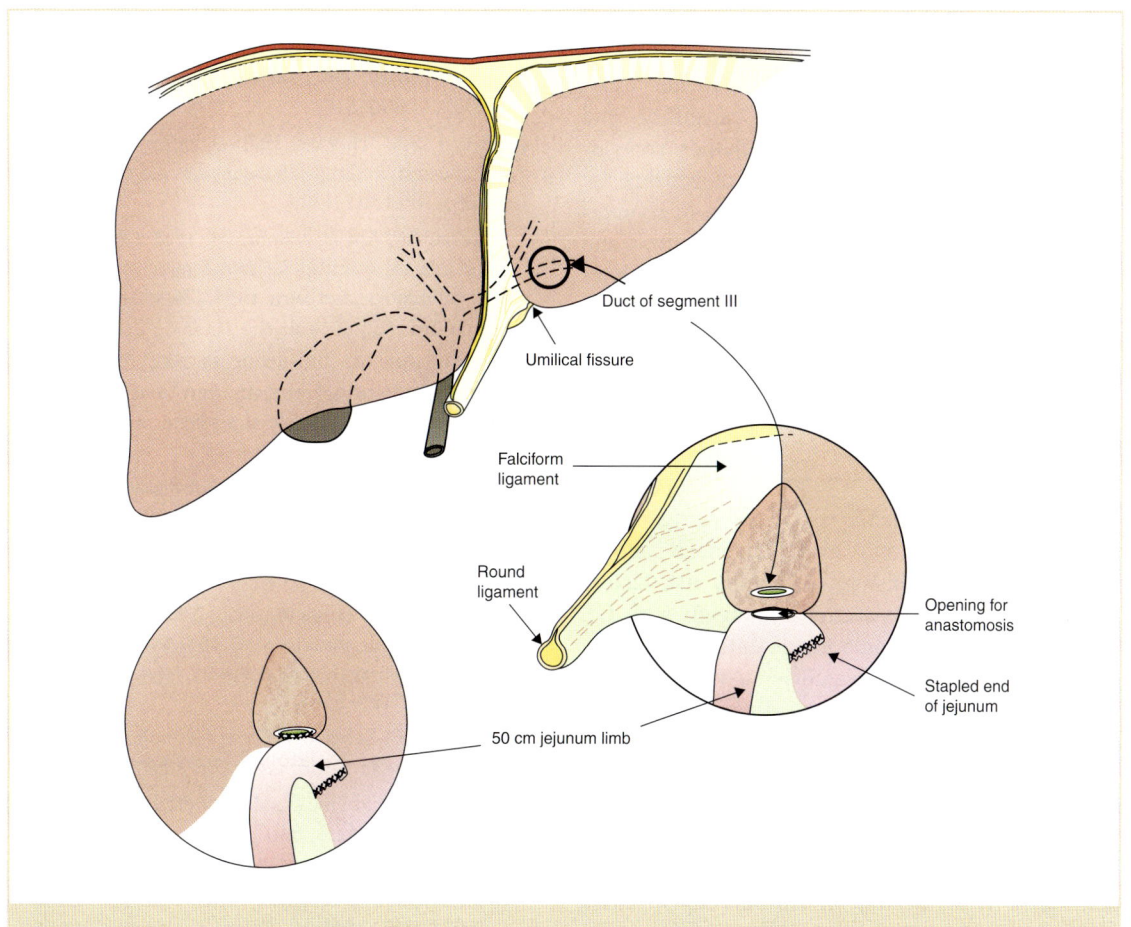

Figure 1-7: The round ligament approach to construct a segment III cholangiojejunostomy.

therefore be noted that surgical palliation becomes a far more attractive option in situations where long-term survival might be expected, as in the case of locally advanced disease. When metastatic disease is encountered widely, the risks of operative bypass may outweigh the benefit of surgical bypass, and alternative forms of palliation should be explored.

Nonoperative Palliation

In patients who are deemed unresectable before laparotomy, a nonsurgical approach is preferred in order to palliate symptoms. There are two possible methods for this: endoscopic or percutaneous. Both approaches aim to achieve adequate biliary drainage through the use of stents placed across the obstruction. Over a 92% initial success rate with the percutaneous approach has been reported, which is roughly 10%–15% better than the success with endoscopic approach. Patients undergoing the percutaneous approach for palliation were noted to have similar rates of complications, but a lower rate of repeat instrumentation.[117]

In addition to considering the different types of approach, one needs also to consider the composition of the stent when palliating biliary lesions. Stents can either be plastic or metal, with each having its own relative advantages and disadvantages. Plastic stents are low cost, easy to place, and likewise easily removed.[115] Plastic stents, therefore, can be a good choice in the preoperative or temporary setting. Plastic stents, however, can be narrow and occlude more easily, making them not an ideal choice as a durable long-term solution. In contrast, metal stents are larger in diameter, especially those with self-expanding capability, and less likely to migrate.[118] Multiple studies comparing plastic versus metal stents have shown that the plastic stents require a higher frequency of re-intervention and therefore more re-hospitalizations and greater expense.[119,120] Therefore, in general, for those patients with inoperable hilar cholangiocarcinoma secondary to advance local disease, metal stents are usually preferred.

Summary

Hilar cholangiocarcinoma is a challenging malignancy to diagnose and treat. Diagnosis should include an accurate history to identify risk factors and high-quality cross-sectional imaging with CT or MRI/MRCP to evaluate the extent of disease. A definitive preoperative diagnosis may be difficult to obtain; however, more recent diagnostic modalities such as direct cholangioscopy may help in the future. The only potentially curative therapy for hilar cholangiocarcinoma involves surgical resection. Resection should include not only removal of the extra-hepatic biliary tree but also a concomitant major liver resection in the majority of cases as this leads to the best chance of an R0 resection. Prognosis following resection remains guarded and is associated with lymph node status, tumor grade, and the presence of perineural invasion. Although data on adjuvant therapies such as systemic chemotherapy and radiation therapy are lacking, these should be strongly considered in patients with lymph node metastasis and those with residual disease at the surgical margin (R1/R2). Palliation of patients with inoperable hilar cholangiocarcinoma is critical to maintain quality of life and avoid recurrent bouts of cholangitis. In general, palliation is most effectively achieved through a combination of biliary drainage and chemoradiation therapy.

References

1. Olnes MJ, Erlich R. A review and update on cholangiocarcinoma. *Oncology*. 2004;66:167–179.
2. Ito F, Cho CS, Rikkers LF, Weber SM. Hilar cholangiocarcinoma: current management. *Ann Surg*. 2009;250:210–218.
3. Khan SA, Taylor-Robinson SD, Toledano MB, et al. Changing international trends in mortality rates for liver, biliary and pancreatic tumours. *J Hepatol*. 2002;37:806–813.
4. Khan SA, Thomas HC, Davidson BR, Taylor-Robinson SD. Cholangiocarcinoma. *Lancet*. 2005;366:1303–1314.
5. Nakeeb A, Pitt HA, Sohn TA, et al. Cholangiocarcinoma. A spectrum of intrahepatic, perihilar, and distal tumors. *Ann Surg*. 1996;224:463–473; discussion 473–475.
6. DeOliveira ML, Cunningham SC, Cameron JL, et al. Cholangiocarcinoma: thirty-one-year experience with 564 patients at a single institution. *Ann Surg*. 2007;245:755–762.
7. Klatskin G. Adenocarcinoma of the hepatic duct at its bifurcation within the porta hepatis. An unusual tumor with distinctive clinical and pathological features. *Am J Med*. 1965;38:241–256.
8. Strom BL, Hibberd PL, Soper KA, et al. International variations in epidemiology of cancers of the extrahepatic biliary tract. *Cancer Res*. 1985;45:5165–5168.
9. Shaib Y, El-Serag HB. The epidemiology of cholangiocarcinoma. *Semin Liver Dis*. 2004;24:115–125.
10. Patel T. Worldwide trends in mortality from biliary tract malignancies. *BMC Cancer*. 2002;2:10.
11. Carriaga MT, Henson DE. Liver, gallbladder, extrahepatic bile ducts, and pancreas. *Cancer*. 1995;75:171–190.
12. Bergquist A, Glaumann H, Persson B, Broomé U. Risk factors and clinical presentation of hepatobiliary carcinoma in patients with primary sclerosing cholangitis: a case-control study. *Hepatology*. 1998;27:311–316.
13. Chalasani N, Baluyut A, Ismail A, et al. Cholangiocarcinoma in patients with primary sclerosing cholangitis: a multicenter case-control study. *Hepatology*. 2000;31:7–11.
14. Broome U, Olsson R, Loof L, et al. Natural history and prognostic factors in 305 Swedish patients with primary sclerosing cholangitis. *Gut*. 1996;38:610–615.
15. Aadland E, Schrumpf E, Fausa O, et al. Primary sclerosing cholangitis: a long-term follow-up study. *Scand J Gastroenterol*. 1987;22:655–664.
16. Parkin DM, Srivatanakul P, Khlat M, et al. Liver cancer in Thailand. I. A case-control study of cholangiocarcinoma. *Int J Cancer*. 1991;48:323–328.
17. Chijiiwa K, Koga A. Surgical management and long-term follow-up of patients with choledochal cysts. *Am J Surg*.1993;165:238–242.

18. Lipsett PA, Pitt HA, Colombani PM, et al. Choledochal cyst disease. A changing pattern of presentation. *Ann Surg.* 1994;220:644–652.
19. Ohtsuka T, Inoue K, Ohuchida J, et al. Carcinoma arising in choledochocele. *Endoscopy.* 2001;33:614–619.
20. Nathan H, Pawlik TM, Wolfgang CL, et al. Trends in survival after surgery for cholangiocarcinoma: a 30-year population-based SEER database analysis. *J Gastrointest Surg.* 2007;11:1488–1496; discussion 1496–1497.
21. Khan SA, Davidson BR, Goldin R, et al. Guidelines for the diagnosis and treatment of cholangiocarcinoma: consensus document. *Gut.* 2002;51(suppl 6):VI1–VI9.
22. Jarnagin WR, Shoup M. Surgical management of cholangiocarcinoma. *Semin Liver Dis.* 2004;24:189–199.
23. Wetter LA, Ring EJ, Pellegrini CA, Way LW. Differential diagnosis of sclerosing cholangiocarcinomas of the common hepatic duct (Klatskin tumors). *Am J Surg.* 1991;161:57–62; discussion 62–63.
24. Verbeek PC, van Leeuwen DJ, de Wit LT, et al. Benign fibrosing disease at the hepatic confluence mimicking Klatskin tumors. *Surgery.* 1992;112:866–871.
25. Patel AH, Harnois DM, Klee GG, et al. The utility of CA 19-9 in the diagnoses of cholangiocarcinoma in patients without primary sclerosing cholangitis. *Am J Gastroenterol.* 2000;95:204–207.
26. Ramage JK, Donaghy A, Farrant JM, et al. Serum tumor markers for the diagnosis of cholangiocarcinoma in primary sclerosing cholangitis. *Gastroenterology.* 1995;108:865–869.
27. Choi JY, Kim MJ, Lee JM, et al. Hilar cholangiocarcinoma: role of preoperative imaging with sonography, MDCT, MRI, and direct cholangiography. *AJR Am J Roentgenol.* 2008;191:1448–1457.
28. Burke EC, Jarnagin WR, Hochwald SN, et al. Hilar cholangiocarcinoma: patterns of spread, the importance of hepatic resection for curative operation, and a presurgical clinical staging system. *Ann Surg.* 1998;228:385–394.
29. Gakhal MS, Gheyi VK, Brock RE, Andrews GS. Multimodality imaging of biliary malignancies. *Surg Oncol Clin N Am.* 2009;18:225–239, vii–viii.
30. Park MS, Lee DK, Kim MJ, et al. Preoperative staging accuracy of multidetector row computed tomography for extrahepatic bile duct carcinoma. *J Comput Assist Tomogr.* 2006;30:362–367.
31. Lopera JE, Soto JA, Munera F. Malignant hilar and perihilar biliary obstruction: use of MR cholangiography to define the extent of biliary ductal involvement and plan percutaneous interventions. *Radiology.* 2001;220:90–96.
32. Unno M, Okumoto T, Katayose Y, et al. Preoperative assessment of hilar cholangiocarcinoma by multidetector row computed tomography. *J Hepatobiliary Pancreat Surg.* 2007;14:434–440.
33. Cha JH, Han JK, Kim TK, et al. Preoperative evaluation of Klatskin tumor: accuracy of spiral CT in determining vascular invasion as a sign of unresectability. *Abdom Imaging.* 2000;25:500–507.
34. Aloia TA, Charnsangavej C, Faria S, et al. High-resolution computed tomography accurately predicts resectability in hilar cholangiocarcinoma. *Am J Surg.* 2007;193:702–706.
35. Fulcher AS, Turner MA. HASTE MR cholangiography in the evaluation of hilar cholangiocarcinoma. *AJR Am J Roentgenol.* 1997;169:1501–1505.
36. Guthrie JA, Ward J, Robinson PJ. Hilar cholangiocarcinomas: T2-weighted spin-echo and gadolinium-enhanced FLASH MR imaging. *Radiology.* 1996;201:347–351.
37. Manfredi R, Masselli G, Maresca G, et al. MR imaging and MRCP of hilar cholangiocarcinoma. *Abdom Imaging.* 2003;28:319–325.
38. Manfredi R, Brizi MG, Masselli G, et al. Malignant biliary hilar stenosis: MR cholangiography compared with direct cholangiography. *Radiol Med.* 2001;102:48–54.
39. Reinhold C, Bret PM. Current status of MR cholangiopancreatography. *AJR Am J Roentgenol.* 1996;166:1285–1295.
40. Zidi SH, Prat F, Le Guen O, et al. Performance characteristics of magnetic resonance cholangiography in the staging of malignant hilar strictures. *Gut.* 2000;46:103–106.
41. Yeh TS, Jan YY, Tseng JH, et al. Malignant perihilar biliary obstruction: magnetic resonance cholangiopancreatographic findings. *Am J Gastroenterol.* 2000;95:432–440.
42. Cho ES, Park MS, Yu JS, et al. Biliary ductal involvement of hilar cholangiocarcinoma: multidetector computed tomography versus magnetic resonance cholangiography. *J Comput Assist Tomogr.* 2007;31:72–78.
43. Lee SS, Kim MH, Lee SK, et al. MR cholangiography versus cholangioscopy for evaluation of longitudinal extension of hilar cholangiocarcinoma. *Gastrointest Endosc.* 2002;56:25–32.

44. Vilgrain V. Staging cholangiocarcinoma by imaging studies. *HPB* (Oxford). 2008;10:106–109.
45. Anderson CD, Rice MH, Pinson CW, et al. Fluorodeoxyglucose PET imaging in the evaluation of gallbladder carcinoma and cholangiocarcinoma. *J Gastrointest Surg*. 2004;8:90–97.
46. Kato T, Tsukamoto E, Kuge Y, et al. Clinical role of (18)F-FDG PET for initial staging of patients with extrahepatic bile duct cancer. *Eur J Nucl Med Mol Imaging*. 2002;29:1047–1054.
47. de Bellis M, Sherman S, Fogel EL, et al. Tissue sampling at ERCP in suspected malignant biliary strictures (part 2). *Gastrointest Endosc*. 2002;56:720–730.
48. Dixon JM, Armstrong CP, Duffy SW, Davies GC. Factors affecting morbidity and mortality after surgery for obstructive jaundice: a review of 373 patients. *Gut*. 1983;24:845–852.
49. Blamey SL, Fearon KC, Gilmour WH, et al. Prediction of risk in biliary surgery. *Br J Surg*. 1983;70:535–538.
50. Nakajima M, Akasaka Y, Fukumoto K, et al. Peroral cholangiopancreatosocopy (PCPS) under duodenoscopic guidance. *Am J Gastroenterol*. 1976;66:241–247.
51. Fukuda Y, Tsuyuguchi T, Sakai Y, et al. Diagnostic utility of peroral cholangioscopy for various bile-duct lesions. *Gastrointest Endosc*. 2005;62:374–382.
52. Chen YK, Pleskow DK. SpyGlass single-operator peroral cholangiopancreatoscopy system for the diagnosis and therapy of bile-duct disorders: a clinical feasibility study (with video). *Gastrointest Endosc*. 2007;65:832–841.
53. Hemming AW, Reed AI, Howard RJ, et al. Preoperative portal vein embolization for extended hepatectomy. *Ann Surg*. 2003;237:686–691; discussion 691–693.
54. Abdalla EK, Barnett CC, Doherty D, et al. Extended hepatectomy in patients with hepatobiliary malignancies with and without preoperative portal vein embolization. *Arch Surg*. 2002;137:675–680; discussion 680–681.
55. Madoff DC, Hicks ME, Abdalla EK, et al. Portal vein embolization with polyvinyl alcohol particles and coils in preparation for major liver resection for hepatobiliary malignancy: safety and effectiveness—study in 26 patients. *Radiology*. 2003;227:251–260.
56. Farges O, Belghiti J, Kianmanesh R, et al. Portal vein embolization before right hepatectomy: prospective clinical trial. *Ann Surg*. 2003;237:208–217.
57. Bismuth H, Corlette MB. Intrahepatic cholangioenteric anastomosis in carcinoma of the hilus of the liver. *Surg Gynecol Obstet*. 1975;140:170–178.
58. Jarnagin WR, Fong Y, DeMatteo RP, et al. Staging, resectability, and outcome in 225 patients with hilar cholangiocarcinoma. *Ann Surg*. 2001;234:507–517; discussion 517–519.
59. Chen RF, Li ZH, Zhou JJ, et al. Preoperative evaluation with T-staging system for hilar cholangiocarcinoma. *World J Gastroenterol*. 2007;13:5754–5759.
60. Edge SB, Byrd DR, Compton CC, et al. *AJCC (American Joint Committee on Cancer) Cancer Staging Manual*. New York: Springer; 2010.
61. Kosuge T, Yamamoto J, Shimada K, et al. Improved surgical results for hilar cholangiocarcinoma with procedures including major hepatic resection. *Ann Surg*. 1999;230:663–671.
62. Neuhaus P, Jonas S, Bechstein WO, et al. Extended resections for hilar cholangiocarcinoma. *Ann Surg*. 1999;230:808–818; discussion 819.
63. Launois B, Reding R, Lebeau G, Buard JL. Surgery for hilar cholangiocarcinoma: French experience in a collective survey of 552 extrahepatic bile duct cancers. *J Hepatobiliary Pancreat Surg*. 2000;7:128–134.
64. Seyama Y, Kubota K, Sano K, et al. Long-term outcome of extended hemihepatectomy for hilar bile duct cancer with no mortality and high survival rate. Ann Surg. 2003;238:73–83.
65. Gerhards MF, van Gulik TM, de Wit LT, et al. Evaluation of morbidity and mortality after resection for hilar cholangiocarcinoma--a single center experience. Surgery. 2000;127:395–404.
66. Todoroki T, Kawamoto T, Koike N, et al. Radical resection of hilar bile duct carcinoma and predictors of survival. Br J Surg. 2000;87:306–313.
67. Lillemoe KD, Cameron JL. Surgery for hilar cholangiocarcinoma: the Johns Hopkins approach. J Hepatobiliary Pancreat Surg. 2000;7:115–121.
68. Kawasaki S, Imamura H, Kobayashi A, et al. Results of surgical resection for patients with hilar bile duct cancer: application of extended hepatectomy after biliary drainage and hemihepatic portal vein embolization. Ann Surg. 2003;238:84–92.
69. Nimura Y, Hayakawa N, Kamiya J, et al. Hepatic segmentectomy with caudate lobe resection for bile duct carcinoma of the hepatic hilus. World J Surg. 1990;14:535–543; discussion 544.
70. Kondo S, Hirano S, Ambo Y, et al. Forty consecutive resections of hilar cholangiocarcinoma with no postoperative mortality and no positive ductal

margins: results of a prospective study. Ann Surg. 2004;240:95–101.
71. Ikeyama T, Nagino M, Oda K, et al. Surgical approach to bismuth type I and II hilar cholangiocarcinomas: audit of 54 consecutive cases. Ann Surg. 2007;246:1052–1057.
72. Mizumoto R, Kawarada Y, Suzuki H. Surgical treatment of hilar carcinoma of the bile duct. Surg Gynecol Obstet. 1986;162:153–158.
73. Rea DJ, Munoz-Juarez M, Farnell MB, et al. Major hepatic resection for hilar cholangiocarcinoma: analysis of 46 patients. Arch Surg. 2004;139:514–523; discussion 523–525.
74. Gazzaniga GM, Filauro M, Bagarolo C, Mori L. Surgery for hilar cholangiocarcinoma: an Italian experience. *J Hepatobiliary Pancreat Surg*. 2000;7:122–127.
75. Kitagawa Y, Nagino M, Kamiya J, et al. Lymph node metastasis from hilar cholangiocarcinoma: audit of 110 patients who underwent regional and paraaortic node dissection. *Ann Surg*. 2001;233:385–392.
76. Ito F, Agni R, Rettammel RJ, et al. Resection of hilar cholangiocarcinoma: concomitant liver resection decreases hepatic recurrence. *Ann Surg*. 2008;248:273–279.
77. Hemming AW, Kim RD, Mekeel KL, et al. Portal vein resection for hilar cholangiocarcinoma. *Am Surg*. 2006;72:599–604; discussion 604–605.
78. Munoz L, Roayaie S, Maman D, et al. Hilar cholangiocarcinoma involving the portal vein bifurcation: long-term results after resection. *J Hepatobiliary Pancreat Surg*. 2002;9:237–241.
79. Miyazaki M, Kato A, Ito H, et al. Combined vascular resection in operative resection for hilar cholangiocarcinoma: does it work or not? *Surgery*. 2007;141:581–588.
80. Zhou LX, Xu ZY, Guo JM, Zhang ZW. The role of vascular resection and reconstruction in the treatment of hilar cholangiocarcinoma. *Zhonghua Zhong Liu Za Zhi (Chin J Oncol)*. 2008;30:310–313.
81. Matsuo K, Rocha FG, Ito K, et al. The Blumgart preoperative staging system for hilar cholangiocarcinoma; analysis of resectability and outcomes in 380 patients. *J Am Coll Surg*. 2012;215(3):343–355.
82. Nimura Y, Kamiya J, Kondo S, et al. Aggressive preoperative management and extended surgery for hilar cholangiocarcinoma: Nagoya experience. *J Hepatobiliary Pancreat Surg*. 2000;7:155–162.
83. Nakeeb A, Tran KQ, Black MJ, et al. Improved survival in resected biliary malignancies. *Surgery*. 2002;132:555–563; discussion 563–564.
84. Havlik R, Sbisa E, Tullo A, et al. Results of resection for hilar cholangiocarcinoma with analysis of prognostic factors. *Hepatogastroenterology*. 2000;47:927–931.
85. Meyer CG, Penn I, James L. Liver transplantation for cholangiocarcinoma: results in 207 patients. *Transplantation*. 2000;69:1633–1637.
86. Goldstein RM, Stone M, Tillery GW, et al. Is liver transplantation indicated for cholangiocarcinoma? *Am J Surg*. 1993;166:768–771; discussion 771–772.
87. Rosen CB, Heimbach JK, Gores GJ. Liver transplantation for cholangiocarcinoma. *Transpl Int*. 2010 jul;23(7):692–697.
88. Sudan D, DeRoover A, Chinnakotla S, et al. Radiochemotherapy and transplantation allow long-term survival for nonresectable hilar cholangiocarcinoma. *Am J Transplant*. 2002;2:774–779.
89. Alexander F, Rossi RL, O'Bryan M, et al. Biliary carcinoma. A review of 109 cases. *Am J Surg*. 1984;147:503–509.
90. de Groen PC, Gores GJ, LaRusso NF, et al. Biliary tract cancers. *N Engl J Med*. 1999;341:1368–1378.
91. Nehls O, Klump B, Arkenau HT, et al. Oxaliplatin, fluorouracil and leucovorin for advanced biliary system adenocarcinomas: a prospective phase II trial. *Br J Cancer*. 2002;87:702–704.
92. Penz M, Kornek GV, Raderer M, et al. Phase II trial of two-weekly gemcitabine in patients with advanced biliary tract cancer. *Ann Oncol*. 2001;12:183–186.
93. Knox JJ, Hedley D, Oza A, et al. Combining gemcitabine and capecitabine in patients with advanced biliary cancer: a phase II trial. *J Clin Oncol*. 2005;23:2332–2338.
94. Wagner AD, Buechner-Steudel P, Moehler M, et al. Gemcitabine, oxaliplatin and 5-FU in advanced bile duct and gallbladder carcinoma: two parallel, multicentre phase-II trials. *Br J Cancer*. 2009;101:1846–1852.
95. Charoentum C, Thongprasert S, Chewaskulyong B, Munprakan S. Experience with gemcitabine and cisplatin in the therapy of inoperable and metastatic cholangiocarcinoma. *World J Gastroenterol*. 2007;13:2852–2854.
96. Meyerhardt JA, Zhu AX, Stuart K, et al. Phase-II study of gemcitabine and cisplatin in patients with metastatic biliary and gallbladder cancer. *Dig Dis Sci*. 2008;53:564–570.
97. Murakami Y, Uemura K, Sudo T, et al. Gemcitabine-based adjuvant chemotherapy improves survival after aggressive surgery for hilar cholangiocarcinoma. *J Gastrointest Surg*. 2009;13:1470–1479.

98. Cameron JL, Pitt HA, Zinner MJ, et al. Management of proximal cholangiocarcinomas by surgical resection and radiotherapy. *Am J Surg*. 1990;159:91–97; discussion 97–98.
99. Hayes JK Jr, Sapozink MD, Miller FJ. Definitive radiation therapy in bile duct carcinoma. *Int J Radiat Oncol Biol Phys*. 1988;15:735–744.
100. Pitt HA, Nakeeb A, Abrams RA, et al. Perihilar cholangiocarcinoma. Postoperative radiotherapy does not improve survival. *Ann Surg*. 1995;221:788–797; discussion 797–798.
101. Cheng Q, Luo X, Zhang B, et al. Predictive factors for prognosis of hilar cholangiocarcinoma: postresection radiotherapy improves survival. *Eur J Surg Oncol*. 2007;33:202–207.
102. Sagawa N, Kondo S, Morikawa T, et al. Effectiveness of radiation therapy after surgery for hilar cholangiocarcinoma. *Surg Today*. 2005;35:548–552.
103. Kuvshinoff BW, Armstrong JG, Fong Y, et al. Palliation of irresectable hilar cholangiocarcinoma with biliary drainage and radiotherapy. *Br J Surg*. 1995;82:1522–1525.
104. Moghissi K, Dixon K. Update on the current indications, practice and results of photodynamic therapy (PDT) in early central lung cancer (ECLC). *Photodiagnosis Photodyn Ther*. 2008;5:10–18.
105. Prout GR Jr, Lin CW, Benson R Jr, et al. Photodynamic therapy with hematoporphyrin derivative in the treatment of superficial transitional-cell carcinoma of the bladder. *N Engl J Med*. 1987;317:1251–1255.
106. Gross SA, Wolfsen HC. The role of photodynamic therapy in the esophagus. *Gastrointest Endosc Clin N Am*. 2010;20:35–53, vi.
107. Sibille A, Lambert R, Souquet JC, et al. Long-term survival after photodynamic therapy for esophageal cancer. *Gastroenterology*. 1995;108:337–344.
108. Cunningham SC, Choti MA, Bellavance EC, Pawlik TM. Palliation of hepatic tumors. *Surg Oncol*. 2007 Dec;16(4):277–291.
109. Zoepf T, Jakobs R, Arnold JC, et al. Palliation of nonresectable bile duct cancer: improved survival after photodynamic therapy. *Am J Gastroenterol*. 2005;100:2426–2430.
110. Berr F, Wiedmann M, Tannapfel A, et al. Photodynamic therapy for advanced bile duct cancer: evidence for improved palliation and extended survival. *Hepatology*. 2000;31:291–298.
111. Wiedmann M, Caca K, Berr F, et al. Neoadjuvant photodynamic therapy as a new approach to treating hilar cholangiocarcinoma: a phase II pilot study. *Cancer*. 2003;97:2783–2790.
112. Witzigmann H, Berr F, Ringel U, et al. Surgical and palliative management and outcome in 184 patients with hilar cholangiocarcinoma: palliative photodynamic therapy plus stenting is comparable to r1/r2 resection. *Ann Surg*. 2006;244:230–239.
113. Connor S, Wigmore SJ, Madhavan KK, et al. Surgical palliation for unresectable hilar cholangiocarcinoma. *HPB (Oxford)*. 2005;7:273–277.
114. Traynor O, Castaing D, Bismuth H. Left intrahepatic cholangio-enteric anastomosis (round ligament approach): an effective palliative treatment for hilar cancers. *Br J Surg*. 1987;74:952–954.
115. Singhal D, van Gulik TM, Gouma DJ. Palliative management of hilar cholangiocarcinoma. *Surg Oncol*. 2005;14:59–74.
116. Jarnagin WR, Burke E, Powers C, et al. Intrahepatic biliary enteric bypass provides effective palliation in selected patients with malignant obstruction at the hepatic duct confluence. *Am J Surg*. 1998; 175:453–460.
117. Cheng JL, Bruno MJ, Bergman JJ, et al. Endoscopic palliation of patients with biliary obstruction caused by nonresectable hilar cholangiocarcinoma: efficacy of self-expandable metallic Wallstents. *Gastrointest Endosc*. 2002;56:33–39.
118. Wagner HJ, Knyrim K, Vakil N, Klose KJ. Plastic endoprostheses versus metal stents in the palliative treatment of malignant hilar biliary obstruction. A prospective and randomized trial. *Endoscopy*. 1993;25:213–218.
119. Davids PH, Groen AK, Rauws EA, et al. Randomised trial of self-expanding metal stents versus polyethylene stents for distal malignant biliary obstruction. *Lancet*. 1992;340:1488–1492.
120. Davids PH, Groen AK, Rauws EA, et al. Randomised trial of self-expanding metal stents versus polyethylene stents for distal malignant biliary obstruction. *Lancet*. 1992;340:1488–1492.

CHAPTER 2

Peripheral Cholangiocarcinoma

Sachin Patil & Ronald S. Chamberlain

Cholangiocarcinoma is a rare disease accounting for <2% of all human malignancies.[1] Overall, 2500 new cases are diagnosed every year in the United States.[2] Despite its rarity, cholangiocarcinoma (CC) is the most common malignant tumor arising from the epithelium of the biliary tract, accounting for 15% of all primary liver malignancies,[3] and is second only to hepatocellular carcinoma (HCC), which is the most common hepatic malignancy.[3,4] CC may arise from any part of the biliary tree, and depending on the anatomical location, it is classified into three broad categories: (1) peripheral cholangiocarcinoma (PCC; *intrahepatic tumors*) arising from the intrahepatic bile ducts, (2) hilar CC (*Klatskin tumors*) arising at the confluence of right and left hepatic ducts, and (3) extrahepatic or distal CC arising from the common bile duct.[5] The majority of CC is sporadic; however, there are several identifiable risk factors known to predispose to this neoplasm.[2,5]

PCC is a poorly understood variant of CC. The last 30 years have witnessed a global increase in incidence and mortality of PCC, while the incidence of all other forms of CC has been stable or declined.[6–8] The rarity of PCC presents a great obstacle not only to our understanding of disease pathogenesis and its changing incidence but also to the development of effective treatment approaches. Recent large community-based studies have highlighted important changes in the epidemiology and demographics of PCC; however, these studies offer little insight into novel or improved treatment algorithms.[8–13] Surgery remains the gold standard and only potentially curative modality. The role of adjunct therapeutic modalities such as chemotherapy and radiation therapy (RT) remains investigational.

Surgical Embryology and Anatomy

The extrahepatic biliary duct system develops from the liver bud, a diverticulum of the endoblastic epithelium in the ventral wall of the cephalic portion of the foregut. Development of the liver bud begins around the third week of gestation and is not complete until six weeks after birth. Intrahepatic biliary development begins around the eighth week with the formation of the "ductal plate"; a condensation of the primitive hepatoblast around the largest portal vein branches.[14] The intrahepatic biliary ducts undergo 18–20 orders of branching, of which initial branching orders up to 10 (sometimes 12) can be seen by standard cholangiography.[15] For simplification, intrahepatic bile ducts have been grossly divided into two categories: the "large intrahepatic bile ducts" and the "small intrahepatic bile ducts" (Table 2-1). The liver itself is divided into eight independent functional segments according to the Couinaud classification (Figure 2-1[16]). Each segment has its own vascular inflow and outflow and biliary drainage. In the center of each segment is a branch of the portal vein, hepatic artery, and bile duct, while in the periphery of each segment, there is vascular outflow through one of the three hepatic veins. The liver has a dual blood supply from the portal vein and hepatic arteries, which drain into the hepatic veins. Lymph from the space of Disse (the main source of hepatic lymph), space of Mall, adventitia of sublobular veins, peripheral vascular connective tissue, and the capsule of liver is drained into hilar, celiac, and retroperitoneal lymph nodes (LNs).[17]

Tsuji et al. have described the lymphatic drainage of the liver in detail.[18] Briefly, lymphatic drainage of the liver follows one of three routes: (1) hepatoduodenal (H), (2) cardial (C), or (3) diaphragmatic (D). Route "H" drains along the hepatoduodenal ligament with or without involvement of the hepatic, celiac, or retropancreatic nodes. Route "C" drains into the cardial, lesser curvature, and/or left gastric nodes, whereas route "D" drains along the left phrenic artery to the lateral aortic group of LNs. Routes "H" and "D" are considered primary drainage routes irrespective of the location of hepatic tumors, and route "C" is a possible route for drainage of a peripheral left hepatic lobe tumor or hilar CC.[18]

Location and Pathology

Peripheral cholangiocarcinoma (PCC) arises from the intrahepatic bile duct epithelium beyond the second-order division of the biliary system.[19] It usually occurs in noncirrhotic livers although it is not uncommon to find PCC in cirrhotic livers.[20] In general, 3.3%–40.6% of patients with PCC have associated liver cirrhosis.[21–23] PCC most frequently presents as a large and solitary tumor, but a multinodular or branching mass may be seen in 5% of patients. Based on the gross appearance, PCC is classified into four types[24]: (1) mass-forming (MF) type, (2) periductal infiltrating (PI), (3) intraductal (ID), and (4) MF + PI type. All tumor types typically appear as white and firm lesions with significant desmoplastic stroma, and adenocarcinoma is the most common histological type (90%–95%). Adenosquamous and squamous carcinoma, cholangiocellular carcinoma, mucinous carcinoma, signet-ring cell carcinoma, lymphoepithelioma-like carcinoma, sarcomatous variant, clear cell variant, and mucoepidermoid carcinoma are other histological variants reported by the World Health Organization.[25] Nakajima et al. performed a histopathological study on 102 cases of PCC and proposed a classification system for main PCC histological types (Table 2-2).[26] The pathological features of these subtypes are briefly described in Table 2-3. The gross and histological variants have different biological behaviors, which contribute to their diverse clinical course and outcomes.[27] PCC can spread by both hematogenous and lymphatic routes with a high dissemination rate; 50% of patients with PCC are found to have metastases at autopsy. Hematogenous spread occurs principally

TABLE 2-1: Anatomic Divisions of the Intrahepatic Biliary Ductal System[15,186,187]

Division	Components		Histology
Large intrahepatic bile ducts	First 3–4 orders of division	Right and left hepatic ducts	Lined by columnar cells
	Visible on gross inspection	Segmental ducts	
		Intersegmental/large septal ducts	
Small intrahepatic bile ducts	Intrahepatic biliary tree beginning from the fifth order of division	Small septal ducts	
		Interlobular ducts	Lined by cuboidal cells
	Visible on microscopic examination	Cholangioles	

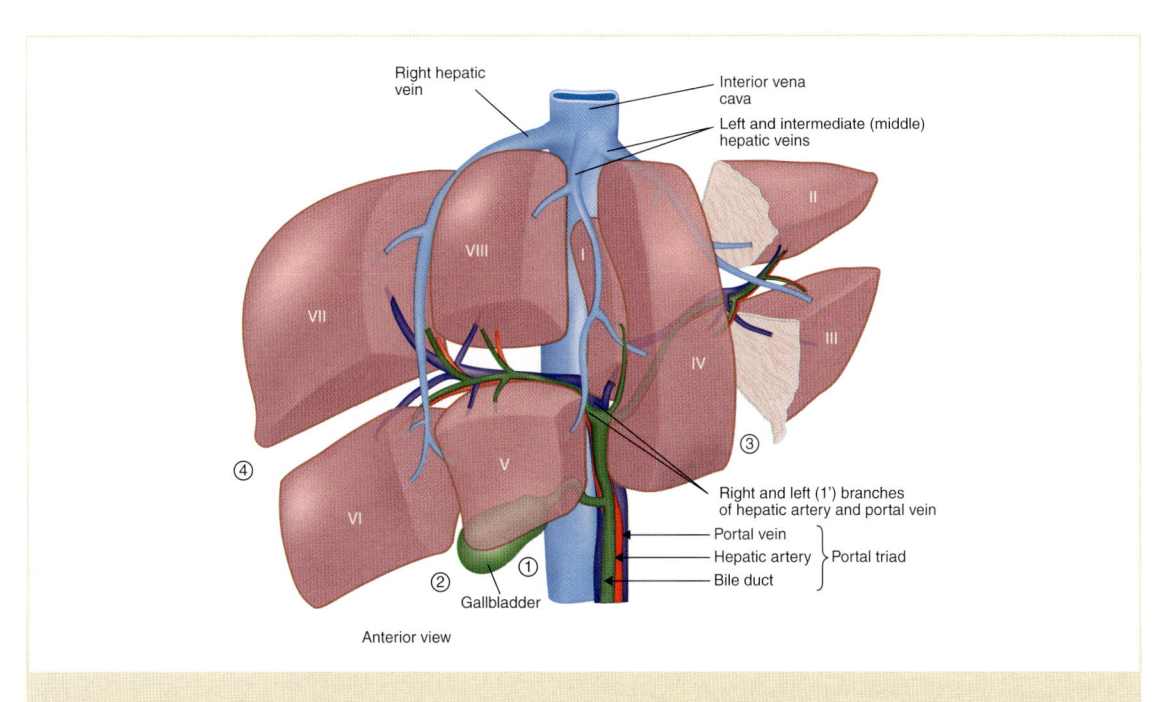

Figure 2-1: Hepatic segmentation. Except for the caudate lobe (segment I), the liver is divided into right and left livers based on the primary (1) division of the portal triad into right and left branches, the plane between the right and left livers being the main portal fissure (1) in which the middle hepatic vein lies. On the visceral surface, this plane is demarcated by the right sagittal fissure. The plane is demarcated on the diaphragmatic surface by an imaginary line (Cantlie line—Cantlie, 1898)* running from the notch for the fundus of the gallbladder to the IVC. The right and left livers are subdivided vertically into medial and lateral sectors by the right portal (2) and left portal (umbilical) (3) fissures, in which the right and left hepatic veins lie. The left portal fissure is demarcated externally by the falciform ligament and the left sagittal fissure. The right portal fissure has no external demarcation. Each division receives a secondary (2) branch of the portal triad (a portal pedicle). (Note: The medial sector of the left liver is a part of the right anatomical lobe; the lateral division of the left liver is the same as the left anatomical lobe.) A transverse plane at the level of the horizontal parts of the right and left branches of the portal triad (4) subdivides three of the four sectors (all but the left medial sector), creating six hepatic segments receiving tertiary branches. The left medial sector is also counted as a hepatic segment, so that the main part of the liver has seven segments (segments II through VIII, numbered clockwise). The caudate lobe (segment I, bringing the total number of segments to eight) is supplied by branches of both right and left divisions and drained by its own minor hepatic veins. Thus, each segment has its own intrasegmental blood supply and biliary drainage. The hepatic veins are intersegmental, draining the portions of the multiple segments adjacent to them.

*Cantlie J: On a new arrangement of the right and left lobes of the liver. Proc Anat Soc Great Britain Ireland 32:4, 1897.

to lungs, bone (mainly vertebrae), adrenals, brain, and other organs. Lung is the most common site of metastases apart from intrahepatic spread.[28] Histological differentiation of PCC from HCC and metastatic adenocarcinoma can be difficult. The histological and immunohistochemical differences among PCC, HCC, and metastatic adenocarcinoma are briefly described in Table 2-4. A thorough systemic staging evaluation is paramount to rule out metastatic adenocarcinoma.

Etiology

A majority of CC arise in the absence of risk factors,[29] and a precise causative factor for PCC remains elusive. Nevertheless, PCC has been associated with a variety of developmental anomalies, genetic factors, inflammatory conditions, and environmental factors (Table 2-5). Most notably, conditions resulting in chronic bile duct inflammation are the most strongly associated risk factors for this neoplasm. Like most gastrointestinal adenocarcinomas, it is hypothesized that PCC follows the classical hyperplasia–adenoma–carcinoma sequence.[30]

Genetic Factors

Several genetic alterations have been observed in PCC including *p53* mutations, tumor suppressor gene methylation, *RAS* mutations, increased expression of *c-erbB-2* and *c-Met* proto-oncogenes, abnormal G1-S cell cycle and altered Transforming growth factor-β/Smad pathway, and increased expression of thymidine phosphorylase leading to increased angiogenesis.[31] Shimonishi et al. have proposed a scheme of genetic events in the hyperplasia–dysplasia–carcinoma process of PCC (Figure 2-2).[32] They hypothesize that chronic inflammation and cholestasis are the initiating events. They observed increased proliferative activity with *c-erbB-2* and *c-MET* overexpression in the hyperplastic biliary epithelium. In the dysplastic cells, they noted increased telomerase activity with increased expression of carcinoembryonic antigen (CEA) and carbohydrate antigen 19-9 (CA 19-9) and decreased expression of sialomucin and sulfomucin. *P53* and *K-ras* mutations with hepatocyte growth factor and interleukin (IL)-6/glycoprotein 130 overexpression were the final events in carcinogenesis.[32]

Parasitic Infection

Pathogenic association between liver fluke infestation, especially *Opisthorchis viverrini* (and less definitively *Clonorchis sinensis*), and CC is suggested by many experimental and epidemiological data sets.[12,31,33] These parasitic infections are endemic in several Asian countries; *O. viverrini* is found primarily in Thailand, Laos, and Cambodia, whereas *C. sinensis* is found in southern China, Korea, Taiwan, Japan, and Vietnam.[12,34] Humans are infected by eating undercooked fish infected with adult worms that then lay eggs in the biliary system. Malignant change in the biliary epithelium after infection with *O. viverrini* has been demonstrated in animal models using Syrian hamsters, particularly if they are fed with nitrosamines.[33] Dietary or endogenous nitrosamine compounds themselves may also be an important cofactor in the process, due to a direct carcinogenic effect on bile duct epithelial cells.[33,35]

Hepatolithiasis

Hepatolithiasis is a common risk factor for CC in many parts of Asia, especially Japan, Taiwan, China, and Korea.[35–38] Nearly 10% of patients with hepatolithiasis in these countries develop CC. Conversely, nearly 70% of CCs in Taiwan manifest with intrahepatic stone disease, whereas in Japan, this figure is only 6%–18%.[35,39,40] There is a reported lag time of approximately eight years between development of hepatolithiasis and CC, and tumors may develop even after complete stone removal.[41] Biliary stones are thought to result in bile stasis, predisposing to recurrent bacterial infections and subsequent inflammation, a potential cofactor for cholangiocarcinogenesis. Biliary intraepithelial neoplasia is considered a precursor lesion in these cases and is typically seen as a microscopic lesion with flat or micropapillary dysplastic epithelium known as biliary dysplasia, atypical biliary epithelium, or carcinoma in situ.[42]

TABLE 2-2: Histological Variants Among 102 Cases of Peripheral Cholangiocarcinoma[26]

Histologic Classification	%
Adenocarcinoma (groups I and II)	
Papillary	26.5
Papillotubular	13.7
Well-differentiated tubular	11.8
Moderately differentiated tubular	26.5
Poorly differentiated tubular	11.8
Other histological variants (group III)	
Adenosquamous carcinoma	2.9
Squamous cell carcinoma	2.9
Mucinous carcinoma	0.98
Anaplastic carcinoma	2.9

Used with permission from Elsevier as adapted from Nakajima et al: Hum Pathol, 1988.

TABLE 2-3: Pathological Features of Peripheral Cholangiocarcinoma (PCC) Subtypes[26,103,189–194]

Subtype	Incidence (% of All PCC)	Gross Morphology	Tumor Behavior
Mass-forming type	40–42	Usually large, up to 15 cm in diameter, well circumscribed, and noncapsulated with wavy or lobulated margins Satellite nodules are a common association (especially around the main tumor)	Tumor invades portal vein early leading to intrahepatic metastases. Later when the tumor enlarges, it tends to involve Glisson's capsule and spread by invasion through lymphatic ducts
Periductal infiltrating type	8–22	It grows along the bile ducts and is elongated, spiculated, or branch like Normally small tumor nodule arising close to the hilum Causes thickening of the bile duct wall with varying degrees of luminal narrowing	Tumor migrates along the portal structures often invading associated vessels Involves Glisson's capsule and lymphatic ducts early in its natural history Invasion of portal venous branches is uncommon
Intraductal type	8–18.8	Usually small, sessile, or polypoid in shape Sometimes presents as a large mass occluding the bile duct Tumors infrequently produce a profuse amount of mucus resulting in partial biliary obstruction	Low rate of lymphatic or intrahepatic metastases, although there may be invasion through the wall of the duct Spreads superficially along the mucosal surface and may result in multiple tumors (papillomatosis) along various bile ducts
Mass-forming + periductal infiltrating type	22.2–31	Combined features of mass-forming and periductal infiltrating type Develops in the central part from relatively larger bile ducts	High incidence of portal vein thrombosis and lymph node metastases

Microscopy

Most PCC are well-differentiated adenocarcinoma displaying a variety of architectural patterns (including tubular, acinar, and trabecular) lined by cuboidal-to-low columnar cells. Tumor cells typically contain vesicular nuclei with nucleoli. Nucleoli are smaller and less eosinophilic than those seen in hepatocellular carcinomas. The cytoplasm may be clear, pale, or eosinophilic, and the cells may be vacuolated. These tumors exhibit a complete range of morphological differentiation, i.e., well differentiated, moderately differentiated, and poorly differentiated. A feature common to all cholangiocarcinomas is the presence of a strong desmoplastic reaction that helps differentiate them from hepatocellular carcinoma. Secretion of mucus may be demonstrable but are rarely bile stained.

TABLE 2-4: Histopathological and Immunohistochemical Differences Between Peripheral cholangiocarcinoma, Hepatocellular carcinoma, and Metastatic Adenocarcinoma[195-198]

	PCC	HCC	Metastatic Adenocarcinoma
Histopathological features	Strong desmoplastic reaction	Presence of sinusoids	Well-formed glands, with prominent necrosis
	Positive for mucin stain	Positive for bile staining	Metastases from colon often contains calcified areas
Immunohistochemical staining features	CK7 +ve	HepPar1 +ve	Metastases from large bowel are CK7 −ve and CK20 +ve
	CK19 +ve	CD10 +ve	
	Galactin 3 +ve	Albumin mRNA +ve	Metastases from breast may be ER/PR +ve
		Claudin 4 +ve	Metastases from lung are TTF1 +ve

Abbreviations: CD10, cluster of differentiation/cluster of designation; CK, cytokeratins; HepPar1, hepatocyte paraffin-1; ER, estrogen receptor; PR, progesterone receptor; TTF1, thyroid transcription factor-1.

TABLE 2-5: Risk Factors Associated with the Development of Cholangiocarcinoma

General risk factors	Advanced age (>65 y) Smoking Obesity Diabetes
Infections	Liver flukes (*Opisthorchis viverrini, Clonorchis sinensis*)[a] Viral infection (human immunodeficiency virus, hepatitis B virus, hepatitis C virus, Epstein–Barr virus)
Toxin exposure	Thoroium oxide (contrast dye) Dioxin Nitrosamines Asbestos Polyvinyl chloride Heavy alcohol consumption
Chronic inflammatory diseases	Primary sclerosing cholangitis[b] Hepatolithiasis (oriental cholangiohepatitis, recurrent pyogenic cholangitis)[a] Liver cirrhosis
Congenital liver anomalies	Fibrocystic liver diseases (e.g., Caroli's disease) Anomalous pancreaticobiliary junction Choledochal cyst
Postsurgical	Biliary-enteric anastomosis

All risk factors listed share the common feature of chronic biliary inflammation.
[a]More common in Eastern countries.
[b]More common in Western countries.

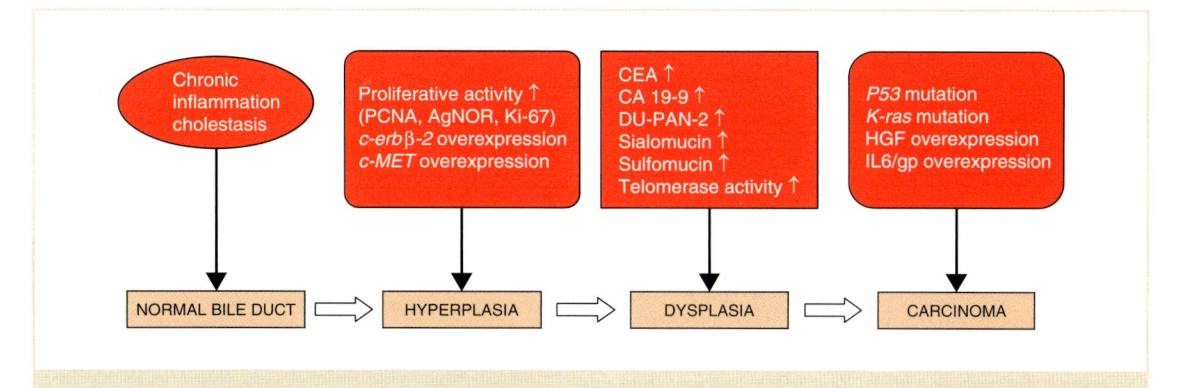

Figure 2-2: Proposed scheme of genetic cellular events in the hyperplasia–dysplasia–carcinoma process of intrahepatic cholangiocarcinogenesis. PCNA, proliferating cell nuclear antigen; AgNOR, argyrophilic nuclear organizer regions; c-erbβ-2, type of tyrosine kinase receptor; c-MET, hepatocyte growth factor receptor; CEA, carcinoembryonic antigen; CA, carbohydrate antigen; DU-PAN-2, pancreatic cancer–associated antigen; P53, tumor suppressor gene; K-ras, Kirsten rat sarcoma viral oncogene; HGF, hepatocyte growth factor; IL-6, interleukin-6. (Used with permission from Springer Science and Business Media LLC as adapted from Shimonishi T, Sasaki M, Nakanuma Y. J Hepatobiliary Pancreat Surg. 2000;7(6):542–550.[32])

Primary Sclerosing Cholangitis

Primary sclerosing cholangitis (PSC) is the most common predisposing condition for PCC in Western countries. CC rates of 8%–40% have been reported among patients with PSC in both follow-up studies and resected specimens.[36] The cumulative risk of developing CC in patients with PSC is 1.5% per annum, with 10%–20% of all PSC patients ultimately developing CC during their lifetime.[11,43] CC in PSC patients typically occurs in the third to fifth decade of life.[44,45] One-third of PSC patients who develop CC do so within two years of diagnosis, and the risk of CC seems unrelated to the duration of the inflammatory disease process.[43,44] Although two-thirds of PSC patients have an inflammatory bowel disease, especially ulcerative colitis,[44] no association between the risk of CC and duration or severity of PSC[35] or the presence, severity, or extent of inflammatory bowel disease has been demonstrated.[44,46]

Fibropolycystic Liver Disease

Congenital abnormalities of the biliary tree such as Caroli's syndrome, congenital hepatic fibrosis, and choledochal cysts (cystic dilatations of the bile ducts) carry a 15% risk of malignant change after the second decade. The overall incidence of CC in patients with untreated congenital biliary cysts is up to 28%,[47,48] and the average age at diagnosis of CC in these patients is 34 years.[49] Despite the high incidence of CC in these patients, the mechanism of carcinogenesis remains unclear, but may be related to biliary stasis, reflux of pancreatic secretion causing chronic inflammation, activation of bile acids, and deconjugation of carcinogens.[50] An alternative mechanism involves polymorphisms of *BSEP, FIC1*, and *MDR3* genes that affect the function of bile salt transporter protein, leading to unbalanced bile content and deconjugation of xenobiotics previously conjugated in the liver.[51-53]

Chemical Carcinogen Exposure

Several chemical toxins have been associated with CC. Promutagenic DNA adducts have been recognized in CC revealing prior exposure to DNA-damaging agents.[54] Thorium dioxide (Thorotrast) is one such chemical that has been strongly associated with the development of CC many years after exposure. Thorotrast was originally used as a radiological contrast agent, but its use was discontinued in 1960s due to its carcinogenic properties.[36,55] Exposure to thorium dioxide carries a risk of CC 300 times that of the unexposed population. Exposure to other chemical carcinogens, such as by-products of the rubber and chemical industries, which include dioxins and nitrosamines,[56] as well as an association with alcohol and smoking[43,46] has been reported, but remains controversial.

Viral Hepatitis

As noted earlier, cirrhosis may be associated with the development of CC.[57,58] Sorensen et al. followed up a cohort of more than 11,000 patients with cirrhosis over six years and showed a 10-fold increased risk of CC compared with the general population.[58] More specifically, hepatitis B virus (HBV) and hepatitis C virus (HCV) have been linked to CC.[59–61] Kobayashi et al. from Japan reported a 1000-fold increased risk of developing CC in patients with HCV.[61] In a case-control study from Korea, 12.5% and 13.8% of patients with CC tested positive for HCV and HBV surface antigen, compared with 3.5% and 2.3% of controls.[59] In a similar study from Italy, 23% and 11.5% of patients with CC tested positive for HCV and HBV compared with 6% and 5.5% of controls.[60] A case-control study within the United States found an adjusted odds ratios of 6.1 for HCV and 5.9 for HIV infection[57] for the development of CC. HCV is a recognized risk factor for HCC and a shared progenitor cell for both hepatocytes and cholangiocytes, supporting a role for HCV in cholangiocarcinogenesis. Additional evidence supporting a link between HCV and CC is the identification of RNA from HCV in CC tissue.[62]

Natural History

Information about natural history of PCC is notably lacking. The absence of specific signs and symptoms of PCC typically leads to a delay from development of initial symptoms to the time of definitive surgical therapy. Delays of between 4.5 and 9 months are common.[22,63,64] A five-year survival of up to 100% among patients with stages I and II disease and 46.9% for patients with stage III disease has been reported. Stage IV disease carries a poor prognosis with one- and three-year survival of 24% and 6%, respectively (Table 2-6). Regardless of stage, survival of patients with PCC who are not candidates for curative interventions is poor with a median survival of 5–14 months[65] and a one-year survival in the range of 11.8%–36.1%.[65–68] Even if resectable, prognosis in patients with both LN metastases and a positive resection margin (R1/R2) is poor with a median survival of only 17 months.[69] Note, even when a R0 resection is achieved, survival of patients is predicted by initial stage of disease at presentation.

Incidence

Over the last 30 years, there has been a worldwide increase in the incidence and mortality rates for PCC reflecting the distribution of local geographic risk factors, in addition to genetic differences among various populations.[36,70] The incidence of PCC is highest in areas of Laos and in north and northeast Thailand, where liver fluke infection is endemic.[34] According to the World Health Organization (1997), the incidence of PCC in Khon Kaen, Thailand, was 88 per 100,000 males and 37 per 100,000 females. The incidence of PCC among all liver cancers was 90% in males and

TABLE 2-6: Survival Among Patients with Peripheral Cholangiocarcinoma According to Stage at Presentation

Author, Year	Stage I 1 y	Stage I 3 y	Stage I 5 y	Stage II 1 y	Stage II 3 y	Stage II 5 y	Stage III 1 y	Stage III 3 y	Stage III 5 y	Stage IV 1 y	Stage IV 3 y	Stage IV 5 y
Isaji, 1999[200]			100			100	46.9		46.9	B-17.6	A-19	A-19
Uenishi, 2001[114]				100	86	86	A-63 B-50	A-31 B-0		A-24	0	0
Okabayashi, 2001[21]		74			48			A-18 B-7				
Jan, 2005[74]		60	45		28.89	17.78		2.65			6.08	

Abbreviations: A, stage IVA without LN or distant metastasis; B, stage IVB with LN and distant metastasis.

94% in females in Kohn Kaen, Thailand, versus 5% in males and 12% in females in Osaka, Japan.[25] The prevalence rate of PCC in the United States is very low at approximately 0.8 per 100,000.[8] The estimated age-adjusted incidence rate for PCC in the United States has increased by 165% over the past three decades.[6] In a review of data from the Surveillance Epidemiology and End Results Registries (SEER; from 1975 to 1999), the incidence of PCC is shown to have increased from 0.32 per 100,000 population to 0.85 per 100,000 population.[6,7] In addition, the increasing incidence has not plateaued as would be expected if the increased incidence was merely due to an advancement in diagnostic modalities such as endoscopic retrograde cholangiopancreatography, magnetic resonance imaging (MRI), or CT, which have become firmly established over this time frame.[10,36,71] In addition, an increase in intrahepatic tumors is greater than the relative decline in extrahepatic tumors.[36,71] These factors suggest that the increasing incidence in PCC is likely a true biologic phenomenon. Interestingly, the unusual increase of PCC in the United States does not seem due to an increase in primary sclerosing cholangitis (PSC), the main known risk factor in the Western world, because the incidence of PSC has not changed. Moreover, PSC is most often associated with the development of intrahepatic tumors in younger patients rather than older age groups where the increased incidence of PCC is not apparent in epidemiological studies.[36,71] To date, although the precise reasons for the increasing incidence of PCC remain elusive, several investigators have hypothesized that risk factors such as HCV infection, chronic nonalcoholic liver disease, and obesity may play a role.[13]

Clinical Presentation and Demographics

Most patients present with nonspecific symptoms such as abdominal pain, jaundice, fever, malaise, and weight loss. Abdominal pain is the most common symptom with jaundice being the second most common (Table 2-7). Although jaundice is usually seen in extrahepatic CC, it can occur in both early and late stages of PCC. In early stages, it is usually

TABLE 2-7: Common Presenting Symptoms Among Patients with Peripheral Cholangiocarcinoma

Author, Year	N	Abdominal Pain (%)	Jaundice (%)	Weight Loss (%)	GI Complaints (%)	Elevated LFTs (%)	No symptoms %
Weber, 2001[105]	53	38	28	4	—[a]	11	19
Valverde, 1999[64]	42	57	2	19	—[a]	—[a]	—[a]
El Rassi, 1999[126]	21	62	19	38	29	—[a]	—[a]
Roayaie, 1998[4]	26	54	—[a]	19	15	—[a]	19
Lieser, 1998[68]	61	67	15	31	30	—[a]	—[a]
Harrison, 1998[108]	32	59	3	—[a]	—[a]	—[a]	—[a]
Yamamoto, 1998[24]	70	19	19	—[a]	—[a]	—[a]	13
Madariaga, 1998[131]	34	71	12	15	34	—[a]	—[a]
Chou, 1997[66]	57	68	15	25	10	—[a]	—[a]
Berdah, 1996[22]	31	35	13	3	13	—[a]	16
Nakeeb, 1996[5]	18	61	0	11	0	0	—[a]
Cherqui, 1995[109]	19	47	26	26	26	—[a]	—[a]
Ohashi, 1994[201]	14	44	21	—[a]	21	—[a]	14

Abbreviations: GI, gastrointestinal; LFTs, liver function tests.
[a]Not mentioned.

due to segmental duct occlusion by tumor; most commonly by an ID growth type. Appearance of jaundice in late stages is generally due to diffuse replacement of liver parenchyma by tumor or by extrahepatic bile duct compression due to metastatic LNs. Of note, nearly one-third of tumors are detected incidentally during routine examination.[72]

Patient age at initial presentation with PCC varies between endemic and nonendemic regions. Patients in endemic regions typically present in the fourth decade of life, whereas patients in nonendemic regions present in the seventh decade of life. PCC is more common in males in all parts of the world (1.7:1) and is nearly always clinically silent until late stages of disease making early diagnosis difficult.

Diagnosis and Workup

Up to one-third of all patients with PCC are found incidentally.[72] All patients presenting with space occupying lesions in the liver require further evaluation. Typically workup includes ultrasound (US), triple phase contrast-enhanced CT scan of the abdomen, and/or MRI with gadolinium enhancement. All radiologic findings should be interpreted cautiously given the overlap among radiological features of PCC, HCC, metastatic liver disease, and benign lesions such as hemangioma, focal nodular hyperplasia, and hepatic adenoma (Table 2-8). Additional workup may include chest X-ray, chest CT, and 18-fluorodeoxyglucose positron emission

TABLE 2-8: Imaging Characteristics for Cholangiocarcinoma According to Morphologic Subtype[88]

Morphologic Subtype	Ultrasonography	Computed Tomography	Magnetic Resonance Imaging
Mass-forming type	Hyperechoic (>3 cm), Hypo or iso-echoic (<3 cm), Peripheral hypoechioc rim (~35% of all tumors)	Homogeneous attenuation Irregular peripheral enhancement Gradual centripetal enhancement	Hyperintense on T2-weighted imaging Hypointense on T1-weighted imaging Peripheral and centripetal enhancement on dynamic contrast-enhanced imaging Associated findings; capsular retraction, satellite nodules, vascular encasement without gross tumor thrombus formation, and hepatolithiasis
Periductal infiltrating type	Small, mass-like lesion or diffuse bile duct thickening with or without obliteration of the bile duct lumen	Diffuse periductal thickening Increased enhancement Abnormally dilated or irregularly narrowed duct	Diffuse periductal thickening with increased enhancement Abnormally dilated or irregularly narrowed duct
Intraductal type	Localized or diffuse duct ectasia with or without an echogenic intraductal polypoid lesion	Tumor appears as hypo- or isoattenuating relative to the surrounding liver on noncontrast CT with enhancement on contrast-enhanced CT Tumor may appear as intraductal polypoid mass or an intraductal cast An associated ductal dilatation that can be diffuse or localized	Diffuse and marked ductal dilatation with an intraductal mass that enhances on contrast-enhanced MR imaging

tomography (FDG-PET). Upper endoscopy may have a role in clarifying locoregional extent of disease and excluding metastases.

Biochemical Investigations and Tumor Markers

Nonspecific derangements in liver function tests (LFTs) can be found with most PCC. Although obstructive jaundice is commonly found in hilar or extrahepatic CC, it is seen in only 2%–28% of patients with PCC. Uniquely, an elevation in the alkaline phosphatase and γ-glutamyl transferase without an increase in bilirubin should raise concern for CC. This LFT is abnormality seen most commonly when there is a segmental ductal tumor causing obstruction without actual biliary involvement.[20,73,74]

Tumor Markers

There are no tumor markers uniquely sensitive enough to be used as a screening tool for PCC, although several may support a clinical suspicion.[75] The most commonly obtained markers are CA 19-9 and CEA. These tumor markers are not specific as they may be elevated in the presence of other malignant (e.g., pancreas and stomach cancer) and benign biliary conditions. Duraker et al. evaluated the role of CEA and CA 19-9 in the screening of benign and malignant pancreatic tumors.[76] Using specific cutoff values for CA 19-9 (29–37 U/mL) and CEA (>5 ng/mL), they reported a sensitivity of 81.3% and 39% for malignant conditions and 24.1% and 8.6% for benign pancreatic conditions, respectively. A specificity of 75.9% for CEA and 91.4% CA 19-9 for detecting pancreatic malignancy was reported.[76] Qin et al. reported a mean serum CA 19-9 concentration of 290.31 ± 5.34 U/L in patients with CC compared with 13.38 ± 2.59 U/L in benign biliary conditions and 12.78 ± 3.69 U/L in healthy individuals ($P < 0.001$).[77] The corresponding mean serum CEA concentrations were 36.46 ± 18.03, 13.84 ± 3.85, and 11.48 ± 3.37 mg/L, respectively ($P < 0.05$).[77] In patients with CC not associated with PSC, serum CA 19-9 value above 100 U/mL had a sensitivity and specificity of 53% and 75%–90%, respectively.[78] In patients with PSC associated CC, serum CA 19-9 levels above 100 U/mL demonstrated a sensitivity and specificity of 75%–89% and 80%–86%, respectively.[46,79,80] In a recent study assessing the value of CA 19-9 (using a cutoff value of 20 U/mL) for diagnosing PSC associated CC, the sensitivity and specificity were 78% and 67%, respectively. The positive and negative predictive values were 23% and 96%, respectively.[81] Serum CA 19-9 combined with ultrasonography, computed tomography (CT), or MRI improved sensitivity for diagnosing CC to 91%, 100%, and 96%, respectively.[81] Patel et al. have reported a positive correlation between CA 19-9 levels and resectability of CC. They noted that a CA 19-9 value of >100 U/mL indicated unresectability with a sensitivity and specificity of 33% and 72%, respectivley.[82] Similarly, Siqueira et al. reported a sensitivity and specificity of 100% and 78.4% for unresectable CC, using a combination of CA 19-9 and CEA with cutoff values of >180 U/mL and >5.2 ng/mL, respectively.[83] Several additional potential tumor markers have been associated with CC including CA-195, CA-242, pancreatic cancer-associated antigen (DU-PAN-2), IL-6, and trypsinogen-2.[75] Human mucin 5, notably subtypes A and C, appear particularly promising for future clinical use with a sensitivity and specificity of 71% and 90%, respectively.[84]

Radiographic Studies

US is the most common initial radiologic investigation for patients presenting with right upper quadrant abdominal pain or jaundice. There are no specific sonographic features to distinguish PCC from other solid intrahepatic mass lesions.[85] Commonly, PCC appears as solitary or multiple mass lesions, but they may also appear as diffuse abnormal liver echotexture displaying hypoechogenicity, hyperechogenicity, or mixed echogenicity.[86] A peripheral hypoechoic rim is seen in about 35% of all PCC and represents either compressed liver parenchyma or proliferating tumor cells.[87] Small tumors (<3 cm) usually appear hypoechoic or isoechoic, whereas large tumors (>3 cm) are usually hyperechoic.[88] There are many overlapping features among PCC, HCC, and metastatic deposits in the liver.[89] Intrahepatic biliary dilatation, atrophy of the liver lobe, turbid appearing mucin, and nodular lesions are highly suggestive of PCC and require evaluation with axial imaging. Transabdominal US cannot appropriately detect intra-abdominal tumor spread and is poor at determining resectability of PCC or other hepatic tumors. Color Doppler US may exhibit a poor signal in PCC in comparison with HCC, which is hypervascular.

Of note, duplex US has a very high sensitivity for detecting portal vein occlusion and infiltration (100% and 83%, respectively).[88]

CT and MRI are considered equivalent in their ability to detect and characterize PCC.[90] CT gives faster results and has significantly few motion artifacts compared with MRI. Moreover, MRI quality is degraded by postembolization susceptibility artifacts.[86] Conversely, MRI has superior contrast resolution compared with CT and may demonstrate satellite lesions and ID tumors earlier.[86] Although certain imaging features of PCC are characteristic, none are specific enough to confirm the diagnosis (Table 2-8).[88] CT characteristics of PCC include an irregular large mass with very low attenuation, slight contrast enhancement usually at the periphery, and focal intrahepatic bile ductal dilatation around the tumor.[91–94] On dynamic CT, the tumor shows low attenuation in the early phase and has increased CT numbers in delayed phase.[94] PCC have a characteristic delayed enhancement from the periphery to center, due to slow uptake of contrast media by interstitial tissue (Figure 2-3).[95–97] MRI characteristics of PCC usually demonstrate an irregular large mass with low intensity on T1-weighted images and high intensity on T2-weighted images, with minimal to moderate tumor rim enhancement of the tumors.[98,99] On dynamic MRI, the tumor shows progressive and concentric filling with contrast material (Figure 2-4).[100]

FDG-PET scanning that detects the focal accumulation of nucleotide tracer 18-fluorodeoxyglucose (FDG) in dividing cells is an emerging staging technique for many cancers. This technique can detect nodular CC as small as 1 cm in diameter, but is less sensitive for infiltrating tumors.[101] The fusion techniques of PET/CT may be applied for more accurate evaluation of small or early PCC, which may not be obvious on routine investigations. FDG-PET has a higher specificity for detecting lymphadenopathy than CT with comparable sensitivity rates. PET may also offer superiority over CT and MRI in detecting distant metastases,[102] especially for detecting N2 level LNs and peritoneal metastases, which are usually noted only at laparoscopy or laparotomy.[103] Kim et al. reported that PET detected distant PCC metastases in 4 of 21 (19%) patients with PCC[103]; however, it is difficult to generalize this finding.

The Role of Percutaneous Biopsy in PCC

Preoperative percutaneous biopsy is not routinely performed to confirm the diagnosis of PCC because sensitivity and specificity are low, and there is some concern of tumor seeding along the needle track.[104] The presence of mucobilia and evidence of perineural tumor spread are highly suggestive of PCC, but these features are rarely appreciated on needle biopsy.[68] The main role of percutaneous biopsy is to confirm a histologic diagnosis prior to beginning adjuvant therapy in unresectable cases or to address a diagnostic dilemma, such as excluding metastases in a patient with a known additional malignancy. In the absence of extrahepatic metastases or bilobar unresectable masses, laparoscopy or laparotomy is the preferred method for histological confirmation with progression to resection if metastases are excluded and the patient is deemed resectable.[68]

Staging of Peripheral Cholangiocarcinoma

No current staging system can stratify patients into specific subgroups that correlate with survival. Two widely used staging systems for PCC are the International Union against Cancer (UICC)/American Joint Committee on Cancer tumor node metastasis (TNM) Staging System and the Liver Cancer Study Group of Japan TNM Staging System (Table 2-9). Jonas et al. compared the fifth and sixth editions of the UICC TNM staging system for PCC and identified several advantages of the sixth edition including grouping of all LN-positive patients into stage IIIc and redefining stage I and II disease categories.[19]

Assessment for Resectability

Radiological imaging is indispensable in both the staging and assessment of resectability for hepatobiliary malignancies. Multivariate analyses have shown that LN metastases, multiple tumors at the initial presentation, symptomatic tumors, and vascular invasion are independent factors associated

Peripheral Cholangiocarcinoma 35

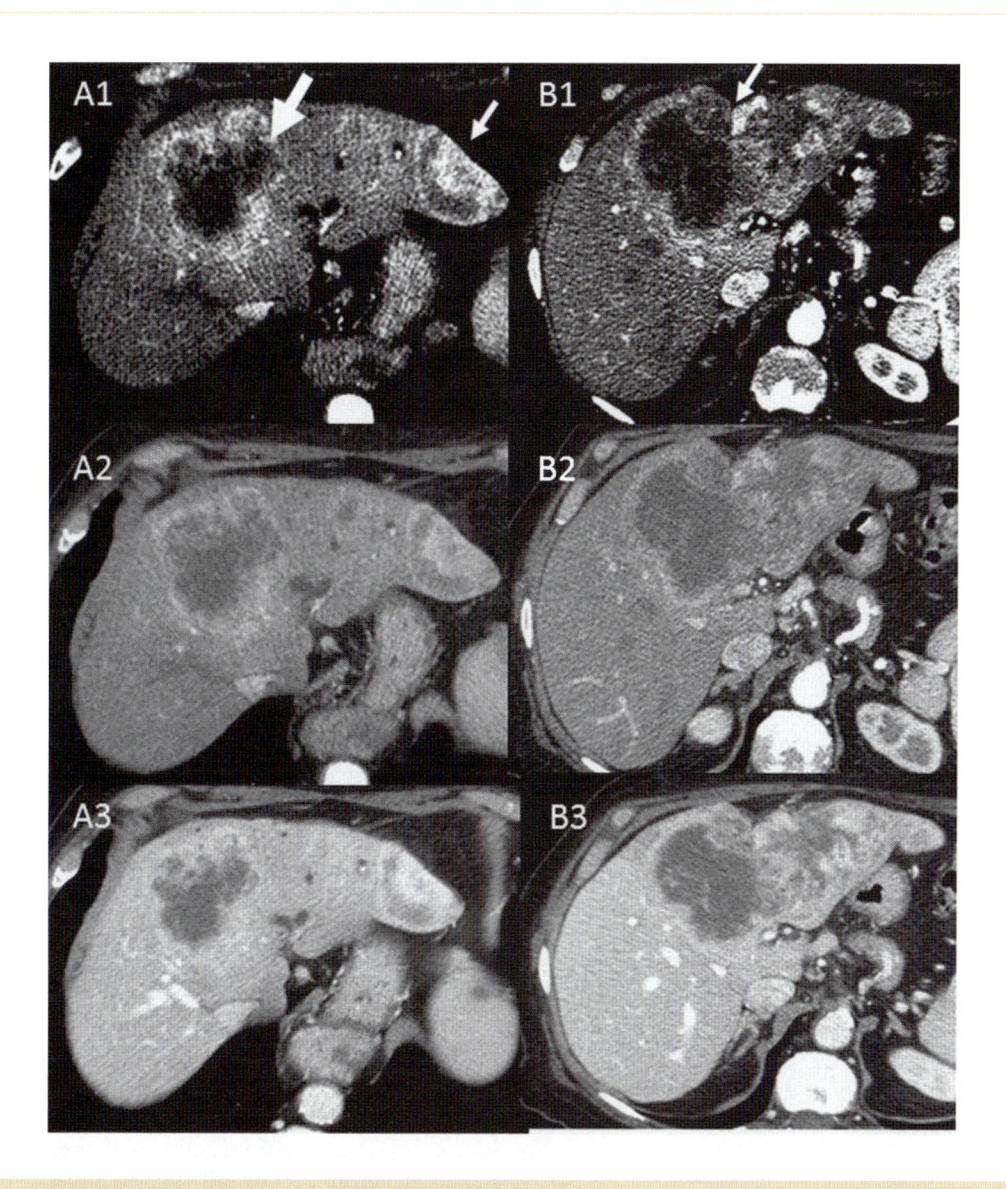

Figure 2-3: Typical CT findings of mass-forming PCC. Two Ct cuts (A) and (B) for a peripheral cholangiocarcinoma, shown in three phases: arterial (1), intermediate (2), and delayed venous (3). Smaller tumors tend to show much arterial enhancement (A1, small arrow), while larger tumors show dark central necrosis and peripheral enhancement (A1, large arrow). Note also the typical umbilicated appearance of the larger tumors (B1, arrow).

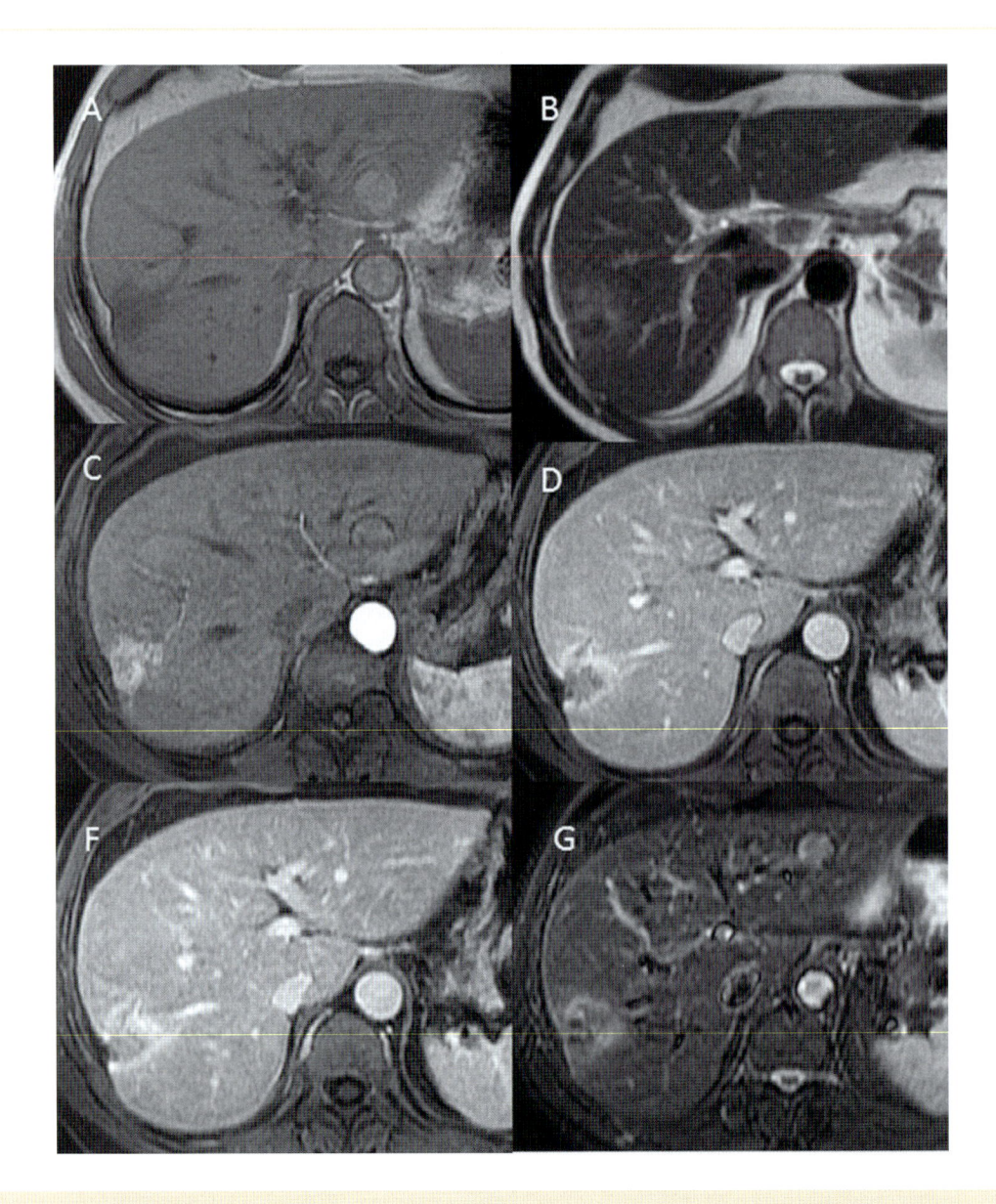

Figure 2-4: Typical MR Imaging features of mass-forming PCC. The tumor is hypointense on T1 images (A), intermediate in intensity on T2 images (B). Contrast enhancement is seen in the arterial phase (C), and centrally washing out in intermediate (D) and late phases (F). It is particularly noticeable in fat-suppressed T2- weighted MR images (G).

TABLE 2-9 Part A: Tumor, Node, and Metastases Staging Systems for Peripheral Cholangiocarcinoma

	UICC/AJCC, Fifth Edition[19]	UICC/AJCC, Sixth Edition[19]	LCSGJ[200]
T stage			
T1	• Solitary < 2 cm, without vascular invasion	Solitary tumor without vascular invasion	Meets following three criteria: 1) Unifocal lesion 2) Size ≤ 2 cm 3) No vascular or serosal involvement
T2	• Solitary < 2 cm, with vascular invasion • Multiple, 1 lobe, <2 cm, without vascular invasion • Solitary >2 cm, without vascular invasion	Solitary tumor with vascular invasion Or Multiple tumors, none >5 cm in the greatest dimension	Two of three T1 criteria satisfied
T3	• Solitary > 2 cm, with vascular invasion • Multiple, 1 lobe, <2 cm, with vascular invasion • Multiple, 1 lobe, >2 cm, with or without vascular invasion	Multiple tumors >5 cm or tumor involving a major branch of the portal or hepatic vein(s)	One of three T1 criteria satisfied
T4	• Multiple, both lobes • Invades major branch of portal or hepatic vein(s) • Invades adjacent organs other than gallbladder • Perforates visceral peritoneum	Tumor(s) with direct invasion of adjacent organs other than the gallbladder or with perforation of visceral peritoneum	No T1 criteria is satisfied
N stage			
N0	Absence of nodal involvement	Absence of nodal involvement	Absence of nodal involvement
N1	Presence of regional lymph node involvement	Presence of regional lymph node involvement	Presence of regional lymph node involvement
M stage			
M0	Absence of metastases	Absence of metastases	Absence of metastases
M1	Presence of metastases	Presence of metastases	Presence of metastases

Abbreviations: UICC, International Union against Cancer; AJCC, American Joint Committee on Cancer; LCSGJ, Liver Cancer Study Group of Japan.

TABLE 2-9 Part B: Tumor, Node, and Metastases Staging Systems for Peripheral Cholangiocarcinoma

UICC/AJCC, Fifth Edition				UICC/AJCC, Sixth Edition				LCSGJ Staging			
	T	N	M		T	N	M		T	N	M
I	T1	N0	M0	Stage I	T1	N0	M0	Stage I	T1	N0	M0
II	T2	N0	M0	Stage II	T2	N0	M0	Stage II	T2	N0	M0
IIIA	T3	N0	M0	Stage IIIA	T3	N0	M0	Stage III	T3	N0	M0
IIIB	T1–3	N1	M0	Stage IIIB	T4	N0	M0	Stage IVA	T4	N0	M0
IVA	T4	Any N	M0	Stage IIIC	Any T	N1	M0	Stage IVB	T1–T4	N1	M0
IVB	Any T	Any N	M1	Stage IV	Any T	Any N	M1		T1–T4	N0,N1	M1

Abbreviations: UICC, International Union against Cancer; AJCC, American Joint Committee on Cancer; LCSGJ, Liver Cancer Study Group of Japan.

with poor postoperative outcomes for nearly all tumors.[85,88] The presence of segmental or lobar atrophy is strongly associated with ipsilateral or contralateral portal vein encasement and unresectability. The accuracy of CT and MRI in detecting hepatic vascular involvement is high, and it is described in approximately 50% of PCC, which more often involve the portal veins than the hepatic veins.[89] Both CT and MRI can demonstrate hepatic arterial involvement with an accuracy of 92.7% and 89%, respectively. Accuracy decreases to 85.5% and 83.6% for detecting portal vein invasion and N2 nodal metastases, respectively.[89] In general, it is important to note that there are significant limitations to the use of all imaging modalities in both PCC staging and assessment of resectability. Satellite nodules are detected only 65% of time[92] and usually only when they are larger than 1 or 2 cm.[89] Okabayashi et al. reported that nearly 37% of satellite lesions, later confirmed by the pathological examination of the resected specimens, were not identified by preoperative CT and intraoperative US.[21]

Diagnostic laparoscopy has an important role in the preoperative assessment of PCC. Weber et al. reported that diagnostic laparoscopy prior to laparotomy spared unnecessary surgery in 6 of 22 (27%) patients with PCC.[105] Similarly, Goere et al. reported a 36% yield and a 67% accuracy for diagnostic laparoscopy in cases of PCC.[106] Although there is no general consensus on which patients with PCC are resectable, criteria for unresectability are less controversial and include the following:

- Medical comorbidities limiting the patients' ability to undergo major surgery
- Significant underlying liver disease prohibiting liver resection
- Bilateral tumor extension to secondary biliary radicals
- Encasement or occlusion of the main portal vein
- Lobar atrophy with contralateral portal vein involvement
- Contralateral tumor extension to secondary biliary radicals
- Evidence of metastases to N2 level LNs
- Presence of distant metastases

Treatment Options for Peripheral Cholangiocarcinoma

There are limited therapeutic options in the management of PCC. Surgical resection with curative intent is the only modality that offers prolonged survival. Despite this fact, Tan et al.[107] have noted that only 12% patients with PCC undergo surgical resection, which underscores the biologic aggressiveness of the disease, but may also point to a therapeutic nihilism, which biases the clinical approach to this neoplasm. For patients deemed inoperable, a variety of palliative therapies have been used, although limited data exist to suggest an advantage of one modality over another. The role of neoadjuvant and adjuvant chemotherapy and radiotherapy remains investigational and unproven.

Surgery for PCC

The ultimate goal in the treatment of PCC is complete resection of the tumor with negative margins (R0 resection). The extent of resection depends on the location of the tumor, vascular involvement, and LN status. To achieve tumor-free margins, hepatic resections are tailored according to local tumor burden. In general, lobectomy or extended hepatic resection is commonly required to achieve R0 margins, although they are associated with increased rate of morbidity and mortality.[27] The resectability rate for PCC varies between 50% and 100% and likely reflects selection and treatment bias (Table 2-10).[68,107] The widespread availability of CT and MRI in the preoperative assessment of PCC, as well as the use of laparoscopy and laparoscopic US to avoid negative laparotomy, has resulted in increased resectability rates over time. Ideal candidates for curative resection are those with (1) solitary lesion, (2) no evidence of LN metastases, and (3) those in whom >1 cm tumor-free margin is deemed achievable.[108] Although ideal, these criteria are not universally accepted, and Lang et al. have noted that the presence of satellite lesions is not a contradiction to surgical resection.[27] Moreover, some authors have noted that satellite lesions and the presence of tumor cells within 1 cm from the resected margins do not affect overall survival (OS) after R0 resection (Figure 2-5).[69,109,110] LN metastases and stage of disease at presentation are the only two factors independently associated with a poor outcome after R0 resection,[111] and survival is significantly reduced with LN-positive disease (Table 2-11).

TABLE 2-10: Published Series of Surgical Resection for Peripheral Cholangiocarcinoma Since 1995

Author, Year	N	Overall Resectability N (%)	R0, N (%)	R1, N (%)	R2, N (%)	5-y Survival All	5-y Survival R0	Mortality Rate (%)
Pichlmayr 1995[174]	50	32 (64)	31 (96.9)	1 (3.1)	0	17	N/A	6
Casavilla 1997[175]	54	34 (63)	24 (70.6)	10 (29.4)	0	31	N/A	3.7
Lieser 1998[68]	61	32 (52.4)	28 (87.5)	N/A	4 (12.5)	N/A	45	0
Madariaga 1998[131]	34	34 (100)	24 (70.6)	10 (29.4)	0	35	51	6
Valverde 1999[64]	35	29 (82.9)	29 (100)	N/A	N/A	22	N/A	3.3
Inoue 2000[113]	88	52 (59)	36 (69.2)	16 (30.8)	N/A	36	55	2
Weber 2001[105]	53	33 (62)	20 (61)	13 (39.3)	N/A	31	N/A	3
DeOliveira 2007[127]	44	44 (100)	20 (45.5)	24 (54.5)	N/A	N/A	N/A	4
Li 2009[112]	136	79 (58.1)	65 (82.2)	14 (17.7)	N/A	N/A	N/A	2.2

N, total number of patients R0, tumor-free resection margin; R1, microscopically positive resection margin; R2, macroscopically positive resection margin; N/A, not available.

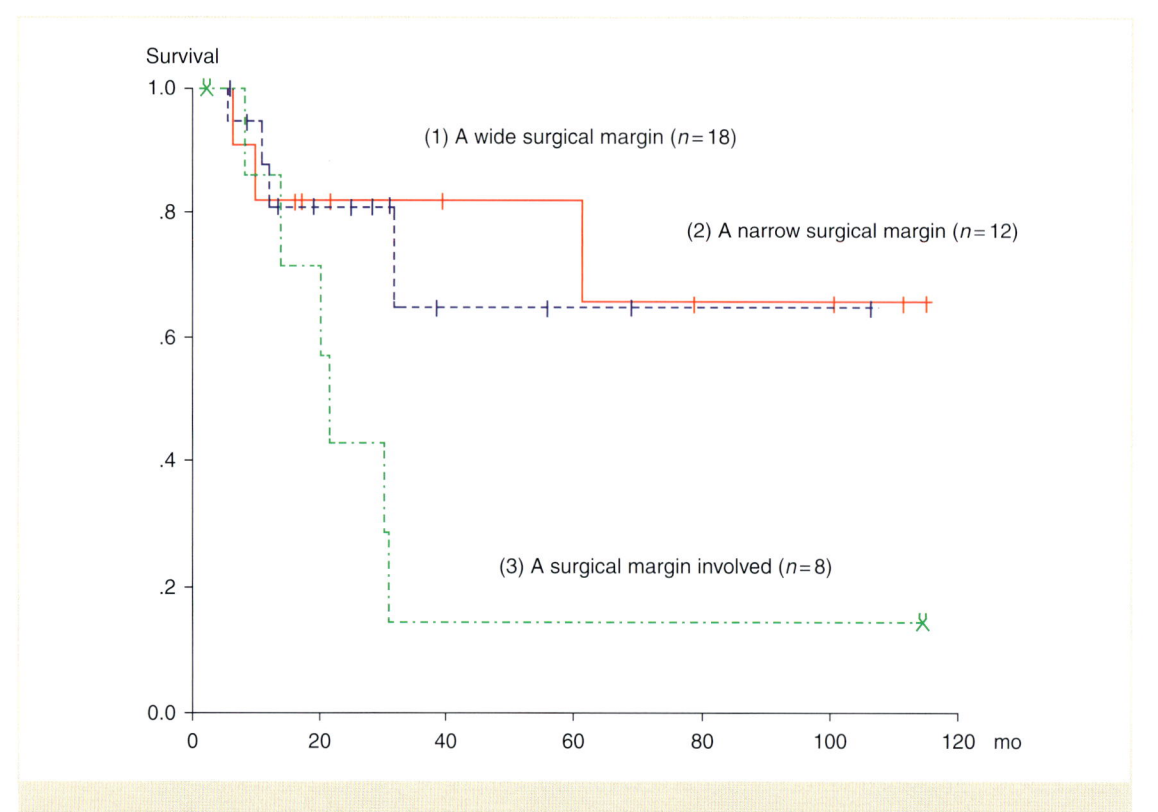

Figure 2-5: Overall survival among 38 patients of peripheral cholangiocarcinoma according to surgical margin status, without lymph node metastasis. The statistically significant differences revealed were as follows: wide surgical margin (>5 mm) vs. narrow surgical margin (≤5 mm), $P < 0.8252$; wide surgical margin (>5 mm) vs. positive surgical margin, $P < 0.0396$; narrow surgical margin (≤5 mm) vs. positive surgical margin, $P < 0.0373$. (Adapted with permission from Wiley from Shimada et al.[69])

TABLE 2-11: Published Reports of Lymph Node Metastases on Survival In Patients with Peripheral Cholangiocarcinoma Undergoing Tumor-Free Resected Margins (R0)

Author, Year	R0 Resection With Negative Lymph Nodes				R0 Resection With Positive Lymph Nodes			
	N	1 y	3 y	5 y	N	1 y	3 y	5 y
Nozaki 1998[203]	32	61.3	37.6	37.6	15	53.3	13.3	6.7
Lang 2005[27]	12	94	82		4	Three patients are alive at 7, 21, and 30 mo		
Lang 2009[115]	38	93	58	33	15	53	27	20
Li 2009[112]	41	76.4	51.4	30	12	50	0	0
Jonas 2009[19]	98	79		37.8	40	Only two patients survived beyond 3 y and one reached 5 y		

Abbreviations: DFS, disease-free survival; LN, lymph nodes; R0, tumor-free resected margins.

TABLE 2-12: Reports of Extended Hepatic Resections and Survival in Patients with Peripheral Cholangiocarcinoma Since 1992

Author, Year	Total, N	Extended, N (%)	Survival (%) 1 y	3 y	5 y	Median Survival (mo)
Yamamoto, 1992[124]	20	9 (45)	64.5	37.6	37.6	N/A
Cherqui, 1995[109]	14	8 (57)	58	N/A	N/A	14
Casavilla, 1997[175]	34	15 (44)	60	37	31	N/A
Chu, 1997[204]	39	8 (21)	57.3	23.9	15.9	12.2
Harrison, 1998[108]	32	16 (50)	76	56	42	59
Madariaga, 1998[131]	34	18 (53)	67	40	35	19
Roayaie, 1998[4]	16	11 (69)	86	64	21	42.9
Valverde, 1999[64]	29	20 (69)[a]	86	63	22	N/A
Weimann, 2000[176]	95	N/A	64	31	21	17.7
Inoue, 2000[113]	52	23 (44)	63	36	36	18
Weber, 2001[105]	33	15 (45)	83	55	31	37.4
Kawarada, 2002[205]	37	19 (51)	54.1	34	23.9	31.5
Lang, 2009[115]	83	65 (78.3)	71	38	21	26

Abbreviation: N/A, not available.
[a]Survival was analyzed for 28 patients.

Noncurative Resection (R1 and R2 resection)

In general, there is no role for palliative surgery or resection in PCC. However, a positive surgical margin is usually an outcome rather than an intent of surgical therapy. Microscopically positive resection margin (R1 status) is found in 3%–54.5% of hepatic resections for PCC (Table 2-12), and as such, an intraoperative frozen section should be performed routinely. Microscopically positive margins are usually seen in tumors close to major vessels and those with satellite nodules.[112] Whether an R1 resection will yield a similar outcome as an R0 resection is unclear. Tamandl et al. reported a median recurrence-free survival of 11.4 months for patients with negative margins and 9.9 months for patients with R1 resection ($P < 0.88$). The median OS was 27.2 months for patients with R0 resection and not reached in the R1 group ($P < 0.35$).[110] Shimada et al. reported a five-year and median survival of 56.8% and 62 months for patients undergoing R0 resection compared with 16.7% and 20 months for patients with a positive resection margins, respectively ($P < 0.06$).[69] On the contrary, Lang et al. reported a median and one- and three-year survival rates of 46 months, 94%, and 82%, respectively, in patients with negative resection margins compared with a median survival of five months and a one-year survival rate of 22% in patients with a positive resection margins ($P < 0.004$).[27] Similarly, Uenishi et al. reported a one-, three-, and five-year survival of 77.8%, 66.7%, and 66.7%, respectively, for patients with R0 margins compared with a 46.8%, 5.8%, and 0% for patients with a positive resection margins ($P < 0.003$).[113]

The Role of Extended Hepatectomy and Aggressive Resection

Improvement in imaging and surgical techniques has led to an increasingly aggressive surgical approach to PCC. Large or advanced-stage tumors previously deemed unapproachable are now treated with resection of the extrahepatic biliary tract, vascular hilar structures, vena cava, and diaphragm along with extended hepatectomy. A review of published series since 1992 reveals that between 21% and 78.3% of patients with PCC required extended hepatic resections (Table 2-16). Val-verde et al. reported on a group of 42 patients with stage III and IV disease and found that 63% required resection of four or more hepatic segments, and in 21.4% of patients, the resection was extended to include the inferior vena cava, diaphragm, and/or common bile duct.[64] An R0 resection was achieved in all but one patient who was found to have peritoneal deposits at the time of resection. Although an R0 resection may be achievable, it is important to note that aggressive surgical treatment is associated with considerable morbidity and mortality. Postoperative morbidity rates ranged from 56% to 63% in patients undergoing extended or radical resections compared with 45% for patients with PCC undergoing less aggressive surgery. Postoperative mortality rates range between 6% and 9.6% following radical resections of PCC.[22,27,114] Despite their increased morbidity and mortality, more aggressive approach, hepatic resection is associated with increased OS. Li et al. reported that stage IV patients treated with aggressive surgical resection had a median survival of 14 months in comparison with three months for those who did not undergo aggressive resection.[111] Importantly, patients undergoing extended resections had a higher incidence of LN metastases (80%) compared with patients who did not require extended resections (34.2%), and this may explain the decreased survival even when a R0 resection was achieved.[63]

The Significance of the Number and Site of Involved Lymph Nodes in Pcc

There is a mixed opinion regarding the significance of the number and sites of LN involvement in PCC. Suzuki et al. and Nakagawa et al. have suggested that only one tumor nodule and one LN metastases or one tumor nodule with just two LNs involved may offer a better prognosis.[72,115] However, Uenishi et al. found no correlation between postoperative survival and the number of positive LNs.[113] More recently, Tamandl et al. reported that patients with a LN ratio (ratio of the number of positive LNs to the total number of LNs harvested) of >0.2 had a poor prognosis in regard to OS and recurrence.[116] There is no reported difference in the OS between patients with regional or distant LN metastases.[116,117]

Routine LN Sampling or Dissection

PCC is associated with a high incidence of LN metastases in comparison with HCC.[118] The incidence of LN metastases in PCC varies between 17% and 62% and carries a poor prognosis (Figure 2-6).[117,119] Currently, there is no consensus regarding the role of LN dissection in patients with PCC,[115,117,120,121] and selection criteria are not well established. Currently, there is no role for routine perihepatic LN sampling in patients with PCC. The LN positivity rate in patients of PCC without preoperative and intraoperative evidence of enlarged LNs is low.[122,123] Grobmyer et al. reported that in patients with primary and metastatic liver cancer with nonpalpable LNs, the incidence of metastases to perihepatic LNs was as low as 1%.[123] Similarly, Shimada et al. reported a therapeutic benefit of only 4% with prophylactic LN dissection in patients with MF type of PCC, as only 3 of 13 patients for whom LN dissection was not done went on to develop recurrence within the LNs.[119] Although some subtypes such as the MF+PI tumor may be at a higher risk, there is no sufficient data available to clearly define groups of patients with PCC who may benefit from LN dissection. That said, significant effort should be made to examine LN metastases prior to embarking on major resection, which may be associated with significant morbidity in patients with positive LN without any survival advantage. Chou et al. reported that patients with hilar LN metastases (N = 11) had a median survival of five months compared with 36 months in patients without LN metastases (N = 8).[66,124] Similarly El Rassi et al. noted a one-year survival rate of 80% for LN-negative patients compared with 50% in patients with LN-positive disease.[125] No patient in the latter group survived two years, compared with a two- and three-year survival of 25% and 35%, respectively, for LN-negative patients.[125] DeOliveira et al.[126]

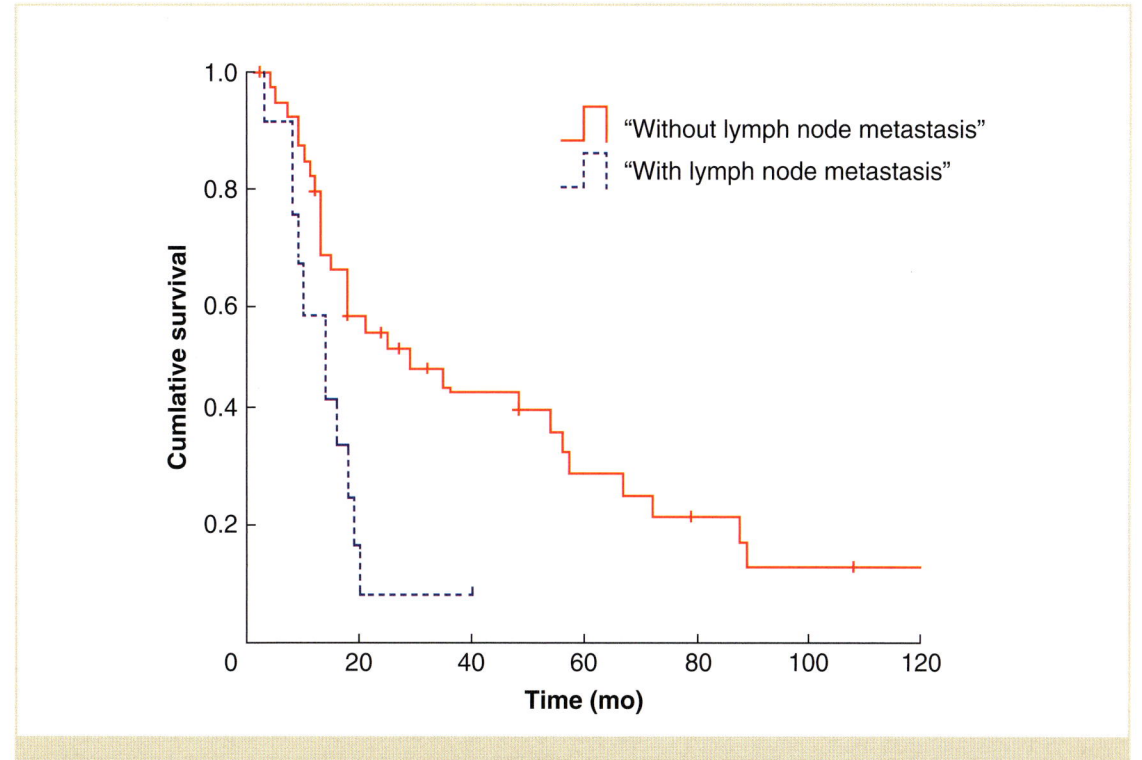

Figure 2-6: Survival outcomes among peripheral cholangiocarcinoma patients with (N = 12) and without (N = 41) lymph node metastasis after curative resection (P < 0.013). (Adapted from Li et al.[111])

reviewed 564 patients with CC (including 44 patients with PCC) and reported that although LN dissection was often performed in patients with PCC, it was not done routinely. In this group, 29% of patients with PCC were found to have LN metastases with a hazard ratio (HR) of 3.47 (1.18–10.27) and 1.04 (0.24–4.60) on univariate and multivariate analysis. The median and five-year survival for patients with PCC was 28 months and 40%, respectively. These authors concluded that based on their own experience and a review of literature, there is insufficient evidence to perform routine LN dissection in patients with PCC.[126]

Outcomes of Surgical Resection

R0 surgical resection offers the only chance of long-term survival with acceptable mortality for patients with PCC.[127] The reported five-year OS for PCC ranges between 17% and 36%; whereas five-year survival after R0 resections is between 45% and 55%, respectively. Although decreased, the five-year survival rates for the patients requiring extended hepatic resections are also acceptable and range from 15.9% to 42% (Table 2-12). Yamamoto et al. have reported a five-year OS of 10% in patients requiring extensive surgery for PCC compared with 53% in patients undergoing nonextended R0 resection.[63] LN-positive PCC and stage III and IV disease are associated with a decreased OS even when R0 resection can be achieved.[109,128] Lang et al. reported a five-year survival of only 20% in PCC patients with LN metastases after R0 curative resection.[27] Similarly, Valverde et al. reported a median survival of only 30 months for patients with stage III disease, 26 months for stage IVa disease, and 2 months for stage IVb disease following R0 surgical resection.[64] Patients with unresectable disease have a one-year survival of approximately 15.7%, while survival among unresected patients is unaffected by stage of disease.[68]

Adjuvant Therapy

The role of adjuvant therapy in the treatment of patients who had undergone an R0 resection for PCC remains investigational, although its use is not uncommon. Adjuvant therapy is typically reserved for PCC patients with recurrence or in patients with R1/R2 resection.[20,129] Despite this practice, published reports reveal no impact on OS following adjuvant therapy.[4,114,130] Madariaga et al. treated 24 of the 32 (75%) PCC patients with adjuvant therapy, which included RT ($N = 6$), chemotherapy ($N = 15$), or both ($N = 3$). These authors reported no difference in survival of the patients with or without adjuvant therapy ($P = 0.42$).[130]

Palliative Therapy

Palliative Chemotherapy

The role of palliative chemotherapy in advanced cases of PCC and CC is not firmly established. The rarity of PCC has required most clinical trials to enroll patients with all types of biliary tract tumors, and the number of patients with PCC has normally been quite small. Moreover, the lack of randomization and small study size makes it impossible to perform comparison between published results. Currently, there is no consensus regarding best agent or regimen for unresectable or metastatic PCC. Several chemotherapeutic agents have been shown to have activity in the palliative setting for advanced CC of all types. These agents include 5-fluorouracil (5-FU/leucovorin), mitomycin-C, cisplatin, doxorubicin, and gemcitabine. Gemcitabine and 5-FU have been extensively studied as single agents or in combination chemotherapy regimens.[130] 5-FU has an overall response rate (RR) of 0%–40% and a median survival advantage of 2–12 months when used as single-agent 5-FU-based chemotherapy.[123,132–141] When gemcitabine is used as a single agent, the overall RR and median survival were 8%–60% and 6.3–16 months, respectively.[142–149] In a retrospective review of 304 patients with unresectable biliary tract cancer (including 93 patients with PCC), Yonemoto et al. identified gemcitabine as the most effective chemotherapeutic agent. Among patients with all types of CC treated with gemcitabine-based chemotherapy, the partial response (PR), stable disease (SD), and progressive disease (PD) rates were 6.9%, 50%, and 39.7%, respectively.[150] Patients treated with 5-FU-based chemotherapy by those same authors had PR, SD, and PD rates of 0%, 36.7%, and 36.7%, respectively. Most importantly those authors observed a 50% reduction in the overall mortality of patients treated with gemcitabine.[150] Among patients with unresectable PCC treated by these authors, they observed a median survival of 8.44 months with a PR and PD rates of 3.2% and 96.7%, respectively. No patient experienced a complete response.[150]

Results of combination chemotherapy are unfortunately no more promising. Combination therapy with 5-FU and cisplatin produced a median survival of 11 months,[132] whereas combinations with gemcitabine resulted in a median survival ranging from 5 to 15.4 months.[131] The combination of gemcitabine with cisplatin has yielded the most favorable results, mostly among patients with a good performance status and adequate hepatic function. In gemcitabine/cisplatin-treated patients, the PR ranged from 27.5% to 50% with a median survival in the range of 5 to 11.3 months.[132,151,152] When gemcitabine is combined with oxaliplatin, Andre et al. reported an overall RR of 36% with a median survival of 15.4 months.[133] Combination of gemcitabine with other agents such as capecitabine, irinotecan, and docetaxel has demonstrated minimal increased activity versus gemcitabine alone.[134,153,154]

It is important to note that extrahepatic CC has a superior response to chemotherapy compared with PCC. The RR among patients with extrahepatic CC ranges from 10% to 40%, whereas PCC had a RR in the range of 6% to 10%. Conversely, the RR does not correlate with increased median survival, which is in the range of 5–10 months for all types of CC (Table 2-13). Slupski et al. have reported the only complete response in a patient with disseminated PCC to lungs and liver.[151] The patient was treated with nine cycles of PIAF (doxorubicin, cis-platinum, 5-FU, and interferon alpha-2A) and reported disease free at 30 months following liver resection.[151]

Regional Intra-Arterial Chemotherapy

Hepatic intra-arterial chemotherapy, such as transcatheter arterial chemoembolization (TACE) or transcatheter arterial chemoinfusion (TACI), has been shown to be safe and potentially effective

TABLE 2-13: Combination Chemotherapy Trials for Advanced PCC

Author, Year	Chemotherapy Regimen	Patients With Cholangiocarcinoma						Patients With PCC					
		N	Response Rate (%)	Median Survival (mo)	Partial Response (%)	Stable Disease (%)	Progression (%)	N	Response Rate (%)	Median Survival (mo)	Partial Response (%)	Stable Disease (%)	Progression (%)
Sanz-Altamira, 1998[153]	Carboplatin + 5-FU + LV	14	21.4	5				4		9	25	25	50
Ducurex, 1998[134]	5-FU + cisplatin	25	25	10	24			6					
Lee, 2004[135]	Epirubicin + cisplatin + 5-FU infusion	24	40	8	39.5	23.2		20	10	4.97	10	45	45
Park, 2006[154]	Epirubicin + cisplatin + oral 5-FU	43	40	8	39.5	23.2		15					
Furuse, 2006[155]	UFT + doxorubicin	24	12.5	7.6	12.5	54.1	29.2	10		11	20		
Feisthammel, 2007[206]	Irinotecan + folinic acid + 5-FU	30	10	6.3	10	10	80	17	6	5.3	5.8	5.8	88.2

Abbreviations: 5-FU, 5-flurouracil; LV, Leucovorin; PCC, peripheral cholangiocarcinoma; UFT, uracil/tegafur.

TABLE 2-14: Selected Reports of Intra-Arterial Chemotherapy Trials for Patients with Advanced Peripheral Cholangiocarcinoma

Author, Year	N	Chemotherapy Regimen	Survival Median (mo)	1 y (%)	2 y (%)	3 y (%)	PR (%)	Response SD (%)	PD (%)
Transarterial chemoinfusion									
Tanaka 2002[206]	11	5-FU-based chemotherapy	21[a]	91	51	20		18	18
Vogl 2006[159]	11[b]	Gemcitabine infusion	13.5					75	25
Combined systemic and regional chemotherapy									
Cantore 2005[208]	30[c]	Systemic 5-FU infusion + Hepatic intra-arterial epirubicin and cisplatin infusion	13.2	54	20		36.3	40	20
Kirchoff 2005[158]	8	Systemic gemcitabine chemotherapy + TACE (doxorubicin + cisplatin + starch microspheres)	12				37.5	62.5	
Poggi 2009[162]	9	Embolization with oxaliplatin preloaded hepaspheres followed by intra-arterial chemotherapy with oxaliplatin + gemcitabine	30				44	56	
Transarterial chemoembolization (TACE)									
Burger 2005[163]	17	Cisplatin ± embolic particle	23						
Vogl 2006[159]	12[d]	Hepatic intra-arterial gemcitabine infusion + Spherex	20.2					92	8
Herber 2007[209]	15	Lipidol + mitomycin C	16.3	54.5	27.5	27.5			
Gusani 2008[160]	42	Gemcitabine-based chemotherapy followed by embolization with embospheres	13.8[e]					47.6	33.3

Abbreviations: ChT = chemotherapy; 5-FU = fluorouracil; PR, partial response; SD, stable disease; PD, progressive disease; TACE, transcatheter arterial chemoembolization.
[a]Value calculated from the data given in the published article.
[b]Study group included three patients with metastatic adenocarcinoma pancreas.
[c]Study group included five patients with carcinoma gall bladder.
[d]Study group included four patients with metastatic adenocarcinoma pancreas.
[e]Median survival time measured from initiation of TACE treatment.

approach for the treatment of patients with unresectable, primary, and metastatic hepatic malignancies.[155,156] Intra-arterial chemotherapy is typically delivered by either continuous arterial infusion or arterial chemoembolization. When either approach is used, it is normally combined with systemic chemotherapy. Although it is associated with reduced systemic toxicity, both TACE and TACI can result in a progressive rarefaction of the intrahepatic arteries and bile ducts and is a major limitation of this approach.[157] The major advantage of regional intra-arterial infusion of chemotherapeutic agent is that it allows very high local drug concentration to be achieved in the liver (and tumor). Those drug levels are normally 10–100 times higher than that achieved by systemic administration,[158] and by eliminating blood supply to the tumor, it may also prevent washout of chemotherapeutic agents resulting in even higher drug concentrations to the tumor cells over a longer duration.[159] The majority of intra-arterial chemotherapy studies, particularly among patients with CC, are nonrandomized and involve only small number of patients. Moreover, no standard protocol has been followed regarding intra-arterial chemotherapy; hence, it is difficult to compare results. Irrespective of these problems, a median survival of 12–30 months has been reported with a one-year survival of 54.5%–91% and three-year survival of 20%–27.5% (Table 2-14). Aliberti et al. compared the results of TACE versus systemic chemotherapy in a small group of 20 patients with unresectable PCC.[160] Patients consenting to TACE were enrolled in the TACE only group, while the reminder of the patients were allocated to the systemic chemotherapy group. Eleven patients were treated with TACE using slow-releasing doxorubicin-eluting beads, and nine patients received systemic chemotherapy with various combinations of 5-FU, cisplatin, and doxorubicin. TACE achieved a mean reduction of tumor volume of 45% (range: 30%–69%) compared with baseline measurements. At the end of the study, 8 of 11 patients in the TACE group were alive with a median survival of 13 months and only 1 of 9 patients in the systemic chemotherapy group was alive with a median survival of 7 months.[160] When treatment for both lobes of the liver was required, TACE was divided into two sessions with 15–20 days between treatments to avoid liver failure.[160] When compared with systemic therapy, adverse effects of chemotherapeutic agents were significantly reduced when administered by TACE (Table 2-15).[161] In patients undergoing TACE,

TABLE 2-15: Adverse Events Associated with TACE and Systemic Chemotherapy in Patients Treated with a Combined Approach[160]

Adverse Events[a]	OEM-TACE Group (%) All Grades	G3	Systemic Chemotherapy Group (%) All Grades	G3	p
Pain	42	9	25	—	<0.042[b]
Nausea and vomiting	30	—	72	16	<0.001[b]
Asthenia	3	—	25	9	<0.001[c]
Peripheral neuropathy	4	—	40	16	<0.001[c]
Leukopenia	4	—	25	9	<0.001[c]
Cholangitis	7	1	—	—	<0.058[c]
Hypertensive crisis	1	1	—	—	n.s.
Elevated AST and ALT	30	—	16	—	<0.053[c]

With permission from Springer Science and Business Media reproduced from Poggi G, Amatu A, Montagna B, et al. OEM-TACE: a new therapeutic approach in unresectable intrahepatic cholangiocarcinoma. *Cardiovasc Intervent Radiol.* 2009;32(6): 1187–1192.
Abbreviations: ALT, alanine aminotransferase; AST, aspartamine aminotransferase; G3, grade 3; n.s., not significant; OEM-TACE, oxaliplatin-eluting microspheres-transcatheter arterial chemoembolization.
[a]Classified by Common Terminology Reporting Criteria (CTCAE 3.0)
[b]Chi-square test
[c]Fisher test.

adverse events consisted of fever, nausea, vomiting, diarrhea, hypertension, tachycardia, and right upper quadrant pain, the so called postembolization syndrome. These events persisted for hours to a few days and were managed conservatively.[159,162]

Palliative Radiation Therapy

The efficacy of adjuvant RT for PCC has not been evaluated in a prospective randomized trial. Shinohara et al. retrospectively analyzed the SEER database from 1988 to 2003 and identified 3839 patients with PCC who received RT as primary treatment or in the postoperative setting.[163] These authors reported that adjuvant RT following surgery was associated with an improved median survival (11 months) compared with radiation alone (7 months) and was associated with a 9.3% reduction in the risk of death. When patients treated with radiation were compared with the no treatment group, median survival was seven months in the former group versus three months in the later. Most importantly, among patients treated with surgery alone, the median survival and reduction in mortality were comparable with patients treated with RT alone (six months and 38%, respectively). On multivariate analysis, local (HR = 0.51, confidence interval [CI]: 0.46–0.56) and regional disease (HR = 0.66, CI: 0.60–0.73) was associated with a better outcome in comparison with distant disease (HR = 1), $P < 0.0001$.[163] Zeng et al. reported on a series of 75 patients with PCC in which 38 patients received adjuvant external beam radiation therapy (EBRT). A median total dose of 50 Gy (range: 30–60 Gy) was given in daily doses of 2 Gy/fraction five times a week after a median delay of 352 days (range: 75–1007 days) following surgery. The criteria by which the patients were selected to receive EBRT were not clearly delineated; nevertheless, they reported a better OS following EBRT for both resectable and nonresectable PCC patients compared with those who did not receive EBRT (Table 2-16).[65] Patients with LN recurrence following surgery also had better OS after EBRT compared with those not receiving EBRT.[65]

Advanced radiation techniques including selective internal radiation therapy (SIRT) with Yttrium-90 (^{90}Y) microspheres has more recently emerged as a viable therapeutic option for the treatment of a variety of primary and liver tumor.[164–167] SIRT has been shown safe and is associated with minimal side effects.[168,169] Ibrahim et al. reported on 24 patients with unresectable PCC, who underwent SIRT with ^{90}Y microspheres. The median OS was 14.9 months. Survival benefits were primarily observed in patients without cancer-related symptoms, no portal vein thrombosis, and with peripheral tumor patterns. Complete (100%) tumor necrosis was achieved in two patients, and one patient was down-staged to permit surgical resection.[168] Saxena et al. have reported on a group of 25 patients with unresectable PCC treated with ^{90}Y radioembolization. In their study, PR or SD was observed in 74% of patients. The median OS from diagnosis was 20.4 months, and median survival after ^{90}Y SIRT was 9.3 months with one- and three-year survival rates of 40% and 13%, respectively.[169] Similar to Ibrahim et al., these authors noted improved survival in patients with peripheral type of tumor and among those without cancer-related symptoms.[168]

In summary, further research is required to establish patient selection criteria, ideal mode, method,

TABLE 2-16: Clinical Efficacy of Radiotherapy in the Treatment of Patients with Peripheral Cholangiocarcinoma[65]

Survival Rates	External Beam Radiotherapy			Nonexternal Beam Radiotherapy		
	All Pts	Resectable Tumor	Unresectable Tumor	All Pts	Resectable Tumor	Unresectable Tumor
1 y (%)	50		36.1	24.8		19
2 y (%)	11.8		19	5.5		4.7
Median survival (days)		468	356		211	212

dose, and role for RT in the treatment of patients with PCC. Despite the lack of conclusive evidence, however, patients who undergo an R1 or R2 resection should be considered for adjuvant radiotherapy. The role of adjuvant radiotherapy in PCC patients undergoing an R0 resection is less clear and is not advocated outside of a clinical trial.

Role of Transplantation

Although liver transplantation (LTx) was initially thought to be an ideal treatment for PCC, subsequent studies have yielded poor outcomes and a high incidence of recurrence; leading nearly all transplant centers to view PCC as a contraindication to LTx outside of a clinical trial.[170–173] Among centers that are performing LTx for PCC, most patients have unresectable advanced T stage disease in the absence of LN or systemic metastases.[173–182] Transplant candidates typically have low tumor stage, with tumor located in unfavorable location and with decreased liver reserve (advanced cirrhosis).[183] The reported overall five-year survival following LTx in PCC patients is between 0% and 42% (Table 2-17). Interestingly, O'Grady et al. has suggested that it is inappropriate to consider LTx for patients with <50% chance of five-year survival, which would exclude all PCC patients, even though a five-year survival of 42% following LTx for PCC is not oncologically trivial.[180,184]

Interest in LTx for patients with CC has recently gained new light after De Vreede et al. reported a disease-free survival of 92% after a median follow-up of 37 months. In this study, a group of 19 patients with unresectable hilar CC without intrahepatic or

TABLE 2-17: Selected Reports of Liver Transplant Among Patients with Peripheral Cholangiocarcinoma

Author, Year	N	Median Survival (mo)	Overall Survival (%) 1 y	3 y	5 y	Tumor Recurrence (%)
Registry data						
ELTR, 2000[183]	186	—	58	38	29	—
CTTR Database,[a] 2000[177]	207	23	72	48	23	51
UNOS/OPTN,[a] 2008[177]	280	Nonretransplant pts (n = 258) = 35.63 Retransplant pts (n = 22) = 16	74	—	38	—
Single-center data						
O'Grady 1988[179]	13	13	38	10	10	46.1
Pichlmayr 1995[174]	22	—	20.8	0	0	—
Casavilla 1997[175]	20	Stage I + II = 21.1 Stage III + IV = 19.2	70	29	18	59.3
Weimann 2000[176]	24	5.5	21	4	0	62.5
Shimoda 2001[180]	16	—	62	39	—	53.8
Robles 2004[181]	23	—	77	65	42	35
Sotiropoulos 2008[182]	10	32.2	70	50	33	—

Abbreviations: ELTR, European Liver Transplant Registry; CTTR, Cincinatti Transplant Tumor Registry; UNOS/OPTN, United Network for Organ Sharing/Organ Procurement and Transplantation Network; N, number of patients.
[a]Study included both hilar and peripheral type of cholangiocarcinomas.

extrahepatic metastases were enrolled and treated with LTx and neoadjuvant chemoradiotherapy. All patients except one had early stage disease (stage I or II).[185] In a follow-up report from the same institution, five-year post-LTx survival was 82%, among a group of 38 patients with hilar CC treated in this manner.[186] Despite the promise of these two reports, in point of fact, the published median survival for PCC after LTx is between 5.5 and 35.63 months with recurrence rates in the range of 35%–62.5% (Table 2-17). More recently, Sotiropoulos et al. reported on the outcome of LTx among 10 patients with PCC. The median survival was 25.3 months, with a one-, three-, and five-year survival rates of 70%, 50%, and 33%, respectively. Tumor recurrence was observed in two patients, who ultimately succumbed to disease. These authors concluded that patients with PCC associated with liver cirrhosis and patients with PCC without involvement of the hilar bifurcation are those most likely to benefit from LTx.[181] In summary, the role of LTx in PCC is very controversial regardless of performance within a clinical trial. It is our view that LTx should be considered only in PCC patients with unresectable low tumor stage, in the absence of LN and distant metastasis and always combined with systemic chemotherapy.

Recurrence

PCC is associated with a high rate of recurrence even after R0 resection. Overall 38%–89% of PCC patients will recur with a median time to recurrence ranging from 12 to 20 months. A two-year disease-free interval is achieved in only 9%–20% of patients. Lang et al. reported a 62.6% recurrence rate in the setting of an R0 resection.[114] The liver remnant was the most common site of recurrence, and hepatic recurrence occurred in 38%–70% of patients. Other commonly reported sites of recurrence include LNs, lung, and bone (Table 2-18). In a review of 53 patients with PCC, Weber et al. identified three factors independently associated with recurrence: (1) the presence of multiple tumors, (2) vascular invasion, and (3) tumor size.[105] Madariaga et al. reviewed 34 patients with PCC and identified that the presence of multiple tumors, incomplete resection margins, and mean tumor size of >5 cm were independently associated with a high rate of recurrence.[130]

TABLE 2-18: Site and Time to Recurrence Among Patients with Peripheral Cholangiocarcinoma[209]

Parameters	%
Recurrence rate	38–89
2-y disease-free survival	9–20
Median time to recurrence	12–20 mo
Sites of recurrence	
Liver	38–70
Retroperitoneum/lymph node	5–12
Lung	4–33
Bone	6–13
Other	9–20

Summary

PCC is a rare disease with an increasing global incidence and mortality rate. PCC exhibits aggressive behavior, and more than 80% of patients succumb to the disease within a year of diagnosis if untreated. Most patients present with nonspecific symptoms, contributing to a delay in diagnosis. Although certain imaging features of PCC are characteristic, there are no features specific for CC. Curative resection is the only modality of treatment, which provides prolonged survival; however, there are no clear surgical selection criteria. Although resectability rates are increasing, recurrence is high even after an R0 resection. The role of neoadjuvant, adjuvant, and palliative chemotherapy is poorly defined, and additional randomized trials are needed. Liver transplantation may offer hope to a small subset of patients, but ethical issues and limited organ availability leave LTX in this setting very controversial.

References

1. Parker SL, Tong T, Bolden S, Wingo PA. Cancer statistics, 1996. *CA Cancer J Clin*. 1996;46(1):5–27.
2. de Groen PC, Gores GJ, LaRusso NF, et al. Biliary tract cancers. *N Engl J Med*. 1999;341(18): 1368–1378.

3. Olnes MJ, Erlich R. A review and update on cholangiocarcinoma. *Oncology*. 2004;66(3):167–179.
4. Roayaie S, Guarrera JV, Ye MQ, et al. Aggressive surgical treatment of intrahepatic cholangiocarcinoma: predictors of outcomes. *J Am Coll Surg*. 1998;187(4):365–372.
5. Nakeeb A, Pitt HA, Sohn TA, et al. Cholangiocarcinoma. A spectrum of intrahepatic, perihilar, and distal tumors. *Ann Surg*. 1996;224(4):463–473.
6. Shaib YH, Davila JA, McGlynn K, El-Serag HB. Rising incidence of intrahepatic cholangiocarcinoma in the United States: a true increase? *J Hepatol*. 2004;40(3):472–477.
7. Patel T. Worldwide trends in mortality from biliary tract malignancies. *BMC Cancer*. 2002;2:10.
8. McLean L, Patel T. Racial and ethnic variations in the epidemiology of intrahepatic cholangiocarcinoma in the United States. *Liver Int*. 2006;26(9):1047–1053.
9. Wood R, Brewster DH, Fraser LA, et al. Do increases in mortality from intrahepatic cholangiocarcinoma reflect a genuine increase in risk? Insights from cancer registry data in Scotland. *Eur J Cancer*. 2003;39(14):2087–2092.
10. Taylor-Robinson SD, Toledano MB, Arora S, et al. Increase in mortality rates from intrahepatic cholangiocarcinoma in England and Wales 1968-1998. *Gut*. 2001;48(6):816–820.
11. Chapman RW. Risk factors for biliary tract carcinogenesis. *Ann Oncol*. 1999;10(suppl 4):308–311.
12. Parkin DM, Srivatanakul P, Khlat M, et al. Liver cancer in Thailand. I. A case-control study of cholangiocarcinoma. *Int J Cancer*. 1991;48(3):323–328.
13. Welzel TM, Graubard BI, El-Serag HB, et al. Risk factors for intrahepatic and extrahepatic cholangiocarcinoma in the United States: a population-based case-control study. *Clin Gastroenterol Hepatol*. 2007;5(10):1221–1228.
14. Roskams T, Desmet V. Embryology of extra- and intrahepatic bile ducts, the ductal plate. *Anat Rec (Hoboken)*. 2008;291(6):628–635.
15. Ludwig J, Ritman EL, LaRusso NF, et al. Anatomy of the human biliary system studied by quantitative computer-aided three-dimensional imaging techniques. *Hepatology*. 1998;27(4):893–899.
16. Moore KL, Dalley AF. *Clinically Oriented Anatomy*. 5th ed. Baltimore, MD: Lippincott Williams & Wilkins; 2006:294.
17. Castaing D. Surgical anatomy of the biliary tract. *HPB (Oxford)*. 2008;10(2):72–76.
18. Tsuji T, Hiraoka T, Kanemitsu K, et al. Lymphatic spreading pattern of intrahepatic cholangiocarcinoma. *Surgery*. 2001;129(4):401–407.
19. Jonas S, Thelen A, Benckert C, et al. Extended liver resection for intrahepatic cholangiocarcinoma: a comparison of the prognostic accuracy of the fifth and sixth editions of the TNM classification. *Ann Surg*. 2009;249(2):303–309.
20. Aljiffry M, Walsh MJ, Molinari M. Advances in diagnosis, treatment and palliation of cholangiocarcinoma: 1990–2009. *World J Gastroenterol*. 2009;15(34):4240–4262.
21. Okabayashi T, Yamamoto J, Kosuge T, et al. A new staging system for mass-forming intrahepatic cholangiocarcinoma: analysis of preoperative and postoperative variables. *Cancer*. 2001;92(9):2374–2383.
22. Berdah SV, Delpero JR, Garcia S, et al. A western surgical experience of peripheral cholangiocarcinoma. *Br J Surg*. 1996;83(11):1517–1521.
23. Ishikawa K, Sasaki A, Haraguchi N, et al. A case of an alpha-fetoprotein-producing intrahepatic cholangiocarcinoma suggests probable cancer stem cell origin. *Oncologist*. 2007;12(3):320–324.
24. Yamamoto M, Takasaki K, Yoshikawa T, et al. Does gross appearance indicate prognosis in intrahepatic cholangiocarcinoma? *J Surg Oncol*. 1998;69(3):162–167.
25. Nakanuma Y, Sripa B, Vatanasapt V, Leong AS-Y, Ponchon T, Ishak KG. et al. Intrahepatic cholangiocarcinoma. In: Hamilton Stanley R, Aaltonen Lauri A, eds. *World Health Organization Classification of Tumors, WHO Pathology and Genetics of Tumors of the Digestive System*. Lyon: IARC Press; 2000.
26. Nakajima T, Kondo Y, Miyazaki M, Okui K. A histopathologic study of 102 cases of intrahepatic cholangiocarcinoma: histologic classification and modes of spreading. *Hum Pathol*. 1988;19(10):1228–1234.
27. Lang H, Sotiropoulos GC, Fruhauf NR, et al. Extended hepatectomy for intrahepatic cholangiocellular carcinoma (ICC): when is it worthwhile? Single center experience with 27 resections in 50 patients over a 5-year period. *Ann Surg*. 2005;241(1):134–143.
28. Crawford JM. Liver and biliary tract. In: Kumar V, Fausto N, Abbas A, eds. *Pathologic Basis of Diseases*. 7th ed. Philadelphia, PA: Harcourt Bruce and Company 2004:650–655.
29. Malhi H, Gores GJ. Review article: the modern diagnosis and therapy of cholangioc-

30. Bartlett DL. Intrahepatic cholangiocarcinoma: a worthy challenge. *Cancer J*. 2009;15(3): 255–256.
31. Watanapa P. Cholangiocarcinoma in patients with opisthorchiasis. *Br J Surg*. 1996;83(8): 1062–1064.
32. Shimonishi T, Sasaki M, Nakanuma Y. Precancerous lesions of intrahepatic cholangiocarcinoma. *J Hepatobiliary Pancreat Surg*. 2000;7(6):542–550.
33. Thamavit W, Bhamarapravati N, Sahaphong S, et al. Effects of dimethylnitrosamine on induction of cholangiocarcinoma in Opisthorchis viverrini-infected Syrian golden hamsters. *Cancer Res*. 1978;38(12):4634–4639.
34. Watanapa P, Watanapa WB. Liver fluke-associated cholangiocarcinoma. *Br J Surg*. 2002;89(8):962–970.
35. Khan SA, Thomas HC, Davidson BR, Taylor-Robinson SD. Cholangiocarcinoma. *Lancet*. 2005;366(9493):1303–1314.
36. Shaib Y, El-Serag HB. The epidemiology of cholangiocarcinoma. *Semin Liver Dis*. 2004;24(2):115–125.
37. Zhou YM, Yin ZF, Yang JM, et al. Risk factors for intrahepatic cholangiocarcinoma: a case-control study in China. *World J Gastroenterol*. 2008;14(4):632–635.
38. Lee TY, Lee SS, Jung SW, et al. Hepatitis B virus infection and intrahepatic cholangiocarcinoma in Korea: a case-control study. *Am J Gastroenterol*. 2008;103(7):1716–1720.
39. Chen MF. Peripheral cholangiocarcinoma (cholangiocellular carcinoma): clinical features, diagnosis and treatment. *J Gastroenterol Hepatol*. 1999;14(12):1144–1149.
40. Okuda K, Nakanuma Y, Miyazaki M. Cholangiocarcinoma: recent progress. Part 1: epidemiology and etiology. *J Gastroenterol Hepatol*. 2002;17(10):1049–1055.
41. Ahrendt SA, Nakeeb A, Pitt HA. Cholangiocarcinoma. *Clin Liver Dis*. 2001;5(1):191–218.
42. Zen Y, Adsay NV, Bardadin K, et al. Biliary intraepithelial neoplasia: an international interobserver agreement study and proposal for diagnostic criteria. *Mod Pathol*. 2007;20(6):701–709.
43. Bergquist A, Ekbom A, Olsson R, et al. Hepatic and extrahepatic malignancies in primary sclerosing cholangitis. *J Hepatol*. 2002;36(3):321–327.
44. Broome U, Olsson R, Loof L, et al. Natural history and prognostic factors in 305 Swedish patients with primary sclerosing cholangitis. *Gut*. 1996;38(4):610–615.
45. Pitt HA, Dooley WC, Yeo CJ, Cameron JL. Malignancies of the biliary tree. *Curr Probl Surg*. 1995;32(1):1–90.
46. Chalasani N, Baluyut A, Ismail A, et al. Cholangiocarcinoma in patients with primary sclerosing cholangitis: a multicenter case-control study. *Hepatology*. 2000;31(1):7–11.
47. Scott J, Shousha S, Thomas HC, Sherlock S. Bile duct carcinoma: a late complication of congenital hepatic fibrosis. Case report and review of literature. *Am J Gastroenterol*. 1980;73(2):113–119.
48. Lipsett PA, Pitt HA, Colombani PM, et al. Choledochal cyst disease. A changing pattern of presentation. *Ann Surg*. 1994;220(5): 644–652.
49. Simeone DM. Gallbladder and biliary tree: anatomy and structural anomalies. In: Yamada T, ed. *Textbook of Gastroenterology*. Philadelphia, PA: Lippincott Willimas and Wilkins; 1999:2244–2257.
50. Ohtsuka T, Inoue K, Ohuchida J, et al. Carcinoma arising in choledochocele. *Endoscopy*. 2001;33(7):614–619.
51. van Mil SW, Klomp LW, Bull LN, Houwen RH. FIC1 disease: a spectrum of intrahepatic cholestatic disorders. *Semin Liver Dis*. 2001;21(4):535–544.
52. Jacquemin E. Role of multidrug resistance 3 deficiency in pediatric and adult liver disease: one gene for three diseases. *Semin Liver Dis*. 2001;21(4):551–562.
53. Thompson R, Strautnieks S. BSEP: function and role in progressive familial intrahepatic cholestasis. *Semin Liver Dis*. 2001;21(4):545–550.
54. Khan SA, Carmichael PL, Taylor-Robinson SD, et al. DNA adducts, detected by 32P postlabelling, in human cholangiocarcinoma. *Gut*. 2003;52(4):586–591.
55. Sahani D, Prasad SR, Tannabe KK, et al. Thorotrast-induced cholangiocarcinoma: case report. *Abdom Imaging*. 2003;28(1):72–74.
56. Hardell L, Bengtsson NO, Jonsson U, et al. Aetiological aspects on primary liver cancer with special regard to alcohol, organic solvents and

acute intermittent porphyria—an epidemiological investigation. *Br J Cancer.* 1984;50(3):389–397.

57. Shaib YH, El-Serag HB, Davila JA, et al. Risk factors of intrahepatic cholangiocarcinoma in the United States: a case-control study. *Gastroenterology.* 2005;128(3):620–626.

58. Sorensen HT, Friis S, Olsen JH, et al. Risk of liver and other types of cancer in patients with cirrhosis: a nationwide cohort study in Denmark. *Hepatology.* 1998;28(4):921–925.

59. Shin HR, Lee CU, Park HJ, et al. Hepatitis B and C virus, *Clonorchis sinensis* for the risk of liver cancer: a case-control study in Pusan, Korea. *Int J Epidemiol.* 1996;25(5):933–940.

60. Donato F, Gelatti U, Tagger A, et al. Intrahepatic cholangiocarcinoma and hepatitis C and B virus infection, alcohol intake, and hepatolithiasis: a case-control study in Italy. *Cancer Causes Control.* 2001;12(10):959–964.

61. Kobayashi M, Ikeda K, Saitoh S, et al. Incidence of primary cholangiocellular carcinoma of the liver in japanese patients with hepatitis C virus-related cirrhosis. *Cancer.* 2000;88(11):2471–2477.

62. Yin F, Chen B. Detection of hepatitis C virus RNA sequences in hepatic portal cholangiocarcinoma tissue by reverse transcription polymerase chain reaction. *Chin Med J (Engl).* 1998;111(12):1068–1070.

63. Yamamoto M, Takasaki K, Yoshikawa T. Extended resection for intrahepatic cholangiocarcinoma in Japan. *J Hepatobiliary Pancreat Surg.* 1999;6(2):117–121.

64. Valverde A, Bonhomme N, Farges O, et al. Resection of intrahepatic cholangiocarcinoma: a Western experience. *J Hepatobiliary Pancreat Surg.* 1999;6(2):122–127.

65. Zeng ZC, Tang ZY, Fan J, et al. Consideration of the role of radiotherapy for unresectable intrahepatic cholangiocarcinoma: a retrospective analysis of 75 patients. *Cancer J.* 2006;12(2):113–122.

66. Chou FF, Sheen-Chen SM, Chen YS, et al. Surgical treatment of cholangiocarcinoma. *Hepatogastroenterology.* 1997;44(15):760–765.

67. Kiefer MV, McNally M, Robertson M, et al. CAM/Ethiodol/PVA chemoembolization of intrahepatic cholangiocarcinoma. *J Vasc Interv Radiol.* 2009;20(2):S117.

68. Lieser MJ, Barry MK, Rowland C, et al. Surgical management of intrahepatic cholangiocarcinoma: a 31-year experience. *J Hepatobiliary Pancreat Surg.* 1998;5(1):41–47.

69. Shimada K, Sano T, Sakamoto Y, et al. Clinical impact of the surgical margin status in hepatectomy for solitary mass-forming type intrahepatic cholangiocarcinoma without lymph node metastases. *J Surg Oncol.* 2007;96(2):160–165.

70. Tullo A, D'Erchia AM, Honda K, et al. New p53 mutations in hilar cholangiocarcinoma. *Eur J Clin Invest.* 2000;30(9):798–803.

71. Khan SA, Taylor-Robinson SD, Toledano MB, et al. Changing international trends in mortality rates for liver, biliary and pancreatic tumours. *J Hepatol.* 2002;37(6):806–813.

72. Suzuki S, Sakaguchi T, Yokoi Y, et al. Clinicopathological prognostic factors and impact of surgical treatment of mass-forming intrahepatic cholangiocarcinoma. *World J Surg.* 2002;26(6):687–693.

73. Suh KS, Roh HR, Koh YT, et al. Clinicopathologic features of the intraductal growth type of peripheral cholangiocarcinoma. *Hepatology.* 2000;31(1):12–17.

74. Jan YY, Yeh CN, Yeh TS, et al. Clinicopathological factors predicting long-term overall survival after hepatectomy for peripheral cholangiocarcinoma. *World J Surg.* 2005;29(7):894–898.

75. Khan SA, Davidson BR, Goldin R, et al. Guidelines for the diagnosis and treatment of cholangiocarcinoma: consensus document. *Gut.* 2002;51(suppl 6):VI1–VI9.

76. Duraker N, Hot S, Polat Y, et al. CEA, CA 19-9, and CA 125 in the differential diagnosis of benign and malignant pancreatic diseases with or without jaundice. *J Surg Oncol.* 2007;95(2):142–147.

77. Qin XL, Wang ZR, Shi JS, et al. Utility of serum CA19-9 in diagnosis of cholangiocarcinoma: in comparison with CEA. *World J Gastroenterol.* 2004;10(3):427–432.

78. Lamerz R. Role of tumour markers, cytogenetics. *Ann Oncol.* 1999;10(suppl 4):145–149.

79. Maestranzi S, Przemioslo R, Mitchell H, Sherwood RA. The effect of benign and malignant liver disease on the tumour markers CA19-9 and CEA. *Ann Clin Biochem.* 1998;35(pt 1):99–103.

80. Nichols JC, Gores GJ, LaRusso NF, et al. Diagnostic role of serum CA 19-9 for cholangiocarcinoma in patients with primary sclerosing cholangitis. *Mayo Clin Proc.* 1993;68(9):874–879.

81. Charatcharoenwitthaya P, Enders FB, Halling KC, Lindor KD. Utility of serum tumor markers, imaging, and biliary cytology for detecting cholangiocarcinoma in primary scle-

rosing cholangitis. *Hepatology*. 2008;48(4): 1106–1117.
82. Patel AH, Harnois DM, Klee GG, et al. The utility of CA 19-9 in the diagnoses of cholangiocarcinoma in patients without primary sclerosing cholangitis. *Am J Gastroenterol*. 2000;95(1):204–207.
83. Siqueira E, Schoen RE, Silverman W, et al. Detecting cholangiocarcinoma in patients with primary sclerosing cholangitis. *Gastrointest Endosc*. 2002;56(1):40–47.
84. Bamrungphon W, Prempracha N, Bunchu N, et al. A new mucin antibody/enzyme-linked lectin-sandwich assay of serum MUC5AC mucin for the diagnosis of cholangiocarcinoma. *Cancer Lett*. 2007;247(2):301–308.
85. Uenishi T, Yamazaki O, Yamamoto T, et al. Serosal invasion in TNM staging of mass-forming intrahepatic cholangiocarcinoma. *J Hepatobiliary Pancreat Surg*. 2005;12(6): 479–483.
86. Sainani NI, Catalano OA, Holalkere NS, et al. Cholangiocarcinoma: current and novel imaging techniques. *Radiographics*. 2008;28(5):1263–1287.
87. Wernecke K, Henke L, Vassallo P, et al. Pathologic explanation for hypoechoic halo seen on sonograms of malignant liver tumors: an in vitro correlative study. *AJR Am J Roentgenol*. 1992;159(5):1011–1016.
88. Chung YE, Kim MJ, Park YN, et al. Varying appearances of cholangiocarcinoma: radiologic-pathologic correlation. *Radiographics*. 2009;29(3):683–700.
89. Vilgrain V, Van Beers BE, Flejou JF, et al. Intrahepatic cholangiocarcinoma: MRI and pathologic correlation in 14 patients. *J Comput Assist Tomogr*. 1997;21(1):59–65.
90. Okami J, Dono K, Sakon M, et al. Patterns of regional lymph node involvement in intrahepatic cholangiocarcinoma of the left lobe. *J Gastrointest Surg*. 2003;7(7):850–856.
91. Choi BI, Park JH, Kim YI, et al. Peripheral cholangiocarcinoma and clonorchiasis: CT findings. *Radiology*. 1988;169(1):149–153.
92. Ros PR, Buck JL, Goodman ZD, et al. Intrahepatic cholangiocarcinoma: radiologic-pathologic correlation. *Radiology*. 1988;167(3):689–693.
93. Itai Y, Araki T, Furui S, et al. Computed tomography of primary intrahepatic biliary malignancy. *Radiology*. 1983;147(2):485–490.
94. Honda H, Onitsuka H, Yasumori K, et al. Intrahepatic peripheral cholangiocarcinoma: two-phased dynamic incremental CT and pathologic correlation. *J Comput Assist Tomogr*. 1993;17(3):397–402.
95. Takayasu K, Ikeya S, Mukai K, et al. CT of hilar cholangiocarcinoma: late contrast enhancement in six patients. *AJR Am J Roentgenol*. 1990;154(6):1203–1206.
96. Yoshikawa J, Matsui O, Kadoya M, et al. Delayed enhancement of fibrotic areas in hepatic masses: CT-pathologic correlation. *J Comput Assist Tomogr*. 1992;16(2):206–211.
97. Itai Y, Ohtomo K, Kokubo T, et al. CT of hepatic masses: significance of prolonged and delayed enhancement. *AJR Am J Roentgenol*. 1986; 146(4):729–733.
98. Tani K, Kubota Y, Yamaguchi T, et al. MR imaging of peripheral cholangiocarcinoma. *J Comput Assist Tomogr*. 1991;15(6):975–978.
99. Hamrick-Turner J, Abbitt PL, Ros PR. Intrahepatic cholangiocarcinoma: MR appearance. *AJR Am J Roentgenol*. 1992;158(1):77–79.
100. Fan ZM, Yamashita Y, Harada M, et al. Intrahepatic cholangiocarcinoma: spin-echo and contrast-enhanced dynamic MR imaging. *AJR Am J Roentgenol*. 1993;161(2):313–317.
101. Anderson CD, Rice MH, Pinson CW, et al. Fluorodeoxyglucose PET imaging in the evaluation of gallbladder carcinoma and cholangiocarcinoma. *J Gastrointest Surg*. 2004; 8(1):90–97.
102. Kim YJ, Yun M, Lee WJ, et al. Usefulness of 18F-FDG PET in intrahepatic cholangiocarcinoma. *Eur J Nucl Med Mol Imaging*. 2003;30(11):1467–1472.
103. Kim TK, Choi BI, Han JK, et al. Peripheral cholangiocarcinoma of the liver: two-phase spiral CT findings. *Radiology*. 1997;204(2): 539–543.
104. Colli A, Cocciolo M, Mumoli N, et al. Peripheral intrahepatic cholangiocarcinoma: ultrasound findings and differential diagnosis from hepatocellular carcinoma. *Eur J Ultrasound*. 1998;7(2):93–99.
105. Weber SM, Jarnagin WR, Klimstra D, et al. Intrahepatic cholangiocarcinoma: resectability, recurrence pattern, and outcomes. *J Am Coll Surg*. 2001;193(4):384–391.
106. Goere D, Wagholikar GD, Pessaux P, et al. Utility of staging laparoscopy in subsets of biliary cancers: laparoscopy is a powerful diagnostic tool in patients

with intrahepatic and gallbladder carcinoma. *Surg Endosc.* 2006;20(5):721–725.
107. Tan JC, Coburn NG, Baxter NN, Kiss A, Law CH. Surgical management of intrahepatic cholangiocarcinoma–a population-based study. Ann Surg
108. Harrison LE, Fong Y, Klimstra DS, et al. Surgical treatment of 32 patients with peripheral intrahepatic cholangiocarcinoma. *Br J Surg.* 1998;85(8):1068–1070.
109. Cherqui D, Tantawi B, Alon R, et al. Intrahepatic cholangiocarcinoma. Results of aggressive surgical management. *Arch Surg.* 1995;130(10):1073–1078.
110. Yamamoto M, Takasaki K, Otsubo T, et al. Recurrence after surgical resection of intrahepatic cholangiocarcinoma. *J Hepatobiliary Pancreat Surg.* 2001;8(2):154–157.
111. Tamandl D, Herberger B, Gruenberger B, et al. Influence of hepatic resection margin on recurrence and survival in intrahepatic cholangiocarcinoma. *Ann Surg Oncol.* 2008;15(10):2787–2794.
112. Li SQ, Liang LJ, Hua YP, et al. Long-term outcome and prognostic factors of intrahepatic cholangiocarcinoma. *Chin Med J (Engl).* 2009;122(19):2286–2291.
113. Inoue K, Makuuchi M, Takayama T, et al. Long-term survival and prognostic factors in the surgical treatment of mass-forming type cholangiocarcinoma. *Surgery.* 2000;127(5):498–505.
114. Uenishi T, Hirohashi K, Kubo S, et al. Histologic factors affecting prognosis following hepatectomy for intrahepatic cholangiocarcinoma. *World J Surg.* 2001;25(7):865–869.
115. Lang H, Sotiropoulos GC, Sgourakis G, et al. Operations for intrahepatic cholangiocarcinoma: single-institution experience of 158 patients. *J Am Coll Surg.* 2009;208(2):218–228.
116. Nakagawa T, Kamiyama T, Kurauchi N, et al. Number of lymph node metastases is a significant prognostic factor in intrahepatic cholangiocarcinoma. *World J Surg.* 2005;29(6):728–733.
117. Tamandl D, Kaczirek K, Gruenberger B, et al. Lymph node ratio after curative surgery for intrahepatic cholangiocarcinoma. *Br J Surg.* 2009;96(8):919–925.
118. Uenishi T, Kubo S, Yamazaki O, et al. Indications for surgical treatment of intrahepatic cholangiocarcinoma with lymph node metastases. *J Hepatobiliary Pancreat Surg.* 2008;15(4):417–422.
119. Ercolani G, Grazi GL, Ravaioli M, et al. The role of lymphadenectomy for liver tumors: further considerations on the appropriateness of treatment strategy. *Ann Surg.* 2004;239(2):202–209.
120. Shimada K, Sano T, Nara S, et al. Therapeutic value of lymph node dissection during hepatectomy in patients with intrahepatic cholangiocellular carcinoma with negative lymph node involvement. *Surgery.* 2009;145(4):411–416.
121. Uenishi T, Yamazaki O, Horii K, et al. A long-term survivor of intrahepatic cholangiocarcinoma with paraaortic lymph node metastasis. *J Gastroenterol.* 2006;41(4):391–392.
122. Shimada M, Yamashita Y, Aishima S, et al. Value of lymph node dissection during resection of intrahepatic cholangiocarcinoma. *Br J Surg.* 2001;88(11):1463–1466.
123. Konstadoulakis MM, Roayaie S, Gomatos IP, et al. Fifteen-year, single-center experience with the surgical management of intrahepatic cholangiocarcinoma: operative results and long-term outcome. *Surgery.* 2008;143(3):366–374.
124. Grobmyer SR, Wang L, Gonen M, et al. Perihepatic lymph node assessment in patients undergoing partial hepatectomy for malignancy. *Ann Surg.* 2006;244(2):260–264.
125. Chou FF, Sheen-Chen SM, Chen CL, et al. Prognostic factors of resectable intrahepatic cholangiocarcinoma. *J Surg Oncol.* 1995;59(1):40–44.
126. El Rassi ZE, Partensky C, Scoazec JY, et al. Peripheral cholangiocarcinoma: presentation, diagnosis, pathology and management. *Eur J Surg Oncol.* 1999;25(4):375–380.
127. DeOliveira ML, Cunningham SC, Cameron JL, et al. Cholangiocarcinoma: thirty-one-year experience with 564 patients at a single institution. *Ann Surg.* 2007;245(5):755–762.
128. Ribero D, Pinna AD, Guglielmi A, et al. Surgical approach for long-term survival of patients with intrahepatic cholangiocarcinoma: a multi-institutional analysis of 434 patients. *Arch Surg.* 2012;20:1–7.
129. Yamamoto J, Kosuge T, Takayama T, et al. Surgical treatment of intrahepatic cholangiocarcinoma: four patients surviving more than five years. *Surgery.* 1992;111(6):617–622.
130. Jarnagin WR, Shoup M. Surgical management of cholangiocarcinoma. *Semin Liver Dis.* 2004;24(2):189–199.

131. Madariaga JR, Iwatsuki S, Todo S, et al. Liver resection for hilar and peripheral cholangiocarcinomas: a study of 62 cases. *Ann Surg*. 1998;227(1):70–79.
132. Thongprasert S. The role of chemotherapy in cholangiocarcinoma. *Ann Oncol*. 2005; 16(suppl 2):ii93–ii96.
133. Choi CW, Choi IK, Seo JH, et al. Effects of 5-fluorouracil and leucovorin in the treatment of pancreaticbiliary tract adenocarcinomas. *Am J Clin Oncol*. 2000;23(4):425 428.
134. Ducreux M, Rougier P, Fandi A, et al. Effective treatment of advanced biliary tract carcinoma using 5-fluorouracil continuous infusion with cisplatin. *Ann Oncol*. 1998;9(6):653–656.
135. Lee MA, Woo IS, Kang JH, et al. Epirubicin, cisplatin, and protracted infusion of 5-FU (ECF) in advanced intrahepatic cholangiocarcinoma. *J Cancer Res Clin Oncol*. 2004;130(6):346–350.
136. Falkson G, MacIntyre JM, Moertel CG. Eastern Cooperative Oncology Group experience with chemotherapy for inoperable gallbladder and bile duct cancer. *Cancer*. 1984;54(6): 965–969.
137. Takada T, Kato H, Matsushiro T, et al. Comparison of 5-fluorouracil, doxorubicin and mitomycin C with 5-fluorouracil alone in the treatment of pancreaticbiliary carcinomas. *Oncology*. 1994;51(5):396–400.
138. Gebbia V, Majello E, Testa A, et al. Treatment of advanced adenocarcinomas of the exocrine pancreas and the gallbladder with 5-fluorouracil, high dose levofolinic acid and oral hydroxyurea on a weekly schedule. Results of a multicenter study of the Southern Italy Oncology Group (G.O.I.M.). *Cancer*. 1996;78(6):1300–1307.
139. Patt YZ, Jones DV Jr, Hoque A, et al. Phase II trial of intravenous flourouracil and subcutaneous interferon alfa-2b for biliary tract cancer. *J Clin Oncol*. 1996;14(8):2311–2315.
140. Ellis PA, Norman A, Hill A, et al. Epirubicin, cisplatin and infusional 5-fluorouracil (5-FU) (ECF) in hepatobiliary tumours. *Eur J Cancer*. 1995;31A(10):1594–1598.
141. Taieb J, Mitry E, Boige V, et al. Optimization of 5-fluorouracil (5-FU)/cisplatin combination chemotherapy with a new schedule of leucovorin, 5-FU and cisplatin (LV5FU2-P regimen) in patients with biliary tract carcinoma. *Ann Oncol*. 2002;13(8):1192–1196.
142. Raderer M, Hejna MH, Valencak JB, et al. Two consecutive phase II studies of 5-fluorouracil/leucovorin/mitomycin C and of gemcitabine in patients with advanced biliary cancer. *Oncology*. 1999;56(3):177–180.
143. Gebbia V, Giuliani F, Maiello E, et al. Treatment of inoperable and/or metastatic biliary tree carcinomas with single-agent gemcitabine or in combination with levofolinic acid and infusional fluorouracil: results of a multicenter phase II study. *J Clin Oncol*. 2001;19(20): 4089–4091.
144. Alberts SR, Al-Khatib H, Mahoney MR, et al. Gemcitabine, 5-fluorouracil, and leucovorin in advanced biliary tract and gallbladder carcinoma: a North central cancer treatment group phase II trial. *Cancer*. 2005;103(1):111–118.
145. Doval DC, Sekhon JS, Gupta SK, et al. A phase II study of gemcitabine and cisplatin in chemotherapy-naive, unresectable gall bladder cancer. *Br J Cancer*. 2004;90(8):1516–1520.
146. Thongprasert S, Napapan S, Charoentum C, Moonprakan S. Phase II study of gemcitabine and cisplatin as first-line chemotherapy in inoperable biliary tract carcinoma. *Ann Oncol*. 2005;16(2):279–281.
147. Andre T, Tournigand C, Rosmorduc O, et al. Gemcitabine combined with oxaliplatin (GEMOX) in advanced biliary tract adenocarcinoma: a GERCOR study. *Ann Oncol*. 2004;15(9):1339–1343.
148. Kuhn R, Hribaschek A, Eichelmann K, et al. Outpatient therapy with gemcitabine and docetaxel for gallbladder, biliary, and cholangiocarcinomas. *Invest New Drugs*. 2002;20(3): 351–356.
149. Bhargava P, Jani CR, Savarese DM, et al. Gemcitabine and irinotecan in locally advanced or metastatic biliary cancer: preliminary report. *Oncology (Williston Park)*. 2003;17(9 suppl 8):23–26.
150. Knox JJ, Hedley D, Oza A, et al. Gemcitabine concurrent with continuous infusional 5-fluorouracil in advanced biliary cancers: a review of the Princess Margaret Hospital experience. *Ann Oncol*. 2004;15(5):770–774.
151. Yonemoto N, Furuse J, Okusaka T, et al. A multicenter retrospective analysis of survival benefits of chemotherapy for unresectable biliary tract cancer. *Jpn J Clin Oncol*. 2007;37(11):843–851.
152. Slupski MW, Szczylik C, Jasinski MK. Unexpected response to systemic chemotherapy in case of primarily nonresectable advanced disseminated intrahepatic cholangiocarcinoma. *World J Surg Oncol*. 2007;5:36.
153. Sanz-Altamira PM, Ferrante K, Jenkins RL, et al. A phase II trial of 5-fluorouracil, leucovorin, and

carboplatin in patients with unresectable biliary tree carcinoma. *Cancer*. 1998;82(12):2321–2325.

154. Park SH, Park YH, Lee JN, et al. Phase II study of epirubicin, cisplatin, and capecitabine for advanced biliary tract adenocarcinoma. *Cancer*. 2006;106(2):361–365.

155. Furuse J, Okusaka T, Funakoshi A, et al. Early phase II study of uracil-tegafur plus doxorubicin in patients with unresectable advanced biliary tract cancer. *Jpn J Clin Oncol*. 2006;36(9):552–556.

156. Kim JH, Yoon HK, Sung KB, et al. Transcatheter arterial chemoembolization or chemoinfusion for unresectable intrahepatic cholangiocarcinoma: clinical efficacy and factors influencing outcomes. *Cancer*. 2008;113(7):1614–1622.

157. Lopez RR Jr, Pan SH, Lois JF, et al. Transarterial chemoembolization is a safe treatment for unresectable hepatic malignancies. *Am Surg*. 1997;63(10):923–926.

158. Kirchhoff T, Zender L, Merkesdal S, et al. Initial experience from a combination of systemic and regional chemotherapy in the treatment of patients with nonresectable cholangiocellular carcinoma in the liver. *World J Gastroenterol*. 2005;11(8):1091–1095.

159. Vogl TJ, Schwarz W, Eichler K, et al. Hepatic intraarterial chemotherapy with gemcitabine in patients with unresectable cholangiocarcinomas and liver metastases of pancreatic cancer: a clinical study on maximum tolerable dose and treatment efficacy. *J Cancer Res Clin Oncol*. 2006;132(11):745–755.

160. Gusani NJ, Balaa FK, Steel JL, et al. Treatment of unresectable cholangiocarcinoma with gemcitabine-based transcatheter arterial chemoembolization (TACE): a single-institution experience. *J Gastrointest Surg*. 2008;12(1):129–137.

161. Aliberti C, Benea G, Tilli M, Fiorentini G. Chemoembolization (TACE) of unresectable intrahepatic cholangiocarcinoma with slow-release doxorubicin-eluting beads: preliminary results. *Cardiovasc Intervent Radiol*. 2008;31(5):883–888.

162. Poggi G, Amatu A, Montagna B, et al. OEM-TACE: a new therapeutic approach in unresectable intrahepatic cholangiocarcinoma. *Cardiovasc Intervent Radiol*. 2009;32(6):1187–1192.

163. Burger I, Hong K, Schulick R, et al. Transcatheter arterial chemoembolization in unresectable cholangiocarcinoma: initial experience in a single institution. *J Vasc Interv Radiol*. 2005;16(3):353–361.

164. Shinohara ET, Mitra N, Guo M, Metz JM. Radiation therapy is associated with improved survival in the adjuvant and definitive treatment of intrahepatic cholangiocarcinoma. *Int J Radiat Oncol Biol Phys*. 2008;72(5):1495–1501.

165. Kulik LM, Carr BI, Mulcahy MF, et al. Safety and efficacy of 90Y radiotherapy for hepatocellular carcinoma with and without portal vein thrombosis. *Hepatology*. 2008;47(1):71–81.

166. Salem R, Lewandowski RJ, Atassi B, et al. Treatment of unresectable hepatocellular carcinoma with use of 90Y microspheres (TheraSphere): safety, tumor response, and survival. *J Vasc Interv Radiol*. 2005;16(12):1627–1639.

167. Gates VL, Atassi B, Lewandowski RJ, et al. Radioembolization with Yttrium-90 microspheres: review of an emerging treatment for liver tumors. *Future Oncol*. 2007;3(1):73–81.

168. Gaba RC, Lewandowski RJ, Kulik LM, et al. Radiation lobectomy: preliminary findings of hepatic volumetric response to lobar yttrium-90 radioembolization. *Ann Surg Oncol*. 2009;16(6):1587–1596.

169. Ibrahim SM, Mulcahy MF, Lewandowski RJ, et al. Treatment of unresectable cholangiocarcinoma using yttrium-90 microspheres: results from a pilot study. *Cancer*. 2008;113(8):2119–2128.

170. Saxena A, Bester L, Chua TC, et al. Yttrium-90 radiotherapy for unresectable intrahepatic cholangiocarcinoma: a preliminary assessment of this novel treatment option. *Ann Surg Oncol*. 2010;17(2):484–491.

171. Penn I. Hepatic transplantation for primary and metastatic cancers of the liver. *Surgery*. 1991;110(4):726–734.

172. Goldstein RM, Stone M, Tillery GW, et al. Is liver transplantation indicated for cholangiocarcinoma? *Am J Surg*. 1993;166(6):768–771.

173. Busuttil RW, Farmer DG. The surgical treatment of primary hepatobiliary malignancy. *Liver Transpl Surg*. 1996;2(5 suppl 1):114–130.

174. Pichlmayr R, Weimann A, Oldhafer KJ, et al. Role of liver transplantation in the treatment of unresectable liver cancer. *World J Surg*. 1995;19(6):807–813.

175. Casavilla FA, Marsh JW, Iwatsuki S, et al. Hepatic resection and transplantation for peripheral cholangiocarcinoma. *J Am Coll Surg*. 1997;185(5):429–436.

176. Weimann A, Varnholt H, Schlitt HJ, et al. Retrospective analysis of prognostic factors after liver resection and transplantation for cholangiocellular carcinoma. *Br J Surg.* 2000;87(9):1182–1187.
177. Meyer CG, Penn I, James L. Liver transplantation for cholangiocarcinoma: results in 207 patients. *Transplantation*. 2000;69(8):1633–1637.
178. Becker NS, Rodriguez JA, Barshes NR, et al. Outcomes analysis for 280 patients with cholangiocarcinoma treated with liver transplantation over an 18-year period. *J Gastrointest Surg.* 2008;12(1):117–122.
179. O'Grady JG, Polson RJ, Rolles K, et al. Liver transplantation for malignant disease. Results in 93 consecutive patients. *Ann Surg.* 1988;207(4):373–379.
180. Shimoda M, Farmer DG, Colquhoun SD, et al. Liver transplantation for cholangiocellular carcinoma: analysis of a single-center experience and review of the literature. *Liver Transpl.* 2001;7(12):1023–1033.
181. Robles R, Figueras J, Turrion VS, et al. Spanish experience in liver transplantation for hilar and peripheral cholangiocarcinoma. *Ann Surg.* 2004;239(2):265–271.
182. Sotiropoulos GC, Kaiser GM, Lang H, et al. Liver transplantation as a primary indication for intrahepatic cholangiocarcinoma: a single-center experience. *Transplant Proc.* 2008;40(9):3194–3195.
183. European Liver Transplant Registry. *Data Analysis Booklet 05/1968–12/2000*. Paris: ELTR; 2000:46–48.
184. Pascher A, Jonas S, Neuhaus P. Intrahepatic cholangiocarcinoma: indication for transplantation. *J Hepatobiliary Pancreat Surg.* 2003;10(4):282–287.
185. O'Grady JG. Treatment options for other hepatic malignancies. *Liver Transpl.* 2000;6(6 suppl 2):S23–S29.
186. De Vreede, Steers JL, Burch PA, et al. Prolonged disease-free survival after orthotopic liver transplantation plus adjuvant chemoirradiation for cholangiocarcinoma. *Liver Transpl.* 2000;6(3):309–316.
187. Rea DJ, Heimbach JK, Rosen CB, et al. Liver transplantation with neoadjuvant chemoradiation is more effective than resection for hilar cholangiocarcinoma. *Ann Surg.* 2005;242(3):451–458.
188. Healey JE Jr, Schroy PC. Anatomy of the biliary ducts within the human liver; analysis of the prevailing pattern of branchings and the major variations of the biliary ducts. *AMA Arch Surg.* 1953;66(5):599–616.
189. Hobsley M. Intra-hepatic anatomy; a surgical evaluation. *Br J Surg.* 1958;45(194):635–644.
190. Rosai J. Tumors and tumor like conditions of liver. In: Rosai J, ed. *Ackerman's Surgical Pathology*. 9th ed. St Louis, Missouri; 2004:992–1035.
191. Sasaki A, Aramaki M, Kawano K, et al. Intrahepatic peripheral cholangiocarcinoma: mode of spread and choice of surgical treatment. *Br J Surg.* 1998;85(9):1206–1209.
192. Yoon KH, Ha HK, Kim CG, et al. Malignant papillary neoplasms of the intrahepatic bile ducts: CT and histopathologic features. *AJR Am J Roentgenol.* 2000;175(4):1135–1139.
193. Weinbren K, Mutum SS. Pathological aspects of cholangiocarcinoma. *J Pathol.* 1983;139(2):217–238.
194. Lim JH. Cholangiocarcinoma: morphologic classification according to growth pattern and imaging findings. *AJR Am J Roentgenol.* 2003;181(3):819–827.
195. Lee WJ, Lim HK, Jang KM, et al. Radiologic spectrum of cholangiocarcinoma: emphasis on unusual manifestations and differential diagnoses. *Radiographics.* 2001;21 Spec No:S97–S116.
196. Quaglia A, Bhattacharjya S, Dhillon AP. Limitations of the histopathological diagnosis and prognostic assessment of hepatocellular carcinoma. *Histopathology.* 2001;38(2):167–174.
197. Lodi C, Szabo E, Holczbauer A, et al. Claudin-4 differentiates biliary tract cancers from hepatocellular carcinomas. *Mod Pathol.* 2006;19(3):460–469.
198. Dennis JL, Hvidsten TR, Wit EC, et al. Markers of adenocarcinoma characteristic of the site of origin: development of a diagnostic algorithm. *Clin Cancer Res.* 2005;11(10):3766–3772.
199. Oien KA, Dennis JL, Evans TRJ. Metastatic adenocarcinoma of unknown origin. In: Kirkham N, Shepherd NA, eds. *Progress in Pathology*. Cambridge University Press; 2007:135–162.
200. Isaji S, Kawarada Y, Taoka H, et al. Clinicopathological features and outcome of hepatic resection for intrahepatic cholangiocarcinoma in Japan. *J Hepatobiliary Pancreat Surg.* 1999;6(2):108–116.
201. Ohashi K, Nakajima Y, Tsutsumi M, et al. Clinical characteristics and proliferating activity of intrahepatic cholangiocarcinoma. *J Gastroenterol Hepatol.* 1994;9(5):442–446.

202. Yang J, Yan LN. Current status of intrahepatic cholangiocarcinoma. *World J Gastroenterol.* 2008;14(41):6289–6297.

203. Nozaki Y, Yamamoto M, Ikai I, et al. Reconsideration of the lymph node metastasis pattern (N factor) from intrahepatic cholangiocarcinoma using the International Union Against Cancer TNM staging system for primary liver carcinoma. *Cancer.* 1998;83(9):1923–1929.

204. Chu KM, Lai EC, Al-Hadeedi S, et al. Intrahepatic cholangiocarcinoma. *World J Surg.* 1997;21(3):301–305.

205. Kawarada Y, Yamagiwa K, Das BC. Analysis of the relationships between clinicopathologic factors and survival time in intrahepatic cholangiocarcinoma. *Am J Surg.* 2002;183(6):679–685.

206. Feisthammel J, Schoppmeyer K, Mossner J, et al. Irinotecan with 5-FU/FA in advanced biliary tract adenocarcinomas: a multicenter phase II trial. *Am J Clin Oncol.* 2007;30(3):319–324.

207. Tanaka N, Yamakado K, Nakatsuka A, et al. Arterial chemoinfusion therapy through an implanted port system for patients with unresectable intrahepatic cholangiocarcinoma—initial experience. *Eur J Radiol.* 2002;41(1):42–48.

208. Cantore M, Mambrini A, Fiorentini G, et al. Phase II study of hepatic intraarterial epirubicin and cisplatin, with systemic 5-fluorouracil in patients with unresectable biliary tract tumors. *Cancer.* 2005;103(7):1402–1407.

209. Herber S, Otto G, Schneider J, et al. Transarterial chemoemboliztion (TACE) for inoperable intrahepatic cholangiocarcinoma. *Cardiovasc Intervent Radiol.* 2007;30(6):1156–1165.

210. Martin R, Jarnagin W. Intrahepatic cholangiocarcinoma. Current management. *Minerva Chir.* 2003;58(4):469–478.

CHAPTER 3

Gallbladder Cancer

Anu Behari & Vinay K. Kapoor

Gallbladder cancer (GBC) is the most common malignancy of the biliary tract worldwide. Despite advances in imaging which permit earlier diagnosis, increasing experience with extensive surgical resections which can now be performed more safely, GBC remains a disease with a grim prognosis with overall survival rates of less than 10% at five years.[1,2]

Epidemiology

GBC has several well-known epidemiological characteristics.

GBC is the commonest biliary tract malignancy worldwide. It was as late as 1977, in the ninth edition of the International Classification of Diseases that GBC received its due recognition as a separate entity (156). Before that (eighth edition 1967), GBC was clubbed with cancers of the extrahepatic bile duct and ampulla.

GBC shows striking variations in its geographical distribution. It is rare in the United States, United Kingdom, Western Europe, Australia, and New Zealand with incidence rates in women approximately 1.0 per 100,000 each year.[3] In the United States, it is the fifth most common cancer of the gastrointestinal tract after colorectal, pancreas, stomach, and esophagus cancer. GBC is more common in certain geographical areas including Central and South America with high incidence rates in females (Peru 12.9, Chile 12.0, and Colombia 9.8), central and eastern Europe (Hungary 9.2 and Poland 8.7), and Japan. Chile has one of the highest incidence rates of GBC in the world (12.0) and is the leading cause of cancer deaths in females.[4,5] It is estimated that in the United States incidence rates in women are 1.2 per 100,000 per year and about 3000 deaths occur each year due to gallbladder and other biliary cancers.

GBC is common in some ethnic groups with high incidence rates reported in Native American Indian and Mexican American populations in the southwest United States. In New Zealand, Maoris have higher incidence of GBC than non-Maoris.[6]

India has a population of more than one billion and incidence rates in women are Delhi (North) 9.8, Bhopal (Central) 3.9, Mumbai (West) 2.6, and Chennai (South) 0.9 per 100,000 per year. In India with an expected average national incidence rate of 5 per 100,000 per year, as many 50,000 deaths each year can be expected to be due to GBC.[4,7]

GBC is more common in north India when compared to the south. In Delhi in north India, it is the fourth most common cancer (following breast 30, cervix 22, and ovary 10) and the most common gastrointestinal cancer in women. Incidence rates in women in north India (9.8 per 100,000 per year) are one of the highest in the world.[4,7] Even Indians who have migrated abroad such as to the UK, Singapore, Kuwait, or Fiji carry a high risk. Therefore, GBC has been called an "Indian" disease.[8] In north India, GBC has been reported to be the most common cause of malignant surgical obstructive jaundice.[9] GBC is also common in the entire northern parts of the Indian subcontinent (Pakistan, north India, and Bangladesh). In Pakistan, GBC is the third most common cancer in women after breast and oral cavity.[10] In Bangladesh, it is the most common hepato-biliary pancreatic cancer (HK Chowdhary Personal communication).

These geographic/regional variations in incidence rates may be explained either by racial ethnic variations in susceptibility to GBC or by environmental factors.

Risk Factors

Age and Sex

Incidence of GBC increases steadily with age in both sexes. Female preponderance is one of the distinguishing epidemiological features of GBC with incidence in females being two to six times that of males. In women, parity is a risk factor for both gallstones and GBC. A positive association between number of live births and risk of GBC has been reported.[11] Younger age at menarche, early age at first pregnancy, higher number of pregnancies, and prolonged fertility have been proposed as factors that may enhance the risk of cancer of the biliary tract.[12]

Gallstones

Gallstones are present in majority of patients with GBC—more than 90% in Chile, about 60%–70% in India, and 50%–60% in Japan. Older autopsy studies report a 3% incidence of GBC in patients with gallstones as compared to <0.2% in those without gallstones.[3] The epidemiology of GBC and gallstones shows striking parallels; both showing increasing incidence with age, female preponderance, and identical interethnic variations.

Patients with gallstones have sevenfold higher risk of GBC than normal population.[13] The risk of GBC in patients with gallstones is variable and is dependent on race and sex as well as the duration of exposure to gallstones.[14] It is higher in populations with high GBC incidence rates. Native Americans with gallstones have been estimated to have 21 times higher risk of developing GBC than those without gallstones.[14] Risk of GBC has been reported to increase with increasing size of gallstone(s). Patients with larger stones (>3 cm) have about 10 times higher risk of having GBC than those with smaller (<1 cm) stones. Two studies[15,16] reported a higher risk of GBC in patients with larger gallstones; a third study,[17] however, did not find any correlation between gallstones size and risk of GBC. A higher incidence of GBC has been reported in patients with Mirizzi's syndrome. Redaelli et al. found a 28% coincidental cases of GBC in patients with Mirizzi's syndrome as compared to a 2% incidence in patients with gallstones alone.[18] In our experience the coincident occurrence of GBC with Mirizzi's syndrome was 5.3%.[19] Increased gallstones/gallbladder volume ratio is associated with a higher risk of GBC.[20] The type of gallstones may also be important—more than 80% of gallstones in north India, where GBC is common, are cholesterol gallstones.[21] In south India, where GBC is much less common, majority (>60%) of gallstones are pigment and only 5% are cholesterol gallstones.[22]

Unexpected GBC is reported more often in the setting of acute cholecystitis than gallstones alone. In one series, as many as one-third of incidentally detected GBC had presented as acute cholecystitis, and age >70 years and a clinical diagnosis of empyema were the two most significant risk factors for incidental GBC.[23]

Despite the strong association between gallstones and GBC, a causal association remains to be proven and it is important to remember that only a small number of patients with gallstones later develop cancer and approximately 10%–40% of patients with GBC have no stones.

Bacterial Infection

It has been postulated that bacterial infection associated with gallstones might result in the formation, in bile, of local high concentrations of carcinogens. Significantly higher levels of secondary bile acids (lithocholic and deoxycholic) in bile and a higher incidence of positive bile cultures have been reported in patients with GBC as compared to patients with gallstones and normal controls.[24-26] Of patients with GBC, those with positive bile cultures have been reported to have significantly higher levels of secondary bile acids as compared to those with negative cultures.[24]

Salmonella typhi establishes itself in the gallbladder after an acute infection, and the patient becomes an asymptomatic carrier. Typhoid carriers have a higher risk of developing and dying of hepatobiliary cancers including GBC.[27–29]

Chemical Carcinogens

Reporting from north India, an area of high incidence of GBC and high concentrations of heavy metals in drinking water, Shukla et al. found significantly higher mean concentrations of heavy metals such as cadmium, chromium, and lead in bile from patients with GBC as compared to those with gallstones alone.[30] Bile from patients with GBC has been reported to have significantly higher levels of 4-hydroxynonenal—a major product of liver microsomal lipid peroxidation, which is washed away from hepatocytes along with bile and, if retained in the gallbladder for a prolonged period, may lead to tumorigenesis.[31]

Porcelain Gallbladder

Earlier series reported a very high but variable incidence of 13%–61% of GBC in patients with porcelain gallbladder. More recently, reporting on 44 patients with porcelain gallbladder, Stephen et al. found no GBC in 17 patients with complete intramural calcification as compared to a 7% incidence of GBC in 27 patients with selective mucosal calcification (odds ratio of 13.89 [$P = 0.01$]).[32] It is unknown whether the calcification of the gallbladder wall per se or the fact that it represents a later stage of inflammatory changes in the gallbladder wall of patients with long-standing gallstones is responsible for the high risk.

Anomalous Pancreaticobiliary Ductal Junction

Anomalous pancreaticobiliary ductal junction is considered to be a risk factor for carcinoma of the biliary tract; the associated reflux of pancreatic juice into the biliary tree is thought to cause chronic inflammation and metaplasia of the bile duct epithelium. The incidence of neoplasia in these patients varies between 12% and 67%. Patients with anomalous pancreaticobiliary ductal junction with no associated choledochal cyst have been reported to have a 50% incidence of GBC as compared to 5% in those with anomalous pancreaticobiliary ductal junction and choledochal cyst.[33] GBC associated with anomalous pancreaticobiliary ductal junction is believed to differ from GBC associated with gallstones in its molecular biology.[34]

Gallbladder Polyps

Gallbladder polyps are found in 0.004%–13% of gallbladders removed.[35] Most of the polypoid lesions are benign with cholesterol polyps constituting the majority. The possibility of a polyp being malignant increases with the age of the patient, increasing size of the lesion, when the lesion is sessile rather than pedunculated, single rather than multiple, and is associated with gallstones. A cholecystectomy is thus indicated in the above situations, especially if the patient is symptomatic and/or the lesion is showing a rapid increase in size on serial ultrasound examinations.[36] It has been proposed that a polypoid lesion less than 18 mm is potentially an early stage cancer and can be resected laparoscopically whereas a larger polyp may be an advanced cancer and should be removed by an extended cholecystectomy (EC).[37]

Adenomyomatosis

Segmental adenomyomatosis has been reported to be associated with a higher (6.4%) incidence of GBC than the diffuse type (3.1%).[38]

Miscellaneous

Patients with a cholecystoenteric fistula have been reported to have 15% incidence of GBC.[39]

A strong association has been observed between the risk of GBC and high body weight, especially among women. There are reports of a positive association with total calorie intake, high carbohydrate intake, and an inverse association with dietary fiber intake and micronutrients in vegetables and fruits, vitamin C and vitamin E.[40]

The relationship between GBC and xanthogranulomatous cholecystitis, which is a variant of chronic cholecystitis and can mimic GBC, remains elusive. In a study from north India, Rao et al. reported a 6% incidence of GBC in 435 patients with xanthogranulomatous cholecystitis.[41]

Clinical Features

There are no signs and symptoms that are specific for GBC, and the clinical picture depends upon the stage of the disease. Early GBC may present clinically exactly like benign gallstone disease. Physical examination in patients with early GBC is essentially normal. Early GBC is, thus, an elusive disease.[42] In two studies from areas with a high incidence of GBC, where the index of suspicion is high, none of the early GBC were diagnosed clinically and almost half of these were diagnosed after histopathological examination.[42,43] Some of the patients with long-standing symptoms of gallstones may notice a change in nature of symptoms from intermittent episodes of biliary colic to a more continuous dull aching pain in the right upper quadrant of abdomen at times with radiation to back.

Symptoms in later stages usually represent adjacent organ involvement—pain (continuous, dull aching, in the right upper abdomen [due to liver infiltration], which may radiate to the back), jaundice (due to biliary obstruction), early satiety, postprandial fullness, nausea and vomiting (due to duodenal infiltration or malignant gastroparesis which may be present in as many as 40% of patients), anorexia, and weight loss; a gallbladder mass may be palpable. In patients with surgical obstructive jaundice, if the gallbladder is palpable (distended), the obstruction is more likely to be due to a growth at the lower end of the common bile duct (CBD) (periampullary or pancreatic cancer); a cancer in the neck of gallbladder causing mucocele is an exception to this "rule."

Pruritus is a very distressing symptom in patients with GBC and biliary obstruction and may interfere with sleep and impairs quality of life. These are all, however, features of advanced GBC.
A special mention should be made of jaundice as it is an ominous sign that portends advanced disease, most unlikely to be cured by surgical intervention.[45] At times, the jaundice may be painless and progressive, mimicking periampullary cancers.

Patients with metastatic disease may have a nodular liver, ascites, umbilical nodule, and enlarged left supraclavicular lymph nodes. Peritoneal deposits in pelvis may be detected on per-rectal/per-vaginal examination.

GBC may have unusual (atypical) presentations such as acute cholecystitis, mucocele, and empyema due to a mass in the neck of the gallbladder resulting in obstruction of the cystic duct, gastrointestinal bleeding (upper and lower) due to duodenal/colonic infiltration, intestinal obstruction due to peritoneal dissemination, and so forth.[46] A large gallbladder mass with extensive liver infiltration may undergo central necrosis, which can cause fever, tachycardia, and tenderness; leukocytosis may be present and ultrasound and Computed tomography (CT) show a mass with irregular margins and central liquefaction—all features of a liver abscess. Advanced GBC may infiltrate right half of transverse colon and cause intestinal obstruction. Peritoneal dissemination may cause uncorrectable small bowel obstruction.[46]

Timing of Diagnosis

Obvious

Clinically obvious GBC is usually advanced—disease beyond the gallbladder wall and lymph nodes beyond hepato-duodenal ligament (HDL).

Suspected (on Imaging)

An irregular/localized thickening of the gallbladder wall or a single large sessile gallbladder polyp should be treated as "suspected" GBC.

Unsuspected

GBC suspected for the first time during cholecystectomy (for presumed gallstone disease)—can be confirmed by peroperative (intraoperative) fine needle aspiration cytology (FNAC), imprint cytology, or frozen section examination.

Incidental

Incidental GBC should be defined as one which was not suspected preoperatively (clinically or on imaging) or peroperatively (at laparotomy/laparoscopy or on opening the gallbladder) and is detected for the first time on histopathological examination of a gallbladder removed with a presumed diagnosis of gallstones. It is not the same as unsuspected GBC.

Missed

Some patients who have undergone cholecystectomy for presumed gallstones present some months later with jaundice and/or gastro-duodenal obstruction. These are patients in whom GBC was missed at the time of cholecystectomy as the gallbladder was not subjected to histological examination (and sometimes an early GBC is missed even on histology).

The manner of presentation of GBC seems to vary in different geographical areas. Areas where GBC is highly prevalent and clinical index of suspicion is high, preoperative diagnosis is usually obvious after preliminary imaging. Rates of "true" incidental GBC, discovered after histological examination of a gallbladder removed for presumed benign gallstone disease, are, therefore, usually low. In Western countries, where GBC is an uncommon disease and experience with management is limited to few tertiary care referral centers, a postoperative diagnosis after cholecystectomy, followed by referral for further treatment, is more common. Such incidental detection rates are reported to be as high as 47%, and there is an impression that increasing rates of laparoscopic cholecystectomy may play a role.[47,48]

Diagnosis

Routine laboratory investigations usually do not identify any findings that may be specific to and diagnostic of GBC. The diagnosis of GBC rests primarily on imaging, ultrasound, contrast enhanced computerized tomography, and magnetic resonance imaging being the primary imaging modalities employed. Cross-sectional imaging usually reveals one of the following patterns: (1) focal or diffuse mural thickening, (2) intraluminal polypoidal mass originating from gallbladder wall, and (3) a subhepatic mass replacing or obscuring the gallbladder and often infiltrating the adjacent liver.[49]

Ultrasound

Being readily available and noninvasive, an abdominal ultrasound is the first investigation that is usually done for common abdominal complaints and which may not only diagnose but also help to stage GBC.

Ultrasound findings in GBC include a mass replacing gallbladder, localized thickening of gallbladder wall, and a polypoidal intraluminal mass.[50,51] Protruding masses are better detected on ultrasound whereas flat lesions causing diffuse thickness of gallbladder wall are difficult to diagnose on ultrasound. Presence of gallstones also makes diagnosis of early lesions difficult—detection is better and earlier in the absence of gallstones. Ultrasound is, however, a poor investigation for detection of early GBC. Findings in early GBC include echogenic mucosa, discontinuous mucosa, and submucosal echolucency.[52,53] Loss of interface between the gallbladder wall and liver parenchyma suggests liver invasion. Intrahepatic biliary radical dilatation on ultrasound indicates biliary obstruction. Ultrasound can detect small amount of ascites.

Ultrasound is poor for staging of GBC; it often under-stages the disease, especially adjacent organ involvement like hepatic, duodenal, and colonic infiltration, lymph node spread, and liver metastases.

The overall accuracy of ultrasound for staging is about 40%.[51,54,55]

Ultrasound is also helpful to guide aspiration of ascitic fluid, which can then be subjected to cytological examination for malignant cells and to perform FNAC of gallbladder mass, liver metastases, and enlarged lymph nodes.

Endovascular, intraportal, ultrasound has been used to detect HDL invasion in neck tumors.

Chest X-Ray

Rarely, patients with GBC may have blood-borne pulmonary metastases. All patients with GBC should have at least a chest X-ray before any expensive investigations, for example CT, or before an operation is performed.

Contrast Enhanced Computed Tomography

A spiral, contrast-enhanced, multidetector thin-slice CT scan is essential for staging the disease and to assess resectability. Polypoidal lesions enhance homogenously whereas infiltrative lesions show irregular enhancement with areas of necrosis. CT is highly sensitive for detecting liver infiltration and metastases but sensitivity for detecting lymph nodal spread is low. Involved lymph nodes are large (>10 mm), round (cf. oval normal lymph nodes), and show ring-like or heterogeneous enhancement. CT with good oral/rectal and IV contrast can suggest duodenal and colonic involvement—proximity, compression, and infiltration which can be confirmed by upper gastrointestinal endoscopy or colonoscopy. Duodenal infiltration in GBC is seen on postero-superior wall of the first part of duodenum (cf. pancreatic cancer, where it is seen on medial wall of the second part of duodenum). Omental infiltration and small surface deposits on the liver and peritoneum are usually missed on CT (as also on ultrasound).

Magnetic resonance imaging

The role of magnetic resonance imaging in GBC is evolving. GBC appears hypointense on T1 weighted images and hyperintense on T2 weighted images. Magnetic resonance imaging (along with magnetic resonance cholangiography and magnetic resonance angiography) may give information provided by CT, cholangiography (endoscopic retrograde cholangiography/percutaneous transhepatic cholangiography), and angiography about biliary and vascular invasion. In a study assessing MR findings in GBC, sensitivity for direct hepatic invasion was 100%, and was 92% for lymph node metastasis.[56]

Positron Emission Tomography

Positron emission tomography is sensitive for diagnosis of GBC but can be falsely positive in patients with acute cholecystitis. In a recent report from the Memorial Sloan Kettering Cancer Center,[57] positron emission tomography scan detected unsuspected metastases (not detected on CT) in 7 out of 31 patients with GBC and thus avoided an unnecessary laparotomy. While evaluating the efficacy of integrated (18) F-fluorodeoxyglucose positron emission tomography-CT in determining occult metastatic or residual locoregional disease in patients with incidental GBC, Shukla et al. concluded that in patients with incidental GBC without metastatic disease, positron emission tomography-CT and multi-detector contrast-enhanced helical CT seem to have roles complementing each other. Positron emission tomography-CT was able to detect occult metastatic or residual locoregional disease in some of these patients, and seems to be useful in the preoperative diagnostic algorithm of patients whose multi-detector contrast-enhanced helical CT is normal or indicates locally advanced disease.[58]

Cholangiography

GBC in neck or cystic duct of the gallbladder may directly infiltrate common hepatic duct/common bile duct (CHD/CBD) and cause high or mid-CBD obstruction. Tumors in fundus or body of the gallbladder with liver infiltration may cause changes (distortion, stricture, or obliteration) of intrahepatic ducts in segments IV and V. Cholangiography is useful to evaluate hilar block with no mass on ultrasound or CT (to differentiate GBC from cholangiocarcinoma), to evaluate mid-CBD obstruction on ultrasound (to differentiate GBC from Mirizzi's syndrome) and to evaluate postcholecystectomy jaundice (to differentiate missed GBC from choledocholithiasis and benign biliary stricture).

Diagnostic cholangiography today will be magnetic resonance cholangiography. Endoscopic retrograde cholangiography or percutaneous transhepatic cholangiography should be performed only when a therapeutic intervention is planned to relieve biliary obstruction and jaundice.

Therapeutic endoscopic retrograde cholangiography/percutaneous transhepatic cholangiography may be indicated in patients with GBC who have surgical obstructive jaundice.

1. To bring bilirubin down by endoscopic or percutaneous stenting before a major liver resection is performed and prior to chemoradiotherapy
2. To palliate jaundice (and associated pruritus) by endoscopic or percutaneous stenting in unresectable cases
3. To control uncontrolled cholangitis not responding to parenteral antibiotics

Doppler Ultrasound

Doppler is useful for evaluation of hepatic artery and portal vein in patients with GBC at neck causing biliary obstruction that indicates involvement of the HDL. Involvement of main hepatic artery and portal vein usually indicates unresectability unless resection and reconstruction of these vessels is performed.

Angiography

Conventional angiography was used earlier to detect involvement of vessels (portal vein, hepatic artery) in the HDL; it has now been replaced by Doppler ultrasound, contrast enhanced computed tomography, CT angiography, and MR angiography.

Upper Gastrointestinal Endoscopy

Upper gastrointestinal endoscopy should be performed in patients with possibly resectable disease but with suspicion of duodenal involvement on imaging (e.g., CT). Duodenal infiltration on upper gastrointestinal endoscopy usually indicates unresectability (unless pancreatico-duodenectomy [PD] is planned). Upper gastrointestinal endoscopy is also performed in patients with symptoms of gastric outlet obstruction to differentiate between mechanical obstruction and malignant gastroparesis.

Endoscopic Ultrasound

Endoscopic ultrasound is useful for diagnosis of early GBC and for accurate T and N staging.[59] Endoscopic ultrasound-guided FNAC of enlarged lymph nodes may be performed to confirm if enlarged lymph nodes are malignant.

Ascitic Fluid Cytology

Patients with GBC may have ascites. This may be nutritional—associated with pedal edema and low serum albumin level. Ascites may also be malignant—due to peritoneal dissemination. Ultrasound- or CT-guided ascitic fluid aspiration and cytology should be performed to rule out malignant ascites as patients with peritoneal dissemination and malignant ascites have a very poor prognosis and should not undergo surgery.

Laparoscopy

Staging laparoscopy may reveal peritoneal/omental/ovarian and pelvic deposits that were not seen on ultrasound or CT. A cake-like rolled-up omentum may also be seen on laparoscopy. It may also reveal surface liver metastases undetected on imaging. If no dissemination is found, minimal dissection may be performed to assess local infiltration into the HDL, duodenum, and colon. We strongly recommend that staging laparoscopy should be performed before laparotomy, as it may avoid an unnecessary laparotomy in as many as one-fourth to one-third of cases.[60]

Laparoscopic Ultrasound

Laparoscopic ultrasound may help to detect intrahepatic space occupying lesions not detected on preoperative ultrasound or CT. It may also assess infiltration of HDL, duodenum, and colon better than laparoscopy alone.

Tumor Markers

GBC is known to produce α-fetoprotein, carcinoembryonic antigen, and carbohydrate antigen 19-9 but their role in screening, diagnosis, prognosis, or follow-up is not well established.

Tissue Diagnosis

A preoperative positive cytological diagnosis is not essential if the lesion is apparently resectable on imaging and the patient is being planned for surgery because in case of suspicion of GBC, even if cytology is negative, it is advisable to go ahead with an extended cholecystectomy (EC). Such a policy will result in a few extended cholecystectomies being performed for benign disease such as chronic cholecystitis or xanthogranulomatous cholecystitis, but this is acceptable because EC is a no-mortality, low-morbidity procedure. Also, if a positive cytology is insisted upon in every case before EC, many early GBCs will be denied appropriate resection and cure.

FNAC is a simple, safe, and reliable method to obtain tissue diagnosis. It can be performed under US/CT guidance from a gallbladder mass and thick-walled gallbladder; FNAC is almost 100% specific (no false-positive). False-negative results due to inadequate smear are, however, common and necessitate repeat procedure. FNAC has been reported to have a very high sensitivity (90%) and specificity (100%) for diagnosis in advanced GBC.[61] A recent study reported a sensitivity, specificity, and positive predictive value of 73%, 100%, and 100% of ultrasound-guided FNAC in gallbladder masses.[62]

Tissue diagnosis is essential in patients with advanced or metastatic disease who are not being considered for surgery. FNAC can also be performed from enlarged abdominal lymph nodes, liver nodules, enlarged supraclavicular lymph nodes, and umbilical nodule.

FNAC can be performed intraoperatively also for peroperative tissue diagnosis, which is essential if resection is not planned. Liver metastases, peritoneal, omental, or pelvic deposits, enlarged lymph nodes, and gallbladder may also be subjected to frozen section histological examination to confirm tissue diagnosis intraoperatively. Imprint cytology is of immense use for an intraoperative diagnosis where frozen section facilities are not available. At laparotomy, a suspected enlarged lymph node or liver/omental/peritoneal deposit may be removed, bisected, and touched on a glass slide and subjected to imprint cytology. A suspicious gallbladder may be removed, opened, and mucosal surface touched on a glass slide for imprint cytology. Also, imprint cytology is quicker than frozen section.

Differential Diagnosis

Early GBC is difficult to differentiate from gallstone disease as patients with early GBC have symptoms of associated gallstones only and the cancer per se is asymptomatic. In patients with gallstones, recent change in character of pain from intermittent biliary colic to continuous dull ache may suggest GBC.

Xanthogranulomatous cholecystitis may mimic GBC in clinical presentation, imaging, and even operative findings and can be nearly impossible to differentiate from GBC. It may coexist with GBC and so even a pre/intraoperative cytological diagnosis of XGC does not rule out presence of GBC.[41]

Hilar block due to cholangiocarcinoma, Mirizzi's syndrome, and portal lymphadenopathy may present in an identical manner to GBC with surgical obstructive jaundice. Identification of a mass in the neck of gallbladder favors a diagnosis of GBC but sometimes this may be very difficult.

Malignant ascites in GBC resembles that due to any other advanced intra-abdominal cancer.

Postcholecystectomy jaundice due to missed GBC may be differentiated from that due to a bile duct injury and benign biliary stricture in that the postoperative course after cholecystectomy is usually uneventful and the biliary obstruction is high (Bismuth Type III or IV).[63]

"Thick-Walled" Gallbladder

The gallbladder wall >3 mm (on ultrasound) is described as thick. Diffuse and uniform thickening of the gallbladder wall could be present in acute cholecystitis, chronic cholecystitis, xanthogranulomatous cholecystitis and, rarely, GBC. In areas where both gallstone disease and GBC are common, this can be a frequent dilemma. In a prospective evaluation of 60 diffuse thick-walled gallbladders, 30 were found to be due to chronic cholecystitis, 28 due to xanthogranulomatous cholecystitis, and only 2 were due to GBC. These two were indistinguishable from the rest even at surgery.[64] A diffuse thick-walled gallbladder can be approached laparoscopically though conversion rate will be higher. Irregular or localized thickening of gallbladder wall should raise suspicion of GBC and should be further investigated by CT. Such cases are better managed as suspected GBC by open operation. Provision should be made for intraoperative FNAC, imprint cytology, and/or frozen section to assist intraoperative decision making.

Staging Systems

The original staging system proposed by Nevin et al.[65] is no longer followed. The tumor node metastasis system proposed by the International Union Against Cancer (UICC) and the American Joint Committee on Cancer (AJCC) is the most commonly followed staging system. GBC was not included in the AJCC–UICC tumor node metastasis classification till 1982. The AJCC–UICC proposed the tumor node metastasis classification and staging system in 1987. The UICC–AJCC staging system (Table 3-1) was published in the fifth edition in 1997, revised in the sixth edition in 2002, and again in the seventh edition in 2010.[66-68] The Japanese surgeons have long followed the staging system proposed by the Japanese Society for Biliary Surgery.

Nevin Stage Grouping (No Longer Followed)

Stage I Intramucosal only
Stage II Extends to the muscularis
Stage III Extends through the serosa
Stage IV Transmural involvement and cystic lymph nodes involved
Stage V Direct extension to liver and/or distant metastases

Summary of Changes (From Fifth [1997] to Sixth [2002] Edition)

- The T and N classifications were changed in an effort to separate locally invasive tumors into potentially resectable (T3) and unresectable (T4).
- There was no longer a distinction between T3 and T4 based on the depth of liver invasion.
- Lymph node metastasis was now classified as stage IIB, and stage IIA was reserved for large, invasive tumors (resectable), without lymph node metastasis.
- Stage grouping was changed to allow stage III to signify locally unresectable disease and stage IV to indicate metastatic disease.

In the most recent seventh edition (2010)
The cystic duct is now included in this classification scheme.

- The N classification now distinguishes hilar nodes (N1: lymph nodes adja-cent to the cystic duct, bile duct, hepatic artery, and portal vein) from other regional nodes (N2: celiac, periduodenal, and peripancreatic lymph nodes and those along the superior mesenteric artery).
- Stage groupings have been changed to better correlate with surgical resectability and patient outcome; locally unresectable T4 tumors have been reclassified as stage IV.
- Lymph node metastasis is now classified as stage IIIB (N1) or stage IVB (N2).

TABLE 3-1: UICC–AJCC Staging System for Gallbladder Cancer

AJCC Fifth Edition 1997	AJCC Sixth Edition 2002	AJCC Seventh Edition 2010
T1: Tumor invades lamina propria or muscle	T1: Tumor invades lamina propria or muscle	T1: Tumor invades lamina propria or muscle
T1a: Tumor invades lamina propria T1b: Tumor invades muscle layer	T1a: Tumor invades lamina propria T1b: Tumor invades muscle layer	T1a: Tumor invades lamina propria T1b: Tumor invades muscle layer
T2: Tumor invades perimuscular connective tissue; no extension beyond serosa or into liver	T2: Tumor invades perimuscular connective tissue; no extension beyond serosa or into liver	T2: Tumor invades perimuscular connective tissue; no extension beyond serosa or into liver
T3: Tumor perforates the serosa (visceral peritoneum) or directly invades one adjacent organ, or both (extension 2 cm or less into liver)	T3: Tumor perforates the serosa (visceral peritoneum) and/or directly invades the liver and/or one other adjacent organ or structure, such as the stomach, duodenum, colon, pancreas, omentum, or extrahepatic bile ducts	T3: Tumor perforates the serosa (visceral peritoneum) and/or directly invades the liver and/or one other adjacent organ or structure, such as the stomach, duodenum, colon, pancreas, omentum, or extrahepatic bile ducts
T4: Tumor extends more than 2 cm into liver and/or into two or more adjacent organs (stomach, duodenum, colon, pancreas, omentum, extrahepatic bile ducts, any involvement of liver)	T4: Tumor invades main portal vein or hepatic artery or invades multiple extrahepatic organs or structures	T4: Tumor invades main portal vein or hepatic artery or invades multiple extrahepatic organs or structures
N1: Metastasis in cystic duct, pericholedochal, and/or hilar lymph nodes (i.e., in the HDL)	N1: Regional lymph node metastasis	N1: Metastases to nodes along the cystic duct, common bile duct, hepatic artery, and/or portal vein
N2: Metastasis in peripancreatic (head only), periduodenal, periportal, celiac, and/or superior mesenteric lymph nodes	N2: Excluded	N2: Metastases to peri-aortic, pericaval, superior mesenteric artery, and/or celiac artery lymph nodes

Abbreviations: AJCC, American Joint Committee on Cancer; HDL, hepato-duodenal ligament; UICC, International Union Against Cancer.

We had suggested two major changes in the AJCC–UICC classification.[69]

1. Involvement of muscle layer should be classified as T2 (instead of T1b) as it merits an EC (cf. simple cholecystectomy for T1a lamina propria).
2. Involvement of distant (celiac, superior mesenteric, para-aortic, and aorto-caval) lymph nodes (LNs) indicates poor prognosis. These LNs were earlier (AJCC–UICC fifth edition 1997) classified as N2 (cf. LNs in HDL being classified as N1). We had proposed that these LNs be classified as N3 (instead of N2) as their involvement indicates poor prognosis akin to metastatic (M1) disease.

Pathology

Macroscopically, GBC may be papillary-pedunculated, nodular nonpedunculated, and papillary infiltrative, nodular infiltrative, infiltrative (no elevation) filling up form, massive types or special types.[70]

Microscopically, most (about 90%) are adenocarcinomas; the remaining are squamous or adenosquamous; carcinoid, sarcoma, melanoma, and lymphoma have been rarely reported in GBC.

Spread: Surgical Implications

GBC spreads directly and by lymphatic, vascular, intraperitoneal, perineural, and intraductal routes to liver and other adjacent organs (common bile duct, duodenum, colon, and omentum) as well to regional lymph nodes and distant sites.[71]

The liver is invaded directly as well as by lymphatic and venous pathways and is involved in 34%–95% of patients with GBC. Microscopic angiolymphatic invasion of portal tracts has been described as a major mode of hepatic involvement. Japanese surgeons differentiate between invasion toward the gallbladder bed (gallbladder bed type) from invasion toward the hepatic hilum (hilar type). The former have an expansive tumor margin as against an infiltrative one in the hilar type. It has been observed that GBC invades the liver bed contiguously forming an expansive mass in the bed type, whereas it invades the loose connective tissue in the hepatic hilum with lymphatic and perineural invasion in the hepatic hilar type.[72,73] While the expansive tumor margin can be taken care of by an extended hepatectomy, the hepatic hilar type are extremely difficult to resect with negative surgical margins.

Bile duct involvement in GBC results from both direct tumor extension as well as perineural and lymphatic routes. Shimizu et al. explored the pathological manner of involvement of HDL and described four types of spread: direct extramural spread (type I), continuous intramural spread (type II), distant spread separated from the primary tumor (type III), and spread of cancer cells from metastatic lymph nodes (type IV). More than one type of spread was often present. Invasion of the HDL was present in 24 of 44 patients without preoperative obstructive jaundice and in 2 of 13 patients with stage IB disease. Patients with types II, III, and IV spread into the HDL had significantly better survival than those with type I spread. The authors concluded that since preoperative diagnosis of this invasion is difficult, strong consideration should be given to resection of the extrahepatic bile ducts and lymph nodes.[74]

Invasion of the HDL constitutes one of the major reasons for unresectability in GBC. This is due to the spread into interstitial tissue, lymphatic permeation, venous invasion, and perineural invasion, which occur in 75% of cases with involvement of HDL. Extensive infiltration into the HDL precludes curative resection. Unsuspected microscopic invasion of HDL is present in a large number of tumors.[74] Also, patients with severe involvement of HDL have been reported to have a high chance of para-aortic lymph node involvement and are unlikely to have a cure with radical resections.[75]

The venous drainage of gallbladder takes place either over 2–20 smaller vessels directly into the liver parenchyma of the gallbladder bed, or over a robust gallbladder vein that terminates in the ascending portal branch of liver segments V and VIII.

Lymph flow in the gallbladder occurs from the mucosa via the lymphatic channels in the muscular layer and in the subserosal layer to the lymph nodes at the neck of the gallbladder. The lymph flow to the right of the HDL (the pericholedochal, posterior pancreatico-duodenal, and then inter-aortic nodes) the so-called "cholecysto-retropancreatic pathway" is the main route of spread, and the left route (pericholedochal, lymph nodes along the hepatic artery to the common hepatic artery, retroportal or celiac, and inter or left lateral para-aortic nodes) the "cholecystocoeliac pathway" comprises an alternative route.[76] Ito et al. also describe the "cholecysto-mesenteric pathway."[77] The right and the left routes communicate at the lymph nodes around the pancreatic head. Direct lymphatic channels from the retropancreatic lymph nodes to the para-aortic nodes have been described. Most studies indicate that the hepatic hilar nodes are not an important draining area in GBC, but Lin et al. reported involvement of hepatic hilar nodes in 35% of their patients.

Incidence of lymph node involvement increases with increasing transmural spread of primary tumor. T1a tumors do not have nodal metastases. In T1b tumors, however, nodal spread may be present in as many as 11% of patients.[78] The rates of LN involvement as relating to depth of tumor in the gallbladder as reported in various series are summarized in Table 3-2.[75,76,79] A high incidence of para-aortic node involvement has also been seen in patients with severe involvement of HDL.[75] Though the rationale for lymph node dissection in GBC is sound, whether

TABLE 3-2: Frequency of Lymph node Involvement in GBC

Series	Overall (%)	pT1 (%)	pT2 (%)	pT3/T4 (%)
Kondo[72,29] (n = 60)	73 (38% para-aortic node involvement)	—	57	80
Shimada Cancer[75] (n = 41)	63	0	62	81
Tsukada Cancer[76] (n = 111)	54	0	46	79

removal of regional lymph nodes provides any therapeutic benefit is still unclear. The fact that variable extents of lymph node dissections done for a heterogeneous group of patients with different stages of disease have been retrospectively analyzed in most of these reports makes it even more difficult to draw any definite conclusions.

Four percent of all and as many as 19% of papillary variant of GBC may have intraductal spread into distal biliary tracts. Perineural spread occurs in about 20% of patients and is a predictor of poor prognosis. GBC also has a propensity to spread in the peritoneal cavity resulting in peritoneal, omental, ovarian, and pelvic deposits. Blood-borne metastases occur to liver, lungs, and bones. Rare sites of metastasis include umbilicus, left supraclavicular, and axillary lymph nodes.

The primarily locoregional mode of spread of GBC makes it theoretically amenable to surgical resection at least in the early stages.

Management

Most centers in the Western world, except groups such as the Memorial Sloan Kettering Cancer Center, New York USA, have traditionally had a pessimistic attitude and nihilistic approach toward GBC. This, coupled with the rarity of and lack of familiarity with GBC, sometimes results in inadequate and incomplete treatment of even early—potentially resectable and possibly curable—GBC, for example, simple cholecystectomy only for T1b or T2 tumors.[80] Most Japanese centers, on the other hand, have an aggressive approach even for advanced GBC. The supraradical resectional procedures including major hepatectomy, pancreaticoduodenectomy, adjacent organ resections, vascular resections, hepato-duodenal ligamentectomy, extensive retroperitoneal lymphadenectomy, and so forth performed by various Japanese groups are, however, associated with high mortality (still in double figures) and major morbidity and have resulted in anecdotal long-term survivors only. We have advocated a "Buddhist" Indian "middle path" (between Western pessimism and Japanese aggression) for management of GBC. This includes an aggressive surgical approach for management of early (resectable, curable) GBC and conservative, nonsurgical (endoscopic or radiological) palliation for advanced GBC.[81]

Complete removal of the primary tumor along with its area of locoregional spread, before distant metastases have occurred, provides the only chance of cure in a patient with GBC. The ability to achieve a complete tumor resection largely depends upon the stage of the disease at presentation. By and large, treatment for GBC still remains largely palliative as in most patients the disease is either metastatic or locally advanced at the time of diagnosis. Management, therefore, depends upon the stage of the disease and manner of presentation and whether the patient has already been subjected to a cholecystectomy as well as performance status and comorbidities of the patient. Those with obviously metastatic or unresectable, locally advanced disease can only be offered symptomatic relief. In GBC, this usually means management of pain, jaundice, pruritus, cholangitis, and gastric outlet obstruction, usually by nonsurgical means (vide infra). Potentially curative surgery is offered to the minority of patients, in whom investigations reveal disease amenable to surgical extirpation (Figure 3-1).

Suspected GBC

In a patient in whom the diagnosis of GBC is suspected preoperatively, further management should proceed systematically to rule out metastatic disease and to stage the locoregional extent of disease to decide resectability (Figure 3-1). In patients with nonmetastatic disease, factors that usually determine

Hepatobiliary Cancer

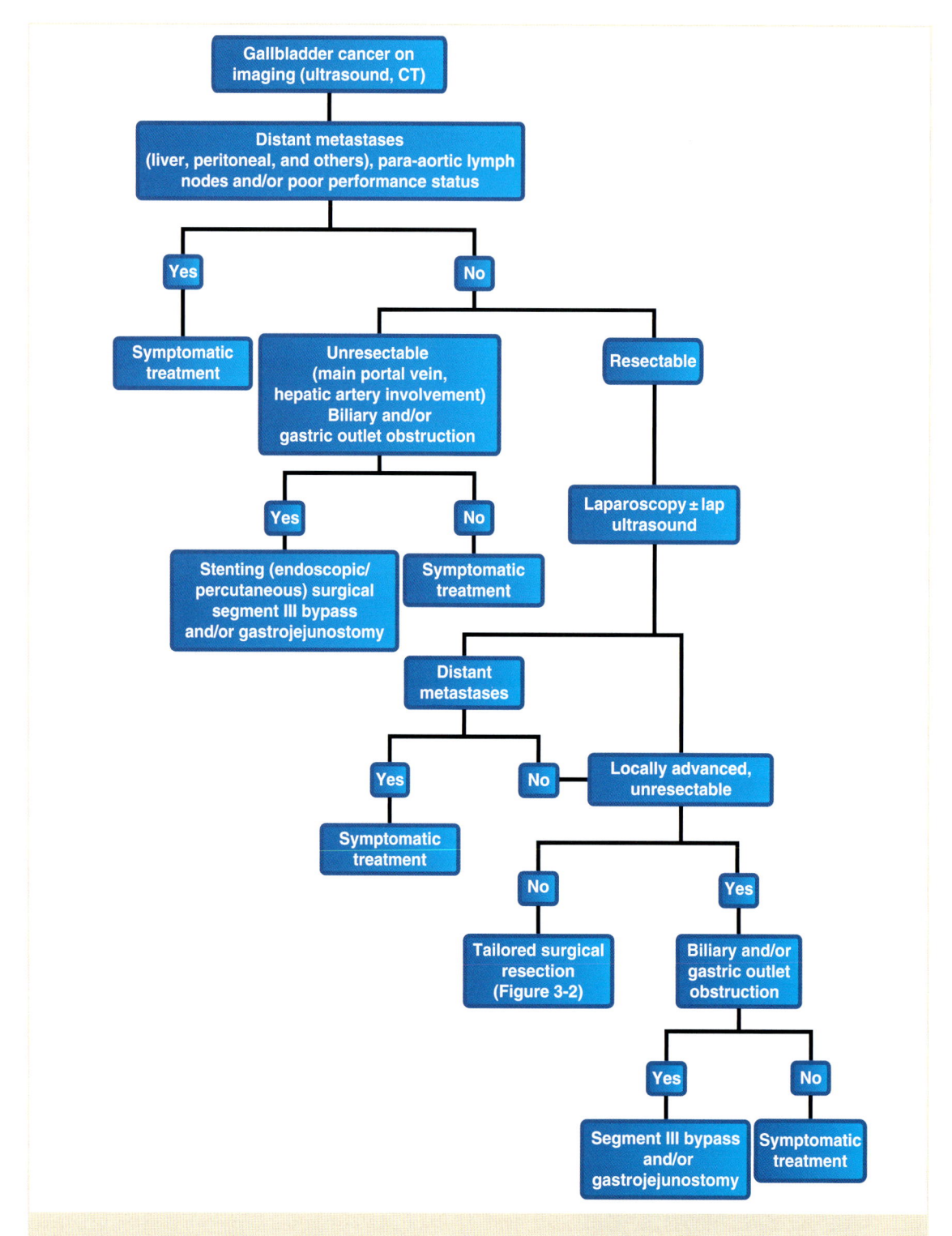

Figure 3-1: Algorithm for management of patient with suspected gallbladder cancer prior to surgery.

chances as well as the extent of a potentially curative surgical resection include the size and location (fundus, body, and neck), of the primary tumor, extent of nodal involvement (limited to hepatoduodenal ligament (HDL), or distant viz. celiac, superior mesenteric, para-aortic), involvement of common bile duct, hepatic artery, and portal vein. The performance status of the patient and comorbidities remain important considerations as before any major surgical procedure.

Though the exact extent of resection may vary from extended Cholecystectomy (EC) to hepatopancreatico-duodenectomy (Figure 3-2), the aim is to stay ahead of the spreading tumor front on the hepatic, nodal, HDL and adjacent organ fronts. The basic components of a potentially curative surgical resection include

1. En bloc cholecystectomy
2. Liver resection
   In tumors located in the fundus or body of the gallbladder and with no or minimal liver infiltration, a 2 cm, nonanatomic wedge of the liver around the gallbladder bed or a formal segment IVb+5 resection is enough to provide a negative surgical margin on the hepatic front. For tumors with more extensive liver infiltration and for tumors at or near the neck, which are close to or involve the right portal pedicle, an extended right hepatectomy (IV, V, VI, VII, and VIII) or a right hepatectomy with IVb resection is needed to provide clear margins. Some Japanese surgeons have advocated the so-called "Taj Mahal" or central mesohepatectomy for similar lesions.[82] Patients with jaundice need preoperative biliary drainage (endoscopic or percutaneous) before a major liver resection is performed, as the commonest cause of death after a major hepatectomy is liver failure. In patients in whom an extended right hepatectomy is planned, preoperative right portal vein embolization is performed to induce right lobe atrophy and left lobe hypertrophy to increase residual liver volume and reduce the risk of postoperative liver failure.[83] Selective embolization of PV branch to segment IV may also be added because segment is also removed in extended right hepatectomy. Before portal vein embolization is performed, patient

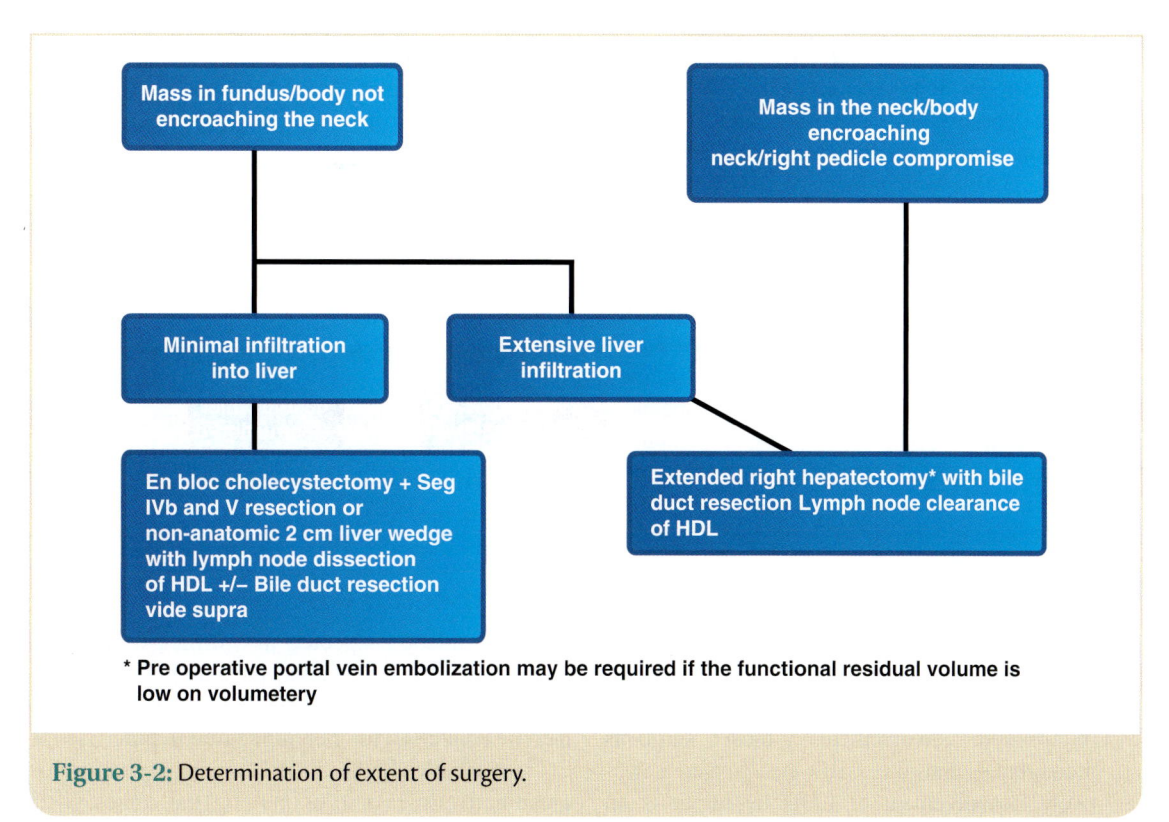

* Pre operative portal vein embolization may be required if the functional residual volume is low on volumetery

Figure 3-2: Determination of extent of surgery.

should be made anicteric by endoscopic biliary stenting. It may be advisable to perform a staging laparoscopy before portal vein embolization to rule out peritoneal dissemination. Surgery should be performed at least two to three weeks after portal vein embolization.

3. Lymph node dissection

   The likelihood of presence of tumor in regional lymph nodes in a significant number of patients with GBC (Table 3-2) provides the rationale for lymph node clearance as an integral component of surgery for GBC. There is, however, a lack of consensus on the exact extent as well as the effect of lymph node clearance on long-term survival. The terms "portal lymph node dissection," "extended lymph node dissection," and "radical lymph node dissection" have all been used to describe varying extents of nodal dissection.[84] Most surgeons, especially in the West, do what has been called "standard lymph node dissection" that includes clearance of nodes with skeletonization of HDL. This involves removal of cystic (12c), pericholedochal (12b), hilar (12h), proper hepatic artery (12a), periportal (12p), postero-superior pancreaticoduodenal (13a), and common hepatic artery lymph nodes with skeletonization of hepatic artery, portal vein, and bile duct. Japanese surgeons (and in recent years some centers in the West) have been more aggressive with lymph node dissections, routinely removing nodes posterior to head of pancreas along with celiac, superior mesenteric, and even para-aortic nodes. Some groups go to the extent of doing a pancreatico-duodenal resection to achieve R0 resections in carefully selected patients.[85–87] Addition of pancreatico-duodenal resection, especially in a patient who is undergoing an extended hepatic resection, definitely increases morbidity and mortality of the procedure while definite benefits in terms of prolongation of survival have been difficult to achieve. Obviously, patient selection is crucial.[88]

4. CBD excision

   Though some authors recommend routine excision of CBD to take care of unsuspected, microscopic involvement[74] most surgeons recommend that the CBD be excised selectively.[89] Involvement of CBD by tumor is an important predictor of poor prognosis irrespective of the extent of resection, and CBD excision has been reported to be associated with higher morbidity.[90] CBD excision is required for tumors of gallbladder neck or cystic duct, to facilitate nodal clearance in a bulky HDL, and during reresection for incidental GBC when the cystic duct margin is positive. Some surgeons remove the CBD as a routine during reresection because it is nearly impossible to differentiate involvement due to tumor from postoperative scarring of tissues.

5. Adjacent involved organ resection (colon, stomach, and first part of duodenum)

   Segmental resection of involved colon, distal stomach, and occasionally a disc of duodenum can be done when the extent of local infiltration by tumor allows complete removal. A PD may be added if the extent of duodenal infiltration dictates it. More often a PD is added to facilitate lymph nodal clearance around the pancreatic head when it is assessed that this will lead to an R0 resection in a patient who is considered fit to withstand addition of another major procedure (vide supra). *Right upper quadrantectomy* (major hepatectomy, PD, distal gastrectomy, right hemicolectomy, and right nephrectomy) has also been reported for advanced GBC.

6. Vascular resections

   Major hepatic resection, with resection and reconstruction of HDL structures (CBD, hepatic artery, and portal vein) and PD, has been performed by some Japanese groups to achieve negative surgical margins. Results of these studies, however, indicate that though technically feasible vascular resections add to operative difficulty and time, are associated with higher morbidity and mortality, and do not confer any significant long-term survival advantage.[91–93]

Unsuspected GBC

GBC should be suspected in a difficult cholecystectomy—dense adhesions, unclear plane in gallbladder bed; laparoscopic cholecystectomy should then be converted to open procedure if expertise for EC is available (Figure 3-3). If during operation for presumed (clinical and/or imaging) gallstones, GBC

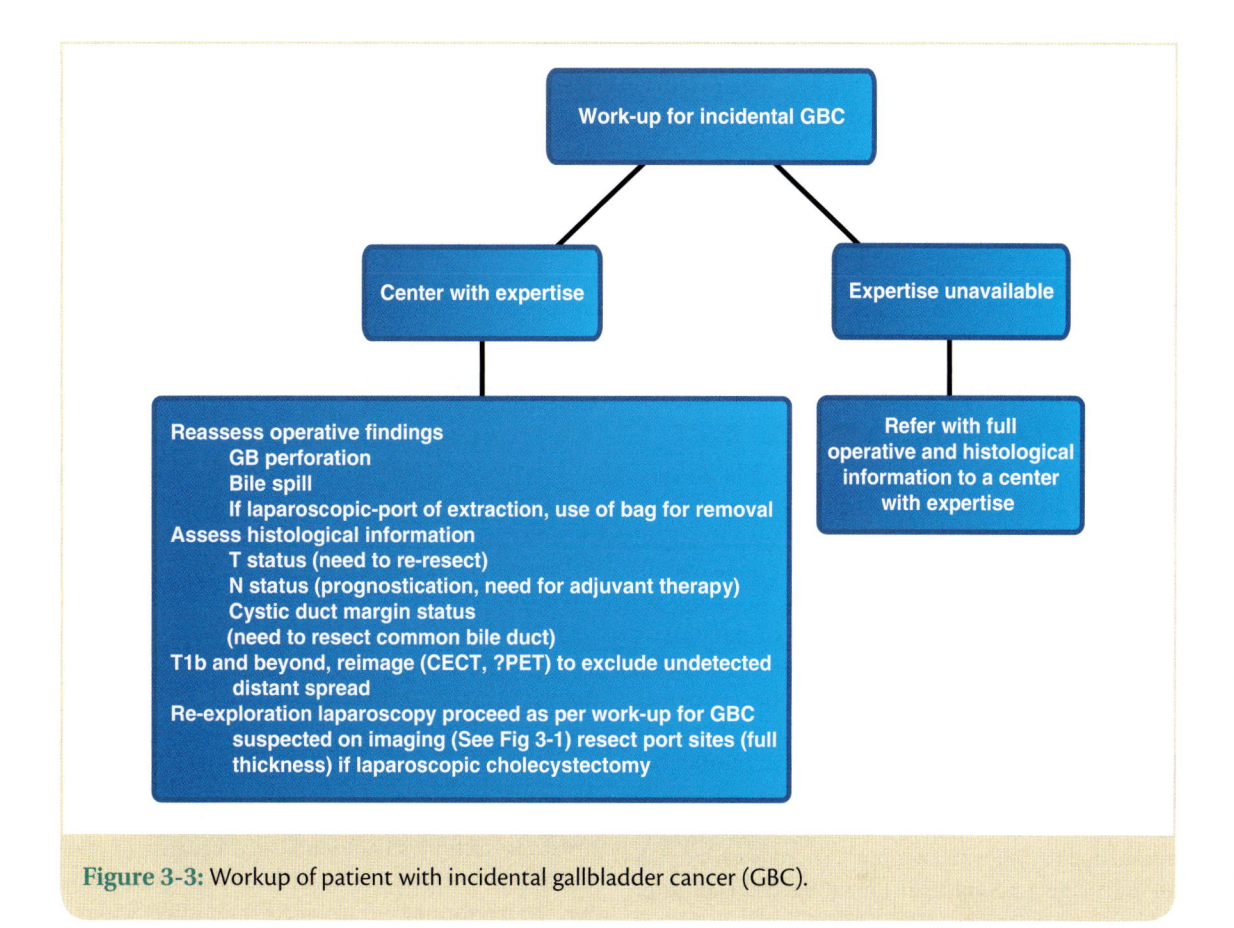

```
                    ┌─────────────────────────┐
                    │ Work-up for incidental GBC │
                    └─────────────────────────┘
                         /              \
           ┌──────────────────┐   ┌──────────────────┐
           │ Center with expertise │   │ Expertise unavailable │
           └──────────────────┘   └──────────────────┘
```

Reassess operative findings
  GB perforation
  Bile spill
  If laparoscopic-port of extraction, use of bag for removal
Assess histological information
  T status (need to re-resect)
  N status (prognostication, need for adjuvant therapy)
  Cystic duct margin status
  (need to resect common bile duct)
T1b and beyond, reimage (CECT, ?PET) to exclude undetected distant spread
Re-exploration laparoscopy proceed as per work-up for GBC suspected on imaging (See Fig 3-1) resect port sites (full thickness) if laparoscopic cholecystectomy

Refer with full operative and histological information to a center with expertise

Figure 3-3: Workup of patient with incidental gallbladder cancer (GBC).

is suspected the approach depends on the available expertise. If, as is likely to be the case, expertise for proper curative resection for GBC is not available, the gallbladder should not be mobilized, it should be covered with omentum (to prevent duodenum and colon from getting adherent), and the patient should be referred to a center with expertise. If GBC is suspected after the gallbladder has been removed and specimen opened, the subhepatic fossa should be thoroughly irrigated with sterile water (to kill any viable tumor cells), gallbladder bed should be covered with omentum, and the patient referred to a center with expertise to complete the EC.

Incidental GBC

Patients with incidental GBC (GBC detected on histological examination of gallbladder after cholecystectomy for presumed gallstone disease) should be advised to undergo reoperation for completion extended cholecystectomy except when disease was confined to mucosa (T1a) in which case simple cholecystectomy alone may be adequate. Reoperation for completion extended cholecystectomy should be performed in T1a lesions also if the cystic lymph node removed along with the gallbladder was positive (N1) or if the gallbladder neck/cystic duct margin was positive. To provide the benefit of doubt to the patients, reoperation should be advised if T stage is not available.

Patient should be thoroughly examined (supraclavicular lymph nodes, port-site/incision metastases, umbilical nodule, ascites, pelvic deposits) and investigated (chest X-ray, ultrasound, CT, positron emission tomography, staging laparoscopy) to look for distant metastases which, if present, contraindicate reoperation.

Completion extended cholecystectomy involves resection of 2 cm nonanatomical wedge of liver in gallbladder fossa (or formal resection of segment IVB and V) and lymph nodal dissection in the HDL, behind duodenum and pancreas head, and along hepatic artery to the right of celiac axis. If cholecystectomy was performed laparoscopically, all ports must be excised full thickness (skin to peritoneum) to prevent port site metastases. Port site metastases are most common at the port of extraction, but they are seen at other ports also.[94]

Since bile spill is common during LC, these patients should receive chemotherapy.

The approach to management of patients with GBC depending upon the timing of presentation is summarized in Figures 3-1 through 3-4.

GBC and Laparoscopic Surgery

Laparoscopic cholecystectomy (LC) has become the gold standard for management of symptomatic gallstones. Recently reports of laparoscopic radical cholecystectomy for GBC have also appeared in the literature.[95,96] This is technically possible but the follow-up in the small number of patients is too short to allow valid conclusions regarding its long-term efficacy. Till such evidence becomes available, laparoscopic cholecystectomy should be contraindicated if there is preoperative (clinical or imaging) suspicion of GBC and patient should be given the benefit of chance of cure by an appropriate open surgical resection.[97] There is a high risk of port site and intraperitoneal metastases after LC for unsuspected GBC. High intraperitoneal pressure, gas currents, chimney effect, and bile spill are possible causes. Gallbladder perforation and bile spill are more common during LC. Port site metastases are more common when tumor has reached serosa but have been seen in early lesions also. Following the report of Wibbenmeyer et al.[98] regarding dissemination of early GBC following LC, several other reports have confirmed the same. Port site metastases can occur even if gallbladder did not get opened during LC and there was no bile spill.[94] Port site metastases can be prevented/reduced by several methods, for example, gasless laparoscopy, irrigation with sterile water to kill shed malignant cells, extraction in a bag (to prevent contamination of port of extraction and the resultant port site metastases), and deflating the abdomen before taking out trocars. Aretxabala of Chile (an area with very high incidence rates for GBC) recommends extraction of all gallbladders in a plastic bag as an early GBC may not be apparent even at operation.

The only way to detect early GBC is to open, wash, and examine every gallbladder removed for presumed gallstones in the operation theatre itself and subject any suspicious area (mucosal ulceration, nodule, irregularity, and thickening) to frozen section or imprint cytology. It goes without saying that all removed gallbladders must be subjected to a thorough histological examination to detect an unsuspected GBC. Some reports advise against routine histopathological examination of gallbladder as a wasteful exercise and advocate selective histopathological examination of suspected gallbladders only.[99] These recommendations are from areas where GBC is not common and should not be followed. All gallbladders removed for presumed gallstones must be sent for routine histopathological examination (even if they look normal on gross appearance) as this is the only way that early, resectable and curable incidental GBC can be discovered.[100]

Noncurative Simple Cholecystectomy

In a patient who is found to have metastatic disease or positive distant lymph nodes at laparotomy, EC or a major resection is contraindicated because of poor prognosis. A noncurative simple cholecystectomy may be performed, if technically feasible without going through gross tumor. This, when combined with postoperative chemoradiotherapy, may improve survival (as compared to no resection) and may palliate pain and prevent possible future complications of acute cholecystitis and empyema.

Management of Port Site Metastases

In patients who have been operated, metastases in incision scar/port sites are not uncommon. If a patient presents with a late port site recurrence, CT should be done to evaluate the extent of disease. If CT reveals it to be an isolated localized recurrence, it may be resectable.[101,102] Laparoscopy should then be performed to rule out peritoneal dissemination. In the absence of peritoneal dissemination on laparoscopy, the port site recurrence should be widely excised including all layers of abdominal wall from skin to peritoneum and the residual defect may require repair with a mesh and skin flap. Port site recurrence, however, usually indicates metastatic disease and has a poor prognosis, even after its excision.

Results of Surgery and Prognosis

The results of surgery for GBC are determined primarily by the stage of disease and biology of the tumor.[103,104] Together, these two factors determine the feasibility of a curative surgical resection and its outcome. In a recent analysis of 4424 patients with GBC from Japan, Kayahara et al. reported five-year survival rates for stages I, II, III, IVA, and IVB (fifth edition) to be 83%, 70%, 45%, 23%, and 9%, respectively.[103] The importance of achieving a complete (R0) resection in improving survival has been widely reported.[105–110] Spread of disease beyond the gallbladder and increasing involvement of adjacent structures as well as presence of nodal metastases decrease the likelihood of an R0 resection.

For stage I disease, many series report more than 90% five-year survival following simple cholecystectomy.[111–113] It is generally accepted that simple cholecystectomy is adequate for T1a lesions. For T1b lesions, however, controversy persists. While some report good result after simple cholecystectomy,[111,112] others recommend an EC because of the pattern of recurrence in T1b lesions following simple cholecystectomy.[114,115] For tumors reaching the perimuscular connective tissue (T2), the survival advantage provided by EC is clearly evident in a number of reports (Table 3-3).[116–124]

For patients with more advanced lesions, which require major hepatic resections usually with CBD resection and occasionally a pancreatico-duodenectomy and combined vascular resection, the results are better than what they were a decade earlier yet far from ideal (Table 3-4).[72,73,83,125–128] Ouchi et al. reported that no patient with serosal disease survived more than five years even after major resections.[129] In the series by Yamaguchi et al., none of the patients with T3 or T4 lesions survived for five years.[130] Some large, transmural tumors without nodal metastases may represent a subgroup of biologically different cancers, which can be resected completely and have a better prognosis.[121] More recent experience suggests that there is a definite survival advantage of nonresected advanced GBC, especially when negative surgical margins are achieved. This, however, is achieved at the expense of a high morbidity and mortality, and increased length of hospital stay. Addition of extended hepatectomy, associated portal vein or hepatic artery resection, CBD excision, and pancreatico-duodenectomy contributes significantly to increase in morbidity and mortality.[73,90,92,131] Many series club cholangiocarcinoma with GBC when

TABLE 3-3: Results of Extended Cholecystectomy for T2 Disease

Series	Number of Patients	Procedure	5-y Survival (%)
Shirai[117]	35	SC	40.5
	10	EC	90
Yamaguchi[118]	25	SC	36
Oertli[119]	17	SC	24
Matsumoto[120]	09	EC	100
Bartlett[121]	08	EC	88
Paquet[122]	05	EC	80
De Aretxabala[123]	18	SC	20
	20	EC	70
Fong[124]	16	SC	19
	37	EC	61

Abbreviations: EC, extended cholecystectomy; SC, simple cholecystectomy.

TABLE 3-4: Results of Major Resections in Gallbladder Cancer

Author	Number	Morbidity (%)	Mortality (%)	Survival (5 y)	Actual longterm survivors	Recurrence (%)
Nimura[125]	14	92	25	—	—	—
Nakamura[126]	7	71	0	2 y: 28%	1	100
Miyazaki[73]	44 (all stage III/IV)	45	20	R0: 20% R1: 0%	R0: 2 R1: 1	—
Kondo[91]	N = 80 (60 stage III/V)	51	18	III: 33% IVM0: 17%, M1: 3%	9	—
Shimizu[127]	79 (all stage IV)	48	11	14%	—	—
Muratore[128]	70 70 (T1, T2, T3, T4)	33	6	III: 36% IV: 0%	All dead within 2 y	
D'Angelica[90]	109 T1: 4 T2: 37 T3: 61 T4: 2 67%N0	53	5	42% stage and histological grade and CBD involvement	27	
Nagino[83]	90 All T3/T4		18	17%	5	

discussing extensive hepatic resections for biliary tract cancer, thus making it difficult to extract information about results for GBC alone. A careful perusal of these makes it clear that results for GBC are worse than those for cholangiocarcinoma.[83] Most patients with advanced GBC have a combination of several poor prognosticators, which is reflected in the good results being limited to a highly select subgroup of patients. Perineural invasion has been reported to be common in advanced GBC and has been reported to have a significant negative impact on prognosis.[132]

Involvement of lymph nodes is one of the most important predictors of a poor prognosis in GBC. Whether removing involved lymph nodes only provides better staging or it also helps in prolonging survival remains unanswered, and various reports from literature offer conflicting opinions (Table 3-5).[105,121,133–138] Many reports, mainly from the West,[121,133] and our center[105] report a dismal prognosis once lymph nodes are involved irrespective of whether they are dissected and removed or not. Some reports from Japan show that though the prognosis becomes poorer with lymph node involvement, at least in patients with nodal involvement limited to cystic and pericholedochal nodes, if a curative resection is performed, considerable improvement in survival can be expected.[75,135,136] Recent reports from Japan suggest that the number of involved lymph nodes rather than their exact location may be a better determinant of prognosis, and improvement in survival may be expected if R0 resection is possible.[137,138] Two patients in one series survived for more than five years despite having involvement of para-aortic nodes that were removed during a radical lymphadenectomy.[137] Such patients are, however, exceptions rather than the rule and on the whole there

TABLE 3-5: Results of Surgery (5-y survival) Depending Upon Nodal Status

Series	N0	N+
Behari[105]	58%	0%
Benoist[133]	43%	0%
Okamoto[134]	37%	0%
Bartlett[121]		0%
Chijiwa[135]		50% for N1 after R0 0% for N2
Shirai[117]	89% for R0 85% overall	69% for R0 45% overall
Shimada[75]	N0 and N1: 85.4%	N2: 33% Coeliac, SMA, para-aortic: 0%
Sakata[137]	81%	1 LN: 62%, 2-3 LN: 43% ≥4 LN: 15%
Endo[138]	pN1: 19.2%, pN2: 10%, >N2: 0%	1 LN: 33% 2 or more LN: 0%

is agreement on the dismal prognostic significance of para-aortic node involvement, which is considered to be almost similar to that of metastatic disease.[75,139]

Presence of biliary infiltration is an important predictor of poor prognosis—majority of patients with GBC and jaundice being unresectable.[45] Miyazaki et al. observed that curative resection was possible in 14 out of 15 patients with hepatic invasion alone but this could be done in only 7 out of 26 patients with bile duct involvement.[73] Kaneoka et al. studied the issue of HDL involvement in GBC and found that no patient with bile duct involvement survived five years, and the three-year survival in patients who had both bile duct and lymph node involvement was a dismal 3%.[107] In a recent report from Memorial Sloan Kettering Cancer Center, D'angelica et al. found CBD involvement to be an independent predictor of poor prognosis and CBD resection as an independent determinant of increased morbidity following extended hepatic resections.[90]

Predictors of prognosis in GBC are summarized in Table 3-6. Increasing large series of patients treated by a radical surgical approach are being reported.[140–142] There is no doubt that surgical treatment is essential for long-term survival of these patients.

Palliation

Most patients with GBC have advanced unresectable disease. Majority of patients with advanced GBC have biliary obstruction causing jaundice, pruritus, and cholangitis. Though cure cannot be offered to majority of these patients, they need palliation of these distressing symptoms. Patients with advanced unresectable disease survive for a median of less than six months. Surgical bypass provides a onetime palliation without the need of repeated hospital visits, admissions, and interventions. Nonsurgical (endoscopic or radiological) palliation in the form of biliary stenting, however, is preferable if facilities and expertise are available.

Biliary obstruction in patients with advanced GBC may be relieved by therapeutic endoscopic or radiological intervention or surgical biliary bypass.[142,143] Endoscopic stenting (ES) is indicated in patients with GBC who have biliary obstruction resulting in pruritus and cholangitis not responding to antibiotics (oral and parenteral). Role of ES to decrease high bilirubin alone is debatable; reduction of bilirubin may provide palliation in terms of relief of anorexia and a feeling of well-being. A single stent is adequate if confluence is patent; in presence of confluence block, both right and left hepatic ducts need to be stented. If right sectoral (anterior and posterior) or segmental (especially segment V) ducts are involved, percutaneous radiological (multiple) stenting is preferable to ES. Biliary obstruction in GBC is usually high, either due to direct infiltration of the CHD/CBD or because of its compression by enlarged metastatic lymph nodes at porta hepatis. Common hepatic duct is, therefore, not available/suitable for bypass and left hepatic duct, though available, is not preferred as the biliaryenteric anastomosis will be too close to the tumor and may soon get blocked as a result of tumor infiltration. Intrahepatic segment III duct (Figure 3-4) is, therefore, used for creating bilio-enteric anastomosis (BEA) (cholangiojejunostomy) to a Roux-en-Y

TABLE 3-6: Predictors of prognosis

Predictors of Good Prognosis	Predictors of Poor Prognosis
Node negative disease	Node positive disease, especially beyond HDL, para-aortic nodal involvement
R0 resection	Involvement of bile duct by tumor
Papillary histology	Portal vein involvement
	Hepatic artery involvement
	Severe HDL involvement
	High-grade tumor, perineural spread, lymphatic invasion
	Bile/tumor spill during cholecystectomy

Abbreviation: HDL, hepato-duodenal ligament.

loop of jejunum. This can be approached at the base of the round ligament at the junction of inferior surface of segments III and IV or by performing a hepatotomy to the left of falciform ligament on the anterior surface of segment III. The same Roux-en Y limb may be used to decompress a distended gallbladder in a "triple bypass."[144]

Therapeutic gastrojejunostomy should be performed in symptomatic patients with mechanical gastric outlet obstruction (as demonstrated on upper gastro-intestinal endoscopy (UGIE) or CT). Anticipatory gastrojejunostomy may be performed in patients without symptoms of gastric outlet obstruction but with duodenal infiltration (as seen on CT or UGIE or at operation and impending or incipient gastric outlet obstruction). Prophylactic gastrojejunostomy (patients with no symptoms of gastric outlet obstruction and no duodenal infiltration on CT, UGIE, or at operation) is not indicated.[145] Gastrojejunostomy should not be performed in patients without overt or

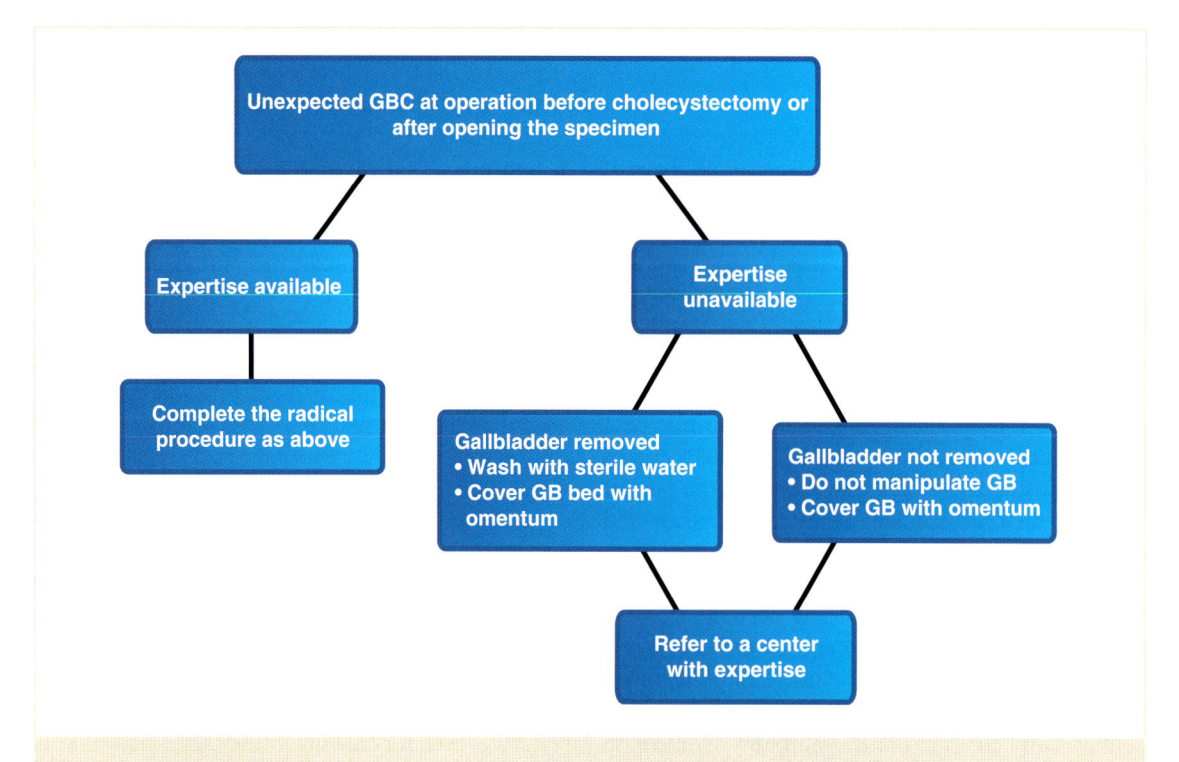

Figure 3-4: Management algorithm for patient with unsuspected gallbladder cancer during surgery prior to cholecystectomy or after obtaining specimen.

impending duodenal infiltration but with symptoms of gastric stasis due to malignant gastroparesis and delayed gastric emptying. More and more patients with gastric outlet obstruction are now being treated with gastro-duodenal stenting as an alternative to gastrojejunostomy. This can be performed endoscopically or fluoroscopically. Though expensive, it is an easier option. In unresectable cases, ileo–(distal) transverse colonic anastomosis may palliate intestinal (colonic) obstruction if present. Extensive peritoneal dissemination can cause small bowel obstruction, which may be difficult to palliate.

Intractable pain in patients with unresectable locally advanced GBC may be relieved by celiac plexus block. This may be performed at laparotomy or by image (ultrasound, CT, and endoscopic ultrasound) guided percutaneous posterior approach using two 15–20 cm long needles with image intensifier. Twenty to thirty milliliters of 50%–75% alcohol is injected on either side of the coeliac axis.

Radiotherapy and Chemotherapy

Many factors make it difficult to draw any conclusions regarding the place of radiotherapy and/or chemotherapy in management of GBC, both in the primary and adjuvant setting.

The relative rarity of GBC makes it difficult and time consuming to accrue patients in adequate numbers for randomized trials. Since majority of patients with GBC present in advanced stages of the disease, most of them are suitable for only palliative care. Most studies of radiotherapy as well as chemotherapy in GBC consist of small, single institution series, often club GBC with cholangiocarcinoma and other biliary tract cancers, and are retrospective. Several different protocols of radiation and different chemotherapy regimes are often assessed in the same study. The stage distribution is heterogeneous, and there is an inherent bias toward selection of patients with better performance status.

Patterns of recurrence following surgery provide a guide to the possible role of adjuvant modalities. At the Memorial Sloan Kettering Cancer Center, 97 patients underwent potentially curative resection for GBC, follow-up was available in 80 patients, 53 (66%) patients had recurrence at a median of 12 months. Sixty-two percent of recurrences occurred within 12 months and 88% within 24 months. Seventy-two percent of recurrences were distant, 17% were local and 11% regional.[146] The authors concluded that an adjuvant therapeutic strategy targeting only locoregional disease, such as radiotherapy, is unlikely to have a significant impact in the overall management of GBC.

Both radiotherapy and chemotherapy have been mainly used in patients with locally advanced, unresectable disease with a primarily palliative intent. Despite anecdotal reports of significant response rates, no chemotherapy or radiotherapy options tested to date have shown any substantial activity. Because of the proximity of liver and other upper abdominal viscera, which have poor tolerance to radiotherapy, intraoperative radiotherapy and brachytherapy have been reported to be more useful in GBC. Todoroki et al. reported an improvement in survival with addition of intraoperative radiotherapy in patients with R1 resection; it was not required in patients with R0 resection and was not useful in patients with R2 resection.[106] Intraluminal brachytherapy using Indium 142 through tubes placed intraoperatively or percutaneously may help to keep stents patent longer.

Earlier studies of chemotherapy in GBC reported the use of mainly 5FU, alone or in combination, with low response rates of 0%–10% with single agent therapy and better response rates though at the expense of higher toxicity with combination therapy.[147–149] More recently Gemcitabine alone or in combination with Cisplatin or Oxaliplatin and 5FU or Capecitabine is appearing more promising. Addition of Cisplatin and Oxaliplatin, however, increases the toxicity significantly (>20%–50% grade 3 toxicity). In a recent systemic review of the role of Gemcitabine in GBC and cholangiocarcinoma, the authors could not find any RCTs addressing the issue and from the 13 single-arm studies included in the review concluded that surgery remains the treatment of choice for GBC. For patients who are not considered for surgery with curative intent but who are willing and able to tolerate treatment with chemotherapy, Gemcitabine, either alone or in combination with a fluoropyrimidine (such as 5FU or Capecitabine), appears to be a reasonable alternative to best supportive care, although this conclusion has not been confirmed with an RCT.[150] That Gemcitabine alone or in combination is usually well tolerated has been shown by several studies and, because of the absence of any effective alternative therapies, is offered to patients with advanced unresectable GBC.[151,152] Its role in the adjuvant setting is still largely unclear.

Takada et al. reported their experience with 140 patients with GBC allocated randomly to either the 5FU and Mitomycin (MF group) or the control group (surgery alone). All patients were followed for five years. After ineligible patients were excluded, 112 patients with GBC (69 in the MF group and 43 in the control group) were studied. The five-year survival rate was significantly better in the MF group (26%) compared with the control group (14%) ($P = 0.0367$). Similarly, the five-year disease-free survival (DFS) rate of patients with GBC was 20% in the MF group, which was significantly higher than the 12% DFS rate reported in the control group ($P = 0.0210$). The most commonly reported adverse drug reactions were anorexia, nausea/emesis, stomatitis, and leukopenia, none of which were noted to be serious.[153]

No other large randomized trials addressing the issue of adjuvant radiotherapy and/or chemotherapy are available. Small experiences with Gemcitabine in the neoadjuvant setting have been reported but the evidence is still far from conclusive.[155]

It has been proposed that adjuvant chemo/radiotherapy should be given after surgical resection in patients with node-positive and stage III disease as well as in patients who have had a noncurative simple cholecystectomy.[155] Chemotherapy may also be indicated in patients with incidental GBC when bile spill occurred during initial laparoscopic cholecystectomy.

Prior to chemotherapy, jaundice, if present, should be palliated by endoscopic/percutaneous stenting and there should be no infection at the time of starting therapy.

Therapy targeted against biomarkers such as growth factor receptors is being tried in hepatobiliary cancers including GBC, but their role in GBC is not yet established.

Prevention

Prophylactic Cholecystectomy for Asymptomatic Gallstones

Prophylactic cholecystectomy for asymptomatic gallstones detected incidentally on ultrasound is a matter of great debate and huge controversy. Data from the West do not support prophylactic cholecystectomy for asymptomatic gallstones to prevent GBC because of the extremely low risk of GBC in these populations.[156,157] Large studies addressing the natural history of asymptomatic gallstones in high incidence populations are not available although there is evidence to suggest that this may be different. In Chile, many surgeons recommend prophylactic cholecystectomy for asymptomatic gallstones, even without hard data to support it. Considering the uniformly dismal prognosis of GBC, unless diagnosed early and the absolute prevention that cholecystectomy offers, a case has been made for prophylactic cholecystectomy, especially in young healthy women from northern India, when they are diagnosed to have asymptomatic gall stones.[158] Considering the prevalence rate of 4%, offering prophylactic cholecystectomy as above even in one state (e.g., Uttar Pradesh with an estimated population of 150 million) would mean a staggering cost and the logistics would be unmanageable to say the least. To add the 0.4% incidence of bile duct injury to these numbers adds another dimension that cannot be ignored.[159]

Future

It is important that the etiology of GBC be found to enable primary prevention interventions to be instituted. Etio-pathogenesis, especially the role of gallstones in the causation of GBC, needs to be elucidated in detail. Markers need to be identified for those patients with asymptomatic gallstones who are at highest risk for developing GBC and who are candidates for selective prophylactic cholecystectomy (secondary prevention).

References

1. Arnaud JP, Casa C, Georgeac C, et al. Primary carcinoma of the gallbladder–review of 143 cases. *Hepatogastroenterology*. 1995;42(6):811–815.
2. Batra Y, Pal S, Dutta U, et al. Gallbladder cancer in India: a dismal picture. *J Gastroenterol Hepatol*. 2005;20(2):309–314.
3. Diehl AK. Epidemiology of gallbladder cancer: a synthesis of recent data. *J Natl Cancer Inst*. 1980;65(6):1209–1214.
4. Randi G, Franceschi S, La Vecchia C. Gallbladder cancer worldwide: geographical distribution and risk factors. *Int J Cancer*. 2006;118:1591–1602.

5. Roa I, Araya JC, Villaseca M, et al. Gallbladder cancer in a high risk area: morphological features and spread patterns. *Hepatogastroenterology*. 1999;46(27):1540–1546.
6. Koea J, Phillips A, Lawes C, et al. Gall bladder cancer, extrahepatic bile duct cancer and ampullary carcinoma in New Zealand: demographics, pathology and survival. *ANZ J Surg*. 2002;72(12):857–861.
7. National Cancer Registry Programme. Two-year Report of the Population Based Cancer Registries; 1997–1998.
8. Kapoor VK. An Indian meets the American Indians. *Natl Med J India*. 2009;22(4):204–205.
9. Sikora SS, Kapoor R, Pradeep R, et al. Palliative surgical treatment of malignant obstructive jaundice. *Eur J Surg Oncol*. 1994;20(5):580–584.
10. Bhurgri Y, Bhurgri A, Hasan SH, et al. Cancer patterns in Karachi division (1998–1999). *J Pak Med Assoc*. 2002;52(6):244–246.
11. Lambe M, Trichopoulos D, Hsieh CC, et al. Parity and cancers of the gall bladder and the extrahepatic bile ducts. *Int J Cancer*. 1993;54(6):941–944.
12. Moerman CJ, Berns MP, Bueno de Mesquita HB, Runia S. Reproductive history and cancer of the biliary tract in women. *Int J Cancer*. 1994;57(2):146–153.
13. Levin B. Gallbladder carcinoma. *AnnOncol*. 1999;10(suppl 4):129–130.
14. Lowenfels AB, Lindström CG, Conway MJ, Hastings PR. Gallstones and risk of gallbladder cancer. *J Natl Cancer Inst*. 1985;75(1):77–80.
15. Diehl AK. Gallstone size and the risk of gallbladder cancer. *JAMA*. 1983;250:2323–2329.
16. Lowenfels AB, Walker AM, Althaus DP, et al. Gallstone growth, size, and risk of gallbladder cancer: an interracial study. *Int J Epidemiol*. 1989;18:50–54.
17. Moerman CJ, Lagerwaard FJ, Bueno de Mesquita HB, et al. Gallstone size and the risk of gallbladder cancer. *Scand J Gastroenterol*. 1993;28(6):482–486.
18. Redaelli CA, Büchler MW, Schilling MK, et al. High coincidence of Mirizzi syndrome and gallbladder carcinoma. *Surgery*. 1997;121(1):58–63.
19. Prasad TL, Kumar A, Sikora SS, et al. Mirizzi syndrome and gallbladder cancer. *J Hepatobiliary Pancreat Surg*. 2006;13(4):323–326.
20. Vitetta L, Sali A, Little P, Mrazek L. Gallstones and gall bladder carcinoma. *Aust N Z J Surg*. 2000;70(9):667–673.
21. Choudhuri G, Agarwal DK, Negi TS. Polarizing microscopy of partially dissolved gallstone powder: a simple technique for studying gallstone composition. *J Gastroenterol Hepatol*. 1995;10(3):241–245.
22. Jayanthi V, Palanivelu C, Prasanthi R, et al. Composition of gallstones in Coimbatore District of Tamil Nadu State. *Indian J Gastroenterol*. 1998;17(4):134–135.
23. Lohsiriwat V, Vongjirad A, Lohsiriwat D. Value of routine histopathologic examination of three common surgical specimens: appendix, gallbladder, and hemorrhoid. *World J Surg*. 2009;33(10):2189–2193.
24. Pandey M, Vishwakarma RA, Khatri AK, et al. Bile, bacteria, and gallbladder carcinogenesis. *J Surg Oncol*. 1995;58(4):282–283.
25. Shukla VK, Tiwari SC, Roy SK. Biliary bile acids in cholelithiasis and carcinoma of the gall bladder. *Eur J Cancer Prev*. 1993;2(2):155–160.
26. Csendes A, Becerra M, Burdiles P, et al. Bacteriological studies of bile from the gallbladder in patients with carcinoma of the gallbladder, cholelithiasis, common bile duct stones and no gallstones disease. *Eur J Surg*. 1994;160(6–7):363–367.
27. Welton JC, Marr JS, Friedman SM. Association between hepatobiliary cancer and typhoid carrier state. *Lancet*. 1979;1(8120):791–794.
28. Caygill CP, Hill MJ, Braddick M, Sharp JC. Cancer mortality in chronic typhoid and paratyphoid carriers. *Lancet*. 1994;343(8889):83–84.
29. Shukla VK, Singh H, Pandey M, et al. Carcinoma of the gallbladder–is it a sequel of typhoid? *Dig Dis Sci*. 2000;45(5):900–903.
30. Shukla VK, Prakash A, Tripathi BD, et al. Biliary heavy metal concentrations in carcinoma of the gall bladder: case-control study. *BMJ*. 1998;317(7168):1288–1289.
31. Shukla VK, Shukla PK, Pandey M, et al. Lipid peroxidation product in bile from patients with carcinoma of the gallbladder: a preliminary study. *J Surg Oncol*. 1994;56(4):258–262.
32. Stephen AE, Berger DL. Carcinoma in the porcelain gallbladder: a relationship revisited. *Surgery*. 2001;129(6):699–703.
33. Chijiwa K, Kimura H, Tanaka M. Malignant potential of the gallbladder in patients with anomalous pancreaticobiliary junction: the difference in risk between patients with and without choledochal cyst. *Int Surg*. 1995;80(1):61–64.

34. Lazcano-Ponce EC, Miquel JF, Muñoz N, et al. Epidemiology and molecular pathology of gallbladder cancer. *CA Cancer J Clin*. 2001;51;349–364.
35. Aretxabala X de, Rossi RL, Oberfield RA, et al. Gallbladder cancer. In: Pitt HA, CarrLocke DL, Ferruci JT, eds. *Hepatobiliary and Pancreatic Diseases: The Team Approach to Management*. Boston, MA: Little, Brown and Company; 1995:295–304.
36. Kwon W, Jang JY, Lee SE, et al. Clinicopathologic features of polypoid lesions of the gallbladder and risk factors of gallbladder cancer. *J Korean Med Sci*. 2009;24(3):481–487. Epub 2009 Jun 12.
37. Kubota K, Bandai Y, Noie T, et al. How should polypoid lesions of the gallbladder be treated in the era of laparoscopic cholecystectomy? *Surgery*. 1995;117(5):481–487.
38. Ootani T, Shirai Y, Tsukada K, Muto T. Relationship between gallbladder carcinoma and the segmental type of adenomyomatosis of the gallbladder. *Cancer*. 1992;69(11):2647–2652.
39. Berliner SD, Burson LC. One-stage repair for cholecyst-duodenal fistula and gallstone ileus. *Arch Surg*. 1965;90:313–316.
40. Zatonski WA, La Vecchia C, Przewozniak K, et al. Risk factors for gallbladder cancer: a Polish case-control study. *Int J Cancer*. 1992;51(5):707–711.
41. Rao RV, Kumar A, Sikora SS, et al. Xanthogranulomatous cholecystitis: differentiation from associated gall bladder carcinoma. *Trop Gastroenterol*. 2005;26(1):31–33.
42. Kapoor VK, Pradeep R, Haribhakti SP, et al. Early carcinoma of the gallbladder: an elusive disease. *J Surg Oncol*. 1996;62(4):284–287.
43. de Aretxabala X, Roa I, Araya JC, et al. Operative findings in patients with early forms of gallbladder cancer. *Br J Surg*. 1990;77(3): 291–293.
44. Singh B, Kapoor VK, Sikora SS, et al. Malignant gastroparesis and outlet obstruction in carcinoma gall bladder. *Trop Gastroenterol*. 1998;19(1):37–39.
45. Hawkins WG, DeMatteo RP, Jarnagin WR, et al. Jaundice predicts advanced disease and early mortality in patients with gallbladder cancer. *Ann Surg Oncol*. 2004;11(3):310–315.
46. Haribhakti SP, Awasthi S, Pradeep R, et al. Carcinoma gallbladder: atypical presentations and unusual associations. *Trop Gastroenterol*. 1997;18(1):32–34.
47. Shih SP, Schulick RD, Cameron JL, et al. Gallbladder cancer: the role of laparoscopy and radical resection. *Ann Surg*. 2007;245(6):893–901.
48. Butte JM, Matsuo K, Gönen M, et al. Gallbladder cancer: differences in presentation, surgical treatment, and survival in patients treated at centers in three countries. *J Am Coll Surg*. 2011;212(1):50–61. Epub 2010 Nov 12.
49. Gore RM, Yaghmai V, Newmark GM, et al. Imaging benign and malignant disease of the gallbladder. *Radiol Clin North Am*. 2002; 40(6):1307–1323.
50. Franquet T, Montes M, Ruiz de Azua Y, et al. Primary gallbladder carcinoma: imaging findings in 50 patients with pathologic correlation. *Gastrointest Radiol*. 1991;16(2): 143–148.
51. Bach AM, Loring LA, Hann LE, et al. Gallbladder cancer: can ultrasonography evaluate extent of disease? *J Ultrasound Med*. 1998;17(5):303–309.
52. Wibbenmeyer LA, Sharafuddin MJ, Wolverson MK, et al. Sonographic diagnosis of unsuspected gallbladder cancer: imaging findings in comparison with benign gallbladder conditions. *AJR Am J Roentgenol*. 1995;165(5):1169–1174.
53. Onoyama H, Yamamoto M, Takada M, et al. Diagnostic imaging of early gallbladder cancer: retrospective study of 53 cases. *World J Surg*. 1999;23(7):708–712.
54. Pandey M, Sood BP, Shukla RC, et al. Carcinoma of the gallbladder: role of sonography in diagnosis and staging. *J Clin Ultrasound*. 2000;28(5):227–232.
55. Haribhakti SP, Kapoor VK, Gujral RB, Kaushik SP. Staging of carcinoma of the gallbladder–an ultrasonographic evaluation. *Hepatogastroenterology*. 1997;44(17): 1240–1245.
56. Schwartz LH, Black J, Fong Y, et al. Gallbladder carcinoma: findings at MR imaging with MR cholangiopancreatography. *J Comput Assist Tomogr*. 2002;26(3):405–410.
57. Corvera CU, Blumgart LH, Akhurst T, et al. 18F-fluorodeoxyglucose positron emission tomography influences management decisions in patients with biliary cancer. *J Am Coll Surg*. 2008;206(1):57–65. Epub 2007 Oct 1.
58. Shukla PJ, Barreto SG, Arya S, et al. Does PET-CT scan have a role prior to radical re-resection for incidental gallbladder cancer? *HPB (Oxford)*. 2008;10(6):439–445.
59. Mitake M, Nakazawa S, Naitoh Y, et al. Endoscopic ultrasonography in diagnosis of the extent of

gallbladder carcinoma. *Gastrointest Endosc.* 1990;36(6):562–566.
60. Agrawal S, Sonawane RN, Behari A, et al. Laparoscopic staging in gallbladder cancer. *Dig Surg.* 2005;22(6):440–445. Epub 2006 Feb 10.
61. Zargar SA, Khuroo MS, Mahajan R, et al. US-guided fine-needle aspiration biopsy of gallbladder masses. *Radiology.*1991;179(1): 275–278.
62. Iqbal M, Gondal KM, Qureshi AU, Tayyab M. Comparative study of ultrasound guided fine needle aspiration cytology with open/laparoscopic biopsy for diagnosis of carcinoma gallbladder. *J Coll Physicians Surg Pak.* 2009;19(1):17–20.
63. Sharma A, Behari A, Sikora SS, et al. Post-cholecystectomy biliary strictures: not always benign. *J Gastroenterol Hepatol.* 2008; 23:63–66.
64. Srikanth G, Kumar A, Khare R, et al. Should laparoscopic cholecystectomy be performed in patients with thick-walled gallbladder? *J Hepatobiliary Pancreat Surg.* 2004;11(1):40–44.
65. Nevin JE, Moran TJ, Kay S, King R. Carcinoma of the gallbladder: staging, treatment, and prognosis, *Cancer.* 1976;37:141–148.
66. Fleming ID, Cooper JS, Henson DE, et al. *AJCC Cancer Staging Manual.* 5th ed. New York, NY: Springer; 1997.
67. Greene FL, Page DL, Fleming ID, et al. *AJCC Cancer Staging Manual.* 6th ed. New York, NY: Springer; 2002.
68. Edge SB, Byrd DR, Compton CC, et al. eds. *AJCC Cancer Staging Manual.* 7th ed. New York, NY: Springer; 2010.
69. Kapoor VK, Sonawane RN, Haribhakti SP, et al. Gall bladder cancer: proposal for a modification of the TNM classification. *Eur J Surg Oncol.* 1998;24(6):487–491.
70. Sumiyoshi K, Nagai E, Chijiiwa K, Nakayama F. Pathology of carcinoma of the gallbladder. *World J Surg.* 1991;15(3):315–321.
71. Fahim RB, McDonald JR, Richards JC, Ferris DO. Carcinoma of the gallbladder: a study of its modes of spread. *Ann Surg.* 1962;156:114–124.
72. Kondo S, Nimura Y, Kamiya J, et al. Mode of tumor spread and surgical strategy in gallbladder carcinoma. *Langenbecks Arch Surg.* 2002;387(5–6):222–228. Epub 2002 Oct 2.
73. Miyazaki M, Itoh H, Ambiru S, et al. Radical surgery for advanced gallbladder carcinoma. *Br J Surg.* 1996;83(4):478–481.
74. Shimizu Y, Ohtsuka M, Ito H, et al. Should the extrahepatic bile duct be resected for locally advanced gallbladder cancer? *Surgery.* 2004;136(5):1012–1017; discussion 1018.
75. Shimada H, Endo I, Fujii Y, et al. Appraisal of surgical resection of gallbladder cancer with special reference to lymph node dissection. *Langenbecks Arch Surg.* 2000;385(8):509–514.
76. Tsukada K, Kurosaki I, Uchida K, et al. Lymph node spread from carcinoma of the gallbladder. *Cancer.* 1997;80(4):661–667.
77. Ito M, Mishima Y, Sato T. An anatomical study of the lymphatic drainage of the gallbladder. *Surg Radiol Anat.* 1991;13(2):89–104.
78. Lee SE, Jang JY, Lim CS, et al. Systematic review on the surgical treatment for T1 gallbladder cancer. *World J Gastroenterol.* 2011;17(2):174–180.
79. Kondo S, Nimura Y, Hayakawa N, et al. Regional and para-aortic lymphadenectomy in radical surgery for advanced gallbladder carcinoma. *Br J Surg.* 2000;87(4):418–422.
80. Jensen EH, Abraham A, Habermann EB, et al. A critical analysis of the surgical management of early-stage gallbladder cancer in the United States. *J Gastrointest Surg.* 2009;13(4):722–727. Epub 2008 Dec 13.
81. Kapoor VK. Advanced gallbladder cancer: Indian "middle path." *J Hepatobiliary Pancreat Surg.* 2007;14(4):366–373. Epub 2007 Jul 30.
82. Kawarada Y, Isaji S, Taoka H, et al. S4a + S5 with caudate lobe (S1) resection using the Taj Mahal liver parenchymal resection for carcinoma of the biliary tract. *J Gastrointest Surg.* 1999;3(4):369–373.
83. Nagino M, Kamiya J, Nishio H, et al. Two hundred forty consecutive portal vein embolizations before extended hepatectomy for biliary cancer: surgical outcome and long-term follow-up. *Ann Surg.* 2006;243(3):364–372.
84. Shirai Y, Wakai T, Hatakeyama K. Radical lymph node dissection for gallbladder cancer: indications and limitations. *Surg Oncol Clin N Am.* 2007;16(1):221–232. Review.
85. Shirai Y, Ohtani T, Tsukada K, et al. Combined pancreaticoduodenectomy and hepatectomy for patients

86. Sasaki R, Takahashi M, Funato O, et al. Hepatopancreatoduodenectomy with wide lymph node dissection for locally advanced carcinoma of the gallbladder: long-term results. *Hepatogastroenterology*. 2002;49: 912–915.
87. Araida T, Yoshikawa T, Azuma T, et al. Indications for pancreatoduodenectomy in patients undergoing lymphadenectomy for advanced gallbladder carcinoma. *J Hepatobiliary Pancreat Surg*. 2004;11:45–49.
88. Nishio H, Nagino M, Ebata T, et al. Aggressive surgery for stage IV gallbladder carcinoma; what are the contraindications? *J Hepatobiliary Pancreat Surg*. 2007;14(4): 351–357. Epub 2007 Jul 30.
89. Shukla PJ, Barreto SG. Systematic review: should routine resection of the extra-hepatic bile duct be performed in gallbladder cancer? *Saudi J Gastroenterol*. 2010;16(3):161–167.
90. D'Angelica M, Dalal KM, DeMatteo RP, et al. Analysis of the extent of resection for adenocarcinoma of the gallbladder. *Ann Surg Oncol*. 2009;16(4):806–816. Epub 2008 Nov 5.
91. Kondo S, Nimura Y, Hayakawa N, et al. Extensive surgery for carcinoma of the gallbladder. *Br J Surg*. 2002;89(2):179–184.
92. Kondo S, Nimura Y, Kamiya J, et al. Factors influencing postoperative hospital mortality and long-term survival after radical resection for stage IV gallbladder carcinoma. *World J Surg*. 2003;27(3):272–277. Epub 2003 Feb 27.
93. Chijiiwa K, Kai M, Nagano M, et al. Outcome of radical surgery for stage IV gallbladder carcinoma. *J Hepatobiliary Pancreat Surg*. 2007;14(4):345–350. Epub 2007 Jul 30.
94. Paolucci V, Schaeff B, Schneider M, Gutt C. Tumor seeding following laparoscopy: international survey. *World J Surg*. 1999;23(10):989–995; discussion 996–997.
95. Gumbs AA, Hoffman JP. Laparoscopic completion radical cholecystectomy for T2 gallbladder cancer. *Surg Endosc*. 2010;24(12): 3221–3223. Epub 2010 May 25.
96. Kim EK, Lee SK, Kim WW. Does laparoscopic surgery have a role in the treatment of gallbladder cancer? *J Hepatobiliary Pancreat Surg*. 2002;9(5):559–563.
97. Weiland ST, Mahvi DM, Niederhuber JE, et al. Should suspected early gallbladder cancer be treated laparoscopically? *J Gastrointest Surg*. 2002;6(1):50–56; discussion 56–57.
98. Wibbenmeyer LA, Wade TP, Chen RC, et al. Laparoscopic cholecystectomy can disseminate in situ carcinoma of the gallbladder. *J Am Coll Surg*. 1995;181(6):504–510.
99. Bazoua G, Hamza N, Lazim T. Do we need histology for a normal-looking gallbladder? *J Hepatobiliary Pancreat Surg*. 2007;14(6):564–568.
100. Behari A, Kapoor VK. Does gallbladder cancer divide India? *Indian J Gastroenterol*. 2010; 29(1):3–7.
101. Nakagawa S, Tada T, Furukawa H, et al. Late-type recurrence at the port site of unexpected gallbladder carcinoma after a laparoscopic cholecystectomy: report of a case. *Surg Today*. 2000;30(9): 853–855.
102. Suzuki K, Kimura T, Hashimoto H, et al. Port site recurrence of gallbladder cancer after laparoscopic surgery: two case reports of long-term survival. *Surg Laparosc Endosc Percutan Tech*. 2000;10(2):86–88.
103. Kayahara M, Nagakawa T, Nakagawara H, et al. Prognostic factors for gallbladder cancer in Japan. *Ann Surg*. 2008;248(5):807–814.
104. Pawlik TM, Choti MA. Biology dictates prognosis following resection of gallbladder carcinoma: sometimes less is more. *Ann Surg Oncol*. 2009;16(4):787–788. Epub 2009 Jan 23.
105. Behari A, Sikora SS, Wagholikar GD, et al. Longterm survival after extended resections in patients with gallbladder cancer. *J Am Coll Surg*. 2003;196(1):82–88.
106. Todoroki T, Kawamoto T, Takahashi H, et al. Treatment of gallbladder cancer by radical resection. *Br J Surg*. 1999;86(5):622–627.
107. Kaneoka Y, Yamaguchi A, Isogai M, et al. Hepatoduodenal ligament invasion by gallbladder carcinoma: histologic patterns and surgical recommendation. *World J Surg*. 2003;27(3):260–265. Epub 2003 Feb 27.
108. Ogura Y, Mizumoto R, Isaji S, et al. Radical operations for carcinoma of the gallbladder: present status in Japan. *World J Surg*. 1991;15(3):337–343.
109. Schauer RJ, Meyer G, Baretton G, et al. Prognostic factors and long-term results after surgery for gallbladder carcinoma: a retrospective study of 127 patients. *Langenbecks Arch Surg*. 2001;386(2):110–117.

110. Kai M, Chijiiwa K, Ohuchida J, et al. A curative resection improves the postoperative survival rate even in patients with advanced gallbladder carcinoma. *J Gastrointest Surg*. 2007;11(8):1025–1032.
111. Shirai Y, Yoshida K, Tsukada K, et al. Early carcinoma of the gallbladder. *Eur J Surg*. 1992;158(10):545–548.
112. Wakai T, Shirai Y, Yokoyama N, et al. Early gallbladder carcinoma does not warrant radical resection. *Br J Surg*. 2001;88(5):675–678.
113. de Aretxabala X, Roa I, Hepp J, et al. Early gallbladder cancer: is further treatment necessary? *J Surg Oncol*. 2009;100(7):589–593.
114. Wagholikar GD, Behari A, Krishnani N, et al. Early gallbladder cancer. *J Am Coll Surg*. 2002;194(2):137–141.
115. Shukla PJ, Barreto G, Kakade A, Shrikhande SV. Revision surgery for incidental gallbladder cancer: factors influencing operability and further evidence for T1b tumours. *HPB (Oxford)*. 2008;10(1):43–47.
116. Wakai T, Shirai Y, Hatakeyama K. Radical second resection provides survival benefit for patients with T2 gallbladder carcinoma first discovered after laparoscopic cholecystectomy. *World J Surg*. 2002;26(7):867–871. Epub 2002 Apr 18.
117. Shirai Y, Yoshida K, Tsukada K, Muto T. Inapparent carcinoma of the gallbladder. An appraisal of a radical second operation after simple cholecystectomy. *Ann Surg*. 1992;215(4):326–331.
118. Yamaguchi K, Tsuneyoshi M. Sub-clinical gallbladder carcinoma. *Am J Surg*. 1992;163(4):382–386.
119. Oertli D, Herzog U, Tondelli P. Primary carcinoma of the gallbladder: operative experience during a 16 year period. *Eur J Surg*. 1993;159(8):415–420.
120. Matsumoto Y, Fujii H, Aoyama H, et al. Surgical treatment of primary carcinoma of the gallbladder based on the histologic analysis of 48 surgical specimens. *Am J Surg*. 1992;163(2):239–245.
121. Bartlett DL, Fong Y, Fortner JG, et al. Long-term results after resection for gallbladder cancer. Implications for staging and management. *Ann Surg*. 1996;224(5):639–646.
122. Paquet KJ. Appraisal of surgical resection of gallbladder carcinoma with special reference to hepatic resection. *J Hepatobiliary Pancreat Surg*. 1998;5(2):200–206.
123. de Aretxabala XA, Roa IS, Burgos LA, et al. Curative resection in potentially resectable tumours of the gallbladder. *Eur J Surg*. 1997;163(6):419–426.
124. Fong Y, Jarnagin W, Blumgart LH. Gallbladder cancer: comparison of patients presenting initially for definitive operation with those presenting after prior noncurative intervention. *Ann Surg*. 2000 Oct;232(4):557-69.
125. Nimura Y, Hayakawa N, Kamiya J, et al. Hepatopancreatoduodenectomy for advanced carcinoma of the biliary tract. *Hepatogastroenterology*. 1991;38(2):170–175.
126. Nakamura S, Nishiyama R, Yokoi Y, et al. Hepatopancreatoduodenectomy for advanced gallbladder carcinoma. *Arch Surg*. 1994;129(6):625–629.
127. Shimizu H, Kimura F, Yoshidome H, et al. Aggressive surgical approach for stage IV gallbladder carcinoma based on Japanese Society of Biliary Surgery classification. *J Hepatobiliary Pancreat Surg*. 2007;14(4):358–365. Epub 2007 Jul 30.
128. Muratore A, Polastri R, Capussotti L. Radical surgery for gallbladder cancer: current options. *Eur J Surg Oncol*. 2000;26(5):438–443.
129. Ouchi K, Owada Y, Matsuno S, Sato T. Prognostic factors in the surgical treatment of gallbladder carcinoma. *Surgery*. 1987;101:731–737.
130. Yamaguchi K, Chijiiwa K, Saiki S, et al. Retrospective analysis of 70 operations for gallbladder carcinoma. *Br J Surg*. 1997; 84(2):200–204.
131. Ebata T, Nagino M, Nishio H, et al. Right hepatopancreatoduodenectomy: improvements over 23 years to attain acceptability. *J Hepatobiliary Pancreat Surg*. 2007;14(2): 131–135. Epub 2007 Mar 27.
132. Yamaguchi R, Nagino M, Oda K, et al. Perineural invasion has a negative impact on survival of patients with gallbladder carcinoma. *Br J Surg*. 2002;89(9):1130–1136.
133. Benoist S, Panis Y, Fagniez P-L. Long-term results after curative resection for carcinoma of the gallbladder. *Am J Surg*. 1998;175:118–122.
134. Okamoto A, Tsuruta K, Ishiwata J, et al. Treatment of T3 and T4 carcinomas of the gallbladder. *Int Surg*. 1996;81(2):130–135.
135. Chijiiwa K, Tanaka M. Carcinoma of the gallbladder: an appraisal of surgical resection. *Surgery*. 1994;115:751–756.
136. Shirai Y, Yoshida K, Tsukada K, et al. Radical surgery for gallbladder carcinoma. Long-term results. *Ann Surg*. 1992;216(5):565–568.
137. Sakata J, Shirai Y, Wakai T, et al. Number of positive lymph nodes independently determines the prognosis after resection in patients with

gallbladder carcinoma. *Ann Surg Oncol.* 2010;17(7): 1831–1840. Epub 2010 Jan 15.

138. Endo I, Shimada H, Tanabe M, et al. Prognostic significance of the number of positive lymph nodes in gallbladder cancer. *J Gastrointest Surg.* 2006;10(7):999–1007.

139. Shirai Y, Sakata J, Wakai T et al. "Extended" radical cholecystectomy for gallbladder cancer: long-term outcomes, indications, and limitations. *World J Gastroenterol.* 2012, 18(34):4736–4743.

140. Lim H, Seo DW, Park DH, et al. Prognostic factors in patients with gallbladder cancer after surgical resection: analysis of 279 operated patients. *J Clin Gastroenterol.* 2012 (Epub ahead of print).

141. Shen CM, Niu GC, Cui W, et al. The improvement of surgical treatment for patients with gallbladder cancer: analysis of 208 consecutive cases over the past decade. *J Gastrointest Surg.* 2012;16(12):2239–2246. Epub 2012 Oct 12.

142. Vij JC, Govil A, Chaudhary A, et al. Endoscopic biliary endoprosthesis for palliation of gallbladder carcinoma. *Gastrointest Endosc.* 1996;43(2 Pt. 1): 121–123.

143. Kapoor VK, Pradeep R, Haribhakti SP, et al. Intrahepatic segment III cholangiojejunostomy in advanced carcinoma of the gallbladder. *Br J Surg.* 1996;83(12):1709–1711.

144. Saxena R, Sikora SS, Kaushik SP. Atriple bypass procedure for advanced carcinoma of the neck of gallbladder.*Br J Surg.* 1995; 82(3):394–395.

145. Sikora SS, Kapoor VK. Bypass for malignant duodenal obstruction–politics of change: therapeutic. Selective! Prophylactic? *Indian J Gastroenterol.* 1999;18(3):99–100.

146. Jarnagin WR, Ruo L, Little SA, et al. Patterns of initial disease recurrence after resection of gallbladder carcinoma and hilar cholangiocarcinoma: implications for adjuvant therapeutic strategies. *Cancer.* 2003;98(8): 1689–1700.

147. Falkson G, MacIntyre JM, Moertel CG. Eastern Cooperative Oncology Group experience with chemotherapy for inoperable gallbladder and bile duct cancer. *Cancer.* 198;54:965–969.

148. Takada T, Kato H, Matsushiro T, et al. Comparison of 5-fluorouracil, doxorubicin and mitomycin C with 5-fluorouracil alone in the treatment of pancreatic-biliary carcinomas. *Oncology.* 1994;51:396–400.

149. Glimelius B, Hoffman K, Sjoden PO, et al. Chemotherapy improves survival and quality of life in advanced pancreatic and biliary cancer. *Ann Oncol.* 1996;7:593–600.

150. Dingle BH, Rumble RB, Brouwers MC. Cancer Care Ontario's Program in Evidence-Based Care's Gastroin-testinal Cancer Disease Site Group. The role of gemcitabine in the treatment of cholangiocarcinoma and gallbladder cancer: a systematic review. *Can J Gastroenterol.* 2005;19(12):711–716.

151. Doval DC, Sekhon JS, Gupta SK, et al. A Phase II study of gemcitabine and cisplatin in chemotherapy naive, unresectable gall bladder cancer. *Br J Cancer.* 2004;90: 1516–1520.

152. Julka PK, Puri T, Rath GK. A phase II study of gemcitabine and carboplatin combination chemotherapy in gallbladder carcinoma. *Hepatobiliary Pancreat Dis Int.* 2006;5(1): 110–114.

153. Takada T, Amano H, Yasuda H, et al. Is postoperative adjuvant chemotherapy useful for gallbladder carcinoma? A phase III multicenter prospective randomized controlled trial in patients with resected pancreaticobiliary carcinoma. *Cancer.* 2002;95(8): 1685–1695.

154. de Aretxabala X, Roa I, Burgos L, et al. Preoperative chemoradiotherapy in the treatment of gallbladder cancer. *Am Surg.* 1999; 65(3):241–246.

155. Balachandran P, Agarwal S, Krishnani N, et al. Predictors of long-term survival in patients with gallbladder cancer. *J Gastrointest Surg.* 2006;10(6):848–854.

156. Gracie WA, Ransohoff DF. The natural history of silent gallstones: the innocent gallstone is not a myth. *N Engl J Med.* 1982; 307(13):798–800.

157. Friedman GD, Raviola CA, Fireman B. Prognosis of gallstones with mild or no symptoms: 25 years of follow-up in a health maintenance organization. *J Clin Epidemiol.* 1989;42(2):127–136.

158. Mohandas KM, Patil PS. Cholecys-tectomy for asymptomatic gallstones can reduce gall bladder cancer mortality in northern Indian women. *Indian J Gastroenterol.* 2006; 25:147–151.

159. Kapoor VK. Cholecystectomy in patients with asymptomatic gallstones to prevent gall bladder cancer–the case against. *Indian J Gastroenterol.* 2006;25(3):152–154.

SECTION II

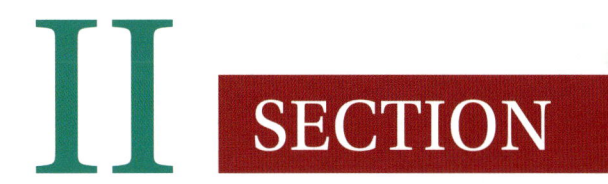

Liver Tumors

Jia-Hong Dong

CHAPTER 4

Benign Liver Lesions

Daniel E. Abbott & David Bentrem

Liver lesions are frequently found in a wide spectrum of patients. The number of benign lesions of the liver identified is increasing as the use of diagnostic imaging increases. The major benign lesions include solid lesions including hepatic adenoma (HA), hemagioma, and focal nodular hyperplasia (FNH) and cystic lesions such as simple cysts, cystadenomas, and echinococcal (Figure 4-1). Oftentimes, the diagnosis is self-evident based on patient history, while other times there exists a significant diagnostic dilemma. Once malignancy has been ruled out, accurate assessment of the hepatic lesion is critical, as therapeutic options range from observation/surveillance to antimicrobial therapy to surgical resection (Table 4-2). Furthermore, adding to challenging diagnostic decision making is the lack of prospective, randomized data to guide management of even more common benign hepatic masses.[1] This chapter is devoted to the characterization, workup, and therapeutic strategies utilized to address the more common benign liver lesions, with mention and key points of more rare disease processes discussed.

Solid Hepatic Masses

Adenoma

Incidence and Characteristics

HAs are by definition benign, though this neoplastic disease is more complex than other benign hepatic lesions. These masses are endocrine-responsive and are essentially a disease of young women who use oral contraceptive pills (OCPs). In women who use OCPs, the annual incidence is 3–4/100,000 women, and the age of incurrence is usually in the third and fourth decades of life. Although this lesion has been found in men, numerous reports place the female:male ratio as high as 11:1 and prior to the routine use of OCPs, this was a rarely described entity.[2,3] With longitudinal investigative study, researchers have demonstrated that the likelihood of developing HA is directly linked to dosage of OCPs and duration of exposure.[4,5] Furthermore, despite the clearly increased risk of long-term OCP use, cessation of oral contraceptives does not always lead to consistent resolution. Although most women will find that their adenomas shrink and/or become less symptomatic, some lesions may actually increase in size. Pregnancy may worsen symptoms of HA, and both enlargement and rupture of HA during pregnancy have been reported, in one case even requiring orthotopic liver transplantation.[4,6,7]

Microscopically, HA is characterized by hepatocyte proliferation. These cells may contain increased fat and/or glycogen, and are most often organized in cords. Although the histologic appearance of HA lacks the usual structures of hepatic veins and portal tracts, this organization may rarely be present in biopsies. In addition, it is difficult to determine whether dysplasia, or even neoplasia in the form of hepatocellular carcinoma, is present in a specimen. Grossly, HAs typically appear as solitary nodules that contain prominent vasculature both within the lesion and on its surface. This surface is usually smooth, variably colored, and may contain a thin pseudocapsule (not a well-organized, structurally sound fibrous capsule).

CYSTIC HEPATIC LESIONS

Simple hepatic cyst
Congenital polycystic disease
Infectious (Echinococcal, Amoebic)
Epidermoid cyst

SOLID HEPATIC LESIONS

Hepatic adenoma
Hemangioma
Hamartoma (biliary or mesenchymal)
Focal Nodular Hyperplasia
Nodular regenerative hyperplasia (adenomatous subtype as well)
Lymphangioma/lymphangiomatosis
Fibroma/neurofibromatosis
Heterotopic rests (e.g., adrenal, pancreatic)

BILIARY LESIONS

Biliary cystadenoma (aka hepatobiliary cystadenoma)
Bile duct adenoma
Biliary papillomatosis
Leiomyomas
Neuroendocrine (gastrin or serotonin secreting) biliary epithelial tumors
Granular cell myoblastoma

Figure 4-1: Benign hepatic and biliary lesions.

The risks of this lesion are two-fold. Firstly, rupture and bleeding are of significant concern, particularly in adenomas > 10 cm. The risk of clinically important hemorrhage, however, does not demonstrate a linear relationship with size, making determination of "at risk" lesions challenging. Some reports have placed the risk of rupture as high as 50%. Furthermore, the consequence of unrecognized or untimely treated hemorrhage may include death, a devastating consequence in this usually young and healthy patient population.

Secondly, it seems clear that there exists a small and finite risk of malignant transformation to hepatocellular carcinoma. The exact risk has not been well established, but can be up to a 15% malignancy rate in patients with HA observed over time. Cessation of OCPs does not in and of itself guarantee against malignant transformation, and this fact must be addressed with each individual patient as they are counseled about the risks and benefits of operative or nonoperative therapy. If observation is chosen, serial serum α-fetal protein may be useful to assess for malignant degeneration.

Physical Exam, Laboratory Testing, and Imaging studies

Patients with HA are more likely to complain of abdominal pain when compared to patients with hemangiomas or nodular lesions, but often these lesions are found incidentally during surgery or imaging for other pathology. Physical examination may demonstrate tenderness in the right upper quadrant, but is entirely nonspecific for this disease process. Likewise, a mass may or may not be appreciated with deep palpation, but again there is no physical finding that reveals the diagnosis of HA versus other liver pathology. As such, diagnosis of HA relies primarily on imaging modalities, and the challenge is distinguishing HA from FNH (Figure 4-2). Laboratory evaluation is marginally helpful, but one may find increases in direct bilirubin (obstruction of biliary radicles) and/or increased alkaline phosphatase. Serum AFP will be normal in the absence of malignant degeneration, and even then cannot be relied upon to completely exclude the diagnosis of cancer.

In terms of imaging, the diagnosis of HA may be made by computed tomography (CT), ultrasound or magnetic resonance (Table 4-1, on CT, preinfusion images reveal a hypodense lesion, while over 90% of adenomas demonstrate peripheral arterial enhancement and continued centripetal flow when intravascular contrast is used. Figure 4-3). Ultrasound can also be utilized, revealing a hyperechoic, well circumscribed mass that may be heterogeneous in appearance due to internal hemorrhage and/or necrosis. One report found that ultrasound-demonstrated intralesion veins without a central artery were able to distinguish HA from FNH.[8] Magnetic resonance imaging (MRI) of HAs are typically hyper- or isointense on T1 imaging, sometimes with early arterial enhancement and on T2-weighted imaging are hyperintense relative to surrounding liver. However, the MR appearance of HA is notoriously variable, and inconsistent fat content or bleeding may confound the diagnosis, limiting the ability to distinguish malignancy from HA.[9,10]

Other, less commonly utilized diagnostic maneuvers include angiography or nuclear scintigraphy. Angiographically, peripheral arterial enhancement and subsequent hypervascularity of the adenoma are

TABLE 4-1: Large Study Series of Adenoma, Focal Nodal Hyperplasia, and Hemangioma

Author, y	N	Lesion	Technique	Outcome	Conclusion
Deneve, 2009[15]	124	Adenoma	119 resection, 5 embolization	25% ruptured; increasing size and recent (6 mos) hormone use predicted rupture; 4% with malignancy, all > 8 cm	Adenomas 4 cm or larger, requiring hormone therapy or symptomatic should be resected
Shen, 2007[54]	86	FNH	All resected	Correct preoperative diagnosis in 59% (MRI most accurate at 77%)	Resection appropriate if symptomatic or diagnostic uncertainty exists
Herman, 2005[34]	249	Hemangioma	Only 3.2% underwent operation	No postoperative complication or death; no morbidity in 78 month follow-up for those observed	Observation of hemangioma is safe; reserve surgery for intractable pain, regional compression or diagnostic uncertainty
Lin, 2004[56]	48	FNH	All resected	2.1% morbidity, no mortality	Observation safe for proven FNH < 5 cm and asymptomatic; otherwise, resection is recommended
Yoon, 2003[35]	115	Hemangioma	52 resections (31 enucleations), 63 observed	25% morbidity, no mortality in resected cohort; 96% with symptom relief	Surgery is safe for symptoms, diagnostic uncertainty; otherwise patients can be observed

Abbreviations: FNH, focal nodular hyperplasia; MRI, magnetic resonance imaging.

typical of an adenoma, in direct contradistinction to FNH, which demonstrate a more central vascular pattern. Scintigraphy is valuable in that these lesions will be "cold" on a scintigram, and this finding favors adenoma rather than FNH. Again, however, this finding is nonspecific and cannot be singularly relied upon.

Indications for Surgery

Although cessation of OCPs for women with HAs may result in resolution, treatment is primarily surgical—to eliminate the risk of rupture and significant bleeding first and foremost, while also eliminating the risk of malignant transformation within the lesion. Surgical intervention is warranted for symptomatic masses that may be either causing pain or obstructing critical structures. Symptomatic relief is very common in patients after surgery, and acceptable morbidity/mortality profiles make resection an attractive therapy.[3,11,12] Generally, the role of angiographic embolization is reserved for bridging prior to definitive surgical therapy (e.g., active bleeding prior to laparotomy) or for unresectable lesions (diffuse or central).

Figure 4-2: Management workup of liver lesion.

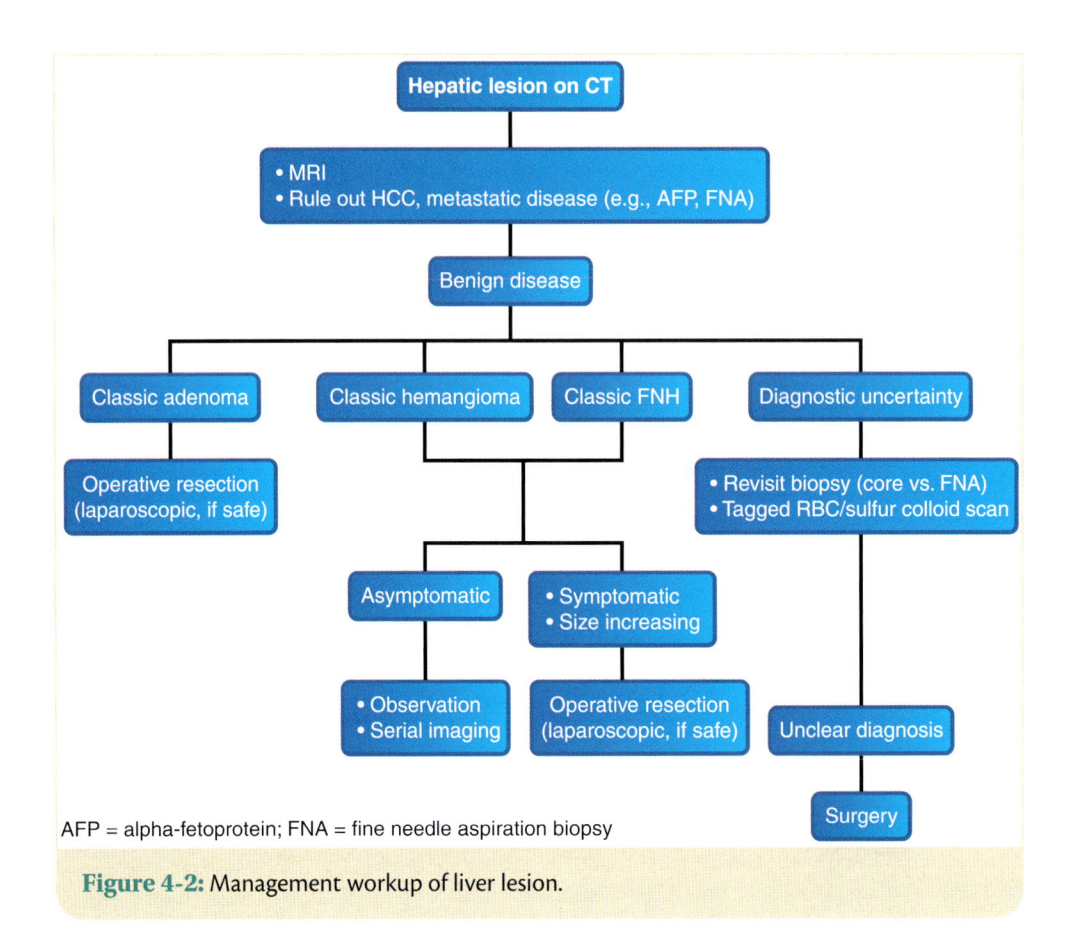

AFP = alpha-fetoprotein; FNA = fine needle aspiration biopsy

The lack of understanding in the natural history of HA makes the optimal treatment of asymptomatic HA unclear. Although some experts suggest cessation of OCPs and surveillance is sufficient, this does not in any way guarantee against malignant degeneration, rupture, or even growth to a symptomatic lesion.[13,14] A large multicenter trial reporting on 124 patients undergoing treatment (119 operative resections and 5 embolized patients) concluded that asymptomatic patients with lesions approaching 4 cm should undergo surgery.[15] Other experts recommend that all HAs be resected once the diagnosis is made. Because recurrence is essentially nonexistent, definitive surgical therapy guards against progression in size, transformation to HCC, and more rare but deadly events including rupture during pregnancy. In addition, a malignancy rate of up to 4%–6% has been reported in specimens resected due to presumed benign pathology.[12,15,16]

An interesting conundrum is found in patients with hepatic adenomatosis (>10 lesions), as complete resection is rarely feasible. One institution encourages resection for lesions > 4 cm due to their predilection for bleeding or malignant transformation[17] and leaving other lesions within the liver parenchyma. Another approach is orthotopic liver transplantation when unresectable disease is present.[12,18,19] The optimal approach is unclear and is likely determined by organ availability and surgeon preference.

Hemangioma

Incidence and Characteristics

Hepatic hemangioma, a purely benign process, is the most common liver mass encountered in large observational studies with a strong 3:1 predilection for females.[20–22] This process demonstrates a large variance in lesion size as well, ranging from small capillary hemangiomata to giant hemangiomata, the cavernous type more commonly problematic in infants. The likely etiology of hemangioma is ectatic vascular malformation and multifocality can be

TABLE 4-2: Imaging Characteristics of Benign Liver Lesions

Entity	CT	MRI	PET	Ultrasound/Doppler
Hemangioma	Peripheral puddling, enhancement of lesion with delayed images	T1: hypointense, T2: hyperintense, peripheral enhancement, excellent sensitivity, specificity	No FDG uptake	Hyperechoic with low flow
Adenoma	Peripheral enhancement with central filling	T1: hyperintense; may have capsule	No FDG uptake (only with malignant transformation)	Hyperechoic, may have anechoic center with hemorrhage, variable flow
FNH	Significant arterial enhancement with low-density central scar	T1: Isodense; T2: Hyperintense central scar; with gadolinium not hypervascularity	No FDG uptake	Variable echoic characteristics; high flow, central arterial signal

Abbreviations: CT, computed tomography; FDG, 18-fluorodeoxyglucose; MRI, magnetic resonance imaging; PET, positron emission tomography.

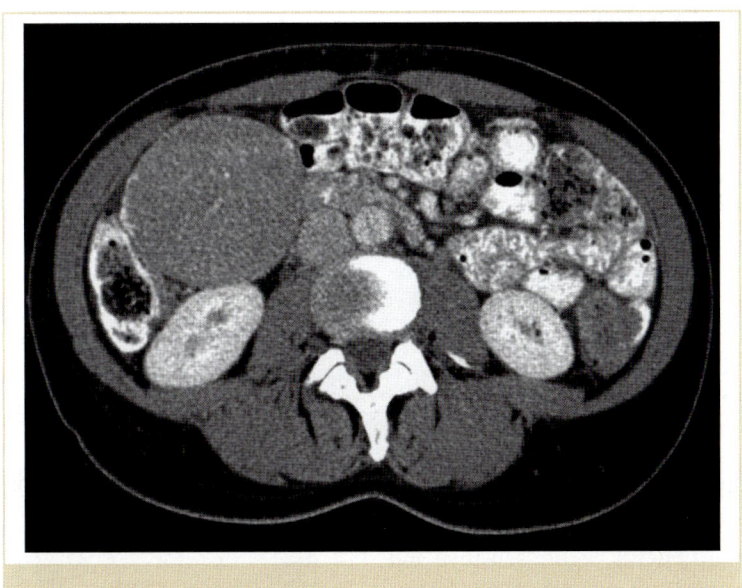

Figure 4-3: Hepatic adenoma demonstrating peripheral enhancement with administration of intravenous contrast.

found in up to 40% of patients.[23] There is no risk of malignant degeneration and a negligible risk of rupture (though there are reports of free rupture into the peritoneal cavity).[24] An association has been made with oral contraceptive use in females, but this link is not well established, as in HA.

Grossly, hemangiomas appear as purplish, thin walled vascular lesions that may contain numerous septae. Furthermore, it may be difficult to discern a thrombosed hemangioma from a primary hepatocellular carcinoma or an involuted and metastatic lesion.[25]

Hemangiomas are frequently asymptomatic and more often incidentally found during routine imaging for other medical conditions, during abdominal surgery, or at autopsy. Symptoms may arise from the following: (1) thrombosis of hemagiomata of all sizes, though cavernous hemangiomata may be particularly symptomatic, (2) mass effect from very large lesions exerting compressive forces and resultant satiety or obstruction, or (3) superficial lesions whose rapid, if temporary, growth may stretch Glisson's capsule and cause right upper quadrant pain.[23] However, Farges demonstrated that up to 54% of patients with hemagioma and abdominal pain ultimately were diagnosed with alternate disease processes to which the pain was attributed,[26] so great care must exercised in the diagnostic process.

Physical Examination, Laboratory Testing, and Imaging Studies

Physical examination will rarely, if ever, indicate the pathologic process of hemangiomata, and liver function tests are, as a rule, normal. Occasionally, laboratory findings may lend evidence to the evolution of this pathologic process. A large hemangioma that may have thrombosed can manifest with thrombocytopenia or anemia when examining a blood count. Specifically, Kasabach–Merritt syndrome describes the clinical scenario of a consumptive coagulopathy and thrombocytopenia from thrombosis of a large, perhaps cavernous hemangioma; this is most often described in children. In addition, an elevation in the direct fraction of bilirubin may result from compression of biliary outflow.

Diagnosis of hemangioma can usually be made by imaging, and proper interpretation of a variety of studies will nearly always result in the correct diagnosis. Hepatic hemangiomas are typically hypodense on precontrast CT, and in the arterial phase, there may be enhancement of the peripheral portions of the lesion. MRI is highly sensitive and specific in the diagnosis of hepatic hemangioma, typically demonstrating a low-signal intensity on T1-weighted images and high-signal intensity on T2-weighted images (Figure 4-4). Specifically, researchers have reported sensitivities and specificities of 73%–100% and 83%–97%, respectively.[12,26–29] When gadolinium is used as an intravenous contrast agent, hemangiomas enhance in a fashion similar to that seen on dynamic CT. A Technicium-labeled red blood cell nuclear medicine study is yet another imaging modality that may be useful and has been noted to be quite specific and posses a 100% positive predictive value in one study.[12] Usually, a hemangioma will fill centripetally with serial, delayed images. Two potential pitfalls of this approach, however, include poor sensitivity in lesions < 2 cm and the rare false positive when these lesions are confused with either primary or secondary malignancies. Finally, some have utilized the more invasive angiographic approach to aid in the diagnostic process. Classically, a hemangioma will exhibit a large feeding vessel with contrast pooling diffusely throughout the lesion. Angiogram is less often used due to the inherent, albeit low, risks of percutaneous vascular access.

However, hemangiomas may at times present a diagnostic challenge in that they can be mistaken for hypervascular malignancies of the liver and can coexist with (and occasionally mimic) other benign and malignant hepatic lesions, including FNH, HA, hepatic cysts, hepatic metastasis, and primary hepatocellular carcinoma, among other entities. With this fact in mind, the use of biopsy for tissue diagnosis in the workup algorithm is controversial and less often used. Although some authors have concluded that this approach is safe,[30,31] there have been other reports of fatal hemorrhage with biopsy using just a fine needle.[32] Ultimately, should there be any diagnostic confusion, it would seem that the safest approach is to incorporate several high quality imaging modalities.

Indications for Surgery

A vast majority of hemangiomas are small and asymptomatic, and multiple studies have confirmed the safety of observation in these patients.[12,21,33]

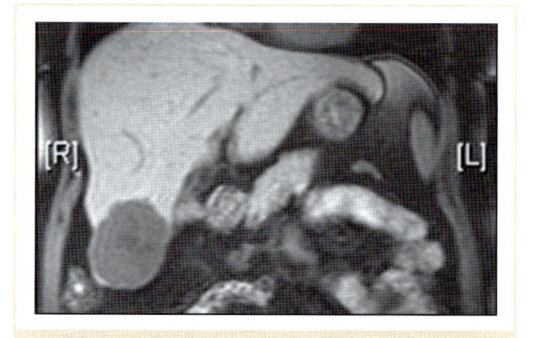

Figure 4-4: Characteristic magnetic resonance imaging image hemangioma.

However, this observational approach must only be applied when the risk of malignancy has been entirely ruled out. Once this has been accomplished, surgical resection is reserved for four clinical scenarios. First, symptomatic lesions refractory to conservative management should be resected. However, abdominal pain is sometimes not eliminated when the hemangioma is removed; this fact must lead to careful counseling and highly thoughtful patient selection, with surgery proceeding only after exclusion of more common and pertinent upper abdominal pathology. Second, the development of Kasabach–Merritt may prompt surgical intervention. Third, rupture with free intraperitoneal hemorrhage is quite rare but necessitates emergent laparotomy, control of bleeding, and resection. Finally, inability to exclude malignancy remains in indication for resection. In a large series of 249 patients with an average follow-up of 78 month, only 3.2% of patients required surgical resection, primarily for right upper quadrant pain.[34] Yet another series from Memorial Sloan Kettering reported on 115 patients with a 45% resection/enucleation rate and symptomatic relief in 96% of patients who underwent resection.[35]

Percutaneous endovascular embolization is a consideration for diffuse lesions, patients with active hemorrhage (utilized as a bridge or definitive therapy) or patients who are poor surgical candidates whose unacceptable operative mortality preclude operative intervention. Liver transplant has also been reported as a viable alternative for unresectable, symptomatic lesions.[36,37] Less well-documented and studied are systemic steroids, interferon α-2a, hepatic artery ligation, and external beam radiation. These may provide symptomatic relief, but care must be taken to counsel the patient that these approaches have widely variable results.

Focal Nodal Hyperplasia

Incidence and Characteristics

FNH was for many years clinically indistinguishable from adenoma. After hemangioma, FNH is the second most common benign hepatic mass, with an approximate incidence of 0.3%.[38] The differences between FNH and HA are currently more well defined, and FNH is becoming increasingly recognized in the population, due predominantly to the use of sophisticated, fine cross-sectional three dimensional imaging. Just as in adenoma, FNH is more commonly diagnosed in women aged 20–40, though on a population-wide basis is more evenly distributed between men and women.

Histologically, FNH is characterized as a vascular malformation that results in hyperplastic hepatic elements that are arranged in a disorganized fashion. Evidence for this assertion is found in the realization of aberrant feeding vessels in up to 60% of lesions, with subsequent increases in sinusoidal pressure.[38,39] Clearly, however, these lesions are not homogenous and do not always conform to this description (i.e., display a very different peripheral vascular pattern) and there is even variation in the clonality of these lesions based on DNA analysis. Grossly, the lesion is characterized by fibrous elements that are interspersed between nodules, most often with a "central scar." This finding is absent in up to 15% of lesions, however, and the absence of this finding, both grossly or on imaging studies, may lead to false assumptions about the character of the lesion.[11,40] Nguyen et al. validate this notion of heterogeneity, histologically classifying 60% of lesions as nonclassical.[41]

OCP use does not increase the risk of developing FNH, but some experts believe OCPs may increase the size of FNH or make them more symptomatic.[42] Contrary to HA, the risk of rupture is exceedingly rare, and in fact nearly all patients afflicted with FNH are asymptomatic and continue to be so with years of follow-up. When a number of large series were analyzed as one, only 14 of 115 patients with the diagnosis of FNH exhibited increasing symptomatology or enlargement.[2,3,12,43–46]

Though the body of literature would not support FNH as either a malignant or premalignant lesion, there are exceptions to this rule. There have been reports of fibrolamellar variant of hepatocellular carcinoma arising within an FNH,[45,47–49] and still other studies bring into question malignant degeneration of FNH in women taking OCPs for a lengthy period of time.[50,51]

Physical Examination, Laboratory Testing, and Imaging Studies

Nearly all patients with FNH are asymptomatic. Only a fraction of patients complain of right upper quadrant pain, and most often, the finding is an incidental one during imaging or surgical intervention for an entirely unrelated reason. Physical examination is likewise nearly always unremarkable. Just as in other benign liver lesions, the only laboratory evaluation that may be abnormal is an elevated bilirubin, due to local mass effect on biliary radicals.

Ultrasound is a reasonable initial diagnostic maneuver. However, most experts agree that there are serious deficits that preclude this imaging modality as a definitive method of diagnosis. The echogenic nature of FNH is variable, at times appearing hypoechogenic and in other instances appearing hyperechogenic. Still yet, one report has demonstrated that the classical "central scar" is visible in only 20% of cases.[52] Perhaps the most pathognomonic finding on ultrasound is that of outwardly radial pulsatile flow emanating from the middle of the lesion with the use of color Doppler. Imaging by CT is the most commonly used modality for diagnosis of FNH. A multiphase contrast infusion is critical to maximize the yield of CT; with early arterial infusion, the entire lesion may become hyperintense with a hypointense "central scar" (Figure 4-5). Delayed portal venous images may then demonstrate a hypervascular central, spokewheel-like appearance when compared to the surrounding liver parenchyma and lesion itself. A third and increasingly appreciated modality is magnetic resonance. Although some authors report that MRI will not demonstrate the classic scar in up to 65% of cases, other researchers have shown a 70% and 98% sensitivity and specificity, respectively, for diagnosing FNH.[11,52,53] FNH usually appears as either hypo- or isointense on T1-weighted images and either iso- or hyperintense on T2 images.

Angiography, with its invasive and often nondiagnostic features, is quickly falling out of favor as infusional, noninvasive imaging (CT and MRI) that become increasingly sophisticated. Another approach, nuclear medicine scintigraphy, is favored by some as an adjunct to some of the forementioned imaging studies when the diagnosis remains in doubt. Proponents of this approach will highlight the radiolabeled uptake of FNH, which can further be augmented by specific tracers taken up by the biliary system. Just as with other modalities, however, this approach is rarely singularly diagnostic, as there can be many false negatives (FNH that is "cold") or false positives (adenomas may also appear "hot").

Biopsies of lesions suspicious for FNH are controversial. The procedure carries a low attendant risk (in contradistinction to hemangioma or adenoma), but may all too often be nondiagnostic or outright misleading. This must be considered before exposing the patient to such an invasive diagnostic maneuver.

Indications for Surgery

Surgery for FNH is often reserved for those patients who are unequivocally symptomatic or for those with diagnostic uncertainty.[54,55] Observation is safe, with most lesions not requiring resection as they are rarely symptomatic.[55] Most patients with FNH will not be symptomatic, so due diligence is critical. Despite the less than clear link between OCPs and FNH, cessation of exogenous estrogens and progesterones may eliminate symptoms in a subcohort of patients, and this no-cost, safe option should be entertained in women taking OCPs. Appropriate serial imaging may be employed if lesion size may be directly linked to the patient's symptoms. Operative resection is safe, however, and in a series of 48 patients with FNH resected, subjects experienced no perioperative mortality, no recurrence with four years follow-up, and a complication rate of only 2.1%.[56]

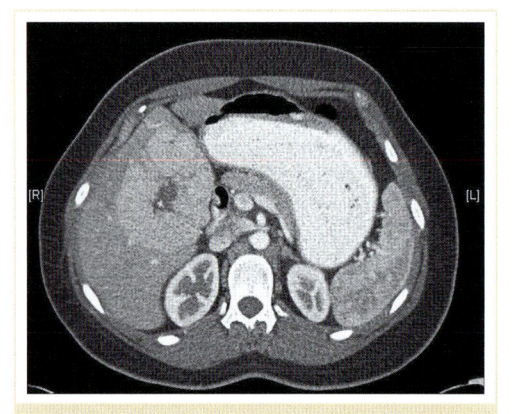

Figure 4-5: Arterial phase computed tomography of hepatic focal nodular hyperplasia; note the pathognomonic central scar of the lesion.

Cystic Hepatic Disease

Cystic hepatic disease is relatively common and generally categorized as either parasitic or nonparasitic. This spectrum of diseases has been greatly impacted

Benign Liver Lesions

by both antimicrobial advances and better proficiency with laparoscopy. Laparoscopic surgery, in general, has rendered many of these diseases increasingly operable with more definitive treatment than with observation or percutaneous drainage, as had been entertained more often in decades past. Below are common hepatic cysts that are encountered worldwide, but the list is by no means exhaustive.

Amebic Cysts

Amoebic cysts, caused by *Entamoeba hystolytica*, are primarily found in developing countries and transmitted in an oral/fecal manner. In the United States, amoebic hepatic cysts are almost exclusively found in immigrants or foreign travelers, though worldwide *Entameoba* is the third most deadly parasite, with over 40 million people harboring disease either in their colon or liver.[57] Patients may be immunocompromised or be malnourished, with establishment of parasite in the liver due to infected portal venous flow. Liquefactant necrosis of hepatocytes spreads peripherally, resulting in a central medium of purulence and blood. The diagnosis of amebic hepatic cyst can be made in a variety of ways, both radiographically and serologically (enzyme immunoassay). Ultrasound is inexpensive, low risk, and may possess 90% accuracy [58], but can also be misleading and requires both expert interpretation and confirmatory testing. CT may also be useful, as densitometric analysis can help to distinguish simple cysts from think purulence to frank blood. The most common confirmatory test, however, is a widely available ELISA that is both expedient and quite sensitive. There is a lag from infection to antibody production, however, and titers may not be positive for over a week after exposure.

Amoebic cysts are routinely treated with antibiotics. Oral metronidazole for 10 days is curative in greater than 90% of patients, though intravenous administration is an excellent alternative if the patient cannot tolerate enteral therapy. Alternative therapies include the following: (1) emetine, which reaches high concentrations in the liver and is much more effective against trophozoites than cysts, (2) choloroquin, which is useful in patients who demonstrate resistance or intolerance to metronidazole or emetine, and (3) diloxanide, which is most commonly used to treat close contacts of those afflicted. Surgery is reserved for patients who fail antimicrobial therapy and does not show a survival benefit when instituted early.[59,60]

Hydatid Cysts

Echinococcal, or hydatid, cysts are caused by the tapeworms *Echinococcus granulosus, Echinococcus multilocularis, Echinococcus vogeli and Echinococcus oligartus*. As the primary host is dog, this disease is global and transmitted in an oral/fecal manner. Embryos translocate across the duodenum, are taken up in the portal venous circulation and are harbored in the liver, more commonly in the right lobe. Two well-documented complications include intraperitoneal rupture (at times precipitating anaphylactic shock) and bile duct fistula formation, which serves as the basis for surgical intervention. Just as in amebic disease, the diagnosis is made with imaging modalities and augmented by serologies. Either by ultrasound or by CT, septations or visible floating walls within the cyst are pathognomonic for *Echinococcal* disease, representing daughter cysts within the cyst proper. CT is especially useful to help delineate the hepatic anatomy when surgical intervention is discussed (Figure 4-6).

Surgery is indicated for large or peripheral cysts, as these are most likely to rupture and cause intraabdominal catastrophe (widespread dissemination that may never be completely cured). Most commonly a pericystectomy is preformed, leaving the unroofed cyst marsupialized and externally drained. Other surgical options include en bloc hepatic resections, closed (without initial intraoperative drainage) or open (drainage followed by cyst wall excision) pericystectomy. Laparoscopic techniques have also been applied.

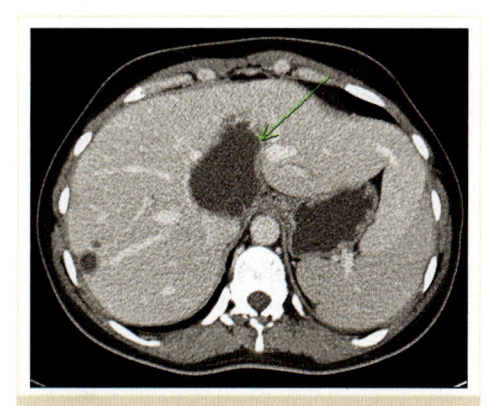

Figure 4-6: Computed tomography in the excretory phase demonstrating an echinococcal cyst in the caudate lobe.

Nonoperative management of hydatid disease is advocated for small, central cysts. The chance of rupture in these is negligible, and serial ultrasound to evaluate progression is safe. The more recent recognition that antihelminth therapy is effective and has given equivocal clinical scenarios a less morbid treatment option when surgery is not clearly indicated. Albendazole and mebendazole are widely utilized, though both require long courses (minimum three months, often times up to 12). Furthermore, although success rates with antimicrobial therapy have been noted to approach 40%, it is unclear if radiologic resolution equates to cure.

Simple Hepatic Cysts

Generally, noninfectious, nonneoplastic cysts can be viewed as: (1) single, (2) multiple, (3) a manifestation of polycystic liver disease, or (4) traumatic cysts. Neoplastic cysts (e.g., cystadenomas) are discussed elsewhere in this chapter. These entities are essentially never life-threatening, and rarely symptomatic. When encountered, however, there are indications for intervention: primarily pain and/or local compression. CT or ultrasound are both reasonable diagnostic strategies, but use of these modalities as lone agents must be used with some caution, as infectious or even neoplastic disease may be missed if aspiration or surgical excision are not utilized.

Aspiration of hepatic cysts is often performed if there are any diagnostic uncertainties. Aspirate of an asymptomatic lesion that demonstrates a normal Ca 19-9 and carcinoembryonic antigen (CEA) is observed unless the patient has strong feelings to the contrary. A lesion with normal cyst fluid CEA and Ca 19-9 but is symptomatic is subjected to intervention. If cyst fluid is high in Ca 19-9 or CEA, biopsy of the lesion is indicated, either percutaneously or laparoscopically, to rule out malignancy, the primary concern being a premalignant cystadenoma or carcinoma.

Traditionally, the treatment of simple nonneoplastic, nonparasitic cysts was either aspiration in association with sclerotherapy (aspiration alone demonstrates nearly 100% recurrence) or open laparotomy with cystectomy or formal hepatic resection. Numerous studies in the last 20 years have advocated sclerotherapy (primarily with alcohol), though this technique has an attendant recurrence of up to nearly 20%. Multiple case series of open partial cystectomy (with or without marsupialization), complete cystectomy, or hepatic resection have led to acceptably low recurrence rates and negligible mortality (0% in some series with many years of follow-up). Laparoscopic intervention, however, has substantially increased the utilization of surgical therapy. Equivalent outcomes are welcomed with shorter hospital stays, less pain, and smaller incisions and have expanded the number of patients who are willing to undergo a definitive surgical excision.

Finally, patients with polycystic liver disease (PCLD) present a unique challenge. Patient selection is critical, with success far more predictable in patients with a few medium to large cysts rather than in patients with numerous, small cysts. Otherwise, patients with polycystic liver disease should forego operation, unless their symptoms are intractable or they have evidence of cyst rupture, hemorrhage, or infection. Complete eradication of cystic disease in polycystic liver disease (PCLD) is frequently unachievable, and exuberant resection may only compromise hepatic function. Laparoscopic excision is a useful tool, particularly with anterior or left-sided lesions that are much more accessible for deroofing, with or without marsupialization.

Benign Biliary Tumors

Benign biliary tract tumors, especially those of extra-hepatic origin, are quite rare. Patients afflicted with biliary tract neoplasms present, as a rule, with obstructive jaundice and are frequently thought to be suffering from a malignant biliary process. This preconception, however, should not blind the clinician to the possibility that a benign tumor may be the inciting factor for obstruction because surgical resection is essentially curative with respect to symptoms, while also eliminating any risk of malignant degeneration.

Biliary Cystadenoma

Biliary cystadenomas (BCA) are defined as benign cystic lesions that are columnar-epithelial lined and possess the capacity to secrete mucous. Also known as intrahepatic bile duct cystadenoma or hepatobiliary cystadenoma, these tumors may contain either serous (more rarely) or mucinous gelatinous material and are most often encapsulated and multilocular (Figure 4-7). Histologically, BCA epithelial lining most closely embodies bile duct characteristics, including occasional findings of neuroendocrine (or occasionally simple endocrine) cells that may lead to neuroendocrine differentiation within the tumor. An example of this phenomenon is the finding of chromagranin or somatostatin staining within the biliary epithelium. In addition, a subtype of BCA that contains mesenchymal stroma is found uniquely in females with histologic features of ovarian-like supportive tissue immunohistochemically confirmed by staining for vimentin, actin, and desmin. This subtype is understood to follow a relatively more benign course when compared to other BCA that do not exhibit specific differentiation patterns.[61] Interestingly, there has also been a report of synchronous pancreatic mucinous neoplasms, leading one to speculate that individual genetic predispositions may predominate on a multiorgan level.[62]

BCA, whether of mucinous or serous subtype, have the potential for malignant degeneration and may develop invasive features. For most patients, long-term follow-up is appropriate. The biliary epithelia of these tumors, whether glandular columnar or simple cuboidal, may display cellular atypia. The entire spectrum of benign to dysplastic BCA epithelia is found, and the finding of any invasive component leads to the appropriate reclassification of a biliary cystadenocarcinoma; oftentimes, this distinction can be very clinically difficult.

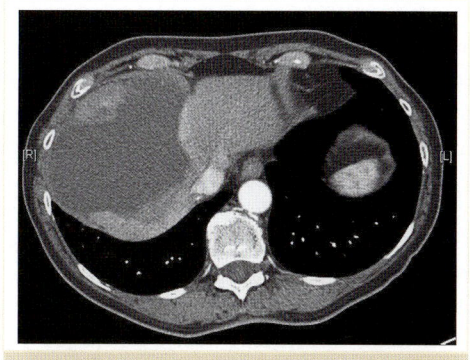

Figure 4-7: Arterial phase computed tomography of hepatic cystadenoma.

Bile Duct Adenoma

Bile duct adenomas, also termed benign cholangioma or cholangioadenoma, are lesions containing normal epithelium lined bile duct-like structures interspersed with lymphocytes and fibrous mesenchyme. Typically, these neoplasms are subcapsular and lack a well-defined capsule themselves. These lesions are benign and may grow up to 2 cm in size.[63] A caveat to their benign phenotype, however, is that these adenomas have premalignant potential. Evidence for this is found in cellular atypia identified within large lesions as well as isolated cases of bile duct adenomas intimately involved with cholangiocarcinoma.

Biliary Microhamartoma

Biliary microhamartomas are very similar to bile duct adenomas in that they are filled with ducts lined with biliary epithelium and supported by a fibrous stroma. They are distinctly different, however, in that they are typically small, multiple, associated with polycystic disease, and often contain bile.[64,65] There is speculation that this entity exists both in sporadic and familial forms, the genetic predisposition broadly associated with polycystic disease throughout the organism. Just as is the case with bile duct adenomas, an association with cholangiocarcinoma has been made, implicating microhamartomas (also known as biliary hamartomas) as precancerous lesions.[66–68]

Biliary Papillomatosis

Billiary papillomas are most often found near the ampulla of Vater, less commonly in the common bile duct and the hepatic ducts. This rare disease may be solitary (associated with a better prognosis), but is more often multiple. It is unclear whether diffuse papillomatosis is itself a benign or malignant condition, but some believe that this condition is essentially a low-grade malignancy.[69,70]

Other Benign Biliary Tumors

The remaining list of even more rare benign biliary neoplasms deserves mention, though their natural history and appropriate treatment are poorly rooted in evidence-based practice due to the infrequency of these disease processes. Granular cell myoblastomas are most frequently found in the extra-hepatic biliary tree, most often afflict African American women and are cured by adequate excision (recurrence has been reported in patients whose local excision was inadequate). Endocrine tumors, which may secrete gastrin or serotonin, can also arise from the common bile duct epithelium, and resection with choledochojejunostomy or hepaticojejunostomy reconstruction is appropriate. Neural tumors are found extremely rarely, with case reports providing our best description of these entities. Leiomyomas, far more commonly found in the upper and mid-gastrointestinal tract, have been reported, but the numbers of bile duct leiomyomas found in the literature are in the single digits.

Treatment of Benign Biliary Lesions

When benign biliary lesions are symptomatic, it is nearly always due to obstructive jaundice secondary to mass effect. Though rare, lesions such as biliary adenoma or papilloma warrant surgical treatment for two reasons. Firstly, endoscopic intervention (i.e., stenting) is only a temporizing measure, certainly not addressing any neoplastic growth that may continue to grow and cause significant symptoms despite mechanical decompression. Furthermore, the considerable risk of cholangitis and the need for stent retrieval and replacement along with its attendant morbidity and cost make such minimally invasive approaches inadequate. Secondly, adequate excision with normal margins around any pathology yields essentially 100% cure, with recurrence of benign disease at resection margins negligible. Such recurrence is found only when initial excision is incomplete, and the initial operation for these benign diseases should be viewed as curative.

Deserving of unique mention is biliary cystadenoma, which is widely recognized to have the ability to undergo malignant transformation. In addition, preoperative discrimination of biliary cystadenoma from cystadenocarcinoma is challenging (if not impossible) and the two related disease processes may very well coexist together (Figure 4-7).[61,71] As such, if the diagnosis of biliary cystadenocarcinoma is entertained, the appropriate therapy is surgical excision with evidence of normal margins.[71,72] Most importantly, the critical principle is not undertreating a presumed cystadenoma.

Surgical Techniques and Respective Outcomes

Just as the natural history of many of these entities are poorly understood due to their relative rarity, so too are a lack of clear data about the optimal technical considerations of hepatic resection for benign disease.[1] Furthermore, individual surgeon experience weighs mightily on whether a laparoscopic or open approach is offered to a patient. As such, discussions of instrumentation, surgical technique, and operative approach to the patient must be considered in proper perspective, with the realization that many (even large) series are essentially observational and descriptive. Note also that although many approaches or devices are discussed singularly, many operations as well as published reports utilize more than one strategy or technology, making interpretation of data challenging.

"Open" Surgery

Refinements in specific techniques have led to incremental advancement in operative blood loss, postoperative complications, and perioperative mortality. Improvements in the understanding of hepatic anatomy and advances in surgical instrumentation (staplers, coagulation devices utilizing radiofrequency [RF]) and operative strategies (low intravascular volume surgery) have each contributed to the movement toward better care of the liver resection patient, though the data do not mandate clear recommendations in many cases (Table 4-3).

Staplers

As stapling devices become more sophisticated and patient use is more widespread, surgeons have accumulated large series of hepatic transections using these instruments. In theory, systematic control of large vascular structures and biliary radicals with reliable, multirow staples provide a consistent, if not time-saving approach, though certainly with the caveat of expense. A retrospective review of 300 patients undergoing either minor (36%) or major (64%) liver resection at a large German center detailed the use of stapling devices for parenchymal transection. A total of 14% of surgeries were performed for benign disease and overall perioperative mortality and morbidity of 4% and 33%, respectively, were reported. The authors' conclusions were that stapler transection of the liver parenchyma was safe and in-line with other large centers' experiences, though this could be questioned, particularly with respect to some large series of laparoscopic liver resections for benign disease (Table 4-3).[73,74–80]

RF Energy

RF energy is gaining increasing traction in the operative management of liver tumors, both benign and malignant. Although a variety of devices exist, the basic tenet of RF technology is heat production between or around electrodes deployed within hepatic parenchyma resulting in tissue coagulation and sealing of even large biliary or vascular structures. Earlier devices utilized monopolar energy with uncontrolled energy release, whereas newer generations of instruments use bipolar energy and can release energy in a much more precise fashion. Proponents of this technique primarily advocate its ability to substantially reduce operative blood loss and perioperative blood transfusion while minimizing the requirement for vascular control.

Laparoscopic Surgery

Yet another and perhaps most pronounced example of increased technical proficiency is the advancement of laparoscopic techniques in hepatic surgery (Table 4-4).[81–84] It has been repeatedly demonstrated that laparoscopic hepatic resection is a feasible and safe surgical practice, and with increased support from the literature regarding (at the very least) comparable outcomes, this has rapidly become accepted as a first-line surgical therapy. Certainly, one must recognize the individual surgeons' expertise, comfort with anatomy, and perhaps most importantly patient selection. Large, central lesions abutting or compressing major vascular or biliary structures are especially hazardous, and one must not let the commonly accepted benefits of laparoscopy outweigh patient-specific risk.

In 1999, Katkhouda detailed 43 patients undergoing laparoscopic resection of benign cystic ($n = 31$) or solid ($n = 12$) hepatic lesions. There were no reported postoperative deaths, and no complications in patients with FNH or adenoma.[85] Particularly for polycystic liver disease, it should be emphasized that large and anteriorly located cysts are optimal for the laparoscopic approach. Likewise, solid lesions in the left lobe or anterior right lobe are particularly favorable for laparoscopic excision.[86] In addition, a Swiss review reports that for uncomplicated but symptomatic liver cysts, laparoscopic deroofing is less morbid than more traditional, open techniques but may also carry a 10%–25% recurrence rate that can be lowered by omentoplasty.[87] It should be recognized, however, that misidentification of a hydatid cyst, for example, as a simple liver cyst with fenestration prior to aspiration can lead to catastrophic spillage and severe perioperative morbidity and disseminated recurrence.

Two Chinese studies report two centers' experience with laparoscopic liver resection for benign solid masses, primarily for patients with hemangiomas. In the first, 14 patients with benign liver lesions underwent successful laparoscopic resection with 0% conversion, perioperative mortality and complication rates.[88] In the other, 18 patients were successfully treated with a laparoscopic hepatic resection, primarily left sided, with essentially no complications reported.[89]

A large multicenter analysis from two high volume liver centers, North-western University (NU) and University of Pittsburgh, demonstrate that laparoscopic hepatic resection compares very favorably to open procedures with regard to outcomes and complications.[90] Of more than 330 cases in the series, only 4 required conversion to an open procedure (none at Northwestern). There was no 30-day mortality, blood transfusion was required in 1% and 4.3% of patients (NU and Pitt, respectively), and bile leaks occurred in about 2% of patients. Length of stay at NU was 1.4 days. No patients required a repeat trip to the operating room. Sixty nine percent of patients in this series had benign liver lesions indicating laparoscopic assisted hepatic resection may be particularly well suited to removal of benign lesions.

Ongoing developments in minimally invasive surgery are providing ever less morbid procedures for treating symptomatic benign tumors. Laparoscopic, single incision and robotic techniques are increasingly popularized.[91–93] Safety and financial data support continued use and development of these techniques in the treatment of patients with benign disease.[94]

TABLE 4-3: Series of Devices for Liver Transection

Author, y	N	Device	Control Method/ Cohort	Operative Time (Mean/min)	Blood Loss (Mean or Median)	Morbidity/Mortality	Author Conclusions
Richter, 2009[74]	96 (32 each cohort)	US dissection, waterjet dissection, dissecting sealer	Compared to each other	Dissecting sealer slowest	No difference in EBL in study cohorts	Overall mortality 4%, similar morbidity profile	Dissecting sealer was more costly, slower
Pai, 2008[75]	384	Habib	None	246 min	305 mL	21% morbidity, 3.4% mortality	Habib is safe and efficacious
Delis, 2008[76]	46	RF	None	Transection time 35 min	100 mL	30% morbidity, no mortality	RF is safe, simple, and useful in cirrhotics
Reddy, 2008[77]	99	VS	CC (N=112)	210 min VS versus 275 min CC	250mL VS vs. 500mL CC	Mortality 2% vs. 4% Morbidity 32% vs. 29% Neither significant	Vascular stapler has comparable safety/ efficacy profile
Ayav, 2007[78]	236	RF (monopolar and bipolar)	None	215 min	157 mL	21% morbidity, 2.1% mortality	RF energy offers acceptable efficacy/ safety profile
Schemmer, 2006[73]	330	Stapler	None	210 min	700 mL	33% morbidity, 4% mortality	Comparable with other large series
Lesurtel, 2005[79]	100	CUSA, Hydrojet, dissecting sealer	CC	CC fastest (3.9 cm/s)	CC smallest EBL (1.5 mL/cm)	Overall 33% morbidity, 4% mortality	CC fastest, lowest EBL, most cost effective
Takayama, 2001[80]	132 (66 each cohort)	Ultrasonic dissector	CC	Transection time 61 vs. 54 min (p = NS)	515 mL vs. 452 mL (p = NS)	Morbidity 20% vs. 14% (p = NS)	Ultrasonic dissector of no benefit; CC provides higher quality hepatectomy

Abbreviations: CC, crush/clamp; CUSA, Cavitron Ultrasonic Surgical Aspirator; EBL, estimated blood loss; NS, not significant; RF, radiofrequency; VS, vascular stapler.

TABLE 4-4: Series of Laparoscopic Liver Resections for Benign Liver Masses (Cystic And Solid)

Author, y	N	Lesions	Operative Time (Mean/min)	Conversion Rate (%)	Mean Blood Loss (mL) or transfusion	Morbidity/Mortality
Cugat, 2009[81]	182	45 cystic, 104 solid	150	8.8	5.5% required transfusion	14.8%, no mortality
Jiang, 2007[89]	18	Hemangioma	185	0	416 mL	No major complications, no mortality
Tarcoveanu, 2006[82]	92	74 cystic, 6 benign, 12 metastatic	—	8.7	—	6.5%, no mortality
Koffron, 2006—NU[90]	197	140 benign, 57 malignant	134	6% hand assisted	1% required transfusion	4.6%, no mortality
Koffron, 2006—Pitt[90]	138	91 benign, 47 malignant	—	50% hand assisted, 2.9% to open	4.3% required transfusion	6.5%, no mortality
Cai, 2004[88]	14	11 hemangioma, 1 FNH, 1 cyst, 1 granuloma	—	0	—	No major complications, no mortality
Descottes, 2003[83]	87	81 solid, 6 cystic	—	9	6% required transfusion (autologous)	5%, no mortality
Descottes, 2000[84]	33	15 cystic, 18 solid (16/18 for adenoma, hemangioma, FNH)	232	3	—	6%, no mortality
Katkhouda, 1999[85]	43	31 cystic, 12 solid (adenoma + FNH)	179	7	156 mL	14.1%, primarily in patients with hydatid disease, no mortality

Abbreviation: FNH, focal nodular hyperplasia.

References

1. Colli A, Fraquelli M, Massironi S, et al. Elective surgery for benign liver tumours. *Cochrane Database Syst Rev*. 2007;(1):CD005164.
2. Kerlin P, Davis GL, McGill DB, et al. Hepatic adenoma and focal nodular hyperplasia: clinical, pathologic, and radiologic features. *Gastroenterology*. 1983;84(5 Pt 1):994–1002.
3. Nagorney DM. Benign hepatic tumors: focal nodular hyperplasia and hepatocellular adenoma. *World J Surg*. 1995;19(1):13–18.
4. Rooks JB, Ory HW, Ishak KG, et al. Epidemiology of hepatocellular adenoma. The role of oral contraceptive use. *JAMA*. 1979;242(7):644–648.
5. Rosenberg L. The risk of liver neoplasia in relation to combined oral contraceptive use. *Contraception*. 1991;43(6):643–652.
6. Athanassiou AM, Craigo SD. Liver masses in pregnancy. *Semin Perinatol*. 1998;22(2):166–177.
7. Santambrogio R, Marconi AM, Ceretti AP, et al. Liver transplantation for spontaneous intrapartum rupture of a hepatic adenoma. *Obstet Gynecol*. 2009;113(2 Pt 2):508–510.
8. Van Hoe L, Baert AL, Gryspeerdt S, et al. Dual-phase helical CT of the liver: value of an early-phase acquisition in the differential diagnosis of noncystic focal lesions. *AJR Am J Roentgenol*. 1997;168(5):1185–1192.
9. Paulson EK, McClellan JS, Washington K, et al. Hepatic adenoma: MR characteristics and correlation with pathologic findings. *AJR Am J Roentgenol*. 1994;163(1):113–116.
10. Mathieu D, Vilgrain V, Mahfouz AE, et al. Benign liver tumors. *Magn Reson Imaging Clin N Am*. 1997;5(2):255–288.
11. Cherqui D, Rahmouni A, Charlotte F, et al. Management of focal nodular hyperplasia and hepatocellular adenoma in young women: a series of 41 patients with clinical, radiological, and pathological correlations. *Hepatology*. 1995;22(6):1674–1681.
12. Weimann A, Ringe B, Klempnauer J, et al. Benign liver tumors: differential diagnosis and indications for surgery. *World J Surg*. 1997;21(9):983–990; discussion 990–991.
13. Knowles DM 2nd, Casarella WJ, Johnson PM, Wolff M. The clinical, radiologic, and pathologic characterization of benign hepatic neoplasms. Alleged association with oral contraceptives. *Medicine (Baltimore)*. 1978;57(3):223–237.
14. Shortell CK, Schwartz SI. Hepatic adenoma and focal nodular hyperplasia. *Surg Gynecol Obstet*. 1991;173(5):426–431.
15. Deneve JL, Pawlik TM, Cunningham S, et al. Liver cell adenoma: a multicenter analysis of risk factors for rupture and malignancy. *Ann Surg Oncol*. 2009;16(3):640–648.
16. Belghiti J, Pateron D, Panis Y, et al. Resection of presumed benign liver tumours. *Br J Surg*. 1993;80(3):380–383.
17. Ribeiro A, Burgart LJ, Nagorney DM, Gores GJ. Management of liver adenomatosis: results with a conservative surgical approach. *Liver Transpl Surg*. 1998;4(5):388–398.
18. Leese T, Farges O, Bismuth H. Liver cell adenomas. A 12-year surgical experience from a specialist hepato-biliary unit. *Ann Surg*. 1988;208(5):558–564.
19. Mueller J, Keeffe EB, Esquivel CO. Liver transplantation for treatment of giant hepatocellular adenomas. *Liver Transpl Surg*. 1995;1(2):99–102.
20. Ishak KG, Rabin L. Benign tumors of the liver. *Med Clin North Am*. 1975;59(4):995–1013.
21. Gilon D, Slater PE, Benbassat J. Can decision analysis help in the management of giant hemangioma of the liver? *J Clin Gastroenterol*. 1991;13(3):255–258.
22. Gandolfi L, Leo P, Solmi L, et al. Natural history of hepatic haemangiomas: clinical and ultrasound study. *Gut*. 1991;32(6):677–680.
23. Tait N, Richardson AJ, Muguti G, Little JM. Hepatic cavernous haemangioma: a 10 year review. *Aust N Z J Surg*. 1992;62(7):521–524.
24. Scribano E, Loria G, Ascenti G, et al. Spontaneous hemoperitoneum from a giant multicystichemangioma of the liver: a casereport. *Abdom Imaging*. 1996;21(5):418–419.
25. Craig JR Peters RL, Edmondson HA. *Tumors of the Liver and Intrahepatic Bile Ducts*. Atlas of tumor pathology, Armed Forces Institute of Pathology. 1989.
26. Farges O, Daradkeh S, Bismuth H. Cavernous hemangiomas of the liver: are there any indications for resection? *World J Surg*. 1995;19(1):19–24.
27. McFarland EG, Mayo-Smith WW, Saini S, et al. Hepatic hemangiomas and malignant tumors: improved differentiation with heavily T2-weighted conventional spin-echo MR imaging. *Radiology*. 1994;193(1):43–47.
28. Lee MG, Baker ME, Sostman HD, et al. The diagnostic accuracy/efficacy of MRI in differentiating hepatic hemangiomas from metastatic colorectal/

breast carcinoma: a multiple reader ROC analysis using a jackknife technique. *J Comput Assist Tomogr*. 1996;20(6):905–913.

29. Soyer P, Dufresne AC, Somveille E, et al. Differentiation between hepatic cavernous hemangioma and malignant tumor with T2-weighted MRI: comparison of fast spin-echo and breath-hold fast spin-echo pulse sequences. *Clin Imaging*. 1998;22(3):200–210.

30. Tung GA, Cronan JJ. Percutaneous needle biopsy of hepatic cavernous hemangioma. *J Clin Gastroenterol*. 1993;16(2):117–122.

31. Heilo A, Stenwig AE. Liver hemangioma: US-guided 18-gauge core-needle biopsy. *Radiology*. 1997;204(3):719–722.

32. Terriff BA, Gibney RG, Scudamore CH. Fatality from fine-needle aspiration biopsy of a hepatic hemangioma. *AJR Am J Roentgenol*. 1990;154(1):203–204.

33. Trastek VF, van Heerden JA, Sheedy PF 2nd, Adson MA. Cavernous hemangiomas of the liver: resect or observe? *Am J Surg*. 1983;145(1):49–53.

34. Herman P, Costa ML, Machado MA, et al. Management of hepatic hemangiomas: a 14-year experience. *J Gastrointest Surg*. 2005;9(6):853–859.

35. Yoon SS, Charny CK, Fong Y, et al. Diagnosis, management, and outcomes of 115 patients with hepatic hemangioma. *J Am Coll Surg*. 2003;197(3):392–402.

36. Chui AK, Vass J, McCaughan GW, Sheil AG. Giant cavernous haemangioma: a rare indication for liver transplantation. *Aust N Z J Surg*. 1996;66(2):122–124.

37. Russo MW, Johnson MW, Fair JH, Brown RS Jr. Orthotopic liver transplantation for giant hepatic hemangioma. *Am J Gastroenterol*. 1997;92(10):1940–1941.

38. Wanless IR, Mawdsley C, Adams R. On the pathogenesis of focal nodular hyperplasia of the liver. *Hepatology*. 1985;5(6):1194–1200.

39. Scoazec JY, Flejou FJ, D'Errico A, et al. Focal nodular hyperplasia of the liver: composition of the extracellular matrix and expression of cell-cell and cell-matrix adhesion molecules. *Hum Pathol*. 1995;1114–2225. vol 26, issue 10

40. Matsushita M, Hajiro K, Suzaki T, et al. Focal nodular hyperplasia of the liver without central scar. *Dig Dis Sci*. 1995;40(11):2407–2410.

41. Nguyen BN, Fléjou JF, Terris B, et al. Focal nodular hyperplasia of the liver: a comprehensive pathologic study of 305 lesions and recognition of new histologic forms. *Am J Surg Pathol*. 1999;23(12):1441–1454.

42. Mathieu D, Zafrani ES, Anglade MC, Dhumeaux D. Association of focal nodular hyperplasia and hepatic hemangioma. *Gastroenterology*. 1989;97(1):154–157.

43. Sorensen TI, Baden H. Benign hepatocellular tumours. *Scand J Gastroenterol*. 1975;10(2):113–119.

44. Knowles DM, Wolff M. Focal nodular hyperplasia of the liver: a clinicopathologic study and review of the literature. *Hum Pathol*. 1976;7(5):533–545.

45. Pain JA, Gimson AE, Williams R, Howard ER. Focal nodular hyperplasia of the liver: results of treatment and options in management. *Gut*. 1991;32(5):524–527.

46. Di Stasi M, Caturelli E, De Sio I, et al. Natural history of focal nodular hyperplasia of the liver: an ultrasound study. *J Clin Ultrasound*. 1996;24(7):345–350.

47. Saul SH, Titelbaum DS, Gansler TS, et al. The fibrolamellar variant of hepatocellular carcinoma. Its association with focal nodular hyperplasia. *Cancer*. 1987;60(12):3049–3055.

48. Muguti G, Tait N, Richardson A, Little JM. Hepatic focal nodular hyperplasia: a benign incidentaloma or a marker of serious hepatic disease? *HPB Surg*. 1992;5(3):171–176; discussion 176–180.

49. Saxena R, Humphreys S, Williams R, Portmann B. Nodular hyperplasia surrounding fibrolamellar carcinoma: a zone of arterialized liver parenchyma. *Histopathology*. 1994;25(3):275–278.

50. Coopersmith CM, Lowell JA, Hassan A, Howard TK. Hepatocellular carcinoma in a patient with focal nodular hyperplasia. *HPB (Oxford)*. 2002;4(3):135–138.

51. Petsas T, Tsamandas A, Tsota I, et al. A case of hepatocellular carcinoma arising within large focal nodular hyperplasia with review of the literature. *World J Gastroenterol*. 2006;12(40):6567–6571.

52. Shamsi K, De Schepper A, Degryse H, Deckers F. Focal nodular hyperplasia of the liver: radiologic findings. *Abdom Imaging*. 1993;18(1):32–38.

53. Vilgrain V, Fléjou JF, Arrivé L, et al. Focal nodular hyperplasia of the liver: MR imaging and pathologic correlation in 37 patients. *Radiology*. 1992;184(3):699–703.

54. Shen YH, Fan J, Wu ZQ, et al. Focal nodular hyperplasia of the liver in 86 patients. *Hepatobiliary Pancreat Dis Int*. 2007;6(1):52–57.
55. Chun Hsee L, McCall JL, Koea JB. Focal nodular hyperplasia: what are the indications for resection? *HPB (Oxford)*. 2005;7(4):298–302.
56. Lin C, Geng L, Chen H, et al. [Focal nodular hyperplasia of the liver: a clinical study of 48 patients]. *Zhonghua Zhong Liu Za Zhi*. 2004;26(9):567–569.
57. Li E, Stanley SL Jr. Protozoa. Amebiasis. *Gastroenterol Clin North Am*. 1996;25(3):471–492.
58. Sepulveda BMN. Clinical manifestations and diagnosis of amebiasis. In: Martinez-Palomo A, ed. *Amebiasis: Human Parasitic Diseases*. Amsterdam: Elsevier; 1986:169–187.
59. Balasegaram M. Management of hepatic abscess. *Curr Probl Surg*. 1981;18(5):282–340.
60. Eggleston FC, Handa AK, Verghese M. Amebic peritonitis secondary to amebic liver abscess. *Surgery*. 1982;91(1):46–48.
61. Devaney K, Goodman ZD, Ishak KG. Hepatobiliary cystadenoma and cystadenocarcinoma. A light microscopic and immunohistochemical study of 70 patients. *Am J Surg Pathol*. 1994;18(11):1078–1091.
62. O'Shea JS, Shah D, Cooperman AM. Biliary cystadenocarcinoma of extrahepatic duct origin arising in previously benign cystadenoma. *Am J Gastroenterol*. 1987;82(12):1306–1310.
63. Allaire GS, Rabin L, Ishak KG, Sesterhenn IA. Bile duct adenoma. A study of 152 cases. *Am J Surg Pathol*. 1988;12(9):708–715.
64. Chung EB. Multiple bile-duct hamartomas. *Cancer*. 1970;26(2):287–296.
65. Thommesen N. Biliary hamartomas (von Meyenburg complexes) in liver needle biopsies. *Acta Pathol Microbiol Scand A*. 1978;86(2):93–99.
66. Homer LW, White HJ, Read RC. Neoplastic transformation of v. Meyenburg complexes of the liver. *J Pathol Bacteriol*. 1968;96(2):499–502.
67. Burns CD, Kuhns JG, Wieman TJ. Cholangiocarcinoma in association with multiple biliary microhamartomas. *Arch Pathol Lab Med*. 1990;114(12):1287–1289.
68. Dekker A, Ten Kate FJ, Terpstra OT. Cholangiocarcinoma associated with multiple bile-duct hamartomas of the liver. *Dig Dis Sci*. 1989;34(6):952–958.
69. Helpap B. Malignant papillomatosis of the intrahepatic bile ducts. *Acta Hepatogastroenterol (Stuttg)*. 1977;24(6):419–425.
70. Ohita H, Yamaguchi Y, Yamakawa O, et al. Biliary papillomatosis with the point mutation of K-ras gene arising in congenital choledochal cyst. *Gastroenterology*. 1993;105(4):1209–1212.
71. Delis SG, Touloumis Z, Bakoyiannis A, et al. Intrahepatic biliary cystadenoma: a need for radical resection. *Eur J Gastroenterol Hepatol*. 2008;20(1):10–14.
72. Vogt DP, Henderson JM, Chmielewski E. Cystadenoma and cystadenocarcinoma of the liver: a single center experience. *J Am Coll Surg*. 2005;200(5):727–733.
73. Schemmer P, Friess H, Hinz U, et al. Stapler hepatectomy is a safe dissection technique: analysis of 300 patients. *World J Surg*. 2006;30(3):419–430.
74. Richter S, Kollmar O, Schuld J, et al. Randomized clinical trial of efficacy and costs of three dissection devices in liver resection. *Br J Surg*. 2009;96(6):593–601.
75. Pai M, Jiao LR, Khorsandi S, et al. Liver resection with bipolar radiofrequency device: habibtrade mark 4X. *HPB (Oxford)*. 2008;10(4):256–260.
76. Delis SG, Bakoyiannis A, Tassopoulos N, et al. Radiofrequency-assisted liver resection. *Surg Oncol*. 2008;17(2):81–86.
77. Reddy SK, Barbas AS, Gan TJ, et al. Hepatic parenchymal transection with vascular staplers: a comparative analysis with the crush-clamp technique. *Am J Surg*. 2008;196(5):760–767.
78. Ayav A, Jiao LR, Habib NA. Bloodless liver resection using radiofrequency energy. *Dig Surg*. 2007;24(4):314–317.
79. Lesurtel M, Selzner M, Petrowsky H, et al. How should transection of the liver be performed? a prospective randomized study in 100 consecutive patients: comparing four different transection strategies. *Ann Surg*. 2005;242(6):814–222; discussion 822–823.
80. Takayama T, Makuuchi M, Kubota K, et al. Randomized comparison of ultrasonic vs clamp transection of the liver. *Arch Surg*. 2001;136(8):922–928.
81. Cugat E, Pérez-Romero N, Rotellar F, et al. Laparoscopic liver surgery: 8 years of multicenter Spanish register. *J Hepatobiliary Pancreat Surg*. 2009;17:262–68.

82. Tarcoveanu E, Georgescu S, Lupaşcu C, et al. [Laparoscopic surgery of the liver, in 92 cases]. *Rev Med Chir Soc Med Nat Iasi*. 2006;110(2):334–346.
83. Descottes B, Glineur D, Lachachi F, et al. Laparoscopic liver resection of benign liver tumors. *Surg Endosc*. 2003;17(1):23–30.
84. Descottes B, Lachachi F, Durand-Fontanier S, et al. [Laparoscopic treatment of solid and cystic tumors of the liver. Study of 33 cases]. *Ann Chir*. 2000;125(10):941–947.
85. Katkhouda N, Hurwitz M, Gugenheim J, et al. Laparoscopic management of benign solid and cystic lesions of the liver. *Ann Surg*. 1999;229(4):460–466.
86. Katkhouda N, Mavor E. Laparoscopic management of benign liver disease. *Surg Clin North Am*. 2000;80(4):1203–1211.
87. Gloor B, Ly Q, Candinas D. Role of laparoscopy in hepatic cyst surgery. *Dig Surg*. 2002;19(6):494–499.
88. Cai XJ, Huang H, Yu H, et al. [Laparoscopic liver resection for benign liver tumors]. *Zhonghua Yi Xue Za Zhi*. 2004;84(20):1698–1700.
89. Jiang WS, Lu BY, Cai XY, et al. [Lap-aroscope hepatectomy for hepatic hemangioma: a report of 18 cases]. *Zhonghua Wai Ke Za Zhi*. 2007; 45(19):1311–1313.
90. Koffron A, Geller D, Gamblin TC, Abecassis M. Laparoscopic liver surgery: shifting the management of liver tumors. *Hepatology*. 2006;44(6):1694–1700.
91. Herman P, Coelho FF, Perini MV, et al. Hepatocellular adenoma: an excellent indication for laparoscopic liver resection. *HPB (Oxford)*. June 2012;14(6):390–395. Epub March 28 2012.
92. Pan M, Jiang Z, Cheng Y, et al. Single-incision laparoscopic hepatectomy for benign and malignant hepatopathy: initial experience in 8 Chinese patients. *Surg Innov*. December 2012;19(4): 446–451. Epub April 2 2012.
93. Choi Gh, Choi SH, Kim SH, et al. Robotic liver resection: technique and results of 30 consecutive procedures. *Surg Endosc*. August 2012; 26(8):2247–2258. Epub February 4 2012.
94. Vanounou T, Steel JL, Nguyen KT, et al. Comparing the clinical and economic impact of laparoscopic versus open liver resection. *Ann Surg Oncol*. April 2010;17(4):998–1009. Epub December 22 2009.

CHAPTER 5

Primary Hepatic Malignancies

Jia-Hong Dong

Primary liver cancer remains a major health problem with great geographic variability. It is currently the sixth most common malignancy with 626,000 new cases per year and is the third most common cause of death from malignancies worldwide.[1] Its incidence is increasing in the United States and Europe.[2] Primary hepatic neoplasms can be broadly classified into hepatocellular, cholangiocellular, or mesenchymal neoplasms according to their cell of origin (Table 5-1). In this chapter, we review the histologic and clinical features of hepatocellular carcinoma and some rare malignant tumors and also present the current approach to diagnosis and management. Intrahepatic cholangiocellular carcinoma is discussed in Ch 2: Peripheral Cholangiocarcinoma.

Hepatocellular Carcinoma

Hepatocellular carcinoma (HCC) accounts for up to 85% of primary hepatic malignancies. It mostly affects patients with liver cirrhosis, and constitutes the leading cause death in these patients.[3–5] The only way to achieve long-term survival is to detect the tumor at an early stage when effective therapy can be applied. During recent years, many advances have been made in diagnosis and treatment of HCC. Progress has largely been due to the understanding the natural history and pathogenesis of HCC, technological achievements, as well as developments in molecular biology.

Epidemiology

The geographic distribution of HCC worldwide is strikingly uneven. Of all the HCC cases, 82% occurred in developing countries (55% in China alone).[1] The areas of high incidence are eastern and southeastern Asia as well as sub-Saharan Africa and Melanesia, where the incidence of HCC ranges from 25 to 52 cases per 100,000 population. In these areas, rates of HCC increase after 20 years of age and peak or stabilize at the age of 50 years and above. The lowest rates of HCC are observed in South Central Asia, Australia, Northern Europe, and America, where the incidence is around 4 to 7 cases per 100,000 population. Recently, a phenomenon of the rise in HCC incidence rates has been documented in several developed countries, mainly due to increased population exposure to environmental risk factors.[6] Decreasing trends were observed in Taiwan, Singapore, India, Sweden, and Spain.[7] The reduction of HCC in most developing countries is attributed to hepatitis B virus (HBV) immunization campaigns and to prevention of nosocomial spread of hepatitis B and C. An excess of HCC incidence in men compared with women has been well documented. The overall ratio in the gender-specific incidence rates is around 2.4 (male:female), much greater in the high-risk areas and less in the low-risk areas.[1]

Etiology

The etiology of HCC, like many other kinds of cancer, has been shown to be multifactorial and

TABLE 5-1: Primary Hepatic Malignancies

Hepatocellular
Hepatocellular carcinoma
Fibrolamellar carcinoma
Hepatoblastoma
Cholangiocellular
Cholangiocarcinoma
Cystoadenocarcinoma
Mesenchymal
Angiosarcoma
Epithelioid hemangioendothelioma
Myofibroblastoma
Embryonal sarcoma
Leiomyosarcoma
Rhabdomyosarcoma
Primary hepatic lymphoma

multistage in nature. The major risk factors for HCC have been well established. Liver cirrhosis is the strongest predisposing factor since 80% of HCCs develop in a cirrhotic liver.[8] Chronic HBV infection is the predominant cause in Asia and Africa and chronic hepatitis C virus (HCV) infection in Japan and Western countries. The risk factors for HCC have been divided into genetic, environmental, and biological factors. They may interact as a group or individually to induce the development of HCC.

Hepatitis B Virus

Epidemiologic, clinical, and experimental studies have shown an etiological association between HBV and HCC. Patients with chronic HBV infection have a 100-fold relative risk for developing HCC, with an annual incidence rate of 2% to 6% in the setting of cirrhosis.[9] Acquisition of HBV infection at birth or during early childhood is the greatest risk for the development of HBV-related HCC since viral infection early in life often becomes persistent as the result of the immaturity of the immune system. The carcinogenic potential of neonatal HBV infection has also been demonstrated in the woodchuck model with HBV infection.[10] Therefore, HBV is the most common carcinogen in Asian and African countries, where HBV infection is prevalent.

Carcinogenesis of HBV has been extensively analyzed, and two pathways have been proposed. One involves chronic necroinflammation of hepatocytes, cellular injury, mitosis, and hepatocyte regeneration. The other evokes direct oncogenic potential of HBV through chromosomal integration (cisactivation) or transactivation of cellular genes.[11] It is likely that both pathways contribute to HBV-related carcinogenesis. The cell cycle can be activated indirectly by compensatory hepatocyte proliferation in response to necrotic inflammation or by overexpression of single or combinations of genes altered by HBV. The integration of HBV DNA into the host cellular DNA may result in transactivation of proto-oncogens, activation of growth factors, and inactivation of tumor suppressor genes, leading to abnormal cell growth.[12,13] In addition, HBV proteins may have a direct effect on cellular functions, and some of these gene products can favor malignant transformation. The in vivo experiments show that expression of HBV x gene in transgenic mice may induce HCC by sensitization of the animals to chemical carcinogens or by altering cellular oncogenes such as c-myc.[14] Several other HBV genes may contribute to hepatic carcinogenesis, including truncated pre-S2/S and a novel spliced transcript of HBV, referred to as the HBV spliced protein.[12]

Hepatitis C Virus

HCV is currently emerging as the leading cause of HCC in developed countries of both the western and eastern hemispheres. The estimated risk for the development of HCC was 17.5-fold greater in HCV carriers than in noncarriers.[15] Around 20%–30% of the estimated 170 million patients with chronic HCV infection worldwide will develop cirrhosis. Once cirrhosis is established, the annual incidence of HCC is of 3%–5%, and one third of them will develop a HCC over their lifetime.[8] In contrast to HBV, HCV mainly establishes persistent infections in adults. The exact mechanisms by which HCV infection causes HCC remain unclear due to the absence of a reliable tissue culture system or a small animal model of HCV infection. The HCV-induced chronic inflammation and the effects of cytokines in liver proliferation and fibrosis are considered as one of the major pathogenic mechanisms. HCV is a single-stranded RNA that does not integrate into the host genome, but HCV-encoded proteins are involved in a wide range of activities, including cell signaling, transcription, cell proliferation, apoptosis, membrane rearrangement, vesicular trafficking, and translational regulation.[16] Both in vitro expression systems and in vivo transgenic mice studies have revealed that HCV gene products, such as core protein, NS3, NS4B, and NS5A, exhibit transformation potential, and several potentially oncogenic pathways can be altered by the expression of HCV proteins.[17–19] In addition, induction of both endoplasmic reticulum stress and oxidative stress by HCV proteins might contribute to liver cell transformation.[16]

Alcohol

Chronic alcohol abuse and alcoholic cirrhosis have long been recognized as a risk factor for the development of HCC. Several studies have suggested that the hepatotoxic effect of alcohol is dose-dependent, and cirrhosis appears to be the basis for alcohol-related HCC. However, it is not certain whether alcohol is a true carcinogen or if it acts as cofactor in the presence of coexistent infection with HBV or HCV. Some epidemiologic studies have shown a high prevalence of HBV and/or HCV markers in patients with HCC who are also alcoholics.[20] In a population-based, case-control study from USA, a synergistic interaction on the risk of HCC has been described between heavy alcohol consumption and viral hepatitis, as well as between heavy alcohol consumption and diabetes.[21] Studies conducted in Greece and Italy have shown that the attributable fractions of heavy alcohol consumption are 15% and 45%, respectively, after adjustment for HBV and HCV serology.[22,23]

Aflatoxin

Exposure to aflatoxins is probably also an important contributor to the high incidence of HCC in the tropical areas, where aflatoxin B1 is a frequent contaminant of grains and legumes. In fact, many epidemiologic studies have shown that the incidence of HCC parallels the prevalence of aflatoxin-contaminated food products.[24] In a case-control study of 18,000 persons of China, the ingestion of aflatoxin increased the relative risk for HCC 3.4 fold. Interestingly, the same study has found that the relative risk for HCC rose to 59 for persons with both aflatoxin and HBV biomarkers.[25] Several animal studies have revealed that HCC may develop in rats feeding with aflatoxin B1 in a dose-dependent pattern, and feeding with aflatoxin may greatly increase the development of HCC in transgenic mice with integrated HBV DNA.[24] There appear to be a multiplicative interaction between aflatoxin ingestion and chronic HBV infection, suggesting different carcinogenic mechanisms. A similar interaction with chronic HCV infection has not been documented. Aflatoxin is a strong mutagen that may result in covalent binding to DNA through epoxidation. However, the exact mechanisms by which aflatoxins cause HCC are not fully understood.

Other risk factors

HCC also develops in patients with autoimmune or metabolic liver diseases, including autoimmune hepatitis, primary biliary cirrhosis, genetic hemochromatosis, porphyria cutanea tarda, tyrosinemia, citrullinemia, glycogenosis, Wilson disease, hereditary fructose intolerance, and α1–antitrypsin deficiency. Male patients with primary biliary cirrhosis have an increased risk of HCC when they develop cirrhosis, with an estimated yearly incidence of 6%.[26] The probability for the development of HCC in patients with genetic hemochromatosis is approximately 5% per year, and combination with age over 55 years, alcohol abuse, and viral hepatitis is associated with a 150-fold increased risk for the development of HCC in these patients.[27] The incidence in Wilson disease and autoimmune hepatitis is poorly defined and apparently is lower than in other etiological groups.

Other factors include dietary factors, chemical compounds, oral contraceptives, tobacco, nonalcoholic fatty liver disease, and nutritional factors. Although some dietary constituents have been suspected carcinogens, including alkaloids of senecio, felce, comfrey, and cycads, most of them have not been proven in human. Thorotrast, a colloidal thorium dioxide, was used as an angiographic contrast in 1930s. It accumulates in the macrophages of the reticuloendothelial system, particularly the liver, and emits high levels of radiation with a long half-life. It has been associated with the development of liver cancer.[28] The association between HCC and oral contraceptives is controversial. Several case-control studies conducted in developed countries have shown relative risks between 1.6 and 5.5 among women who have ever used oral contraceptives.[29] However, a collaborative study conducted by World Health Organization (WHO) found no increased risk for the development of HCC in persons taking oral contraceptives.[30] Growing interest is currently focusing on the associations of liver cancer with tobacco, diabetes mellitus, obesity, and nonalcoholic fatty liver disease. Further studies, however, are needed to clarify and quantify the role of these factors in liver cancer.

Surveillance

Surveillance for HCC has become widely applied on the assumption that early recognition and treatment of HCC may reduce the mortality from the disease. Patients at high risk for developing HCC should be entered into surveillance programs. The at-risk groups of patients include Asian male HBV carriers over the age of 40 years, Asian female HBV over the age of 50 years, African HBV carriers over the age of 20 years, HBV carriers with family history of HCC, and patients with cirrhosis from hepatitis B or C, alcoholic liver disease, genetic hemochromatosis, and primary biliary cirrhosis.[31] Screening tests fall into two categories: serological and radiological. α-Fetoprotein (AFP) has been most intensively investigated as serum marker. Receiver operating curve analysis suggests that a value of 20 ng/mL provides the optimal balance between sensitivity and specificity.[32] However, at this level, the sensitivity is only 60%. This may be inadequately sensitive for general use. Other serological tests for diagnosis of HCC include des-γ-carboxy prothrombin,[33] the ratio of glycosylated AFP to total AFP,[34] α fucosidase,[35] and glypican 3.[36] However, none of these can provide sufficient justification for routine use as a screening test. Abdominal ultrasonography is the most widely used tool for surveillance of HCC. Ultrasonography has been reported to have a sensitivity of between 65% and 80% and a specificity greater than 90% as screening test.[37] Its predictive value for HCC is greater than that of serum AFP (54% vs. 32%).[38,39] The major drawback of ultrasonography for HCC screening is that it is operator dependent. Combination of AFP and ultrasonography may increase detection rate, but increase cost and false-positive rate. The surveillance interval remains controversial. It should be determined by the tumor growth rates and not by the degree of risk. A six-month interval for surveillance has been suggested based on tumor doubling times and is considered cost-effective.[9] A single randomized controlled trial (RCT) has shown a survival benefit in HBV-infected patients who were screened with AFP and ultrasonography every six months.[40] However, there is no similar study showing the benefit for any other cause of liver disease. Aging of patients, deterioration of underlying liver disease, and limited access to curative treatment may hamper the effectiveness of surveillance programs for HCC.

Pathology

Based on the gross appearance (Figure 5-1), HCC can be simply classified as nodular, massive, and diffuse. The nodular type may be solitary or multiple well-circumscribed nodules, the massive type refers to a large tumor mass infiltrating surrounding liver parenchyma with satellite nodules, and the diffuse type is characterized by numerous small tumor nodules with diffuse involvement of the liver. For each type, consideration should be given to the presence of accompanying cirrhosis, tumor encapsulation, and macroscopic invasion of major vessels and bile ducts.

Diagnosis of HCC is usually based on the resemblance between tumor cells and normal hepatocytes in terms of both cytologic appearance and the plate-like pattern of growth. According to the histologic features, HCC can be grouped into trabecular, acinar, compact, and scirrhous types, as well as fibrolamellar carcinoma. The trabecular type is composed of well-formed trabeculae of variable cell layers thick and is separated by sinusoids. Fibrosis is minimal or absent. The acinar or pseudoglandular type is characterized by trabeculae with acinar-like spaces (Figure 5-2). The spaces are not true glands, but represent dilated canaliculi filled with cellular debris, exudate, and macrophages. The compact type is composed of solid sheets of tumor cells with inconspicuous sinusoids. In the scirrhous type, significant fibrous tissue separates cords of tumors cells. The fibrolamellar cancer usually occurs in the noncirrhotic livers and is composed of eosinophilic cells arranged in trabeculae that are surrounded by fibrous bands with lamellar stranding. For each histologic type, different grades of HCC are based on the degree of cell differentiation. The WHO grading system divided HCC into well-differentiated, moderately differentiated,

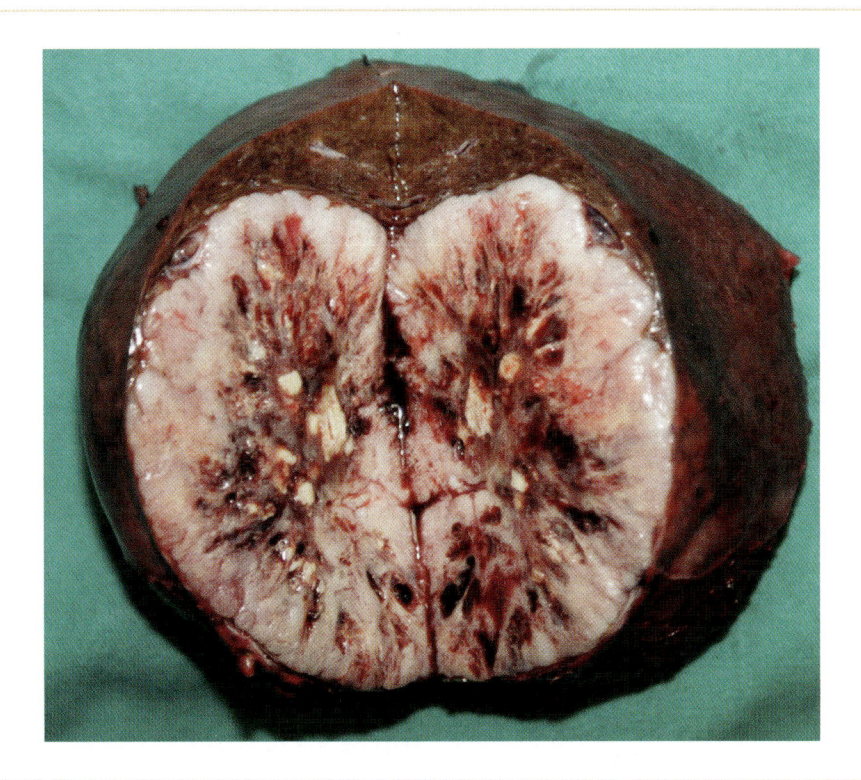

Figure 5-1: Resected specimen of hepatocellular carcinoma in the context of a cirrhotic liver.

poorly differentiated, and undifferentiated types. Despite these classifications and grading of HCC, it is not clear if these variations reflect differences in behavior and influence the prognosis. Combination of HCC and cholangiocarcinoma is composed of a mixture of both HCC and cholangiocarcinoma. These two components may be separate, adjacent to each other, or intimately mixed. One of the explanations for the combined tumor is that hepatocytes and biliary epithelial cells originate from the same pleuripotent progenitor cell.[41] It has been shown that the presence of biliary differentiation is associated with a poor prognosis.[42]

It has been well documented that HCCs develop through a progressive pathway from precancerous lesions to overt malignancies in cirrhotic liver.[43–48] The precancerous lesions proposed by the International Working Party (IWP) of the World Congresses of Gastroenterology comprised microscopic and macroscopic lesions.[49] Microscopic lesions measuring 0.1 cm are referred to dysplastic foci as a cluster of hepatocytes with features of early neoplasia. In particular, small cell dysplasia, consisting of parenchymal cells of smaller size and larger nuclei, is considered direct precursors of HCC.[50] Macroscopic lesions are represented by nodules of more than 0.1 cm in diameter, termed dysplastic nodules (DNs). They can be subclassified into low-grade DNs and high-grade DNs. Low-grade DNs show mild increase in cell density with a monotonous pattern and have no cytologic atypia. Unpaired arteries are sometimes present in small numbers. Low-grade DNs are sometimes vaguely nodular but are often distinct from the surrounding cirrhotic liver due to the presence peripheral fibrous scar. However, it remains difficult to differentiate low-grade DNs and large regenerative nodules, corresponding to nodules of 0.5 cm in diameter, larger than surrounding cirrhotic nodules, without atypia and with no link to neoplasia.[51] Fortunately, this differentiation does not seem to have significant practical consequences at present. High-grade

DNs are characterized by clearly higher cell density than that of surrounding tissue and a higher degree of architectural and/or cytologic atypia.[51] Small cell dysplasia is the most common form of cytologic atypia. Nodule-in-nodule lesions are often present in high-grade DNs. Unpaired arteries are found in most cases, but not in great numbers. High-grade DNs represent borderline lesions of HCC and may be difficult to separate from small well-differentiated HCC (early HCC) (Figure 5-2). Infiltration of the stroma and portal tracts has been employed as a diagnostic criterion to differentiate the two entities. However, recognition of stromal invasion may require experience and the assistance of histochemical and immuohistochemical stains. For instance, cytokeratins 7 or 19 is useful to identify areas of questionable invasion. If such staining indicates a ductular reaction, the focus is considered a pseudoinvasion and does not warrant a diagnosis of HCC.[52]

Currently, the identification of HCC is based not only on a set of cyto-architectural features, but also on a supplement of immunohistology. CD34 immunostaining is useful for visualizing capillarization of sinusoids and for highlighting unpaired arteries. The latter reflects neoangiogenesis, increases in number from early to fully malignant lesions. AFP is a well-established serum marker for diagnosis of HCC, but may not be helpful as tissue marker because of low sensitivity (25% to 30%).[51] Some histochemical markers of malignant transformation have been employed in diagnosis of HCC, including glypican-3 (GPC3), glutamine synthetase (GS), and heat shock protein 70 (HSP70). The immunostaining pattern of GPC3, a cell-surface heparan sulfate proteoglycans that is secreted into the plasma, is usually cytoplasmic but may be membranous or canalicular. It has been shown that GPC3 has a sensitivity of 77% and specificity of 96%, respectively, in the identification of small HCC.[53,54] GS is a catalyst in the synthesis of glutamine from glutamate and ammonia. Of interest, GS is a target gene of β-catenin so that its overexpression is associated with mutations of β-catenin or with activation of this pathway.[55,56] GS immunoreactivity can be seen in 50% of human HCC[57] and has a stepwise increase from precancerous lesions to early HCC to progressed HCC.[58] HSP70 belongs to a class of genes implicated in the regulation of cell cycle, in apoptosis, and in tumorigenesis.[59,60] The immunoreactivity of HSP70 is nucleocytoplasmic and mostly focal with a sensitivity of 70% for identification of CC.[60,61] Using a panel of these three markers,

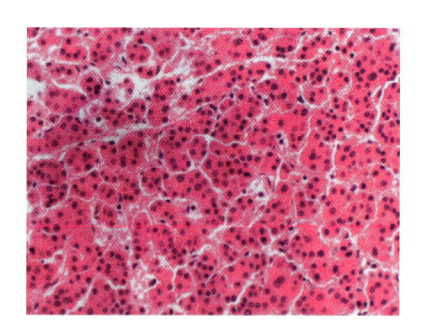

Figure 5-2: Well-differentiated hepatocellular carcinoma composed of trabeculae with various degrees of thickness (hematoxylin and eosin, 100×magficication).

when at least two of them were positive, the sensitivity and specificity for the detection of early HCC were, respectively, 72% and 100%.[61] In addition, new immunohistochemical markers are still under investigation and are likely to prove useful.[62,63]

Diagnosis

HCC usually presents at a very late stage in its natural history because of the lack of symptoms at the early stage. The signs and symptoms are associated with both severity of underlying liver disease and tumor volume. In HCC with normal liver or milder cirrhosis, symptoms related to tumor growth and features of advanced malignancy, such as abdominal distension, weight loss, fever, anorexia, and malaise, are the common findings. In the presence of moderate or severe cirrhosis, clinical presentations of liver failure and portal hypertension, such as ascites, jaundice, tremor, confusion, and encephalopathy, are the predominant features. The right upper quadrant pain occurs in approximately 50% of patients with HCC and varies in intensity from a simple sensation of discomfort through a mild dull ache to a severe unrelenting pain. The onset of acute pain may be triggered by complications related to the tumor, such as spontaneous rupture or intratumoral hemorrhage.

The tests used to diagnose HCC include radiology, biopsy, and AFP serology. An association with chronic liver disease, hypervascularity in arterial phase and washout in venous phase on triphasic computed tomography (CT) and magnetic resonance

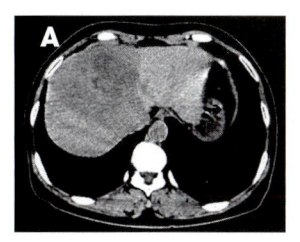

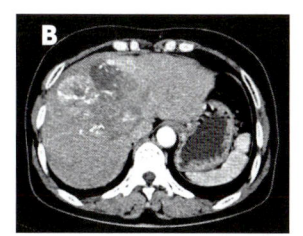

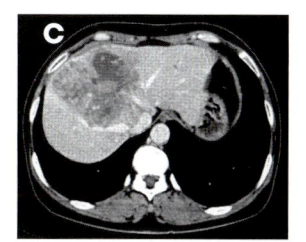

Figure 5-3: Contrast-enhanced computed tomogram. (A) Hepatocellular carcinoma appears as a hypodense mass in the precontrast phase; (B) significantly enhancing tumor in the arterial phase; (C) fast washout in the portal phase.

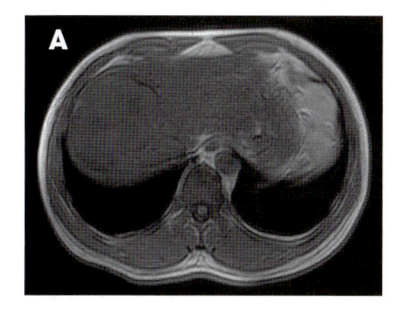

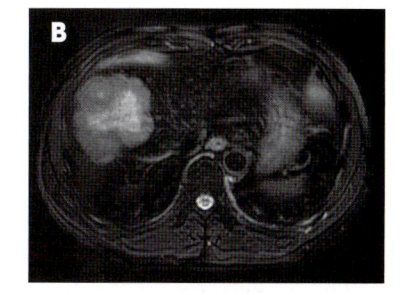

Figure 5-4: Magnetic resonance imaging of an encapsulated hepatocellular carcinoma. (A) a large hypointense heterogeneous mass in the T1-weighted image; (B) hyperintense in the T2-weighted image.

imaging (MRI), and elevated serum level of AFP (>200 ng/mL) are diagnostic for HCC (Figures 5-3 and 5-4). Ultrasound is conventionally used as a screening tool and a guide for percutaneous biopsy due to its wide availability and lack of radiation. In recent studies, however, contrast-enhanced ultrasound shows comparable accuracy and specificity with CT and MRI[64,65] and may be used for noninvasive diagnosis. The American Association for the Study of Liver Disease (AASLD) proposed a set of criteria to establish HCC diagnosis in patients with cirrhosis.[31] The diagnostic algorithm depends on the size of the nodule found on surveillance ultrasound. If the nodule is larger than 2 cm in the setting of cirrhosis and has the typical vascular pattern (i.e., hypervascularity in arterial phase and washout in venous phase) on a dynamic imaging, it should be treated as HCC. For nodules between 1 and 2 cm, HCC may be confidently diagnosed by the coincidental findings of two dynamic imaging techniques showing typical features. Biopsy is recommended if the vascular profile on imaging is not characteristic or is not coincidental among techniques. If the nodule is less than 1 cm, patients should be followed by ultrasound or CT scan at 3–6 monthly intervals because it is difficult to diagnose it with current diagnostic tools. These criteria have been validated[64] and have been increasingly applied in clinical practice. The differential diagnosis of HCC includes DN, adenoma, cholangiocarcinoma, focal nodular hyperplasia, and metastatic carcinoma.

Staging Systems

The staging system is crucial in the management of cancer since it helps to predict the prognosis, to stratify the patients in clinical trials, to allow the exchange of information between institutions, and to guide treatment decisions. HCC represents a particular challenge to develop an ideal staging system. The prognosis of patients and potential treatment approaches are dependent on both the extent of the tumor and the underlying liver function. Nowadays, hepatologists may choose among several different staging systems, but which is the preferred system remains controversial. The variables in each staging system are different, reflecting the heterogeneous methodology and population used to construct the models (Table 5-2).

It is recommended that the staging system takes into account four related aspects: tumor stage, liver function, physical status, and treatment efficacy.[9] The Barcelona Clinic Liver Cancer (BCLC) staging system was developed on the basis of the combination of data derived from several cohort studies and RCTs by the Barcelona group. This classification includes variables related to tumor stage, liver functional status, physical status, and cancer-related symptoms and links the five stages with treatment modalities. It identifies those at very early or early stage who are candidates for curative therapies, those at intermediate or advanced disease stage who may benefit from chemoembolization and new agents, and those at terminal stage with a very poor life expectancy.[8] Currently, attempts to improve the classification and prognosis prediction of HCC are underway. Genomic and proteomic studies will characterize HCC more accurately, such that in future patients with HCC may be classified and treated according to their molecular profile.

Treatment

Historically, the prognosis of patients with HCC has been poor because of late diagnosis, the aggressiveness of the tumor and underlying cirrhosis. However, the success of surveillance programs and the advances in radiologic imaging techniques have led to earlier detection of small HCCs that are amenable to curative treatments. Multiple modalities are currently available to treat HCC. Liver resection, liver transplantation, and local ablation are widely accepted as the curative treatments because these therapies may offer a high rate of complete response in properly selected candidates. Noncurative treatments include transarterial chemoembolization (TACE), radiotherapy, immunotherapy, and systemic chemotherapy. The benefits of treatments should be evaluated through RCTs and meta-analysis. However, virtually no mega-RCTs have compared the efficacy of available treatments, especially for early-stage disease. Any proposed treatment strategy has to be developed based on the analysis of cohort studies of treated individuals. Given the complexity of the disease and the large number of potentially

TABLE 5-2: Variables in Staging Systems for Hepatocellular Carcinoma

Classifications	Tumor stage	α-Fetoprotein	Liver function	Health status
TNM	Number and size of tumor, portal invasion, metastasis	No	No	No
Okuda	50% liver involvement	No	Ascites, albumin, bilirubin	No
CLIP	Number of tumor, 50% liver involvement, portal invasion	400 ng/mL	Child-Pugh	No
BCLC	Number and size of tumor, Okuda, portal invasion, metastasis	No	Child-Pugh, portal hypertension, bilirubin	Performance status
CUPI	TNM	500 ng/mL	Bilirubin, ascites, alkaline phosphatase	Presence of Symptoms
JIS	TNM	No	Child-Pugh	No
GRETCH	Portal invasion	35 μg/L	Bilirubin, alkaline phosphatase	Karnofsky
ER	Estrogen receptor	No	No	No

useful therapies, patients with HCC should be referred to multidisciplinary teams involving surgeons, hepatologists, radiologists, oncologists, and pathologists.

Liver resection

Liver resection is the mainstay of curative therapy for localized HCCs in patients with well-preserved hepatic function. Over the past decades, long-term survival after resection of HCCs has greatly improved. Many large series have reported five-year overall survival rates of approximately 40% to 50% (Table 5-3).[66-80] For early stage HCC, long-term survival may reach a 70% rate in patients with preserved hepatic function.[81-83] Early diagnosis of HCC by better imaging modalities, increased detection of subclinical HCC by screening of high-risk patients, and a reduced perioperative transfusion were identified as the major contributory factors for the improved outcomes.[66] The safety of hepatectomy has also increased with an perioperative mortality of less than 3% and a few major centers have reported a 0 mortality rate in large consecutive series.[84-86] This may be attributed to the substantial advances in patient selection, surgical techniques, and perioperative care.

Currently, a new surgical paradigm, "Precision Liver Surgery", has been proposed for the treatment of a great variety of liver disease including HCC.[87,88] The fundamental philosophy underlying precision liver surgery is scientific determinism. It is a certainty-based surgical practice which covers the entire surgical process, including preoperative evaluation, clinical decision-making, surgical planning, operative manipulation and perioperative management. Its goal is to pursue an optimal recovery which mainly accommodates the three objectives of therapeutic effectiveness, surgical safety, and minimal invasiveness. Through evidence-based decision and controllable surgical intervention, a precise balance has to be sought among maximizing the removal of the target lesion, maximizing the functional liver remnant, and minimizing surgical invasiveness (3M). Accurate preoperative evaluation of tumor status and resectability, functional reserve of future liver remnant, and general conditions of patients is essential for selection of candidates for liver resection. The usual criteria for resectability of HCC include complete oncological removal of the tumor, adequate functional reserve and structural integrity of future liver remnant, and patient's tolerability of surgical invasiveness. Large tumor size alone should not be considered a contraindication for liver resection. Recently, liver resection for HCC with major hepatic vein or portal vein invasion is justified because survival benefits may be expected as compared with nonsurgical treatment.[89]

TABLE 5-3: Selected Series (2001–2010) of Hepatic Resection for HCC with More than 200 Patients

First author, Reference Year	No. of pts.	Cirrhosis	Mortality	5-y OS rate
Zhou[69] 2001	2366	—	2.7%	50%
Kanematsu[70] 2002	303	55%	1.6%	51%
Belghiti[71] 2002	328	50%	6.4%	37%
Wayne[72] 2002	249	73%	6.1%	41%
Ercolani[73] 2003	224	100%	—	42%
Chen[74] 2004	525	91%	2.7%	17%
Wu[75] 2005	426	100%	1.6%	46%–61%[d]
Capussotti[76] 2005	216	100%	8.3%	34%
Hasegawa[88,77] 2005	210	39%	0.0%	35%–66%[d]
Nathan[78] 2009	788	—	—	39%
Yang[79] 2009	481	77%	1.7%	20%–48%[d]
Wang[80] 2010	438	—	7.5%	43%

Abbreviations: OS = overall survival; pts = patients.
[d] Range of 5-y OS among different subgroups.

The major cause of postoperative mortality after liver resection for HCC is hepatic failure due to insufficient remnant liver function. Preoperative prediction of the volume of the functional liver remnant can be accomplished with modern imaging modalities. The resection of up to 80% of the total liver volume is safe and feasible in young patients (≤40 years of age) with normal liver parenchyma.[90] However, liver resection should be conservative in the presence of underlying live disease or in elderly patients. The cirrhotic liver tolerates acute tissue loss poorly because of its impaired function and decreased ability to regenerate.[91]

Currently, there is no consensus on the extent of liver resection in patients with cirrhosis. The evaluation most commonly used relies on the Child-Pugh classification, which is based on a scoring system that includes serum levels of bilirubin and albumin, international normalized ratio, and the presence or absence of ascites and hepatic encephalopathy (Table 5-4).[92] In general, liver resection is offered to Child-Pugh class A and selected Child-Pugh class B patients. However, the predictive value of Child-Pugh classification is not consistent. Not all class A patients have the same degree of liver reserve. Therefore, many centers have employed more sophisticated quantitative liver function tests such as indocyanine green (ICG) clearance test and galactose elimination capacity.[93–96] ICG retention at 15 minutes of less than 14% was identified as the safety limit of major hepatectomy defined as resection of three or more hepatic segments.[97] In contrast, in Western countries, patient selection is usually based on the assessment of the presence of portal hypertension and the serum level of bilirubin.[97] According to the BCLC staging system, the best candidates for hepatectomy are patients with single asymptomatic HCC with preserved liver function, which was defined by the absence of clinically relevant portal hypertension (hepatic venous pressure gradient less than 10 mm Hg, absence of varices or splenomegaly, and platelet count higher than 100,000/mm^3) and normal bilirubin level.[98]

In China, an expert consensus has recently been proposed to assess the hepatic functional reserve and to quantify the safety limit of liver resection, which significantly expands the indications for liver resection, with no increase in post-hepatectomy liver failure (Figure 5-5). According to the Chinese consensus, the safety limit for liver resection depends on the minimal functional liver volume required for body needs, termed the essential functional liver volume (EFLV). The EFLV is based mainly on the standard liver volume and the status of the functional liver reserve. R_{SE}, here, represents the standard ratio of the EFLV to standard liver volume, and R_{SR} represents the standard ratio of the functional volume of liver remnant to standard liver volume. The prerequisite for a safe liver resection is that R_{SR} should be higher than R_{SE}. In detail, R_{SE} should be 0.20 for major hepatectomy in patients with normal liver. For the cirrhotic cases with liver function in Child A class, if ICG R15 is less than 10%, R_{SE} should be 0.40. If ICG R15 ranges from 10% to 20%, R_{SE} should be 0.60, and 0.80 for cases with ICG R15 between 21% and 30%, respectively. Patients can only undergo limited liver resection with ICG R15

TABLE 5-4: Child-Pugh Score[a]

Biochemical and clinical criteria	Points 1	2	3
Total bilirubin (mg/dL)	<2.0	2.0–3.0	>3.0
Albumin (g/L)	>35	28–35	<28
International normalized ratio (INR)	<1.7	1.7–2.2	>2.2
Encephalopathy	None	Grade I or II (or suppressed with medication)	Grade III or IV (or refractory)
Ascites	None	Moderate (or suppressed with medication)	Tense (or refractory)

[a] Patients are grouped into classes according to the cumulative score as follows: grade A (5–6 points, indicating well-compensated disease), grade B (7–9 points, significant functional compromise), and grade C (10–15 points, decompensated disease).

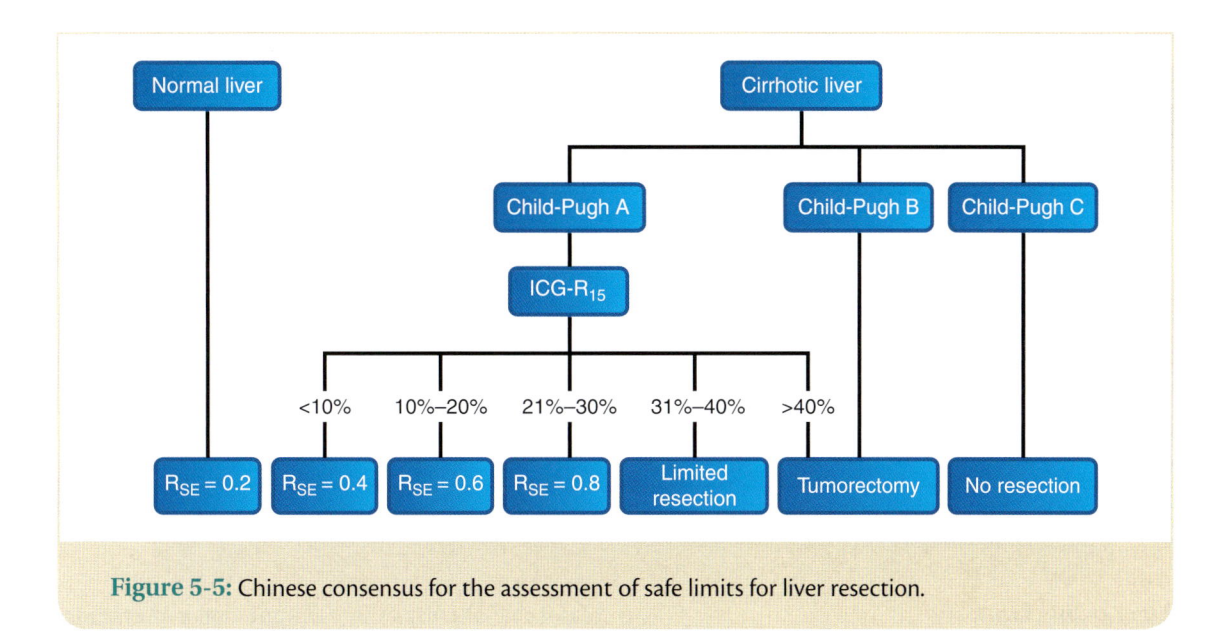

Figure 5-5: Chinese consensus for the assessment of safe limits for liver resection.

ranging from 31% to 40%. When ICG R15 is over 40% or liver function is in Child B class, the tumorectomy becomes the only suitable procedure. Child C class is a contraindication for surgery.

The degree of liver dysfunction does not just influence operative function. The degree of cirrhosis is also a predictor of tumor recurrence.[99] With regard to the BCLC staging system, it should also be noted that well-selected patients with stage C cancer can have good long-term cancer outcomes.[100]

For some unresectable HCC, downstaging treatments including TACE, chemotherapy and radiation therapy can reduce the size and number of tumors to facilitate secondary radical resection.

The major principle of oncologic resection is to eliminate the target lesion en bloc with an adequate tumor-negative margin using tumor-free approaches. The type of hepatectomy performed is dictated by the size and location of the tumor. Liver resection is usually segmental based on Couinaud's segmental hepatic anatomy. Anatomic resection according to the architecture of the portal vein has the potential to remove undetected cancerous foci disseminated from the primary gross tumor through the portal venous system. A few studies have shown that anatomical hepatectomy achieve significantly better overall and disease-free survival than limited hepatectomy in patients with small and solitary HCC.[101–103] Intraoperative ultrasound is a very helpful tool to localize small tumor, detect previously unidentified tumors, and identify parenchymal transection plane combined with injection of dye into the feeding portal branch of tumor-bearing segments. During liver parenchymal transection, a Pringle maneuver may be used to occlude the hepatic inflow to minimize blood loss. To avoid forceful retraction and mobilization of the liver, some centers have utilized the anterior approach, in which the liver is transected from the anterior surface of the liver down to the anterior surface of the inferior vena cava (IVC) after hilar control of the vascular inflow and without prior mobilization of the right lobe containing the tumor. The right lobe is detached from the IVC and the diaphragm after completion of transection. This approach may reduce blood loss, hospital mortality, pulmonary metastasis, and tumorrecurrence as compared with the conventional approach.[104–106] For some unresectable HCC, downstaging treatments including TACE, chemotherapy and radiation therapy can reduce the size and number of tumors to facilitate secondary radical resection.

However, the recurrence rate after hepatectomy remains high (>70% at five years).[82,107–109] Predictors of recurrence are presence of tumor in resection margins, vascular invasion, satellites, and tumor size.[81,110]

Of note, even when recurrence occurs, repeat surgical resection may be a safe and effective option for treatment (Table 5-5).[111–118] Many series have shown that repeat resection can be performed with an operative mortality of less than 3% and with a five-year survival of 40% to 50%.[111–118]

TABLE 5-5: Selected Series of Repeat Hepatic Resection for HCC with More than 20 Patients

First author/Year	No. of pts. (initial resection)	No. of pts. (repeat resection)	Cirrhosis	Minor resections	Mortality	5-y OS rate
Shimada[111] 1998	312	41 (13%)	59%	95%	—	42%
Sugimachi[112] 2001	474	78 (16%)	b	b	0%	47%
Minagawa[113] 2003	334	67 (20%)	69%	91%	0%	56%
Itamoto[114] 2007	483	84 (17%)	67%	87%	0%	50%
Liang[115] 2008	853	44 (5%)	b	82%	0%	28%
Wu[116] 2009	1177	149 (13%)	78%	83%	1%	59%
Nagamo[117] 2009	231	24 (10%)	b	96%	0%	51%
Faber[118] 2011	483	27 (6%)	59%	52%	0%	42%

Abbreviations: OS, overall survival; pts, patients.
[a] Minor resections are defined as ≤ segmentectomy.
[b] Not defined.

Liver transplantation

Theoretically, liver transplantation offers the best chance of cure for HCC patients with cirrhosis since it removes both tumors and preneoplastic lesions that are present in the cirrhotic liver. In addition, it simultaneously cures the underlying liver disease and prevents the development of morbidities associated with portal hypertension and liver failure. In early experiences, however, broad selection criteria led to poor results in terms of recurrence and long-term survival (20% to 40% at five years). The optimal candidates for liver transplantation are patients with early HCC (single HCC < 5 cm or up to three nodules < 3 cm without extrahepatic or vascular spread). This selection criteria (Milan criteria) prompt survival rates of more than 70% at five years and recurrence rates less than 15%.[119] Regarding the stringent selection criteria, expansion of criteria beyond Milan and downstaging HCC to Milan have been attempted in some centers.[120–123] Successful tumor downstaging can be achieved in the majority of carefully selected patients with TACE and radiofrequency ablation (RFA), either alone or in combination.[121] The major drawback of liver transplantation is the shortage of donor organs. The increase of waiting time has led 20% to 50% of the candidates to drop out before receiving transplantation, thus curtailing the outcomes if analyzed according to intention-to-treat. Several strategies have been developed to shorten the waiting times, including giving priority to patients with HCCC, applying adjuvant therapy while on the waiting list and expanding the donor pool. The living donor liver transplantation (LDLT) has emerged as a reasonable alternative to cadaveric donor liver transplantation. It offers a substantial advantage for patients with early-stage HCC who otherwise have to wait for a long time. However, a higher recurrence rate was observed in LDLT despite standard radiological selection criteria based on tumor number and size.[124,125] This may be the result from the selection bias for other clinical characteristics and tumor-enhancing effects of cytokines, growth factors, and transcription factors associated with liver regeneration.[124] More studies are needed to determine whether additional clinical characteristics should be included as selection criteria in LDLT for patients with HCC.

Much debate has involved the relative merits of liver transplantation versus liver resection for patients with small HCC and adequate hepatic reserve. Currently, a resection first with salvage transplantation for recurrence approach is favored, especially for geographic regions with a high incidence of HCC and a low availability of donor livers. Indeed, data comparing liver resection to transplantation are becoming available and indicate similar overall survival rates for primary resection and primary OLT for transplantable HCC (Table 5-6).[126–135]

Local ablation

Local ablative therapy is the therapeutic option for small unresectable HCCs. Treatment modalities include the injection of chemical substances (ethanol and acetic acid) and the modification of local temperature by radiofrequency, microwave, laser, and cryotherapy. Apart from percutaneous intervention

TABLE 5-6: Recent Studies Comparing Longterm Outcome of HCC Patients Treated Primarily with Resection (and Salvage Transplantation) or Primary Liver Transplantation

First author/Year	Primary therapy	Sample Size	5-y OS rate	5-y DFS rate
Lee[126] 2010	Transplantation	78	68%	75%[a]
	Resection	130	52%	50%
Facciuto[127] 2009	Transplantation	119	62%	—
	Resection	60	61%	—
Del Gaudio[128] 2008	Transplantation	147	58%	54%
	Resection	80	66%	41%
Shah[129] 2007	Transplantation	140	64%	78%[a]
	Resection	121	56%	60%
Poon[130] 2007	Transplantation	85	44%	64%[a]
	Resection	228	60%	39%
Margarit[131] 2005	Transplantation	36	50%	—
	Resection	37	78%	—
Bigourdan[132] 2003	Transplantation	17	71%	80%[a]
	Resection	20	36%	40%[a]
Adam[133] 2003	Transplantation	195	61%	58%[a]
	Resection	98	50%	18%
Belghiti[134] 2003	Transplantation	70	—	59%
	Resection	18	—	61%
Figueras[135] 2000	Transplantation	85	60%	60%[a]
	Resection	35	51%	31%

Abbreviations: DFS, disease-free survival; OS, overall survival.
[a]Significant difference as reported in the original study.
[b]Four-year survival rates are reported for patients meeting the Milan criteria.
Source: Adapted from Rahbari NN, Mehrabi A, Mollberg NM, et al.[84] Hepatocellular carcinoma. Current management and perspectives for the future. Ann Surg 2011;253:453–469, Table 3, with permission from Lippincott Williams & Wilkins, US.

under ultrasound guidance, these techniques can also be applied in open or laparoscopic procedure. Percutaneous ablation achieves complete responses in more than 80% of tumors smaller than 3 cm in diameter, but in 50% of tumors of 3 to 5 cm in size.[136] Percutaneous ethanol injection (PEI) and RFA are the two most commonly used techniques for tumor ablation. Long-term studies have shown that five-year survival rate ranged from 40% to 70% in patients with small HCCs after PEI or RFA.[137–139] In several RCTs, RFA was superior to PEI with respect to local recurrence, overall and disease-free survival, especially in tumors > 2 cm.[140–142] However, the major drawback of RFA is its higher rate (up to 10%) of adverse events including pleural effusion and peritoneal bleeding.[143,144] The therapeutic response should be evaluated one month after ablation by a combination of contrast-enhanced imaging (ultrasonography, CT, or MRI) and serum tumor markers. Although not entirely reliable, the absence of enhancement within the neoplastic tissue is considered complete response. The recurrence rate after local ablation is as high as for liver resection. The incidence of local recurrence ranged from 4% to 17% mainly due to the persistence of microscopic satellites around the primary tumor.

Locoregional treatments

Locoregional treatments include transarterial embolization, transarterial chemotherapy, TACE, and transarterial radioembolization. HCC is mostly dependent on the hepatic artery for blood supply, which provides the rationale to support arterial embolization as an effective therapeutic option for HCC. TACE is the most widely used locoregional treatment for unresectable HCCs. It combines the effect of targeted chemotherapy with that of tumor necrosis induced by arterial embolization. The hepatic artery embolization can be achieved by injection of lipiodol (iodized oil) and placement of particles, such as gelfoam, starch microspheres, or metallic coils. Doxorubicin, mitomycin, and cisplatin are the commonly used antitumoral regimens. However, there has not been any standard protocol in the choice of embolization modalities and chemotherapeutic agents. According to conventional WHO criteria, TACE may achieve partial responses in 15% to 55% of patients and significantly delay tumor progression and vascular invasion.[145–148] Response to treatment is associated with a significant improvement in the overall survival of patients. Cumulative meta-analysis of all published RCTs showed modest survival benefits of TACE as compared with control groups.[145] It is interesting to note that the positive RCTs use more strict criteria in the selection of patients for TACE.[146,147] The ideal candidates should be patients with preserved liver function and asymptomatic multinodular tumors without major vascular invasion or extrahepatic spread. Treatment response can be determined by the decrease in the serum level of tumor markers and reduction in tumor burden in dynamic CT or MRI. The postembolization syndrome, which consists of fever, abdominal pain, nausea, vomiting, leukocytosis, and increase in liver enzymes, may be experience in 80% to 90% of TACE procedures. However, it is self-limiting in most patients. TACE may cause acute cholecystitis, biliary tract necrosis, pancreatitis, and gastric erosion or ulcers if the chemoembolization agents are inadvertently injected into these organs. Hepatic failure may also develop after TACE in patients with liver decompensation. Recently, several strategies to improve antitumor activity have been developed, including administration of drug-eluting beads containing chemotherapeutic agents and internal radiation with 131-I-labelled lipiodol or Y-90.[149–151] Further phase III trials are required to determine the benefits of these treatments.

Systemic treatments

The administration of tamoxifen, an estrogen receptor blocker, was initially reported to prolong survival in patients with advanced HCC.[152,153] However, this result has not been confirmed by larger well-designed RCTs.[154–157] A meta-analysis of seven RCTs comparing tamoxifen and conservative management showed neither antitumoral effects nor survival benefit of tamoxifen.[144] Therefore, tamoxifen should not be recommended in advanced HCC. Systemic chemotherapy with conventional agents showed limited antitumoral activity, but unfortunately no impact on patient survival. These drugs such as doxorubicin and cisplatin may produce partial responses in only 10% to 15% of patients and durable remission is rare.[158] Theoretically, combination therapy with different active agents can improve the response rate, but this also carries with it higher toxicity. In a large RCT comparing combination therapy (cisplatin, interferon α, doxorubicin, and fluorouracil) with single-agent therapy (doxorubicin),[159] the response rates were 20.9% for the combination therapy and 10.5% for the single-agent therapy. The median survival of the combination and the single-agent chemotherapies was 8.67 and 6.83 months, respectively, without significant difference between two groups. The combination therapy was associated with a higher rate of morbidity and mortality as compared with the single-agent therapy. There are several other treatment modalities such as octreotide, interferon, external radiation, antiandrogenic therapy, but none have been documented to improve survival.[160–163]

Advances in systemic treatment were underscored by the introduction of molecular targeted therapies in HCC. A number of studies have identified different signaling pathways in the pathogenesis of HCC, providing a potential source of novel molecular targets for new therapies.[164,165] Sorafenib, an oral multikinase inhibitor with activity against several tyrosine kinase and serine/threonine kinases, is the first approved medication for the molecular targeted therapy of HCC. The randomized phased III double-blind placebo-controlled clinical trial has shown significantly increase in survival of three months in patients with advanced HCC treated with sorafenib.[166] This gives hope for further advances in therapy during the exploration of the potential efficacy of sorafenib and other promising agents in combination with other treatment modalities.

Hepatoblastoma

Epidemiology

Hepatoblastoma is the most common malignant tumor of the liver in children, accounting for 79% of liver cancer in children under the age of 15. The incidence of hepatoblastoma is highest in infants (11.2 per million) and falls off rapidly, with most cases occurring before the age of 5.[167] The overall sex ratio ranges from 1.5 to 3.3 (male:female).[167–169] It has been shown that the development of hepatoblastoma was associated with low birth weight.[170–172] Compared with children weighting 2500 g or more, the relative risk of hepatoblastoma among children weighting less than 1000 g, 1000 to 1499 g, 1500 to 1999 g, and 2000 to 2499 g were is 15.64, 2.53, 2.71, and 1.21, respectively, suggesting the lower the birth weight, the higher the risk of hepatoblastoma.[171] In addition, a variety of conditions have been associated with an increased risk for the development of hepatoblastoma, including Bechwith-Wiedemann syndrome, familial polyposis coli, Gardner syndrome, synchronous Wilms tumor, hemihypertrophy, alcohol embryopathy, rhabdomyosarcoma, and congenital anomalies.[173] However, the extent of risk is difficult to determine because of the rarity of hepatoblastoma.

Pathology

Hepatoblastoma occurs as a single mass in around 80% of cases. Histologically, it can be classified as epithelial (56%) and mixed epithelial/mesenchymal (44%).[174] Epithelial hepatoblastoma can be subdivided into four patterns, including fetal epithelial, embryonal and fetal epithelial, macrotrabecular, and small cell undifferentiated. The most common mesenchymal elements are osteoid and cartilage. The tumor cells appear smaller than normal hepatocytes. Hepatoblastoma displays distinct extramedullary hematopoiesis, but no significant ductular differentiation. The fetal histologic subtype or the presence of mesenchymal elements has been shown to be associated with improved prognosis. In contrast, small cell undifferentiated histology is associated with a poor prognosis.[175] Multiple cytogenetic abnormalities have been noted in hepatoblastoma, including a high incidence of trisomies 2, 8, and 20 and rearrangement of chromosome 1q.[176,177]

Diagnosis

The most common presenting feature of the tumor is an enlarging abdominal mass. Accompanying symptoms such as anorexia, abdominal pain, weight loss, nausea, vomiting, and jaundice occur in smaller numbers of cases. The serum level of alpha-fetoprotein is elevated in 90% of cases, and anemia develops in 70%.[178] The levels of bilirubin and liver enzymes are usually normal. Extrahepatic metastasis occurs in 10% to 20% of patients with the lung being the predominant site of metastasis.[179] CT and MRI are helpful in differentiation diagnosis and in evaluating liver lesions and their relationship to vascular structures. There has not been a uniformly accepted staging system for patients with hepatoblastoma. The staging system used in the United States for the Intergroup Hepatoma Studies is based on the resectability of the tumor, that is, complete resection for stage I, microscopic residual tumor for stage II, macroscopic residual, unresectable or tumor rupture for stage III, metastatic tumor for stage IV.[168] The Japanese Society of Pediatric Surgery has adopted a classification based on the TNM staging.[180] The staging proposed by International Society of Pediatric Oncology is based on the number of involved hepatic sectors.[181]

Treatment

Surgical resection offers the only chance of cure for patients with hepatoblastoma and is the treatment of choice in approximately half of patients. The technical details of liver resection in children are similar to those described in adults. Several studies support the effectiveness of chemotherapy combined with surgical resection.[181–184] Preoperative chemotherapy with conventional agents, such as doxorubicin and cisplatin, may result in tumor shrinkage and increase the resectability of hepatoblastoma from 40% to between 60% and 90%.[181] Unfortunately, these chemotherapeutic drugs are associated with significant side effects in children. TACE may offer the advantage of higher tumor concentrations of drugs with lower systemic exposure. However, the potential benefit of TACE over systemic chemotherapy has not been determined.[133] For those unresectable tumors confined in the liver, hepatic transplantation is an effective option with a reported survival of 70% to 80%.[185,186]

Malignancies of Mesenchymal Origin

Primary hepatic malignancies of mesenchymal origin are rare, including angiosarcoma, epithelioid hemangioendothelioma, lymphoma, leiomyosarcoma, rhabdomyosarcoma, fibrosarcoma, and unspecified sarcoma. Most of these tumors occur in adults. These tumors have variable appearances on radiology and present a diagnostic challenge.

Primary Angiosarcoma

Primary angiosarcoma accounts for only 2% of all primary hepatic malignancies, but is the most frequently occurring type of hepatic sarcoma.[187–189] This tumor was found to be associated with environmental or occupational exposure to carcinogens, such as thorium dioxide, vinyl chloride, arsenic, and radiation.[190–192] There was also an association with hemochromatosis and Von Recklinghausen disease.[187] In most reported cases, however, no obvious risk factors can be identified. The gross appearance of hepatic angiosarcoma is characterized by the presence of remarkable necrosis and hemorrhage. Histologically, the tumor is composed of spindle-shaped or pleomorphic malignant endothelial cells. Well-differentiated tumors may have a sinusoidal, papillary, or cavernous form. The sinusoidal pattern is most frequent. The tumor cells are seen to infiltrate the parenchyma and to dissect the hepatocyte cords. Immunostaining with specific antibodies against the phenotype of endothelial cells (CD34, CD31, and factor VIII) helps to establish the diagnosis of angiosarcoma.

Patients with hepatic angiosarcoma usually present late during the course of disease with signs and symptoms of liver disease, pain, and the sensation of abdominal mass. The degree of liver biochemistry derangement tends to reflect the extent of hepatic parenchymal involvement with tumor. The imaging appearance of hepatic angiosarcoma is nonspecific. The diagnosis is best established by tumor biopsy following a suggestive radiologic status. Main differential diagnoses include hemangioma, HCC, and metastases. The clinical course of this malignancy is aggressive, and the prognosis of patients is poor. Surgery has a limited role because most patients have multifocal tumors and extrahepatic metastases at the time of presentation, mostly in the lung and spleen. Liver transplantation is contraindicated due to the high risk for tumor recurrence and short-term survival. The data from European Liver Transplant Registry showed a median survival of only seven months in 17 patients who had undergone liver transplantation for angiosarcoma.[193] The systemic chemotherapy and TACE have been described with very limited value in overall survival improvement.[194,195] This tumor is relatively resistant to radiotherapy.[187]

Epithelioid Hemangioendothelioma

Epithelioid hemangioendothelioma of the liver is a rare vascular tumor with intermediate malignant potential. It occurs most often in adults with a 3:2 preponderance for women.[196] There are no definite risk factors for the development of epithelioid hemangioendothelioma, although liver trauma, oral contraceptive, vinyl chloride, asbestos, and viral hepatitis were implicated.[196,197] The tumor usually consists of multiple nodules that involve both lobes of the liver and range in size from 0.2 to 14 cm.[197] The center of the tumor has a fibrous stoma. Histologically, the tumor is composed of epithelioid and dendritic cells that often contain vacuoles. Immunohistochemically, all tumors were positive for at least one endothelial marker (CD34, CD31, and factor VIII). Two different types have been described.[198] The nodular type is an early manifestation of the disease. The diffuse type reflects advanced-stage disease because of an increase in size and coalescence of the lesions. The most common clinical manifestations are right upper quadrant pain, hepatomegaly, and weight loss. A definitive diagnosis of epithelioid hemangioendothelioma requires histopathologic examination because the imaging findings are not suggestive for vascular tumors.[162] A laparoscopic wedge or core biopsy is sufficient to encompass the architectural features of the tumor, such as the intravascular characteristics.

The natural history of epithelioid hemangioendothelioma is variable and unpredictable, with a clinical course between benign hemangioma and angiosarcoma.[198] Extrahepatic involvement occurs in 30% to 60% of patients and may represent either metastasis or multicentric origin of the tumors.[199] Lung is the most common site of metastases, followed by abdominal lymph nodes, spleen, bone marrow, and peritoneum. The management options for patients with hepatic epithelioid hemangioendothelioma include liver resection, liver transplantation, chemotherapy, radiotherapy, and even follow-up without any therapy. The efficacy of these modalities is difficult to be assessed because of the rarity, heterogeneous status, and variable clinical outcome of the disease. Theoretically, surgical excision is the treatment of choice in patients with limited involvement of the liver. However, liver resection is usually eligible in the majority of patients because of multicentricity of the tumor. For patients with unresectable tumors, liver transplantation remains a reasonable treatment option, even in patients with extrahepatic involvement.[196] The results of liver transplantation are encouraging, with a five-year survival rate of 54.5%.[196] The role of different adjuvant therapies remains to be determined.

diagnosis can be reached only by histopathologic examination.

The prognosis of patients with primary hepatic lymphoma is variable, depending on tumor status, the underlying disease and complications in immunosuppressed patients. Surgery, local ablation, chemotherapy, and radiotherapy, alone or in combination, have been used to the treatment of primary hepatic lymphoma. However, the optimal treatment is still not clear. In localized and resectable tumors, good long-term results have been achieved with surgery alone or combined with chemotherapy.[208,209] The tumors are sensitive to chemotherapy with cyclophosphamide, vincristine, or methotrexate, and multiagent chemotherapy has led to prolonged remissions in some cases.[186]

Primary Hepatic Lymphoma

Primary hepatic lymphoma, which is confined to the liver without involvement of lymph node or bone marrow, is extremely rare. It accounts for about 0.01% of all non-Hodgkin lymphomas.[200,201,202] About 80% of primary hepatic lymphomas are B-cell tumors, whereas the T-cell phenotype accounts for only 8% to 28% of cases.[203] Large cell-type non-Hodgkin lymphoma predominates.[204] The pathogenesis of primary hepatic lymphoma remains unclear. An association between the tumor and immunosuppression has been noted, such as acquired immunodeficiency syndrome, organ transplantation, and chemical immunosuppression.[205,206] In addition, chronic viral infection may be another mechanism of lymphomagenesis, including HCV, Epstein-Barr virus, and herpesvirus.[153,172]

Primary hepatic lymphoma frequently occurs in adults with a four to one male preponderance.[207] Abdominal pain, fever, anorexia, weight loss, night sweats are the presenting clinical features in the majority of patients, but are nonspecific. Unusual presentations include jaundice, ascites, thrombocytopenia, hypercalcemia, and acute liver failure. Liver function test values are altered in 85% of patients, but conventional tumor markers such as AFP and carcinoembryonic antigen are typically negative.[208,209] In most cases, a solitary mass is demonstrated by imaging techniques, although multiple lesions have also been described. There is not a definite characteristic imaging finding for this tumor. The final

References

1. Parkin DM, Bray F, Ferlay J, Pisani P. Global cancer statistics, 2002. *CA Cancer J Clin*. 2005;55:74–108.
2. El-Serag HB, Mason AC. Rising incidence of hepatocellular carcinoma in the United States. *N Engl J Med*. 1999;340:745–750.
3. Fattovich G, Stroffolini T, Zagni I, Donato F. Hepatocellular carcinoma in cirrhosis: incidence and risk factors. *Gastroenterology*. 2004;127:S35–S50.
4. Colombo M, Donato MF. Prevention of hepatocellular carcinoma. *Semin Liver Dis*. 2005;25:155–161.
5. Tsukuma H, Hiyama T, Tanaka S, et al. Risk factors for hepatocellular carcinoma among patients with chronic liver disease. *N Engl J Med*. 1993;328:1797–1801.
6. Bosch FX, Ribes J, Diaz M, Cleries R. Primary liver cancer: worldwide incidence and trends. *Gastroenterology*. 2004;127:S5–S16.
7. McGlynn KA, Tsao L, Hsing AW, et al. International trends and patterns of primary liver cancer. *Int J Cancer*. 2001;94:290–296.
8. Llovet JM, Burroughs A, Bruix J. Hepatocellular carcinoma. *Lancet*. 2003;362:1907–1917.
9. Bruix J, Sherman M, Llovet JM, et al. Clinical management of hepatocellular carcinoma. Conclusions of the Barcelona-2000 EASL conference. European Association for the Study of the Liver. *J Hepatol*. 2001;35:421–430.
10. Rogler CE. Recent advances in hepatitis B viruses and hepatocellular carcinoma. *Cancer Cells*. 1990;2:366–369.

11. Brechot C, Gozuacik D, Murakami Y, Paterlini-Brechot P. Molecular bases for the development of hepatitis B virus (HBV)-related hepatocellular carcinoma (HCC). *Semin Cancer Biol*. 2000;10:211–231.
12. Brechot C. Pathogenesis of hepatitis B virus-related hepatocellular carcinoma: old and new paradigms. *Gastroenterology*. 2004;127:S56–S61.
13. Bonilla Guerrero R, Roberts LR. The role of hepatitis B virus integrations in the pathogenesis of human hepatocellular carcinoma. *J Hepatol*. 2005; 42:760–77.
14. Yen TS. Hepadnaviral X protein: review of recent progress. *J Biomed Sci*. 1996;3:20–30.
15. Donato F, Boffetta P, Puoti M. A meta-analysis of epidemiological studies on the combined effect of hepatitis B and C virus infections in causing hepatocellular carcinoma. *Int J Cancer*. 1998;75:347–354.
16. Liang TJ, Heller T. Pathogenesis of hepatitis C-associated hepatocellular carcinoma. *Gastroenterology*. 2004;127:S62–S71.
17. Ray RB, Steele R, Meyer K, Ray R. Transcriptional repression of p53 promoter by hepatitis C virus core protein. *J Biol Chem*. 1997;272:10983–10986.
18. Moriya K, Fujie H, Shintani Y, et al. The core protein of hepatitis C virus induces hepatocellular carcinoma in transgenic mice. *Nat Med*. 1998;4:1065–1067.
19. Sakamuro D, Furukawa T, Takegami T. Hepatitis C virus nonstructural protein NS3 transforms NIH 3T3 cells. *J Virol*. 1995;69:3893–3896.
20. Di Bisceglie AM, Carithers RL, Jr, Gores GJ. Hepatocellular carcinoma. *Hepatology*. 1998;28: 1161–1165.
21. Yuan JM, Govindarajan S, Arakawa K, Yu MC. Synergism of alcohol, diabetes, and viral hepatitis on the risk of hepatocellular carcinoma in blacks and whites in the U.S. *Cancer*. 2004; 101:1009–1017.
22. Donato F, Tagger A, Chiesa R, et al. Hepatitis B and C virus infection, alcohol drinking, and hepatocellular carcinoma: a case-control study in Italy. Brescia HCC Study. *Hepatology*. 1997;26:579–584.
23. Kuper H, Tzonou A, Kaklamani E, et al. Tobacco smoking, alcohol consumption and their interaction in the causation of hepatocellular carcinoma. *Int J Cancer*. 2000;85:498–502.
24. Wogan GN. Aflatoxin as a human carcinogen. *Hepatology*. 1999;30:573–575.
25. Ross RK, Yuan JM, Yu MC, et al. Urinary aflatoxin biomarkers and risk of hepatocellular carcinoma. *Lancet*. 1992;339:943–946.
26. Howel D, Metcalf JV, Gray J, et al. Cancer risk in primary biliary cirrhosis: a study in northern England. *Gut*. 1999;45:756–760.
27. Fargion S, Fracanzani AL, Piperno A, et al. Prognostic factors for hepatocellular carcinoma in genetic hemochromatosis. *Hepatology*. 1994;20:1426–1431.
28. Doll R, Peto R. The causes of cancer: quantitative estimates of avoidable risks of cancer in the United States today. *J Natl Cancer Inst*. 1981;66:1191–1308.
29. La Vecchia C, Tavani A, Franceschi S, Parazzini F. Oral contraceptives and cancer. A review of the evidence. *Drug Saf*. 1996;14:260–272.
30. Stanford JL, Ray RM, Thomas DB. Combined oral contraceptives and liver cancer. The WHO collaborative study of Neoplasia and steroid contraceptives. *Int J Cancer*. 1989;43:254–259.
31. Bruix J, Sherman M. Management of hepatocellular carcinoma. *Hepatology*. 2005;42:1208–1236.
32. Trevisani F, D'Intino PE, Morselli-Labate AM, et al. Serum alpha-fetoprotein for diagnosis of hepatocellular carcinoma in patients with chronic liver disease: influence of HBsAg and anti-HCV status. *J Hepatol*. 2001;34:570–575.
33. Marrero JA, Su GL, Wei W, et al. Des-gamma carboxyprothrombin can differentiate hepatocellular carcinoma from nonmalignant chronic liver disease in American patients. *Hepatology*. 2003;37:1114–1121.
34. Sato Y, Nakata K, Kato Y, et al. Early recognition of hepatocellular carcinoma based on altered profiles of alpha-fetoprotein. *N Engl J Med*. 1993;328:1802–1806.
35. Giardina MG, Matarazzo M, Morante R, et al. Serum alpha-L-fucosidase activity and early detection of hepatocellular carcinoma: a prospective study of patients with cirrhosis. *Cancer*. 1998;83:2468–2474.
36. Capurro M, Wanless IR, Sherman M, et al. Glypican-3: a novel serum and histochemical marker for hepatocellular carcinoma. *Gastroenterology*. 2003;125:89–97.
37. Bolondi L, Sofia S, Siringo S, et al. Surveillance programme of cirrhotic patients for early diagnosis and treatment of hepatocellular carcinoma: a cost effectiveness analysis. *Gut*. 2001;48:251–259.
38. Colombo M, de Franchis R, Del Ninno E, et al. Hepatocellular carcinoma in Italian patients with cirrhosis. *N Engl J Med*. 1991;325:675–680.
39. Oka H, Tamori A, Kuroki T, et al. Prospective study of alpha-fetoprotein in cirrhotic patients monitored

40. Zhang BH, Yang BH, Tang ZY. Randomized controlled trial of screening for hepatocellular carcinoma. *J Cancer Res Clin Oncol*. 2004;130:417–422.
41. Aterman K. The stem cells of the liver—a selective review. *J Cancer Res Clin Oncol*. 1992;118:87–115.
42. Aishima S, Kuroda Y, Asayama Y, et al. Prognostic impact of cholangiocellular and sarcomatous components in combined hepatocellular and cholangiocarcinoma. *Hum Pathol*. 2006;37:283–291.
43. Sakamoto M, Hirohashi S, Shimosato Y. Early stages of multistep hepatocarcinogenesis: adenomatous hyperplasia and early hepatocellular carcinoma. *Hum Pathol*. 1991;22:172–178.
44. Borzio M, Bruno S, Roncalli M, et al. Liver cell dysplasia is a major risk factor for hepatocellular carcinoma in cirrhosis: a prospective study. *Gastroenterology*. 1995;108:812–817.
45. Le Bail B, Bernard PH, Carles J, et al. Prevalence of liver cell dysplasia and association with HCC in a series of 100 cirrhotic liver explants. *J Hepatol*. 1997;27:835–842.
46. Libbrecht L, Desmet V, Roskams T. Preneoplastic lesions in human hepatocarcinogenesis. *Liver Int*. 2005;25:16–27.
47. Libbrecht L, Craninx M, Nevens F, et al. Predictive value of liver cell dysplasia for development of hepatocellular carcinoma in patients with non-cirrhotic and cirrhotic chronic viral hepatitis. *Histopathology*. 2001;39:66–73.
48. Theise ND, Park YN, Kojiro M. Dysplastic nodules and hepatocarcinogenesis. *Clin Liver Dis*. 2002;6:497–512.
49. Terminology of nodular hepatocellular lesions. International Working Party. *Hepatology*. 1995;22:983–993.
50. Kojiro M, Roskams T. Early hepatocellular carcinoma and dysplastic nodules. *Semin Liver Dis*. 2005;25:133–142.
51. *International Consensus Group for Hepatocellular neoplasia*. Pathologic diagnosis of early hepatocellular carcinoma: a report of the international consensus group for hepatocellular neoplasia. *Hepatology*. 2009;49:658–664.
52. Park YN, Kojiro M, Di Tommaso L, et al. Ductular reaction is helpful in defining early stromal invasion, small hepatocellular carcinomas, and dysplastic nodules. *Cancer*. 2007;109:915–923.
53. Libbrecht L, Severi T, Cassiman D, et al. Glypican-3 expression distinguishes small hepatocellular carcinomas from cirrhosis, dysplastic nodules, and focal nodular hyperplasia-like nodules. *Am J Surg Pathol*. 2006;30:1405–1411.
54. Wang XY, Degos F, Dubois S, et al. Glypican-3 expression in hepatocellular tumors: diagnostic value for preoplastic lesions and hepatocellular carcinomas. *Hum Pathol*. 2006;37:1435–1441.
55. Christa L, Simon MT, Flinois JP, et al. Overexpression of glutamine synthetase in human primary liver cancer. *Gastroenterology*. 1994;106:1312–1320.
56. Zucman-Rossi J, Benhamouche S, Godard C, et al. Differential effects of inactivated Axin1 and activated beta-catenin mutations in human hepatocellular carcinomas. *Oncogene*. 2007;26:774–780.
57. Haussinger D, Sies H, Gerok W. Functional hepatocyte heterogeneity in ammonia metabolism. The intercellular glutamine cycle. *J Hepatol*. 1985;1:3–14.
58. Osada T, Sakamoto M, Nagawa H, et al. Acquisition of glutamine synthetase expression in human hepatocarcinogenesis: relation to disease recurrence and possible regulation by ubiquitin-dependent proteolysis. *Cancer*. 1999;85:819–831.
59. Jolly C, Morimoto RI. Role of the heat shock response and molecular chaperones in oncogenesis and cell death. *J Natl Cancer Inst*. 2000;92:1564–1572.
60. Garrido C, Gurbuxani S, Ravagnan L, Kroemer G. Heat shock proteins: endogenous modulators of apoptotic cell death. *Biochem Biophys Res Commun*. 2001;286:433–442.
61. Di Tommaso L, Franchi G, Park YN, et al. Diagnostic value of HSP70, glypican 3, and glutamine synthetase in hepatocellular nodules in cirrhosis. *Hepatology*. 2007;45:725–734.
62. Llovet JM, Chen Y, Wurmbach E, et al. A molecular signature to discriminate dysplastic nodules from early hepatocellular carcinoma in HCV cirrhosis. *Gastroenterology*. 2006;131:1758–1767.
63. Audard V, Grimber G, Elie C, et al. Cholestasis is a marker for hepatocellular carcinomas displaying beta-catenin mutations. *J Pathol*. 2007;212:345–352.
64. Forner A, Vilana R, Ayuso C, et al. Diagnosis of hepatic nodules 20 mm or smaller in cirrhosis: Prospective validation of the noninvasive diagnostic criteria for hepatocellular carcinoma. *Hepatology*. 2008;47:97–104.
65. Pompili M, Riccardi L, Semeraro S, et al. Contrast-enhanced ultrasound assessment of arterial vascularization of small nodules arising in the cirrhotic liver. *Dig Liver Dis*. 2008;40:206–215.

66. Poon RT, Fan ST, Lo CM, et al. Improving survival results after resection of hepatocellular carcinoma: a prospective study of 377 patients over 10 years. *Ann Surg*. 2001;234:63–70.
67. Grazi GL, Ercolani G, Pierangeli F, et al. Improved results of liver resection for hepatocellular carcinoma on cirrhosis give the procedure added value. *Ann Surg*. 2001;234:71–78.
68. Makuuchi M, Sano K. The surgical approach to HCC: our progress and results in Japan. *Liver Transpl*. 2004;10:S46–S52.
69. Zhou XD, Tang ZY, Yang BH, et al. Experience of 1000 patients who underwent hepatectomy for small hepatocellular carcinoma. *Cancer*. 2001;91:1479–1486.
70. Kanematsu T, Furui J, Yanaga K, et al. A 16-year experience in performing hepatic resection in 303 patients with hepatocellular carcinoma: 1985–2000. *Surgery*. 2002;131:S153–S158.
71. Belghiti J, Regimbeau JM, Durand F, et al. Resection of hepatocellular carcinoma: a European experience on 328 cases. *Hepatogastroenterology*. 2002;49:41–46.
72. Wayne JD, Lauwers GY, Ikai I, et al. Preoperative predictors of survival after resection of small hepatocellular carcinomas. *Ann Surg*. 2002;235:722–730; discussion 30–31.
73. Ercolani G, Grazi GL, Ravaioli M, et al. Liver resection for hepatocellular carcinoma on cirrhosis: univariate and multivariate analysis of risk factors for intrahepatic recurrence. *Ann Surg*. 2003;237:536–543.
74. Chen XP, Qiu FZ, Wu ZD, Zhang BX. Chinese experience with hepatectomy for huge hepatocellular carcinoma. *Br J Surg*. 2004;91:322–326.
75. Wu CC, Cheng SB, Ho WM, et al. Liver resection for hepatocellular carcinoma in patients with cirrhosis. *Br J Surg*. 2005;92:348–355.
76. Capussotti L, Muratore A, Amisano M, et al. Liver resection for hepatocellular carcinoma on cirrhosis: analysis of mortality, morbidity and survival—a European single center experience. *Eur J Surg Oncol*. 2005;31:986–993.
77. Hasegawa K, Kokudo N, Imamura H, et al. Prognostic impact of anatomic resection for hepatocellular carcinoma. *Ann Surg*. 2005;242:252–259.
78. Nathan H, Schulick RD, Choti MA, Pawlik TM. Predictors of survival after resection of early hepatocellular carcinoma. *Ann Surg*. 2009;249:799–805.
79. Yang LY, Fang F, Ou DP, et al. Solitary large hepatocellular carcinoma: a specific subtype of hepatocellular carcinoma with good outcome after hepatic resection. *Ann Surg*. 2009;249:118–123.
80. Wang J, Xu LB, Liu C, et al. Prognostic factors and outcome of 438 Chinese patients with hepatocellular carcinoma underwent partial hepatectomy in a single center. *World J Surg*. 2010;34:2434–2441.
81. Poon RT, Fan ST, Lo CM, et al. Long-term survival and pattern of recurrence after resection of small hepatocellular carcinoma in patients with preserved liver function: implications for a strategy of salvage transplantation. *Ann Surg*. 2002;235:373–382.
82. Llovet JM, Fuster J, Bruix J. Intention-to-treat analysis of surgical treatment for early hepatocellular carcinoma: resection versus transplantation. *Hepatology*. 1999;30:1434–1440.
83. Bruix J, Castells A, Bosch J, et al. Surgical resection of hepatocellular carcinoma in cirrhotic patients: prognostic value of preoperative portal pressure. *Gastroenterology*. 1996;111:1018–1022.
84. Rees M, Plant G, Wells J, Bygrave S. One hundred and fifty hepatic resections: evolution of technique towards bloodless surgery. *Br J Surg*. 1996;83:1526–1529.
85. Torzilli G, Makuuchi M, Inoue K, et al. No-mortality liver resection for hepatocellular carcinoma in cirrhotic and noncirrhotic patients: is there a way? A prospective analysis of our approach. *Arch Surg*. 1999;134:984–992.
86. Fan ST, Lo CM, Liu CL, et al. Hepatectomy for hepatocellular carcinoma: toward zero hospital deaths. *Ann Surg*. 1999;229:322–330.
87. Dong J, Huang Z. Precise liver resection. *Chin J Surg*. 2009;47:1601–1605.
88. Dong JH, Yang SZ, Zeng JP, et al. Precision in Liver Surgery. Semin Liver Dis. 2013;33:189–203.
89. Poon RT, Fan ST, Ng IO, Wong J. Prognosis after hepatic resection for stage IVA hepatocellular carcinoma: a need for reclassification. *Ann Surg*. 2003;237:376–383.
90. Clavien PA, Petrowsky H, DeOliveira ML, Graf R. Strategies for safer liver surgery and partial liver transplantation. *N Engl J Med*. 2007;56:1545–1559.
91. Nagasue N, Yukaya H, Ogawa Y, et al. Human liver regeneration after major hepatic resection. A study of normal liver and livers with chronic hepatitis and cirrhosis. *Ann Surg*. 1987;206:30–39.
92. Pugh RN, Murray-Lyon IM, Dawson JL, et al. Transection of the oesophagus for bleeding oesophageal varices. *Br J Surg*. 1973;60:646–649.

93. Miyagawa S, Makuuchi M, Kawasaki S, Kakazu T. Criteria for safe hepatic resection. *Am J Surg*. 1995;169:589–594.
94. Lau H, Man K, Fan ST, et al. Evaluation of preoperative hepatic function in patients with hepatocellular carcinoma undergoing hepatectomy. *Br J Surg*. 1997;84:1255–1259.
95. Redaelli CA, Dufour JF, Eagner M, et al. Preoperative galactose elimination capacity predicts complications and survival after hepatic resection. *Ann Surg*. 2002;235:77–85.
96. Fan ST, Lai EC, Lo CM, et al. Hospital mortality of major hepatectomy for hepatocellular carcinoma associated with cirrhosis. *Arch Surg*. 1995;130:198–203.
97. Santambrogio R, Kluger MD, Costa M, et al. Hepatic resection for hepatic carcinoma in patients with Child-Pugh's A cirrhosis: is clinical evidence or portal hypertension a contraindication? *HPB (Oxford)*. January 2013;15(1):78–84. Epub 2012 Oct 24.
98. Llovet JM, Fuster J, Bruix J. The Barcelona approach: diagnosis, staging, and treatment of hepatocellular carcinoma. *Liver Transpl*. 2004;10:S115–S120.
99. Hung HH, Lei HJ, Chau GY, et al. Milan criteria, multi-nodularity, and microvascular invasion predict the recurrence patterns of hepatocellular carcinoma after resection. *J Gastrointestinal Surg* 2013;17(4):702–11.
100. Wang JD, Kuo YH, Wang CC, et al. Surgical resection improves the survival of selected hepatocellular carcinoma patients in Barcelona clinic liver cancer Stage C. Dig Liver Dis. 2013;45:510-515.
101. Eguchi S, Kanematsu T, Arii S, et al. Comparison of the outcomes between an anatomical subsegmentectomy and a non-anatomical minor hepatectomy for single hepatocellular carcinomas based on a Japanese nationwide survey. *Surgery*. 2008;143:469–475.
102. Regimbeau JM, Kianmanesh R, Farges O, et al. Extent of liver resection influences the outcome in patients with cirrhosis and small hepatocellular carcinoma. *Surgery*. 2002;131:311–317.
103. Hasegawa K, Kokudo N, Imamura H, et al. Prognostic impact of anatomic resection for hepatocellular carcinoma. *Ann Surg*. 2005;242:252–259.
104. Liu CL, Fan ST, Lo CM, et al. Anterior approach for major right hepatic resection for large hepatocellular carcinoma. *Ann Surg*. 2000;232:25–31.
105. Liu CL, Fan ST, Cheung ST, et al. Anterior approach versus conventional approach right hepatic resection for large hepatocellular carcinoma: a prospective randomized controlled study. *Ann Surg*. 2006;244:194–203.
106. Belghiti J, Guevara OA, Noun R, et al. Liver hanging maneuver: a safe approach to right hepatectomy without liver mobilization. *J Am Coll Surg*. 2001;193:109–111.
107. Okada S, Shimada K, Yamamoto J, et al. Predictive factors for postoperative recurrence of hepatocellular carcinoma. *Gastroenterology*. 1994;106:1618–1624.
108. Shirabe K, Kanematsu T, Matsumata T, et al. Factors linked to early recurrence of small hepatocellular carcinoma after hepatectomy: univariate and multivariate analyses. *Hepatology*. 1991;14:802–805.
109. Poon RT, Fan ST, Lo CM, et al. Intrahepatic recurrence after curative resection of hepatocellular carcinoma: long-term results of treatment and prognostic factors. *Ann Surg*. 1999;229:216–222.
110. Fong Y, Sun RL, Jarnagin W, Blumgart LH. An analysis of 412 cases of hepatocellular carcinoma at a Western center. *Ann Surg*. 1999;229:790–799; discussion 799–800.
111. Shimada M, Takenaka K, Taguchi K, et al. Prognostic factors after repeat hepatectomy for recurrent hepatocellular carcinoma. *Ann Surg*. 1998;227:80–85.
112. Sugimachi K, Maehara S, Tanaka S, Shimada M. Repeat hepatectomy is the most useful treatment for recurrent hepatocellular carcinoma. *J Hepatobiliary Pancreat Surg*. 2001;8:410–416.
113. Minagawa M, Makuuchi M, Takayama T, Kokudo N. Selection criteria for repeat hepatectomy in patients with recurrent hepatocellular carcinoma. *Ann Surg*. 2003;238:703–710.
114. Itamoto T, Nakahara H, Amano H, et al. Repeat hepatectomy for recurrent hepatocellular carcinoma. *Surgery*. 2007;141:589–597.
115. Liang HH, Chen MS, Peng ZW, et al. Percutaneous radiofrequency ablation versus repeat hepatectomy for recurrent hepatocellular carcinoma: a retrospective study. *Ann Surg Oncol*. 2008;15:3484–3493.
116. Wu CC, Cheng SB, Yeh DC, Wang J, P'Eng FK. Second and third hepatectomies for recurrent hepatocellular carcinoma are justified. *Br J Surg*. 2009;96:1049–1057.
117. Nagano Y, Shimada H, Ueda M, et al. Efficacy of repeat hepatic resection for recurrent hepatocellular carcinomas. *ANZ J Surg*. 2009;79:729–733.
118. Faber W, Seehofer D, Neuhaus P, et al. Repeated liver resection for recurrent hepatocellular carcinoma. *J Gastroenterol Hepatol*. 2011;26(7):1189–1194.

119. Mazzaferro V, Regalia E, Doci R, et al. Liver transplantation for the treatment of small hepatocellular carcinomas in patients with cirrhosis. *N Engl J Med*. 1996;334:693–699.
120. Yao FY, Ferrell L, Bass NM, et al. Liver transplantation for hepatocellular carcinoma: comparison of the proposed UCSF criteria with the Milan criteria and the Pittsburgh modified TNM criteria. *Liver Transpl*. 2002;8:765–774.
121. Yao FY, Kerlan RK, Jr, Hirose R, et al. Excellent outcome following down-staging of hepatocellular carcinoma prior to liver transplantation: an intention-to-treat analysis. *Hepatology*. 2008;48:819–827.
122. Cillo U, Vitale A, Grigoletto F, et al. Intention-to-treat analysis of liver transplantation in selected, aggressively treated HCC patients exceeding the Milan criteria. *Am J Transplant*. 2007;7:972–981.
123. Duffy JP, Vardanian A, Benjamin E, et al. Liver transplantation criteria for hepatocellular carcinoma should be expanded: a 22-year experience with 467 patients at UCLA. *Ann Surg*. 2007;246:502–509; discussion 509–511.
124. Lo CM, Fan ST, Liu CL, et al. Living donor versus deceased donor liver transplantation for early irresectable hepatocellular carcinoma. *Br J Surg*. 2007;94:78–86.
125. Fisher RA, Kulik LM, Freise CE, et al. Hepatocellular carcinoma recurrence and death following living and deceased donor liver transplantation. *Am J Transpl*. 2007;7:1601–1608.
126. Lee KK, Kim DG, Moon IS, et al. Liver transplantation versus liver resection for the treatment of hepatocellular carcinoma. *J Surg Oncol*. 2010;101:47–53.
127. Facciuto ME, Rochon C, Pandey M, et al. Surgical dilemma: liver resection or liver transplantation for hepatocellular carcinoma and cirrhosis. Intention-to-treat analysis in patients within and outwith Milan criteria. *HPB (Oxford)*. 2009;11:398–404.
128. Del Gaudio M, Ercolani G, Ravaioli M, et al. Liver transplantation for recurrent hepatocellular carcinoma on cirrhosis after liver resection: University of Bologna experience. *Am J Transpl*. 2008;8:1177–1185.
129. Shah SA, Cleary SP, Tan JC, et al. An analysis of resection vs transplantation for early hepatocellular carcinoma: defining the optimal therapy at a single institution. *Ann Surg Oncol*. 2007;14:2608–2614.
130. Poon RT, Fan ST, Lo CM, et al. Difference in tumor invasiveness in cirrhotic patients with hepatocellular carcinoma fulfilling the Milan criteria treated by resection and transplantation: impact on long-term survival. *Ann Surg*. 2007;245:51–58.
131. Margarit C, Escartin A, Castells L, et al. Resection for hepatocellular carcinoma is a good option in Child-Turcotte-Pugh class A patients with cirrhosis who are eligible for liver transplantation. *Liver Transpl*. 2005;11:1242–1251.
132. Bigourdan JM, Jaeck D, Meyer N, et al. Small hepatocellular carcinoma in Child A cirrhotic patients: hepatic resection versus transplantation. *Liver Transpl*. 2003;9:513–520.
133. Adam R, Azoulay D, Castaing D, et al. Liver resection as a bridge to transplantation for hepatocellular carcinoma on cirrhosis: a reasonable strategy? *Ann Surg*. 2003;238:508–518; discussion 18–19.
134. Belghiti J, Cortes A, Abdalla EK, et al. Resection prior to liver transplantation for hepatocellular carcinoma. *Ann Surg*. 2003;238:885–892; discussion 92–93.
135. Figueras J, Jaurrieta E, Valls C, et al. Resection or transplantation for hepatocellular carcinoma in cirrhotic patients: outcomes based on indicated treatment strategy. *J Am Coll Surg*. 2000;190:580–587.
136. Sala M, Llovet JM, Vilana R, et al. Initial response to percutaneous ablation predicts survival in patients with hepatocellular carcinoma. *Hepatology*. 2004;40:1352–1360.
137. Omata M, Tateishi R, Yoshida H, Shiina S. Treatment of hepatocellular carcinoma by percutaneous tumor ablation methods: ethanol injection therapy and radiofrequency ablation. *Gastroenterology*. 2004;127:S159–S166.
138. Lencioni R, Cioni D, Crocetti L, et al. Early-stage hepatocellular carcinoma in patients with cirrhosis: long-term results of percutaneous image-guided radiofrequency ablation. *Radiology*. 2005;234:961–967.
139. Hasegawa K, Kokudo N, Makuuchi S, et al. Comparison of resection and ablation for hepatocellular carcinoma: a cohort study based on a Japanese nationwide survey. *J Hepatol*. 2013 Apr;58(4):724–9. Epub 2012 Nov 21.
140. Lencioni RA, Allgaier HP, Cioni D, et al. Small hepatocellular carcinoma in cirrhosis: randomized comparison of radio-frequency thermal ablation versus percutaneous ethanol injection. *Radiology*. 2003;228:235–240.
141. Lin SM, Lin CJ, Lin CC, et al. Radiofrequency ablation improves prognosis compared with ethanol injection for hepatocellular carcinoma < or =4 cm. *Gastroenterology*. 2004;127:1714–1723.

142. Shiina S, Teratani T, Obi S, et al. A randomized controlled trial of radiofrequency ablation with ethanol injection for small hepatocellular carcinoma. *Gastroenterology*. 2005;129:122–130.
143. Tateishi R, Shiina S, Teratani T, et al. Percutaneous radiofrequency ablation for hepatocellular carcinoma. An analysis of 1000 cases. *Cancer*. 2005;103:1201–1209.
144. Giorgio A, Tarantino L, de Stefano G, et al. Complications after percutaneous saline-enhanced radiofrequency ablation of liver tumors: 3-year experience with 336 patients at a single center. *AJR Am J Roentgenol*. 2005;184:207–211.
145. Llovet JM, Bruix J. Systematic review of randomized trials for unresectable hepatocellular carcinoma: chemoembolization improves survival. *Hepatology*. 2003;37:429–442.
146. Llovet JM, Real MI, Montana X, et al. Arterial embolisation or chemoembolisation versus symptomatic treatment in patients with unresectable hepatocellular carcinoma: a randomised controlled trial. *Lancet*. 2002;359:1734–1739.
147. Lo CM, Ngan H, Tso WK, et al. Randomized controlled trial of transarterial lipiodol chemoembolization for unresectable hepatocellular carcinoma. *Hepatology*. 2002;35:1164–1171.
148. Bruix J, Sala M, Llovet JM. Chemoembolization for hepatocellular carcinoma. *Gastroenterology*. 2004;127:S179–S188.
149. Varela M, Real MI, Burrel M, et al. Chemoembolization of hepatocellular carcinoma with drug eluting beads: efficacy and doxorubicin pharmacokinetics. *J Hepatol*. 2007;46:474–481.
150. Raoul JL, Guyader D, Bretagne JF, et al. Prospective randomized trial of chemoembolization versus intra-arterial injection of 131I-labeled-iodized oil in the treatment of hepatocellular carcinoma. *Hepatology*. 1997;26:1156–1161.
151. Kulik LM, Carr BI, Mulcahy MF, et al. Safety and efficacy of 90Y radiotherapy for hepatocellular carcinoma with and without portal vein thrombosis. *Hepatology*. 2008;47:71–81.
152. Farinati F, Salvagnini M, de Maria N, et al. Unresectable hepatocellular carcinoma: a prospective controlled trial with tamoxifen. *J Hepatol*. 1990;11:297–301.
153. Martinez Cerezo FJ, Tomas A, Donoso L, et al. Controlled trial of tamoxifen in patients with advanced hepatocellular carcinoma. *J Hepatol*. 1994;20:702–706.
154. Castells A, Bruix J, Bru C, et al. Treatment of hepatocellular carcinoma with tamoxifen: a double-blind placebo-controlled trial in 120 patients. *Gastroenterology*. 1995;109:917–922.
155. Riestra S, Rodriguez M, Delgado M, et al. Tamoxifen does not improve survival of patients with advanced hepatocellular carcinoma. *J Clin Gastroenterol*. 1998;26:200–203.
156. Group C. Tamoxifen in treatment of hepatocellular carcinoma: a randomised controlled trial. *Lancet*. 1998;352:17–20.
157. Chow PK, Tai BC, Tan CK, et al. High-dose tamoxifen in the treatment of inoperable hepatocellular carcinoma: a multicenter randomized controlled trial. *Hepatology*. 2002;36:1221–1226.
158. Leung TW, Johnson PJ. Systemic therapy for hepatocellular carcinoma. *Semin Oncol*. 2001;28:514–520.
159. Yeo W, Mok TS, Zee B, et al. A randomized phase III study of doxorubicin versus cisplatin/interferon alpha-2b/doxorubicin/fluorouracil (PIAF) combination chemotherapy for unresectable hepatocellular carcinoma. *J Natl Cancer Inst*. 2005;97:1532–1538.
160. Kouroumalis E, Skordilis P, Thermos K, et al. Treatment of hepatocellular carcinoma with octreotide: a randomised controlled study. *Gut*. 1998;42:442–447.
161. Llovet JM, Sala M, Castells L, et al. Randomized controlled trial of interferon treatment for advanced hepatocellular carcinoma. *Hepatology*. 2000;31:54–58.
162. Seong J, Park HC, Han KH, Chon CY. Clinical results and prognostic factors in radiotherapy for unresectable hepatocellular carcinoma: a retrospective study of 158 patients. *Int J Radiat Oncol Biol Phys*. 2003;55:329–336.
163. Grimaldi C, Bleiberg H, Gay F, et al. Evaluation of antiandrogen therapy in unresectable hepatocellular carcinoma: results of a European organization for research and treatment of cancer multicentric double-blind trial. *J Clin Oncol*. 1998;16:411–417.
164. Farazi PA, DePinho RA. Hepatocellular carcinoma pathogenesis: from genes to environment. *Nat Rev Cancer*. 2006;6:674–687.
165. Villanueva A, Newell P, Chiang DY, et al. Genomics and signaling pathways in hepatocellular carcinoma. *Semin Liver Dis*. 2007;27:55–76.
166. Llovet JM, Ricci S, Mazzaferro V, et al. Sorafenib in advanced hepatocellular carcinoma. *N Engl J Med*. 2008;359:378–390.
167. Herzog CE, Andrassy RJ, Eftekhari F. Childhood cancers: hepatoblastoma. *Oncologist*. 2000;5: 445–453.

168. Ammann RA, Plaschkes J, Leibundgut K. Congenital hepatoblastoma: a distinct entity? *Med Pediatr Oncol*. 1999;32:466–468.
169. Lee CL, Ko YC. Survival and distribution pattern of childhood liver cancer in Taiwan. *Eur J Cancer*. 1998;34:2064–2067.
170. Ikeda H, Matsuyama S, Tanimura M. Association between hepatoblastoma and very low birth weight: a trend or a chance? *J Pediatr*. 1997;130:557–560.
171. Tanimura M, Matsui I, Abe J, et al. Increased risk of hepatoblastoma among immature children with a lower birth weight. *Cancer Res*. 1998;58:3032–3035.
172. Ribons LA, Slovis TL. Hepatoblastoma and birth weight. *J Pediatr*. 1998;132:750.
173. Stocker JT. Hepatic tumors in children. *Clin Liver Dis*. 2001;5:259–281, viii-ix.
174. Stocker JT. Hepatoblastoma. *Semin Diagn Pathol*. 1994;11:136–143.
175. Haas JE, Muczynski KA, Krailo M, et al. Histopathology and prognosis in childhood hepatoblastoma and hepatocarcinoma. *Cancer*. 1989;64:1082–1095.
176. Sainati L, Leszl A, Stella M, et al. Cytogenetic analysis of hepatoblastoma: hypothesis of cytogenetic evolution in such tumors and results of a multicentric study. *Cancer Genet Cytogenet*. 1998;104:39–44.
177. Parada LA, Limon J, Iliszko M, et al. Cytogenetics of hepatoblastoma: further characterization of 1q rearrangements by fluorescence in situ hybridization: an international collaborative study. *Med Pediatr Oncol*. 2000;34:165–170.
178. Van Tornout JM, Buckley JD, Quinn JJ, et al. Timing and magnitude of decline in alpha-fetoprotein levels in treated children with unresectable or metastatic hepatoblastoma are predictors of outcome: a report from the Children's Cancer Group. *J Clin Oncol*. 1997;15:1190–1197.
179. Brown J, Perilongo G, Shafford E, et al. Pretreatment prognostic factorsfor children with hepatoblastoma—results from the International Society of Paediatric Oncology (SIOP) study SIOPEL 1. *Eur J Cancer*. 2000;36:1418–1425.
180. Morita K, Okabe I, Uchino J, et al. The proposed Japanese TNM classification of primary liver carcinoma in infants and children. *Jpn J Clin Oncol*. 1983;13:361–369.
181. Stringer MD, Hennayake S, Howard ER, et al. Improved outcome for children with hepatoblastoma. *Br J Surg*. 1995;82:386–391.
182. Ortega JA, Krailo MD, Haas JE, et al. Effective treatment of unresectable or metastatic hepatoblastoma with cisplatin and continuous infusion doxorubicin chemotherapy: a report from the Children's Cancer Study Group. *J Clin Oncol*. 1991;9:2167–2176.
183. Ortega JA, Douglass EC, Feusner JH,et al. Randomized comparison of cisplatin/vincristine/fluorouracil and cisplatin/continuous infusion doxorubicin for treatment of pediatric hepatoblastoma: A report from the Children's Cancer Group and the Pediatric Oncology Group. *J Clin Oncol*. 2000;18:2665–2675.
184. von Schweinitz D, Byrd DJ, Hecker H, et al. Efficiency and toxicity of ifosfamide, cisplatin and doxorubicin in the treatment of childhood hepatoblastoma. Study Committee of the Cooperative Paediatric Liver Tumour Study HB89 of the German Society for Paediatric Oncology and Haematology. *Eur J Cancer*. 1997;33:1243–1249.
185. Superina R, Bilik R. Results of liver transplantation in children with unresectable liver tumors. *J Pediatr Surg*. 1996;31:835–839.
186. Reyes JD, Carr B, Dvorchik I, et al. Liver transplantation and chemotherapy for hepatoblastoma and hepatocellular cancer in childhood and adolescence. *J Pediatr*. 2000;136:795–804.
187. Mani H, Van Thiel DH. Mesenchymal tumors of the liver. *Clin Liver Dis*. 2001;5:219–257, viii.
188. Molina E, Hernandez A. Clinical manifestations of primary hepatic angiosarcoma. *Dig Dis Sci*. 2003;48:677–682.
189. Timaran CH, Grandas OH, Bell JL. Hepatic angiosarcoma: long-term survival after complete surgical removal. *Am Surg*. 2000;66:1153–1157.
190. Popper H, Thomas LB, Telles NC, et al. Development of hepatic angiosarcoma in man induced by vinyl chloride, thorotrast, and arsenic. Comparison with cases of unknown etiology. *Am J Pathol*. 1978;92:349–376.
191. Creech JL, Jr, Johnson MN. Angiosarcoma of liver in the manufacture of polyvinyl chloride. *J Occup Med*. 1974;16:150–151.
192. Falk H, Herbert J, Crowley S, et al. Epidemiology of hepatic angiosarcoma in the United States: 1964–1974. *Environ Health Perspect*. 1981;41:107–113.
193. Bonaccorsi-Riani E, Lerut JP. Liver transplantation and vascular tumours. *Transpl Int*. 2010; 23:686–691.
194. Vennarecci G, Ismail T, Gunson B, McMaster P. [Primary angiosarcoma of the liver]. *Minerva Chir*. 1997;52:1141–1146.

195. Stambo GW, Guiney MJ. Hepatic angiosarcoma presenting as an acute intraabdominal hemorrhage treated with transarterial chemoembolization. *Sarcoma*. 2007;2007:90169.
196. Mehrabi A, Kashfi A, Fonouni H, et al. Primary malignant hepatic epithelioid hemangioendothelioma: a comprehensive review of the literature with emphasis on the surgical therapy. *Cancer*. 2006;107:2108–2121.
197. Makhlouf HR, Ishak KG, Goodman ZD. Epithelioid hemangioendothelioma of the liver: a clinicopathologic study of 137 cases. *Cancer*. 1999;85:562–582.
198. Lauffer JM, Zimmermann A, Krahenbuhl L, et al. Epithelioid hemangioendothelioma of the liver. A rare hepatic tumor. *Cancer*. 1996;78:2318–2327.
199. Ishak KG, Sesterhenn IA, Goodman ZD, et al. Epithelioid hemangioendothelioma of the liver: a clinicopathologic and follow-up study of 32 cases. *Hum Pathol*. 1984;15:839–852.
200. Freeman C, Berg JW, Cutler SJ. Occurrence and prognosis of extranodal lymphomas. *Cancer*. 1972;29:252–260.
201. Schweiger F, Shinder R, Rubin S. Primary lymphoma of the liver: a case report and review. *Can J Gastroenterol*. 2000;14:955–957.
202. Aozasa K, Mishima K, Ohsawa M. Primary malignant lymphoma of the liver. *Leuk Lymphoma*. 1993;10:353–357.
203. Lei KI, Chow JH, Johnson PJ. Aggressive primary hepatic lymphoma in Chinese patients. Presentation, pathologic features, and outcome. *Cancer*. 1995;76:1336–1343.
204. Scerpella EG, Villareal AA, Casanova PF, Moreno JN. Primary lymphoma of the liver in AIDS. Report of one new case and review of the literature. *J Clin Gastroenterol*. 1996;22:51–53.
205. Honda H, Franken EA, Jr, Barloon TJ, Smith JL. Hepatic lymphoma in cyclosporine-treated transplant recipients: sonographic and CT findings. *AJR Am J Roentgenol*. 1989;152:501–503.
206. Mohler M, Gutzler F, Kallinowski B, et al. Primary hepatic high-grade non-Hodgkin's lymphoma and chronic hepatitis C infection. *Dig Dis Sci*. 1997;42:2241–2245.
207. Anthony PP, Sarsfield P, Clarke T. Primary lymphoma of the liver: clinical and pathological features of 10 patients. *J Clin Pathol*. 1990;43:1007–1013.
208. Ryan J, Straus DJ, Lange C, et al. Primary lymphoma of the liver. *Cancer*. 1988;61:370–375.
209. Avlonitis VS, Linos D. Primary hepatic lymphoma: a review. *Eur J Surg*. 1999;165:725–729.

CHAPTER 6

Colorectal Cancer Liver Metastases

Peter Kingham & Yuman Fong

Overview

The most common site of blood-borne metastases from colorectal cancers is the liver. Studies have shown that one-quarter of patients with primary colorectal carcinoma present with synchronous hepatic metastasis.[1] In addition, approximately half of patients who have their primary colorectal cancer resected will develop metachronous liver metastasis.[2] Since the early 1980s, studies have shown that resection of colorectal cancer liver metastases can affect survival and potentially cure some patients. Surgical resection of liver metastases has become the standard therapy for patients with isolated liver disease. There have also been recent advances in nonsurgical therapies, such as radiofrequency ablation (RFA) and microwave ablation. These modalities are often used in conjunction with surgical resection or at times instead of surgical resection.

The effective treatment of colorectal liver cancer metastases also consists of chemotherapeutic regimens delivered both systemically and regionally. In patients whom curative resection is not possible, these chemotherapy options can extend life. Despite advances in chemotherapeutic regimens, survival is often less than three years.[3–6] As surgical therapy has become safer and indications for surgery have broadened, five-year survival in patients after a margin-negative hepatic resection is 40%.

This chapter describes the data that have accrued over the last 30 years to justify the use of hepatic resection in patients with hepatic colorectal cancer metastasis. Prognostic variables will be described that help predict which patients are likely to benefit from liver resection. Patient selection for systemic and regional chemotherapy and for liver resection will be reviewed. Advances in surgical techniques, including minimally invasive surgical options, will also be presented. Finally, the morbidity and mortality of liver resections and methods to reduce their sequelae will be considered.

Epidemiology

There are approximately 150,000 new cases of colorectal cancer diagnosed annually in the United States and approximately 60,000 deaths per year.[7] Almost half of all patients with colorectal cancers will develop liver metastases, and in 30% of patients, the liver is the only site of metastases.[1,8,9] In patients with liver metastases, this is the primary determinant of survival.[10]

Natural History

Five-year survival for patients with untreated colorectal cancer liver metastasis is unusual, although patients with solitary or unilobar disease appear to do better than their counterparts.[11,12] The median survival of patients with untreated colorectal liver metastasis is 5–10 months.[13–15] Wood et al. detailed the association between the extent of disease and survival in a retrospective study of 113 patients, where one-year survival was 5.7% in patients with extensive disease, 27% in patients with segmental or unilobular disease, and 60% in patients with a single metastasis.[11]

Wagner et al. retrospectively compared patients considered to have had resectable liver disease with those who did not. They found that three- and five-year survival for patients with resectable disease was 18% and 2%, compared with 4% and 0, respectively, in patients with unresectable disease.[12] A case-control study by Wagner et al. and Adson et al. found similar results when comparing 60 patients who underwent liver resection with 60 patients who did not.[9,16] They reported that patients who underwent resection had 5- and 10-year survivals of 25% and 19%, respectively, whereas no patients who did not undergo resection survived five years. Additional case-control studies have shown similar results. Scheele et al. found that median survival was 30 months in 183 patients who underwent resection of liver metastases compared with 14 months in 62 patients with resectable disease who did not undergo resection.[17] The improved survival seen with resection of colorectal cancer liver metastases has led to surgical resection as the primary therapy for patients with resectable liver metastases.

Results of Resection

Although originally thought of as a systemic process, the rationale for regional therapy with liver resection has developed from the concept that colorectal cancer spreads hematogenously through the portal vein, and the liver is usually the first site of metastases.[18] Liver resection provides a rare opportunity to prevent dissemination of disease from this site. This, combined with the regenerative properties of the liver, has allowed for aggressive surgical resections to treat liver metastases.

Morbidity and Mortality of Liver Resection

Mortality rates with elective liver resections in modern series are often less than 10% and are 3%–5% at high volume centers.[19–28] Complication rates in retrospective series range from 20% to 50% (Table 6-1).[29–34] These rates are high compared with many other surgical resections due to the physiologic sequelae of removing an often significant portion of an organ that is both immunologically and metabolically important. Morbidity rates are reasonable but slightly higher in elderly patients (>70 years old), with 60-day morbidity rates of 32% compared with 28% in patients younger than 70 years.[35] Complications can be divided into liver-specific complications and systemic complications. The most serious liver-specific complication is liver failure. This occurs in up to 8% of major resections.[29,30] Hemorrhage is another potentially life-threatening complication that occurs in less than 3% of cases. More common complications include perihepatic abscesses (2%–10% of patients) and biliary leaks and fistulae (approximately 4% of patients).[29,30]

The most common systemic complication is pulmonary. This likely reflects the cumulative effects of sympathetic pleural effusions and the pulmonary compromise caused by upper abdominal incisions. Up to 5%–10% of pleural effusions may cause enough symptoms to require drainage with tube thoracostomy.[36] Pneumonia can also be seen in 5%–22% of patients.[30] Other causes of mortality include pulmonary emboli and myocardial infarction, which occur in approximately 1% of patients.[29,37]

Most complications are treatable and do not cause extended hospital stays. The median hospital stay in experienced centers is less than two weeks.[33] In a study looking at 1800 liver resections, the median hospital stay was eight days. Only 112 patients required intensive care unit admission.

Long-Term Outcomes

Surgical resection has become the standard therapy for patients with metastatic colorectal cancer isolated to the liver given the long-term results reported in several series (Table 6-2). The first series to demonstrate this was Foster's multi-institutional review in 1978, which showed liver resections were associated with five-year survival rates of approximately 20%, compared with 0 for all other modalities.[38] In more recent studies, five-year survival was 25%–46%, with a median survival of 33–46 months.[19,25,39,40] Several series have published 10-year survival results of 20%–30%.[23,24,28] One series from Memorial Sloan-Kettering Cancer Center (MSKCC) reported actual 10-year survival in 612 patients who had resection of colorectal liver metastases from 1985 to 1994.[41] One hundred two of the 612 patients were actual 10-year survivors. Ninety-seven percent of patients alive at

TABLE 6-1: Complications of liver Resection [Data given as number and percent N(%)]

	Fortner[155]	Scheele[29]	Schlag[30]	Doci[31]	Nordlinger[156]	Cady[34]	Jarnagin[33]	Mala[32]	Coelho[157]	Welsh[158]
Total resections	75	219	122	100	80	244	1803	146	83	252
Liver-related complications										
Hemorrhage	1 (1)	7 (3)	—[a]	3	1 (1)	1	18	4 (3)[b]	—	1 (0.4)
Bile fistula	—	8 (4)	5 (4)	4	—	2	—	2 (1)	11	2 (0.8)
Liver failure	3 (4)	17 (8)	—	3	1 (1)	1	99	—	6	19 (7.5)
Perihepatic abscess	5 (7)	4 (2)	11 (9)	5	2 (3)	1	110	—	—	6 (2.4)
Portal vein thrombosis	1 (1)	—	—	—	—	—	9	1 (<1)	1	—
Renal failure	—	3 (1)	—	1	—	—	—	—	—	—
Infections										
Sepsis	—	—	3 (2)	2	4 (5)	2	39	3 (2)	—	—
Wound	1 (1)	—	7 (6)	—	—	2	94	—	2	2 (0.8)
General complications										
GI bleed	—	—	—	—	—	0	21	—	5	—
DVT	1 (1)	2 (1)	—	—	—	<1	24	—	—	7 (2.8)
Pulmonary embolism	1 (1)	4 (2)	—	—	1 (1)	<1	—	—	—	Included with DVT
Cardiac/MI	1 (1)	2 (1)	6 (5)	1	1 (1)	3	21	1 (<1)	1	6 (2.4)
Pneumonia	3 (4)	—	10 (8)	22	—	1	54	13 (9)	7	—
Pleural effusion	6 (8)	—	—	—	3 (4)	2	154	—	11	—

Abbreviations: DVT, deep vein thrombosis; GI, gastrointestinal; MI, myocardial infarction.
[a]—Data not specified.
[b]One patient reoperated twice for hemorrhage.

TABLE 6-2: Hepatic Resection Results Reported in Modern Series

Study	N	Operative Mortality (%)	Median Survival (mo)	Survival (%) 1-y	3-y	5-y	10-y
Adson[9]	141	3	—	80	42	25	—
Fortner[67]	75	7	—	89	57	35	—
Hughes[62]	607	—	—	—	—	33	—
Schlag[30]	122	4	32	85	40	30	—
Doci[31]	100	5	—	—	28	—	28
Rosen[63]	280	4	—	84	47	25	—
Scheele[20]	434	4	40	85	45	33	20
Fong[23]	1001	2.8	42	89	57	36	22
Minagawa[24]	235	0.85	46	—	51	38	26
Choti[25]	226	1	42	93	57	40	26
Fernandez[159]	100	1	—	86	66	58	—
Pawlik[160]	557	—	74	97	74	58	—
Wei[28]	423	1.6	53	93	—	47	28
Karanjia[161]	283	—	—	90	59	46	—

10 years were disease free at last follow-up. There is also no doubt that surgery alone is a curative treatment for a subset of patients.

Long-term results may also be affected by hospital volume for hepatectomy. One study examined state registries in Maryland and California and found lower morbidity, length of stay, and cost in high-volume centers.[42,43] Fong et al. used the National Medicare Database to show that perioperative outcome correlated with surgical experience. There was a survival advantage in both the perioperative and postoperative periods.[44]

Recurrence and Re-resection

Recurrences after resection of colorectal liver metastases are most commonly found within the liver (approximately 50% of recurrences)[30,45–47] (Table 6-3). The lung is the first site of recurrence in 25% of patients. Recurrence in the colon or rectum occurs in only 10%–20% of cases. In patients with isolated recurrences in the liver, re-resection is often an option. One-third of patients with hepatic recurrences are often eligible for re-resection.[46] Repeat hepatectomies have operative mortality rates that are lower than primary hepatectomies,[48–54] with rates less than 2%. Five-year survival in a recent series was over 40%.[53,54] Complication rates were reported to be 15%–50%.[55] Given the success and safety of repeat hepatectomies, patients with resectable recurrences should be offered this therapy. As ablation technology has improved, the treatment paradigm for these patients has now expanded to include re-resection in combination with ablation, and in unresectable patients, ablation techniques can be considered alone.

Prognostic Variables

Deciding on invasive treatments with significant morbidity and mortality rates requires a thorough analysis of patient prognosis after treatment. Many patient characteristics can assist in predicting outcome after surgery. All patients with liver metastases are considered American Joint Committee on Cancer stage IV, but they are a heterogeneous group. The prognosis, for example, of patients with metachronous tumors with long disease-free intervals is quite different from those with synchronous metastases. Clinical and pathologic variables are associated with the primary tumor and the liver metastases.

Age may be a factor that suggests an increased operative risk, but age and gender have not been found to influence long-term outcome in patients after liver resection.[23,25,56–58] The characteristics of the primary tumor can affect outcome.[23,25,57] The stage of

TABLE 6-3: Location of Initial Recurrence After Resection of Hepatic Colorectal Metastasis

Study	Patients (N)	Recurrence	Liver	Liver and Other	Colon/Rectum	Lung	Lung and Other
Butler[45]	62	30	10 (33)	10 (33)	—	—	—
Ekberg[47]	68	53	19 (28)	25 (47)	8 (15)	3 (6)	12 (23)
Bozetti[2]	45	28	11 (39)	5 (18)	—	5 (17)	—
Nordlinger[156]	80	51	21 (42)	13 (26)	11 (22)	11 (22)	—
Fortner[46]	69	45	8 (12)	–	—	16 (23)	—
Schlag[30]	122	80	17 (14)	55 (45)	–	—	—
Hughes[62]	607	424	149 (35)	42 (10)	33 (8)	73 (17)	–
Abdalla[162]	190		21				
Pawlik[160]	557	225	129 (57)	66 (29)			
Assumpcao[163]	141	80	27 (34)	14 (18)	20 (25)		

the primary tumor, especially nodal status, has a profound effect on survival. In addition, rectal primaries have slightly worse outcome.[29,59] The disease-free interval also affects prognosis, as synchronous tumors have a poorer outcome compared with metachronous lesions.[60] The timing of metachronous lesions is also important, as lesions found within one year of the primary colorectal tumor are associated with worse survival.[61]

Clinical characteristics of the liver tumor are key prognostic variables. Both multiple tumors and bilobar tumors are predictors of long-term outcome.[29,62–65] Although prognosis is better with less than four tumors, resection of even a high number of metastases is better than chemotherapy alone.[62,66,67] However, resection does become more challenging with a greater number of metastases, as in one series by Imamura et al. in which approximately 40% of patients with more than 10 metastases had resections with positive margins.[68] Elevated carcinoembryonic antigen (CEA) >200 ng/mL and tumor size >5 cm are two other factors that are important prognostic variables.[21,62,66] Although both of these factors are important for preoperative prediction of outcome, Fong et al. reported a survival rate of 14% in patients who had tumors greater than 10 cm resected.[56]

Extrahepatic metastases have traditionally been considered a relative contraindication to surgical resection of liver metastases as they are associated with a poor prognosis.[63,69,70] This is changing in some instances due to the success of chemotherapeutic regimens.[71] Small volume lung metastases can be treated with resection, and in selected patients, combined resection of hepatic and pulmonary metastases is associated with prolonged survival.[33,72] Five-year survival was 51% for patients with metastases to the ovary, 30% with metastases to the peritoneum, 28% with metastases to the lung, and 12% with metastases to the portal lymph nodes. Prognostic factors associated with improved survival after resection of both liver and lung metastases include a disease-free interval of >1 year between the first and second metastasis ($P < 0.0001$) and <2 liver lesions ($P < 0.0001$). Direct extension of liver disease to adjacent organs can be often treated with en bloc resection, and these patients should be considered with a different treatment paradigm from those with discrete extrahepatic metastases.[23]

Although resection margin status is another predictor of outcome, there is little consensus as to what optimal margins are. Many studies have shown that positive microscopic or macroscopic margins are associated with poor outcome.[69,73] Most surgeons attempt to achieve at least a 1-cm margin, as when liver micrometastases do occur, they are generally within 5 mm of the tumor's edge.[74] In a review of 1019 patients after hepatectomy, a margin of >1 cm was significant on multivariate analysis ($P < 0.01$), but subcentimeter negative margins were associated with better outcomes than positive margins, suggesting that a subcentimeter margin should not preclude a liver resection.[75] The type of resection that is performed, anatomic versus nonanatomic, has been looked at as a prognostic variable. Liau et al. and Scheele et al. found higher survival rates with anatomic segmental resection.[29,76] Jarnagin et al.

associated these improved outcomes with anatomic resections with lower rates of margin positivity.[33] Wedge resections are often guided by palpation, and due to impaired tactile sense and poor exposure, the specimen can tear at the interface of the tumor and the liver, leaving a positive margin.

The pathologic analysis of liver metastases also provides important prognostic information. Intrabiliary invasion is one such variable that is often overlooked. In one review of 355 patients with resected colorectal liver metastases, Okano et al. reported microscopic bile duct invasion in 42% of patients and macroscopic invasion in 12% of patients.[77] Five-year survival was higher (80%) in patients with well-differentiated tumors with less vascular involvement, compared with those who had poorly differentiated more invasive tumors (57%). Conversely, when there is intrabiliary extension of the tumor that can be diagnosed with imaging or jaundice preoperatively, tumors are often unresectable and there is a 0% five-year survival rate in these unresected patients.[78] The pathologic response to neoadjuvant chemotherapy has shown that chemotherapy is associated with sinusoidal congestion, but these lesions have no impact on postoperative clinical outcome.[79]

Clinical Risk Score

A multitude of clinical factors are associated with improved long-term outcomes. Most of these factors alone are not sufficient enough to preclude surgical resection. Multivariate analyses have been used in two studies to evaluate the importance of these clinical factors. One study by Nordlinger et al. looked at 1500 patients in a multicenter study.[21] Fong et al. examined 1001 patients at MSKCC subjected to resection of colorectal liver metastases.[23] They found seven independent variables that were predictors of prognosis. The five variables available prior to surgery are nodal metastases from the primary cancer, short disease-free interval, largest tumor >5 cm, CEA > 200 ng/mL, and multiple liver metastases (Table 6-4). The two variables available after surgery include extrahepatic disease and positive margin status.

TABLE 6-4: Clinical Risk Score Factors

Largest liver tumor >5 cm
Primary colorectal cancer with positive nodal metastases
Disease-free interval between primary cancer and liver metastases <1 y
>1 liver metastases
Carcinoembryonic antigen >200 ng/mL

Each positive criterion is assigned one point. Overall clinical risk score is the sum of the points.

The five preoperative variables were developed into a scoring system with one point assigned to each variable. This clinical risk score (CRS) has proven useful in reports from several centers in determining optimal candidates for neoadjuvant and adjuvant chemotherapy and for matching patients in trials. In general, with one variable present, five-year survival was reported as 24%–34%. The best prognostic group is patients with 2 or less points. A total of three or four variables identify patients who may benefit from neoadjuvant or adjuvant chemotherapy. If all five variables are present, it is rare to find long-term survivors, and aggressive adjuvant chemotherapy is indicated.

Clinically, the CRS has been verified in Norway and Germany.[32,80] Reissfelder et al. performed a comparative analysis of the MSKCC score, Iwatsuki score, Basingstoke index, Nordlinger score, and Mayo scoring system using 281 patients who underwent resection at a single institution (Table 6-5). Only the MSKCC score ($P = 0.006$) and the Iwatsuki score ($P = 0.01$) provided statistically significant stratification of patients when the scoring systems were used to predict survival.[81] The CRS score has also been applied to the yield from preoperative laparoscopy.[82,83] Patients with a low CRS can avoid unnecessary laparoscopy, and patients with a high CRS who have a higher likelihood of extrahepatic abdominal disease can avoid the morbidity of laparotomy and liver resection. High scores have also been used to justify preoperative 18-fluorodeoxyglucose positron emission tomography (FDG-PET).[84]

There are postoperative molecular pathologic characteristics of liver metastases that are becoming an additional factor for determining risk of recurrence and outcome. Banerjee et al. have reported on

TABLE 6-5: Validation of the Clinical Risk Score : Prediction of Disease-specific Survival with Prognostic Scoring Systems

System	N	Median Time (mo)	95% CI	1 y (%)	3 y (%)	5 y (%)	P
MSKCC score	281	46	42–54	94.6	61.8	33.7	0.006
0	19	56	32–76	94.4	68.8	42	
1	63	49	41–61	93.3	66.1	39.2	
2	100	54	44–59	95.9	69	36	
3	72	31	24–42	94.3	45.6	25.4	
4	22	44	33–61	92.2	58.9	13.2	
5	5	16	2–28	67.4	0	0	
Iwatsuki score	281	46	42–54	94.6	61.8	33.7	0.01
0	26	56	32–72	92.0	68.2	28.5	
1	135	53	43–61	94.7	66.3	41.3	
2	63	43	31–45	93.6	59.2	26.1	
3	54	37	26–53	93.6	50.2	15.7	
4	3	20	16–22	66.6	0	0	
Nordlinger score	281	46	42–54	94.6	61.8	33.7	0.91
Low (0–2)	34	53	32–56	92.3	67.2	31.3	
Medium (3–4)	155	47	41–56	94.8	62.6	34.9	
High (5–7)	92	44	33–59	94.5	56.8	34.5	
Basingstoke Index	281	46	42–54	94.6	61.8	33.7	
0	4	61	18–70	75	50	25.0	
1–5	124	48	42–61	95.1	65.0	37.8	
6–10	85	51	35–59	94.0	59.1	29.1	
11–15	29	36	23–56	96.6	46.8	15.2	
>15	39	44	33–54	92.2	65.1	14.5	
Mayo scoring system	281	46	42–54	94.6	61.8	33.7	0.80
0	27	57	44–73	92.6	75.2	38.5	
1	145	43	37–53	95.1	59.9	31.9	
2	99	51	34–56	93.8	59.1	30.9	
3	10	44	16–22	100	72.9	0	

Abbreviations: 95% CI = 95% confidence interval; MSKCC, Memorial Sloan-Kettering Cancer Center.
Adapted with permission from Springer Science and Business Media from Reissfelder C, Rahbari NN, Koch M et al. Ann Surg Oncol 2009;16(12) 3279–3288.

levels of the transcription factor E2F-1 and tumor thymidylate synthase levels as predictors of tumor response to chemotherapy.[85]

There are also molecular markers of tumor aggressiveness that may be associated with prognosis. Markers such as Ki67, p53, p27, vascular endothelial growth factor, and glucose transporter-1 protein have been described.[86,87] In addition, immune infiltrates, specifically T-cell populations, are potentially a prognostic tool that correlates with survival.[88]

Patient Selection

There have been many advances in radiology in the last 15 years, which have helped assess which patients are optimal candidates for liver resection of colorectal cancer metastases.[89] Preoperative radiologic studies help to reduce the number of unnecessary surgical explorations, and this has helped to improve the selection of patients for surgery and thus outcomes of surgical resection.[26,90–92] Ultrasound, computed tomography (CT) scan, magnetic resonance imaging (MRI), and PET scans have all been used in a multitude of combinations.

Ultrasonography is the least expensive preoperative imaging modality. With an experienced ultrasonographer, this test is useful in determining the relationship between the tumor and nearby hepatic structures, the number of metastases, and the extent of liver involvement. The duplex mode provides the advantage of determining the location of the tumor in relation to the hepatic veins, hilar in-flow vessels, and inferior vena cava. It has replaced the need for angiography in most cases where vascular involvement is in question.[93,94] It is also helpful to diagnose hepatic masses as cysts.

CT scan is the most common preoperative radiologic test. It is useful in examining both the extent and location of disease in the liver, as well as the presence of extrahepatic sites of tumor. Helical CT scans with oral and intravenous contrast are useful for identifying colorectal cancer metastases as they are classically hypovascular. Colorectal metastases generally push structures away from them and do not violate the liver capsule and planes between liver segments.[95] Intravenous contrast should be administered if medically prudent to all patients with concern for liver metastases, and scans should include the chest, abdomen, and pelvis. In patients in whom there is a high suspicion of hepatic metastases with no visible disease on CT scan, CT arterial portography has traditionally been used to investigate for the presence of liver metastases.[96,97] Due to the invasive nature of this examination, MRI scans are more commonly used as the next line of investigation.

CT scans are also helpful in searching for extrahepatic disease. Maithel et al. found that approximately one-third of subcentimeter pulmonary nodules in patients with colorectal liver metastases are metastatic disease.[98] However, these do not alter the three-year disease-specific survival.

MRI scans offer all of the information that CT scans provide and are able to provide additional information, but at a higher cost. Gadolinium-enhanced MRI scans have improved resolution compared with unenhanced MRI.[89] Enhanced MRI scans also have a higher sensitivity than dual-phase CT scans.[99] To evaluate patients with hepatic steatosis, which can be caused by diabetes mellitus, obesity, or chemotherapy, CT scans often have limited ability to detect small tumors. Thus, MRI is recommended for these patients. It is also helpful when there is a question about vascular anatomy that cannot be answered with contrast-enhanced CT scans.

FDG-PET scans are the most important radiologic invention in the past 15 years in treating patients with metastatic colorectal cancer.[100–102] They utilize the glucose analog 18F-FDG to provide information on tumor metabolism. Colorectal metastases are glucose-avid, so there is an increased yield in preoperative staging of patients (Figure 6-1). This improved preoperative staging has improved patient selection,

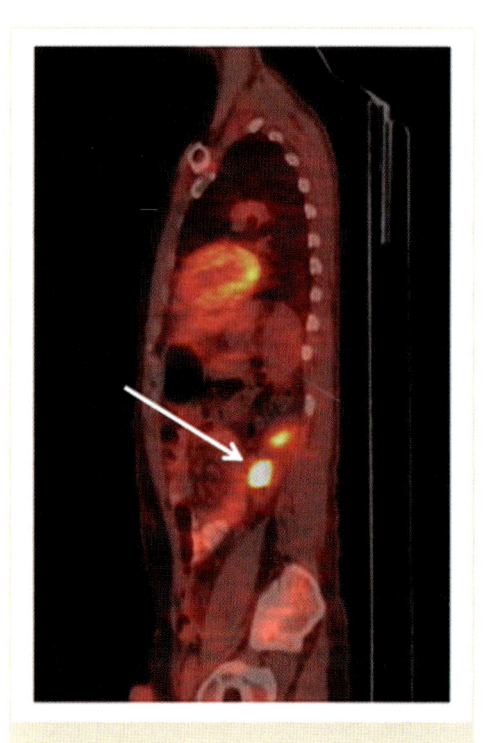

Figure 6-1: A patient with one potentially resectable hepatic metastases in the right lobe of the liver. FDG-PET identified abnormal uptake in the right lung. Patient found with positive retroperitoneal lymph nodes.

and thus, patient survival, recurrence rates, and rates of resectability are all improved after resection.[90] The liver is normally glucose-avid, so CT and MRI scans are superior in detecting liver lesions due to high FDG-PET liver background.[103] Size of colorectal metastases is important in determining the sensitivity of FDG-PET scans. More than 85% of lesions that are >1 cm were identified on FDG-PET scans in one series.[101] On the contrary, small lesions of <1 cm are visible in <20% of PET scans. This number is even smaller (<5%) when patients have been treated with chemotherapy, as glucose uptake is reduced. However, PET scans are useful at identifying sites of disease outside of the liver in the peritoneum, lymph nodes, lungs, and bones. A randomized trial of 150 patients with colorectal liver metastases assigned patients to CT only or CT plus PET-CT with at least three-year follow-up. In the CT-only group, 45% of patients had futile laparotomies compared with 28% in the CT-PET group, with a relative risk reduction of 38% ($P = 0.042$).[104] An important caveat with relying on findings from PET scans is that all glucose-avid tissue, including benign tissue, is identified, so it is important to biopsy extrahepatic sites of increased uptake prior to making treatment decisions.

A common treatment paradigm for preoperative imaging is to utilize CT scans of the abdomen and pelvis along with FDG-PET scanning in high-risk patients. A noncontrast chest CT is included in the CT portion of the FDG-PET scan, precluding the addition of a contrast-enhanced chest CT. MRI and/or ultrasound examinations should be used in patients with fatty livers or when questions arise over anatomic relation of vascular structures.

Laparoscopy is another modality that can assist in staging. It assists in avoiding the morbidity of large laparotomy incisions.[105–107] Both periportal lymph nodes and peritoneum can be examined for disease not identified on imaging studies. In 78% of patients with unresectable disease, laparotomy can be avoided with laparoscopic staging.[108] Avoiding laparotomies shortens the hospital length of stay and time to treatment, lowers the cost, and causes less morbidity.[82] Given that laparoscopy increases the cost of surgery in cases where no disease is found, it should be used in patients who have a high risk of unresectable disease. Patients who have imaging studies suspicious for extrahepatic or unresectable disease are optimal candidates for laparoscopy. The CRS can be used to help stratify patients for laparoscopy, as with a CRS > 2, there is a 42% chance of finding occult metastatic disease, compared with 12% with a CRS < 2.[82]

Portal vein embolization (PVE) can be utilized prior to surgery to improve results of surgical resections in patients with an inadequate future liver remnant (FLR). With a normal liver, patients can often tolerate resection of up to 70% or 80% of their liver.[25,109,110] Patients who require a major resection with liver dysfunction can benefit from contralateral liver hypertrophy. PVE is well tolerated, with 36% of patients in one series having a single-temperature spike postprocedure and 7% with sterile fevers for two to four days.[111] Of the 58 patients in this series, 65% underwent surgical resection a mean of 44 days after PVE. Mean hypertrophy was 24.3% in the left liver with right PVE and 1.5% in the right liver with left PVE. It is unclear whether bevacizumab, a monoclonal antibody against vascular endothelial growth factor, interferes with liver regeneration, as retrospective studies show conflicting results describing the size of the FLR in patients treated with this therapy.[112,113]

Operative Considerations

The optimal timing of resection of synchronous liver metastases and the primary colorectal tumor is debated in the literature. Simultaneous resection avoids the morbidity of a second surgery, and there are no differences in overall survival with immediate resection.[114,115] Overall survival may be improved by delayed resection, due to the improved selection of patients who have not developed additional sites of metastases during the observation period. Five prerequisites for simultaneous resections have been developed by Asbun and Hughes.[116] They include (1) solitary liver metastasis that can be removed with a limited liver resection, (2) an incision suitable for both liver and colon resections, (3) an uncomplicated bowel resection with minimal blood loss, (4) a surgeon who is comfortable with both aspects of the resection, and (5) a patient who is medically fit to undergo both procedures. In high-volume centers, the last two prerequisites are the most applicable. If the colorectal resection and liver resection can be performed simultaneously without increasing morbidity and mortality, it is reasonable to avoid a second surgery, but if one or both resections are extensive, the preference is to perform a staged resection.

As the morbidity of hepatic resections has declined, there has been an increased use of parenchymal-sparing surgical techniques.[117] Over an 11-year period at MSKCC, 440 patients had resection of bilateral liver metastases from colorectal cancer with 90-day mortality of 5.4% and a five-year disease-specific survival of 30%. The trend over the 11 years was for an increased use of wedge resection and a lower number of segments resected.

The operative techniques utilized for resecting hepatic colorectal metastases are similar to traditional resection techniques. A single dose of preoperative prophylactic antibiotics is utilized. Deep vein thromboses are prevented by applying sequential leg compression devices. There are three different types of incisions: subcostal, short midline with an extension to the right 3 cm cephalad from the umbilicus, and long midline. Anesthetic considerations are vital for safe hepatic resections. Low central venous pressure (<5 mm Hg) assists in decreasing bleeding in hepatic venous branches during parenchymal dissection. To help maintain low central venous pressure, 15° of Trendelenburg can be used to help increase venous return and improve cardiac output.

Abdominal exploration is an important facet of all cancer surgeries. It allows for examination of the portocaval, hilar, and celiac axis nodes. Intraoperative ultrasound (IOUS) is also utilized after mobilization of the liver. Lesions found with IOUS can change the operative plan in up to 50% of cases.[118–120]

Although many additional lesions may be identified with this modality, it is uncommon that this changes the operative plan to the point of unresectability.[119] IOUS is a useful adjunct during resection for providing detailed information about the location of the tumors in relation to arterial and biliary structures. Repeated IOUS application can guide the surgeon throughout the resection.[121,122] Results from diagnostic laparotomy are also improved with the addition of IOUS, especially in identifying nodal disease.[83,123–125]

Ablative technologies are increasingly used in conjunction with or in place of surgical resection. Given that up to 60% of patients develop a recurrence after liver resection, most commonly in the liver, ablative techniques have been useful in treating hepatic recurrences (Table 6-6).[126] The question of equivalence between resection and ablation was examined in a retrospective series that looked at 192 patients with only hepatic resection or ablation for colorectal liver metastases.[126,127] In this series, with similar CRSs, number of liver metastases, rate of those who received chemotherapy, and presence of extrahepatic disease, 17% of patients recurred at their ablation site, compared with 2% at the site of resection ($P < 0.001$). It is difficult to compare ablation and resection retrospectively, as there are often many selection biases between these patient populations. Gleisner et al. retrospectively looked at 258 patients with hepatic colorectal metastases who underwent ablation with or without RFA.[128] They found that groups with resection alone and resection combined with RFA were different groups that could not adequately be compared on retrospective analysis.

TABLE 6-6: Local Recurrence and Survival Following Radiofrequency Ablation of Hepatic Colorectal Metastases

Study	N	Method of RFA	Local Recurrence (%)	3-y Survival (%)	5-y Survival (%)
Solbiati[164]	117	Percutaneous	39 (lesions)	46	—[a]
Oshowo[165]	25	Open	33 (patients)	52	—[a]
Abdalla[162]	57	Open	9 (patients)	37	—[a]
Lencioni[166]	423	Percutaneous	25 (lesions)	47	24
Berber[167]	135	Laparoscopic	46 (patients)	34	—[a]
Aloia[168]	30	Open (90%)	37 (patients)	57	27
Abitabile[169]	47	Percutaneous, laparoscopic, open	9	57	21
Otto[170]	28	Percutaneous	32 (patients)	67	48

[a]Data not provided in the manuscript.

Minimally invasive techniques are becoming more common when treating patients with metastatic colorectal metastases.[129] Vibert et al. reported results from 41 patients who underwent laparoscopic resection.[130] Three-year disease-free survival rate was 51% and three-year overall survival was 87%, with median follow-up of 30 months. No randomized, controlled trials have been performed as of yet comparing laparoscopic and open liver resections.

Postoperative Follow-Up

Postoperative care of patients after liver resection involves managing metabolic derangements due to hepatic insufficiency and hepatic regeneration. Hepatic regeneration begins within 12 hours of liver resection, and most regeneration is completed by one week. Early signs of hepatic insufficiency include hypoglycemia and hypoproteinemia. Liver function tests often reveal elevations in alkaline phosphatase, transaminases, and bilirubin. International normalized ratio should be followed, and if it is >1.5, fresh frozen plasma should be given. Platelet counts can also drop, and if they are <50,000/μL, they should be supplemented.

Perioperative Morbidity and Mortality

Morbidity is often related to immunologic and metabolic derangements. Most series report complication rates >20%. General morbidities include pulmonary, cardiac, and infectious complications. Pulmonary complications are frequent given the upper abdominal incision and sympathetic pleural effusions. Pneumonia has been reported in ≤22% of cases.[30,31] Pulmonary embolus is relatively rare (<1% of cases).[31,37] Tube thoracostomy is indicated in ≤10% of patients.[37,131] Myocardial infarctions occur in <1% of patients, as patients are optimized prior to surgery.[29,31,67]

Liver failure is the most serious liver-specific complication. It occurs in up to 8% of patients who undergo major hepatic resections.[29–31,37] Significant hemorrhage occurs in <3% of cases, but when it does occur, it is a major cause of morbidity and mortality. Bile leaks occur in approximately 4% of cases.[29,30] Postoperative abscesses occur in 2%–10% of cases.[29–31,67,131] The median length of hospital stay for patients undergoing major liver resections is less than two weeks. Jarnagin et al. reported a median length of stay of eight days in a series of more than 1800 liver resections, with 112 patients requiring intensive care unit admission.[33]

There is debate in the literature about the appropriate follow-up after surgery. The type and frequency of follow-up have not been shown to affect survival in patients with primary colorectal cancer.[132–134] There are no conclusive data that have demonstrated that follow-up frequency affects survival in patients with hepatic colorectal metastases. Most patients undergo serum CEA level examinations, annual chest X-rays and CT scan of the abdomen and pelvis every three to four months for two years after resection, then every six months for the following five years.

Adjuvant Chemotherapy

Adjuvant systemic chemotherapy has been utilized since the 1980s after studies suggested that chemotherapy could improve outcome.[62,135] More recently, studies have shown that adjuvant chemotherapy improves survival.[136,137] Parks et al. examined patients at MSKCC and Edinburgh Royal Infirmary and compared 518 chemotherapy-naive patients with 274 patients treated with 5-fluorouracil (FU)-based adjuvant chemotherapy.[136] Patients were stratified by CRS. There was an improved survival in patients treated with adjuvant chemotherapy ($P = 0.007$). Portier et al. reported similar results in a randomized multicenter trial that randomized 173 patients after hepatectomy to observation or systemic adjuvant chemotherapy with 5-FU and folinic acid. Patients treated with adjuvant chemotherapy had a five-year disease-free survival rate of 34% compared with 27% in the observation group ($P = 0.03$). Adjuvant chemotherapy was an independent predictor of outcome in this trial.[137]

Patients are now offered several different regimens. Some of these regimens have significant toxicity and offer no clear advantage to 5-FU. Saltz et al. showed in a large randomized trial that 5-FU, leucovorin, and irinotecan in combination caused a significantly higher rate of toxicity with no survival benefit compared with 5-FU and leucovorin alone.[138] Although there are data to support using adjuvant

5-FU and leucovorin, many patients receive more complex regimens. In chemotherapy-naive patients, 5-FU and leucovorin should be offered as the first line in therapy, and this regimen can be broadened to include oxaliplatin- or irinotecan-containing regimens if patients fail to respond.

Hepatic artery infusion is a mode of regional chemotherapy delivery. Most metastatic liver tumors obtain their blood supply from the hepatic arterial supply, compared with normal hepatic tissue that relies on the portal venous system. In addition, because the liver is the most common site of recurrence after liver resection and is the sole site of recurrence in 40% of patients, intra-arterial chemotherapy can also be used in the adjuvant setting.[131] Prospective single-arm trials in the 1990s showed the feasibility and safety of adjuvant regional chemotherapy.[139–141] This treatment was shown to be effective in limiting liver disease in two adjuvant regional chemotherapy trials by Kemeny et al. and Goere et al.[142,143] Given the plethora of additional options for systemic therapy, combining regional floxuridine (FUDR) with irinotecan, oxaliplatin, and bevacizumab is currently utilized. These powerful combinations provide some synergy in the liver and offer treatment of regional and systemic disease (Figure 6-2). Kemeny et al. in 2005 reported a 75% response rate in patients with unresectable hepatic colorectal metastases. Similar results were seen with systemic oxaliplatin and regional FUDR.[144]

Chemotherapy can also be used to downsize tumors in patients with unresectable disease. Bismuth et al. reported on 330 consecutive patients with nonresectable disease.[145] In this group, 53 patients were converted to resectable disease. This series was updated by Adam et al. in 2001, with 13.6% of 701 unresectable patients responding enough to undergo hepatic resection after oxaliplatin, 5-FU, and leucovorin treatment.[146] Similar results have been repeated by many other groups including Ardito et al. in 2012.[147] Clavien et al. showed that hepatic artery infusion pump can be used to convert patients to resectable status.[148]

Neoadjuvant chemotherapy has also been considered. Theoretically, this technique in patients with resectable liver metastases can treat microscopic liver disease and delay surgery to allow for determination of response to chemotherapy, discovery of occult disease, and decrease in the size of the tumors to ease resection. However, there are risks associated with neoadjuvant chemotherapy. Many are toxic to the liver and can affect recovery after hepatectomy. We recommend selective neoadjuvant chemotherapy in patients with a high CRS or who have only recently undergone colonic resection and have not recovered from that surgery. The success of some neoadjuvant regimens has led to the problem of patients with no visible tumor left to resect. Currently, our practice is to utilize IOUS to identify the lesion. If it is sonographically occult, we perform a resection of the area where the tumor was on prior imaging studies.

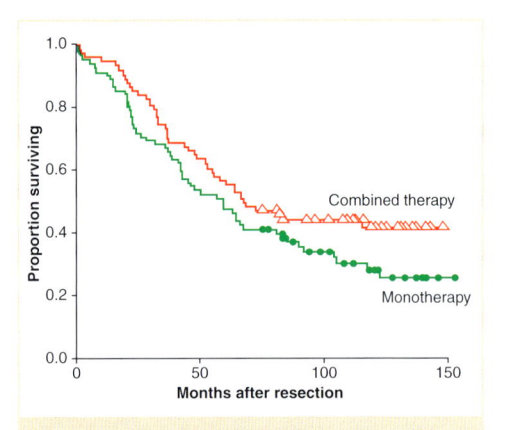

Figure 6-2: Overall survival among patients with metastatic colorectal cancer who were treated with hepatic arterial infusion plus systemic chemotherapy (combined chemotherapy in red) or with systemic therapy alone (monotherapy in green). Used with permission from Massachusetts Medical Society. Kemeny NE. Hepatic arterial infusion after liver resection. *N Engl J Med.* 2005;352(7):734–735.

Liver damage from chemotherapy can be dramatic. In the 1990s, there were reports of liver damage from agents like 5-FU.[149] More modern agents such as bevacizumab, irinotecan, and oxaliplatin cause even greater rates of hepatic toxicity.[150] Chemotherapy-associated hepatic steatohepatitis (CASH) has become a significant clinical entity. The clinical triad associated with it is refractory thrombocytopenia, splenomegaly due to portal hypertension, and hepatic fatty infiltration. CASH can progress to fibrosis and cirrhosis. It is important to identify prior to surgery because PVE may be required to increase the size of the remnant liver in this setting.[151] PVE can provide the surgeon with a glimpse of the regenerative ability of the remnant liver segment.

Modern chemotherapy agents have also been associated with hepatic steatosis and hepatic sinusoidal obstruction.[152–154]

References

1. Bengmark S, Hafstrom L. The natural history of primary and secondary malignant tumors of the liver. I. The prognosis for patients with hepatic metastases from colonic and rectal carcinoma by laparotomy. *Cancer*. 1969;23(1):198–202.
2. Bozzetti F, Doci R, Bignami P, et al. Patterns of failure following surgical resection of colorectal cancer liver metastases. Rationale for a multimodal approach. *Ann Surg*. 1987;205(3):264–270.
3. Kemeny N, Cohen A, Bertino JR, et al. Continuous intrahepatic infusion of floxuridine and leucovorin through an implantable pump for the treatment of hepatic metastases from colorectal carcinoma. *Cancer*. 1990; 65:2446–2450.
4. Saltz L. Irinotecan-based combinations for the adjuvant treatment of stage III colon cancer. *Oncology (Williston Park)*. 2000;14(12 suppl 14):47–50.
5. Cunningham D, Humblet Y, Siena S, et al. Cetuximab monotherapy and cetuximab plus irinotecan in irinotecan-refractory metastatic colorectal cancer. *N Engl J Med*. 2004;351(4):337–345.
6. Baker LH, Talley RW, Matter R, et al. Phase III comparison of the treatment of advanced gastrointestinal cancer with bolus weekly 5-FU vs. methyl-CCNU plus bolus weekly 5-FU. A southwest oncology group study. *Cancer*. 1976;38(1):1–7.
7. Jemal A, Murray T, Ward E, et al. Cancer statistics, 2005. *CA Cancer J Clin*. 2005;55(1):10–30.
8. Charnley RM, Morris DL, Dennison AR, et al. Detection of colorectal liver metastases using intraoperative ultrasonography. *Br J Surg*. 1991; 78(1):45–48.
9. Adson MA, Van Heerden JA, Adson MH, et al. Resection of hepatic metastases from colorectal cancer. *Arch Surg*. 1984;119(6):647–651.
10. Steele G Jr, Osteen RT, Wilson RE, et al. Patterns of failure after surgical cure of large liver tumors. A change in the proximate cause of death and a need for effective systemic adjuvant therapy. *Am J Surg*. 1984;147(4):554–559.
11. Wood CB, Gillis CR, Blumgart LH. A retrospective study of the natural history of patients with liver metastases from colorectal cancer. *Clin Oncol*. 1976;2:285–288.
12. Wagner JS, Adson MA, Van Heerden JA, et al. The natural history of hepatic metastases from colorectal cancer. A comparison with resective treatment. *Ann Surg*. 1984;199(5): 502–508.
13. Jaffe BM, Donegan WL, Watson F, Spratt JS Jr. Factors influencing survival in patients with untreated hepatic metastases. *Surg Gynecol Obstet*. 1968;127(1):1–11.
14. Goslin R, Steele G Jr, Zamcheck N, et al. Factors influencing survival in patients with hepatic metastases from adenocarcinoma of the colon or rectum. *Dis Colon Rectum*. 1982;25(8):749–754.
15. de Brauw LM, van de Velde CJ, Bouwhuis-Hoogerwerf ML, Zwaveling A. Diagnostic evaluation and survival analysis of colorectal cancer patients with liver metastases. *J Surg Oncol*. 1987;34(2):81–86.
16. Wilson SM, Adson MA. Surgical treatment of hepatic metastases from colorectal cancers. *Arch Surg*. 1976;111(4):330–334.
17. Scheele J, Stangl R, Altendorf-Hofmann A. Hepatic metastases from colorectal carcinoma: impact of surgical resection on the natural history. *Br J Surg*. 1990;77(11):1241–1246.
18. Weiss L, Grundmann E, Torhorst J, et al. Haematogenous metastatic patterns in colonic carcinoma: an analysis of 1541 necropsies. *J Pathol*. 1986;150(3):195–203.
19. Younes RN, Rogatko A, Brennan MF. The influence of intraoperative hypotension and perioperative blood transfusion on disease-free survival in patients with complete resection of colorectal liver metastases. *Ann Surg*. 1991;214(2):107–113.
20. Scheele J, Stang R, Altendorf-Hofmann A, Paul M. Resection of colorectal liver metastases. *World J Surg*. 1995;19(1):59–71.
21. Nordlinger B, Guiguet M, Vaillant JC, et al. Surgical resection of colorectal carcinoma metastases to the liver. A prognostic scoring system to improve case selection, based on 1568 patients. Association Francaise de Chirurgie. *Cancer*. 1996;77(7):1254–1262.
22. Jamison RL, Donohue JH, Nagorney DM, et al. Hepatic resection for metastatic colorectal cancer results in cure for some patients. *Arch Surg*. 1997;132(5):505–510.
23. Fong Y, Fortner J, Sun RL, et al. Clinical score for predicting recurrence after hepatic resection for metastatic colorectal cancer: analysis of 1001 consecutive cases. *Ann Surg*. 1999;230(3):309–318.

24. Minagawa M, Makuuchi M, Torzilli G, et al. Extension of the frontiers of surgical indications in the treatment of liver metastases from colorectal cancer: long-term results. *Ann Surg*. 2000;231(4):487–499.

25. Choti MA, Sitzmann JV, Tiburi MF, et al. Trends in long-term survival following liver resection for hepatic colorectal metastases. *Ann Surg*. 2002;235(6):759–766.

26. Belli G, D'Agostino A, Ciciliano F, et al. Liver resection for hepatic metastases: 15 years of experience. *J Hepato-Biliary-Pancreat Surg*. 2002; 9(5):607–613.

27. Mutsaerts EL, van Ruth S, Zoetmulder FA, et al. Prognostic factors and evaluation of surgical management of hepatic metastases from colorectal origin: a 10-year single-institute experience. *J Gastrointest Surg*. 2005;9(2):178–186.

28. Wei AC, Greig PD, Grant D, et al. Survival after hepatic resection for colorectal metastases: a 10-year experience. *Ann Surg Oncol*. 2006;13(5):668–676.

29. Scheele J, Stangl R, Altendorf-Hofmann A, Gall FP. Indicators of prognosis after hepatic resection for colorectal secondaries. *Surgery*. 1991;110:13–29.

30. Schlag P, Hohenberger P, Herfarth C. Resection of liver metastases in colorectal cancer—competitive analysis of treatment results in synchronous versus metachronous metastases. *Eur J Surg Oncol*. 1990;16(4):360–365.

31. Doci R, Gennari L, Bignami P, et al. One hundred patients with hepatic metastases from colorectal cancer treated by resection: analysis of prognostic determinants. *Br J Surg*. 1991;78(7):797–801.

32. Mala T, Bohler G, Mathisen O, et al. Hepatic resection for colorectal metastases: can preoperative scoring predict patient outcome? *World J Surg*. 2002;26(11):1348–1353.

33. Jarnagin WR, Gonen M, Fong Y, et al. Improvement in perioperative outcome after hepatic resection: analysis of 1,803 consecutive cases over the past decade. *Ann Surg*. 2002;236(4):397–406.

34. Cady B, Jenkins RL, Steele GD Jr, et al. Surgical margin in hepatic resection for colorectal metastasis: a critical and improvable determinant of outcome. *Ann Surg*. 1998;227(4):566–571.

35. Adam R, Frilling A, Elias D, et al. Liver resection of colorectal metastases in elderly patients. *Br J Surg*. 2010;97(3):366–376.

36. Coppa GF, Eng K, Ranson JCH, et al. Hepatic resection for metastatic colon and rectal cancer. An evaluation of preoperative and postoperative factors. *Ann Surg*. 1985; 302(2):203–208.

37. Cunningham JD, Fong Y, Shriver C, et al. One hundred consecutive hepatic resections. Blood loss, transfusion, and operative technique. *Arch Surg*. 1994;129(10):1050–1056.

38. Foster JH. Survival after liver resection for secondary tumors. *Am J Surg*. 1978;135(3):389–394.

39. Fong Y, Salo J. Surgical therapy of hepatic colorectal metastasis. *Semin Oncol*. 1999; 26(5):514–523.

40. Karanjia ND, Lordan JT, Fawcett WJ, et al. Survival and recurrence after neo-adjuvant chemotherapy and liver resection for colorectal metastases: a ten year study. *Eur J Surg Oncol*. 2009;35(8):838–843.

41. Tomlinson JS, Jarnagin WR, DeMatteo RP, et al. Actual 10-year survival after resection of colorectal liver metastases defines cure. *J Clin Oncol*. 2007;25(29):4575–4580.

42. Choti MA, Bowman HM, Pitt HA, et al. Should hepatic resections be performed at high-volume referral centers? *J Gastrointest Surg*. 1998;2(1):11–20.

43. Glasgow RE, Showstack JA, Katz PP, et al. The relationship between hospital volume and outcomes of hepatic resection for hepatocellular carcinoma. *Arch Surg*. 1999;134(1):30–35.

44. Fong Y, Gonen M, Rubin D, et al. Long-term survival is superior after resection for cancer in high-volume centers. *Ann Surg*. 2005;242(4):540–544.

45. Butler J, Attiyeh FF, Daly JM. Hepatic resection for metastases of the colon and rectum. *Surg Gynecol Obstet*. 1986;162(2):109–113.

46. Fortner JG. Recurrence of colorectal cancer after hepatic resection. *Am J Surg*. 1988;155(3):378–382.

47. Ekberg H, Tranberg KG, Andersson R, et al. Pattern of recurrence in liver resection for colorectal secondaries. *World J Surg*. 1987; 11(4):541–547.

48. Stone MD, Cady B, Jenkins RL, et al. Surgical therapy for recurrent liver metastases from colorectal cancer. *Arch Surg*. 1990;125(6): 718–721.

49. Bozzetti F, Bignami P, Montalto F, et al. Repeated hepatic resection for recurrent metastases from colorectal cancer. *Br J Surg*. 1992;79(2):146–148.

50. Vaillant JC, Balladur P, Nordlinger B, et al. Repeat liver resection for recurrent colorectal metastases. *Br J Surg*. 1993;80:340–344.

51. Fong Y, Blumgart LH, Cohen A, et al. Repeat hepatic resections for metastatic colorectal cancer. *Ann Surg*. 1994;220(5):657–662.
52. Muratore A, Polastri R, Bouzari H, et al. Repeat hepatectomy for colorectal liver metastases: a worthwhile operation? *J Surg Oncol*. 2001;76(2):127–132.
53. Petrowsky H, Gonen M, Jarnagin W, et al. Second liver resections are safe and effective treatment for recurrent hepatic metastases from colorectal cancer: a bi-institutional analysis. *Ann Surg*. 2002;235(6):863–871.
54. Shaw IM, Rees M, Welsh FK, et al. Repeat hepatic resection for recurrent colorectal liver metastases is associated with favourable long-term survival. *Br J Surg*. 2006;93(4):457–464.
55. Lange JF, Leese T, Castaing D, Bismuth H. Repeat hepatectomy for recurrent malignant tumors of the liver. *Surg Gynecol Obstet*. 1989;169(2):119–126.
56. Fong Y, Cohen AM, Fortner JG, et al. Liver resection for colorectal metastases. *J Clin Oncol*. 1997;15(3):938–946.
57. Lise M, Bacchetti S, Da PP, et al. Patterns of recurrence after resection of colorectal liver metastases: prediction by models of outcome analysis. *World J Surg*. 2001;25(5):638–644.
58. Ohlsson B, Breland U, Ekberg H, et al. Follow-up after curative surgery for colorectal carcinoma. Randomized comparison with no follow-up. *Dis Colon Rectum*. 1995;38(6):619–626.
59. Altendorf-Hofmann A, Scheele J. A critical review of the major indicators of prognosis after resection of hepatic metastases from colorectal carcinoma. *Surg Oncol Clin N Am*. 2003;12(1):165–192, xi.
60. Ballantyne GH, Quin J. Surgical treatment of liver metastases in patients with colorectal cancer. *Cancer*. 1993;71(S12):4252–4266.
61. Bentrem DJ, DeMatteo RP, Blumgart LH. Surgical therapy for metastatic disease to the liver. *Annu Rev Med*. 2005;56:139–156.
62. Hughes KS, Rosenstein RB, Songhorabodi S, et al. Resection of the liver for colorectal carcinoma metastases. A multi-institutional study of long-term survivors. *Dis Colon Rectum*. 1988;31(1):1–4.
63. Rosen CB, Nagorney DM, Taswell HF, et al. Perioperative blood transfusion and determinants of survival after liver resection for metastatic colorectal carcinoma. *Ann Surg*. 1992;216(4):493–504.
64. Bolton JS, Fuhrman GM. Survival after resection of multiple bilobar hepatic metastases from colorectal carcinoma. *Ann Surg*. 2000;231(5):743–751.
65. Kornprat P, Jarnagin WR, Gonen M, et al. Outcome after hepatectomy for multiple (four or more) colorectal metastases in the era of effective chemotherapy. *Ann Surg Oncol*. 2007;14(3):1151–1160.
66. Cady B, Stone MD, McDermott WV Jr, et al. Technical and biological factors in disease-free survival after hepatic resection for colorectal cancer metastases. *Arch Surg*. 1992;127(5):561–568.
67. Fortner JG, Silva JS, Golbey RB, et al. Multivariate analysis of a personal series of 247 consecutive patients with liver metastases from colorectal cancer. I. Treatment by hepatic resection. *Ann Surg*. 1984;199(3):306–316.
68. Imamura H, Seyama Y, Kokudo N, et al. Single and multiple resections of multiple hepatic metastases of colorectal origin. *Surgery*. 2004;135(5):508–517.
69. Gayowski TJ, Iwatsuki S, Madariaga JR, et al. Experience in hepatic resection for metastatic colorectal cancer: analysis of clinical and pathologic risk factors. *Surgery*. 1994;116:703–711.
70. van Ooijen B, Wiggers T, Meijer S, et al. Hepatic resections for colorectal metastases in The Netherlands. A multiinstitutional 10-year study. *Cancer*. 1992;70(1):28–34.
71. Carpizo DR, Are C, Jarnagin W, et al. Liver resection for metastatic colorectal cancer in patients with concurrent extrahepatic disease: results in 127 patients treated at a single center. *Ann Surg Oncol*. 2009;16(8):2138–2146.
72. Miller G, Biernacki P, Kemeny NE, et al. Outcomes after resection of synchronous or metachronous hepatic and pulmonary colorectal metastases. *J Am Coll Surg*. 2007;205(2):231–238.
73. Jenkins LT, Millikan KW, Bines SD, et al. Hepatic resection for metastatic colorectal cancer. *Am Surg*. 1997;63(7):605–610.
74. Kokudo N, Miki Y, Sugai S, et al. Genetic and histological assessment of surgical margins in resected liver metastases from colorectal carcinoma: minimum surgical margins for successful resection. *Arch Surg*. 2002;137(7):833–840.
75. Are C, Gonen M, Zazzali K, et al. The impact of margins on outcome after hepatic resection for colorectal metastasis. *Ann Surg*. 2007;246(2):295–300.
76. Liau KH, Blumgart LH, DeMatteo RP. Segment-oriented approach to liver resection. *Surg Clin North Am*. 2004;84(2):543–561.

77. Okano K, Yamamoto J, Moriya Y, et al. Macroscopic intrabiliary growth of liver metastases from colorectal cancer. *Surgery*. 1999;126(5):829–834.
78. Povoski SP, Klimstra DS, Brown KT, et al. Recognition of intrabiliary hepatic metastases from colorectal adenocarcinoma. *HPB Surg*. 2000;11(6):383–390.
79. Hubert C, Fervaille C, Sempoux C, et al. Prevalence and clinical relevance of pathological hepatic changes occurring after neoadjuvant chemotherapy for colorectal liver metastases. *Surgery*. 2010;147(2):185–194.
80. Merkel S, Bialecki D, Meyer T, et al. Comparison of clinical risk scores predicting prognosis after resection of colorectal liver metastases. *J Surg Oncol*. 2009;100(5):349–357.
81. Reissfelder C, Rahbari NN, Koch M, et al. Validation of prognostic scoring systems for patients undergoing resection of colorectal cancer liver metastases. *Ann Surg Oncol*. 2009;16(12):3279–3288.
82. Jarnagin WR, Conlon K, Bodniewicz J, et al. A clinical scoring system predicts the yield of diagnostic laparoscopy in patients with potentially resectable hepatic colorectal metastases. *Cancer*. 2001;91(6):1121–1128.
83. Grobmyer SR, Fong Y, D'Angelica M, et al. Diagnostic laparoscopy prior to planned hepatic resection for colorectal metastases. *Arch Surg*. 2004;139(12):1326–1330.
84. Schussler-Fiorenza CM, Mahvi DM, Niederhuber J, et al. Clinical risk score correlates with yield of PET scan in patients with colorectal hepatic metastases. *J Gastrointest Surg*. 2004;8(2):150–157.
85. Banerjee D, Gorlick R, Liefshitz A, et al. Levels of E2F-1 expression are higher in lung metastasis of colon cancer as compared with hepatic metastasis and correlate with levels of thymidylate synthase. *Cancer Res*. 2000;60(9):2365–2367.
86. Cao D, Hou M, Guan YS, et al. Expression of HIF-1alpha and VEGF in colorectal cancer: association with clinical outcomes and prognostic implications. *BMC Cancer*. 2009;9:432.
87. Chen YT, Henk MJ, Carney KJ, et al. Prognostic significance of tumor markers in colorectal cancer patients: DNA index, S-phase fraction, p53 expression, and Ki-67 index. *J Gastrointest Surg*. 1997;1(3):266–272.
88. Katz SC, Shia J, Liau KH, et al. Operative blood loss independently predicts recurrence and survival after resection of hepatocellular carcinoma. *Ann Surg*. 2009;249(4):617–623.
89. Bipat S, van Leewen MS, Comans EF, et al. Colorectal liver metastases: CT, MR imaging and PET for diagnosis—meta-analysis. *Radiology*. 2005;237(1):123–131.
90. Strasberg SM, Dehdashti F, Siegel BA, et al. Survival of patients evaluated by FDG-PET before hepatic resection for metastatic colorectal carcinoma: a prospective database study. *Ann Surg*. 2001;233(3):293–299.
91. Valls C, Andia E, Sanchez A, et al. Hepatic metastases from colorectal cancer: preoperative detection and assessment of resectability with helical CT. *Radiology*. 2001;218(1):55–60.
92. Cervone A, Sardi A, Conaway GL. Intraoperative ultrasound (IOUS) is essential in the management of metastatic colorectal liver lesions. *Am Surg*. 2000;66(7):611–615.
93. Gibson RN, Yeung E, Thompson JN, et al. Bile duct obstruction: radiologic evaluation of level, cause, and tumor resectability. *Radiology*. 1986;160(1):43–47.
94. Hann LE, Fong Y, Shriver CD, et al. Malignant hepatic hilar tumors: can ultrasonography be used as an alternative to angiography with CT arterial portography for determination of resectability? *J Ultrasound Med*. 1996;15(1):37–45.
95. Baer HU, Gertsch P, Matthews JB, et al. Resectability of large focal liver lesions. *Br J Surg*. 1989;76(10):1042–1044.
96. Heiken JP, Weyman PJ, Lee JK, et al. Detection of focal hepatic masses: prospective evaluation with CT, delayed CT, CT during arterial portography, and MR imaging. *Radiology*. 1989;171(1):47–51.
97. Soyer P. CT during arterial portography. *Eur Radiol*. 1996;6(3):349–357.
98. Maithel SK, Ginsberg MS, D'Amico F, et al. Natural history of patients with subcentimeter pulmonary nodules undergoing hepatic resection for metastatic colorectal cancer. *J Am Coll Surg*. 2010;210(1):31–38.
99. Ward J, Guthrie JA, Wilson D, et al. Colorectal hepatic metastases: detection with SPIO-enhanced breath-hold MR imaging—comparison of optimized sequences. *Radiology*. 2003;228(3):709–718.
100. Beets G, Penninckx F, Schiepers C, et al. Clinical value of whole-body positron emission tomography with [18F]fluorodeoxyglucose in recurrent colorectal cancer. *Br J Surg*. 1994;81(11):1666–1670.

101. Fong Y, Saldinger PF, Akhurst T, et al. Utility of 18F-FDG positron emission tomography scanning on selection of patients for zresection of hepatic colorectal metastases. *Am J Surg*. 1999;178(4):282–287.
102. Akhurst T, Fong Y. Positron emission tomography in surgical oncology. *Adv Surg*. 2002;36:309–331.
103. Akhurst T, Kates TJ, Mazumdar M, et al. Recent chemotherapy reduces the sensitivity of [18F]fluorodeoxyglucose positron emission tomography in the detection of colorectal metastases. *J Clin Oncol*. 2005; 23(34):8713–8716.
104. Ruers TJ, Wiering B, van dS Jr, et al. Improved selection of patients for hepatic surgery of colorectal liver metastases with (18)F-FDG PET: a randomized study. *J Nucl Med*. 2009;50(7):1036–1041.
105. Babineau TJ, Lewis WD, Jenkins RL, et al. Role of staging laparoscopy in the treatment of hepatic malignancy. *Am J Surg*. 1994;167(1):151–154.
106. Jarnagin WR, Bodniewicz J, Dougherty E, et al. A prospective analysis of staging laparoscopy in patients with primary and secondary hepatobiliary malignancies. *J Gastrointest Surg*. 2000;4(1):34–43.
107. John TG, Greig JD, Crosbie JL, et al. Superior staging of liver tumors with laparoscopy and laparoscopic ultrasound. *Ann Surg*. 1994;220(6):711–719.
108. Potter MW, Shah SA, McEnaney P, et al. A critical appraisal of laparoscopic staging in hepatobiliary and pancreatic malignancy. *Surg Oncol*. 2000;9(3):103–110.
109. Kubota K, Makuuchi M, Kusaka K, et al. Measurement of liver volume and hepatic functional reserve as a guide to decision-making in resectional surgery for hepatic tumors. *Hepatology*. 1997;26(5):1176–1181.
110. Shimamura T, Nakajima Y, Une Y, et al. Efficacy and safety of preoperative percutaneous transhepatic portal embolization with absolute ethanol: a clinical study. *Surgery*. 1997;121(2):135–141.
111. Covey AM, Tuorto S, Brody LA, et al. Safety and efficacy of preoperative portal vein embolization with polyvinyl alcohol in 58 patients with liver metastases. *AJR Am J Roentgenol*. 2005;185(6):1620–1626.
112. Aussilhou B, Dokmak S, Faivre S, et al. Preoperative liver hypertrophy induced by portal flow occlusion before major hepatic resection for colorectal metastases can be impaired by bevacizumab. *Ann Surg Oncol*. 2009;16(6):1553–1559.
113. Zorzi D, Chun YS, Madoff DC, et al. Chemotherapy with bevacizumab does not affect liver regeneration after portal vein embolization in the treatment of colorectal liver metastases. *Ann Surg Oncol*. 2008;15(10):2765–2772.
114. Vogt P, Raab R, Ringe B, Pichlmayr R. Resection of synchronous liver metastases from colorectal cancer. *World J Surg*. 1991;15(1):62–67
115. Brouquet A, Nordlinger B. Surgical strategies to synchronous colorectal liver metastases. *Dig Dis*. 2012;30(suppl 2):132–136.
116. Asbun HJ, Hughes KS. Management of recurrent and metastatic colorectal carcinoma. *Surg Clin North Am*. 1993;73(1):145–166.
117. Gold JS, Are C, Kornprat P, et al. Increased use of parenchymal-sparing surgery for bilateral liver metastases from colorectal cancer is associated with improved mortality without change in oncologic outcome: trends in treatment over time in 440 patients. *Ann Surg*. 2008;247(1):109–117.
118. Parker GA, Lawrence W Jr, Horsley JS III, et al. Intraoperative ultrasound of the liver affects operative decision making. *Ann Surg*. 1989;209(5):569–576.
119. Jarnagin WR, Bach AM, Winston CB, et al. What is the yield of intraoperative ultrasonography during partial hepatectomy for malignant disease? *J Am Coll Surg*. 2001;192(5):577–583.
120. Bismuth H, Castaing D, Garden OJ. The use of operative ultrasound in surgery of primary liver tumors. *World J Surg*. 1987;11(5):610–614.
121. Makuuchi M, Hasegawa H, Yamazaki S, et al. The use of operative ultrasound as an aid to liver resection in patients with hepatocellular carcinoma. *World J Surg*. 1987;11(5):615–621.
122. Torzilli G, Takayama T, Hui AM, et al. A new technical aspect of ultrasound-guided liver surgery. *Am J Surg*. 1999;178(4):341–343.
123. Thaler K, Kanneganti S, Khajanchee Y, et al. The evolving role of staging laparoscopy in the treatment of colorectal hepatic metastasis. *Arch Surg*. 2005;140(8):727–734.
124. Callery MP, Strasberg SM, Doherty GM, et al. Staging laparoscopy with laparoscopic ultrasonography: optimizing resectability in hepatobiliary and pancreatic malignancy. *J Am Coll Surg*. 1997;185(1):33–39.
125. Weitz J, D'Angelica M, Jarnagin W, et al. Selective use of diagnostic laparoscopy prior to planned

hepatectomy for patients with hepatocellular carcinoma. *Surgery*. 2004;135(3):273–281.

126. van der Pool AE, Lalmahomed ZS, de Wilt JH, et al. Local treatment for recurrent colorectal hepatic metastases after partial hepatectomy. *J Gastrointest Surg*. 2009;13(5):890–895.

127. Reuter NP, Woodall CE, Scoggins CR, et al. Radiofrequency ablation vs. resection for hepatic colorectal metastasis: therapeutically equivalent? *J Gastrointest Surg*. 2009; 13(3):486–491.

128. Gleisner AL, Choti MA, Assumpcao L, et al. Colorectal liver metastases: recurrence and survival following hepatic resection, radiofrequency ablation, and combined resection-radiofrequency ablation. *Arch Surg*. 2008;143(12):1204–1212.

129. Nguyen KT, Laurent A, Dagher I, et al. Minimally invasive liver resection for metastatic colorectal cancer: a multi-institutional, international report of safety, feasibility, and early outcomes. *Ann Surg*. 2009;250(5):842–848.

130. Vibert E, Perniceni T, Levard H, et al. Laparoscopic liver resection. *Br J Surg*. 2006;93(1): 67–72.

131. Nordlinger B, Quilichini MA, Parc R, et al. Hepatic resection for colorectal liver metastases. Influence on survival of preoperative factors and surgery for recurrences in 80 patients. *Ann Surg*. 1987;205(3):256–263.

132. Kjeldsen BJ, Kronborg O, Fenger C, Jorgensen OD. A prospective randomized study of follow-up after radical surgery for colorectal cancer. *Br J Surg*. 1997;84(5):666–669.

133. Makela JT, Laitinen SO, Kairaluoma MI. Five-year follow-up after radical surgery for colorectal cancer. Results of a prospective randomized trial. *Arch Surg*. 1995;130(10): 1062–1067.

134. Schoemaker D, Black R, Giles L, Toouli J. Yearly colonoscopy, liver CT, and chest radiography do not influence 5-year survival of colorectal cancer patients. *Gastroenterology*. 1998;114(1):7–14.

135. Pagana TJ. A new technique for hepatic infusional chemotherapy. *Semin Surg Oncol*. 1986;2(2):99–102.

136. Parks R, Gonen M, Kemeny N, et al. Adjuvant chemotherapy improves survival after resection of hepatic colorectal metastases: analysis of data from two continents. *J Am Coll Surg*. 2007;204(5):753–761.

137. Portier G, Elias D, Bouche O, et al. Multicenter randomized trial of adjuvant fluorouracil and folinic acid compared with surgery alone after resection of colorectal liver metastases: FFCD ACHBTH AURC 9002 trial. *J Clin Oncol*. 2006;24(31):4976–4982.

138. Saltz LB, Niedzwiecki D, Hollis D, et al. Irinotecan fluorouracil plus leucovorin is not superior to fluorouracil plus leucovorin alone as adjuvant treatment for stage III colon cancer: results of CALGB 89803. *J Clin Oncol*. 2007;25(23):3456-3461.

139. Curley SA, Roh MS, Chase JL, Hohn DC. Adjuvant hepatic arterial infusion chemotherapy after curative resection of colorectal liver metastases. *Am J Surg*. 1993;166(6): 743–746.

140. Goodie DB, Horton MD, Morris RW, et al. Anaesthetic experience with cryotherapy for treatment of hepatic malignancy. *Anaesth Intensive Care*. 1992;20(4):491–496.

141. Moriya Y, Sugihara K, Hojo K, Makuuchi M. Adjuvant hepatic intra-arterial chemotherapy after potentially curative hepatectomy for liver metastases from colorectal cancer: a pilot study. *Eur J Surg Oncol*. 1991;17(5):519–525.

142. Kemeny N, Huang Y, Cohen AM, et al. Hepatic arterial infusion of chemotherapy after resection of hepatic metastases from colorectal cancer. *N Eng J Med*. 1999;341:2039–2048.

143. Goere D, Benhaim L, Bonnet S, et al. Adjuvant chemotherapy after resection of colorectal liver metastases in patients with high risk of hepatic recurrence: a comparative study between hepatic arterial infusion of oxaliplatin and modern systemic chemotherapy. *Ann Surg*. 2013;257(1):114–120.

144. Kemeny N, Jarnagin WR, Paty P, et al. Phase I trial of systemic oxaliplatin combination chemotherapy with hepatic arterial infusion in patients with unresectable liver metastases from colorectal cancer. *J Clin Oncol*. 2005;23(22):4888–4896.

145. Bismuth H, Adam R, Levi F, et al. Resection of nonresectable liver metastases from colorectal cancer after neoadjuvant chemotherapy. *Ann Surg*. 1996;224(4):509–520.

146. Adam R, Avisar E, Ariche A, et al. Five-year survival following hepatic resection after neoadjuvant therapy for nonresectable colorectal (liver) metastases. *Ann Surg Oncol*. 2001;8(4):347–353.

147. Ardito F, Vellone M, Cassano A, et al. Chance of cure following liver resection for initially unresectable colorectal metastases: analysis of acutal 5-year survival. *J Gastrointest Surg*. 2013;17(2):352–359.

148. Clavien PA, Selzner N, Morse M, et al. Downstaging of hepatocellular carcinoma and

liver metastases from colorectal cancer by selective intra-arterial chemotherapy. *Surgery*. 2002;131(4):433–442.

149. Peppercorn PD, Reznek RH, Wilson P, et al. Demonstration of hepatic steatosis by computerized tomography in patients receiving 5-fluorouracil-based therapy for advanced colorectal cancer. *Br J Cancer*. 1998;77(11):2008–2011.

150. Karoui M, Penna C, min-Hashem M, et al. Influence of preoperative chemotherapy on the risk of major hepatectomy for colorectal liver metastases. *Ann Surg*. 2006;243(1):1–7.

151. Beal IK, Anthony S, Papadopoulou A, et al. Portal vein embolisation prior to hepatic resection for colorectal liver metastases and the effects of periprocedure chemotherapy. *Br J Radiol*. 2006;79(942):473–478.

152. Kooby DA, Fong Y, Suriawinata A, et al. Impact of steatosis on perioperative outcome following hepatic resection. *J Gastrointest Surg*. 2003;7(8):1034–1044.

153. Parikh AA, Gentner B, Wu TT, et al. Perioperative complications in patients undergoing major liver resection with or without neoadjuvant chemotherapy. *J Gastrointest Surg*. 2003;7(8):1082–1088.

154. Rubbia-Brandt L, Audard V, Sartoretti P, et al. Severe hepatic sinusoidal obstruction associated with oxaliplatin-based chemotherapy in patients with metastatic colorectal cancer. *Ann Oncol*. 2004;15(3):460–466.

155. Fortner JG, Silva JS, Maj MC, et al. Multivariate analysis of a personal series of 247 consecutive patients with liver metastases from colorectal cancer. *Ann Surg*. 1984;199: 306–316.

156. Nordlinger B, Parc R, Delva E, et al. Hepatic resection for colorectal liver metastases. *Ann Surg*. 1987;205:256–263.

157. Coelho JC, Claus CM, Machuca TN, et al. Liver resection: 10-year experience from a single institution. *Arq Gastroenterol*. 2004;41(4):229–233.

158. Welsh FKS, Tilney HS, Tekkis PP, et al. Safe liver resection following chemotherapy for colorectal metastases is a matter of timing. *Br J Cancer*. 2007;96(7):1037–1042.

159. Fernandez FG, Drebin JA, Linehan DC, et al. Five-year survival after resection of hepatic metastases from colorectal cancer in patients screened by positron emission tomography with F-18 fluorodeoxyglucose (FDG-PET). *Ann Surg*. 2004;240(3):438–447.

160. Pawlik TM, Scoggins CR, Zorzi D, et al. Effect of surgical margin status on survival and site of recurrence after hepatic resection for colorectal metastases. *Ann Surg*. 2005;241(5): 715–722.

161. Karanjia ND, Lordan JT, Quiney N, et al. A comparison of right and extended right hepatectomy with all other hepatic resections for colorectal liver metastases: a ten-year study. *Eur J Surg Oncol (EJSO)*. January 2009;35(1):65–70.

162. Abdalla EK, Vauthey JN, Ellis LM, et al. Recurrence and outcomes following hepatic resection, radiofrequency ablation, and combined resection/ablation for colorectal liver metastases. *Ann Surg*. 2004;239(6): 818–825.

163. Assumpcao L, Choti MA, Gleisner AL, et al. Patterns of recurrence following liver resection for colorectal metastases: effect of primary rectal tumor site. *Arch Surg*. 2008;143(8):743–749.

164. Solbiati L. Percutaneous radio-frequency ablation of hepatic metastases from colorectal cancer: long-term results in 117 patients1. *Radiology*. 2001;221(1):159–166.

165. Oshowo A. Comparison of resection and radiofrequency ablation for treatment of solitary colorectal liver metastases. *Br J Surg*. 2003;90(10):1240–1243.

166. Lencioni R. Percutaneous radiofrequency ablation of hepatic colorectal metastases: technique, indications, results, and new promises. *Invest Radiol*. 2004;39(11):689–697.

167. Berber E. Predictors of survival after radiofrequency thermal ablation of colorectal cancer metastases to the liver: a prospective study. *J Clin Oncol*. 2005;23(7):1358–1364.

168. Aloia TA. Solitary colorectal liver metastasis: resection determines outcome. *Arch Surg*. 2006;141(5):460–466; discussion 466–467.

169. Abitabile P, Hartl U, Lange J, Maurer CA. Radiofrequency ablation permits an effective treatment for colorectal liver metastasis. *Eur J Surg Oncol (EJSO)*. 2007;33(1):67–71.

170. Otto G, Düber C, Hoppe-Lotichius M, et al. Radiofrequency ablation as first-line treatment in patients with early colorectal liver metastases amenable to surgery. *Ann Surg*. 2010;251(5):796–803.

171. Kemeny NE. Hepatic arterial infusion after liver resection. *N Engl J Med*. 2005;352(7): 734–735.

CHAPTER 7

Metastatic Neuroendocrine Tumors to the Liver

Saboor Khan, David M. Nagorney & Florencia G. Que

Introduction

Neuroendocrine tumors (NETs) encom pass a wide range of neoplasms and clinical behavior depending on their site of origin, hormonal production, and differentiation. First described in 1888 by Lubarsch,[1] the term Karznoid, or carcinoma-like, was introduced by Oberndorfer in 1907 when he described a distinct intestinal tumor that was biologically less aggressive than intestinal adenocarcinoma.[2] The recognition that carcinoid tumors were endocrine related was not widely appreciated until Lembeck was able to extract 5-hydroxytryptamine from a carcinoid tumor.[3]

Neuroendocrine (NE) cells occur throughout the length of the gastrointestinal (GI) tract and are the largest group of hormone-producing cells in the body. NE cells are derived from multipotent stem cells and not, as originally thought, from the migration of neural crest cells. There are at least 13 gut NE cells, which produce various bioactive peptides and amines including serotonin, gastrin, and histamine, stored in vesicles within the cells.

GI-NETs are of significant interest to clinicians and basic scientists. Although there have been marked improvements in the accuracy and earlier diagnosis of these tumors, many patients still present with hepatic metastases. The liver remains second only to regional lymph nodes as the dominant site of metastases from all GI tract malignancies. In contrast to most metastatic GI cancers, which progress rapidly thus significantly effecting duration and quality of life, the clinical course of NETs is in general much slower. The other distinguishing feature is the development of clinical endocrinopathies from overproduction of gut hormones. This small subgroup of patients with metastatic NE malignancies to the liver has become the focus of intensive multimodality therapy.

There are various guidelines published by several professional groups providing information on the investigation, classification, and management of NETs. More recently, North American Neuroendocrine Society has been active in this endeavor.[4] This organization is a collection of scientists, physicians, and surgeons, which represents multiple disciplines.

Classification

Gastroenteropancreatic (GEP) NE tumors historically are divided into two broad types: carcinoid (GI luminal) and noncarcinoid. Traditionally, the biological and biochemical differences have dictated a classification based on the site of origin: foregut (lung, thymus, stomach, duodenum, pancreas, bile duct, gallbladder, and liver), midgut (small intestine, appendix, and proximal colon), and hindgut (distal colon and rectum) occur in the wall submucosally. In contrast, pancreatic neuroendocrine tumors (PNET) have been classified simply whether functional or not.

To distinguish the clinical behavior of NETs, World Health Organization (WHO) (Geneva, Switzerland), on the basis of a consensus conference of pathologists in the year 2000, proposed four subtypes: benign, uncertain, low-grade malignancy, and high-grade malignancy.[5] Each histopathological subtype can be further subclassified as functioning or nonfunctioning. Such histopathological typing of GEP NETs, distinguishing clinical behavior will likely influence interpretation of outcomes after surgical management. Clinically, surgeons addressing metastatic NE cancers to the liver are likely to encounter only low-grade or high-grade malignancy.

The terms carcinoid, islet cell tumors, and NE tumors were used interchangeably throughout the 1980s and 1990s to describe PNETs. In 2000, the WHO chose the terms "NE carcinoma" and "NE tumor" to describe the tumors of the GEP system. The term "carcinoid" in this new classification is limited to describe highly differentiated NE tumors of the GI tract, excluding the pancreas.[6]

A tumor, node, metastases (TNM) classification has been suggested for carcinoids in 2007.[7] Survival stratification by TNM classification has been shown in clinical studies.[8,9] From a liver standpoint, the number and extent of hepatic metastases from NETs have been classified by radiological imaging; single metastasis (type I), isolated metastatic bulk accompanied by smaller deposits (type II), and disseminated metastatic spread (type III).[10]

Management Options

Recent evidence has been evaluated in a consensus paper.[11] Although there are some differences among staging systems and pathology classification systems, many common themes have been recognized, such as the distinction of well-differentiated (low- and intermediate-grade) from poorly differentiated (high-grade) NETs and the significance of proliferative rate in prognostic assessment. Just as importantly, the requirement and guidance on minimum data set for pathological reports has been produced.

Epidemiology

Overall the incidence of GI-NETs is 2.5–5 per 100,000. Using the SEER (Surveillance Epidemiology and End Results)[12] database, the incidence and prevalence of these tumors has increased significantly over the last few decades.[13,14]

NETs are typically diagnosed around 60 years of age. There is a female predominance (60%) and a racial prevalence of African Americans.[14] GI-NETs comprise nearly 75% of all carcinoids with the remainder primarily of bronchopulmonary origin (Table 7-1). Pancreatic NETs occur in 0.5–1 person per 100,000 population. Nonfunctional NETs account for approximately 50% of pancreatic NETs in most series.[15] Interestingly, symptom duration is significantly longer for functional than nonfunctional NETs. The epidemiology of functional PNET varies widely in the clinical setting of the multiple endocrine neoplasia 1 syndrome and is beyond the scope of this chapter.

Natural History and Prognosis

The occurrence of hepatic metastases from NETs is highly variable depending on the primary disease, ranging anywhere from 5%–10% to 75% (for midgut and hindgut NETs). Thus, over half of the patients with a NET will have or may develop hepatic metastases (Table 7-1). The natural history of patients with unresected or unresectable hepatic metastases has been similar. Overall, patients with unresected hepatic metastases from NE cancers have an approximately 30% five-year survival[16] and a median survival of 17 months.[17] As discussed below, resection may impart a survival and symptomatic benefit.[18] Clearly, liver metastases are the most significant factor adversely affecting outcome. Tumor differentiation, the extent of liver disease (50% hepatic replacement versus >75%), and relatively rapid disease progression within the liver are other poor prognostic indicators.[9,18–20] Carcinoid heart disease, which occurs only in the presence of metastatic carcinoid tumor to the liver, independently predicts poor survival (30% survival rate at three years), unless cardiac surgery is undertaken successfully.[21,22]

Diagnosis and Staging of NETs

The diagnosis is based on clinical symptoms, hormone concentration, radiological and nuclear imaging, and histological confirmation, which should be obtained whenever possible.[23]

For symptomatic patients, measurement of circulating peptides and amines (including tumor markers, such as α-fetoprotein, β human chorionic gonadotropin, and carcinoembryonic antigen;

Table 7-1) is helpful on three counts to assist in making the diagnosis, assessing the treatment, and as prognostic indicators.[23–25]

Chromogranin A (CgA) (and synaptophysin) is a large protein that is produced by all cells deriving from the neural crest. Its function is unknown, but it is produced in significant quantities by NET cells, regardless of their secretory status. Plasma CgA may be useful in diagnosis and monitoring disease progression. Chromogranin A has been shown to have a high sensitivity and variable specificity for NETs. Chromogranin A is elevated in 80% of patients with NETs from all sites and seems to correlate with tumor load.[26–28]

TABLE 7-1: Gastroenteropancreatic Neuroendocrine Tumors: Clinical and Biochemical Features

Tumor Type/Site – Incidence 10[6]	Peptide/Amines	Clinical Features	Metastases
Foregut carcinoid Bronchi, thymus, stomach, first part of duodenum, pancreas (2–5)	Serotonin, histamine, ACTH, CRH, GH, 5 HIAA (30%)	Pulmonary obstruction (bronchi), atypical flush, and hormonal syndromes	Liver, lymph nodes, bone
Midgut carcinoid Second part of duodenum, jejunum, ileum, and right colon (4–10)	Serotonin, tachykinins, prostaglandins, bradykinins, and others (70%), 5 HIAA (75%)	Bowel obstruction, typical pink/red flush, wheeze/diarrhea	Liver (60%–80%), lymph nodes
Hindgut carcinoid Transverse colon to rectum (1.5–2.5)	Local production somatostatin, peptide YY, glicentin, neurotensin, serotonin, and other hormones	Incidental finding, local symptoms	Bone metastases (5%–40%)
Insulinoma (1–2)	Insulin, proinsulin	Neuroglucopenia, Whipple's triad	(10%)
Gastrinoma (1–1.5)	Gastrin	Zollinger–Ellison syndrome	(60%–90%)
VIPoma (0.1)	Vasoactive intestinal Peptide	Watery diarrhea, hypokalemia, achlorhydria	(50%–80%)
Glucagonoma (0.01–0.1)	Glucagon	Necrolytic migratory syndrome, diabetes, cachexia	(80%–90%)
Somatostatinoma (<0.1)	Somatostatin	Gall stones, diabetes, steatorrhea, achlorhydria	(60%–70%)
Nonfunctioning tumors (1–2)	Pancreatic polypeptide	Mass effect	(60%–80%)
GRFoma (<0.1)	GRF	Acromegaly	(60%–70%)
ACTHoma (<0.1)	ACTH	Cushing's syndrome	(95%)

Abbreviations: ACTH, adrenocorticotropic hormone, CRH, corticotropin-releasing hormone, GH, growth hormone, 5 HIAA, 5-hydroxyindoleacetic acid

The presence of symptoms, liver metastases, and a positive humoral test is highly suggestive of NET, but histology is necessary for confirmation and will allow proliferation indices to be assessed, which may influence management. The optimum investigations to detect NETs and assess its extent depend on the location. The GI submucosal location makes visualization difficult, whereas luminal primary NETs are perhaps better visualized by endoscopy; solid organ and lymph nodal disease require cross-sectional imaging (computed tomography [CT] and/or magnetic resonance [MR] scan)[29] and, if indicated, endoscopic ultrasound for pancreatic NETs, which has the advantage of biopsy.[23,30] Most NETs express somatostatin receptors (SSTR) and this has led to the development of radiolabeled somatostatin analogs for diagnostic imaging. This is useful in imaging both the primary and metastases.[31,32] Moreover, this aspect is also utilized in management with the development of radiolabeled somatostatin ligand binding as a radio-pharmaceutical treatment strategy (discussed later). More recently, positron emission tomography (PET) (or CT PET) scanning has proven beneficial in the detection and staging of NETs[33,34] and may provide additional value when compared to somatostatin scintiscanning.[35] For addressing hepatic disease, a triple-phase CT and/or liver specific MR scan[36,37] are adequate to assess resectability.

Treatment Strategies

The aim of the treatment should be complete resection, where possible. This applies to primary and metastatic disease.[38,39] Unfortunately for most patients, the presentation is delayed so that cure may not be possible; however, within a multimodality framework, the quality of life may be maintained for a prolonged period of time. Importantly, the focus on palliation and extension of life rather than on complete remission is conceptually a paradigm shift, specific to the management of NET metastases, because most hepatic resections are undertaken for cure in patients with metastatic solid cancers.

Liver-directed Therapies

The relative safety of hepatic resections and ablative procedures has stimulated an interest in the aggressive treatment of NET-related hepatic metastases. Further, due to the indolent nature of most NET tumors, "cytoreduction" can be justified for improving symptom-free survival. This implies removing (surgical resection or ablation) at least 90% of the disease, with the emphasis on minimizing residual disease volume.[40] This concept is particularly applicable to patients with endocrinopathies.[19] However, cytoreduction is also warranted because of relative inefficacy of medical therapies (chemotherapy and radiation). The obvious advantage is that cytoreductive procedures can be repeated and combined with other therapies to gain maximal benefit. As a corollary, the duration of response should be in proportion to the extent of the debulking or cytoreduction of the metastatic NET and the growth rate of the residual NET (Figure 7-1).[17]

Hepatic Resection

The current mainstay of treatment for metastatic GI NE cancers to the liver is resection. Hepatic resection of metastatic NET is recommended if the primary tumor and regional disease are resectable or resected so that there is minimal disease volume in the remnant, frequently quoted as >90%, which is resectable or amenable to ablation.[25] Our initial results in patients with functioning metastases limited to the liver showed that hepatic debulking could be performed safely and overall survival was approximately 75% at four years (Figure 7-1A).[41] There was no significant difference in survival between patients undergoing complete margin-negative (R_0) resection or incomplete conventional resection or resection including extended lymph node dissection (R_{1-2}) (Figure 7-1B). Mean duration of symptom response was nearly two years (Figure 7-1C). Subsequently, our findings in 170 patients with both functioning and nonfunctioning tumors undergoing hepatic resections showed that symptoms resolve in 98% of patients.[42] Median time to symptom recurrence was 45 months, and 59% of patients experienced recurrent symptoms at five years. Overall survival was 61% and 35% at 5 and 10 years, respectively (Figure 7-2A), and was not significantly different for carcinoid versus pancreatic NE patients (Figure 7-2B); also no difference in survival was seen between patients who were or were not symptomatic preoperatively

(Figure 7-2C), and perioperative mortality was 1.2%. Recurrence, however, was 84% at 5 years and 94% at 10 years. Synchronous hepatic disease can be resected together with a pancreatic primary with good results.[43,44]

Reports of minimally invasive resections of NE metastases are also emerging.[45]

The selection criteria for candidacy for operative cytoreduction include resectable/resected primary NET, >90% resectable/ablatable hepatic metastases,

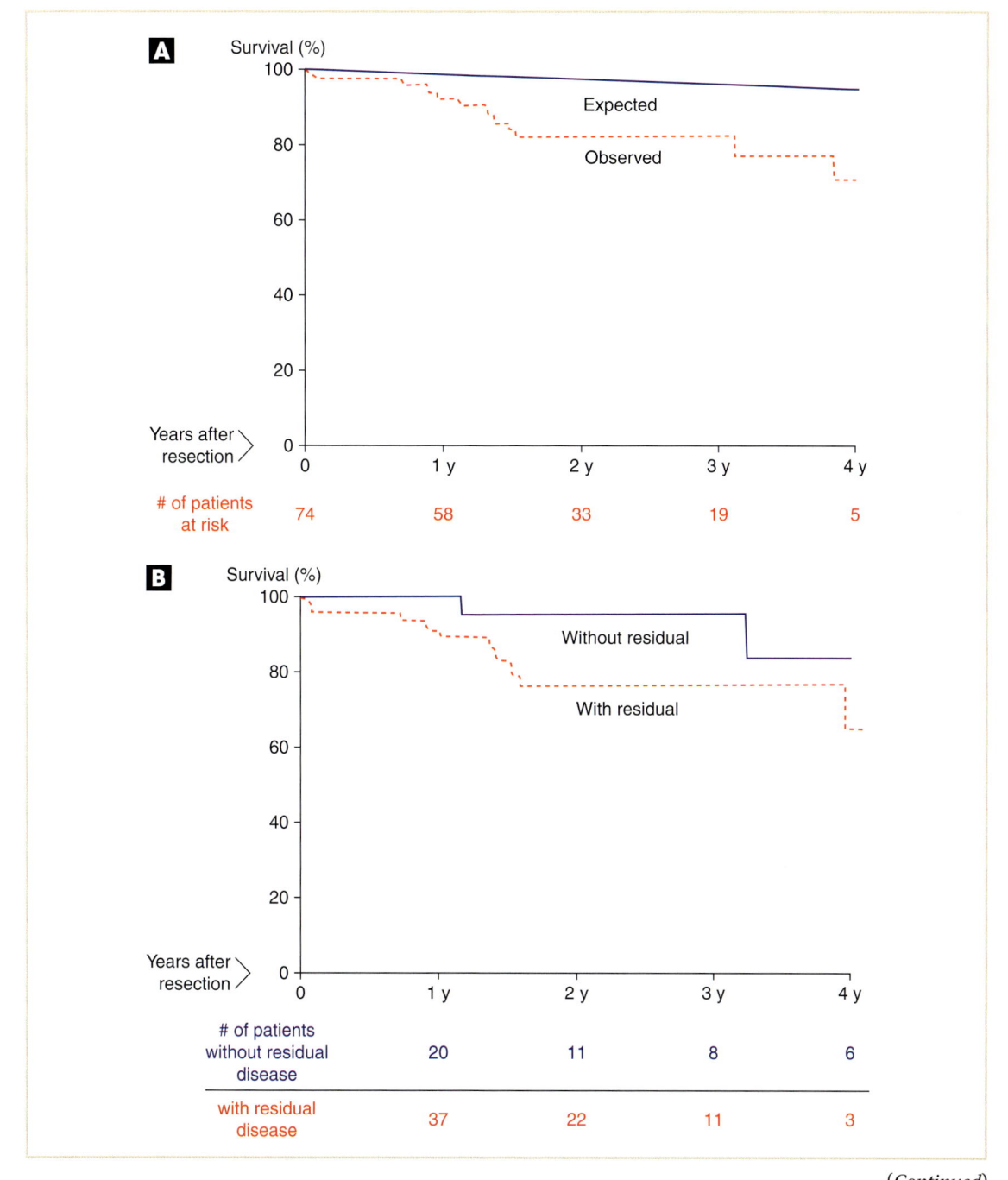

(Continued)

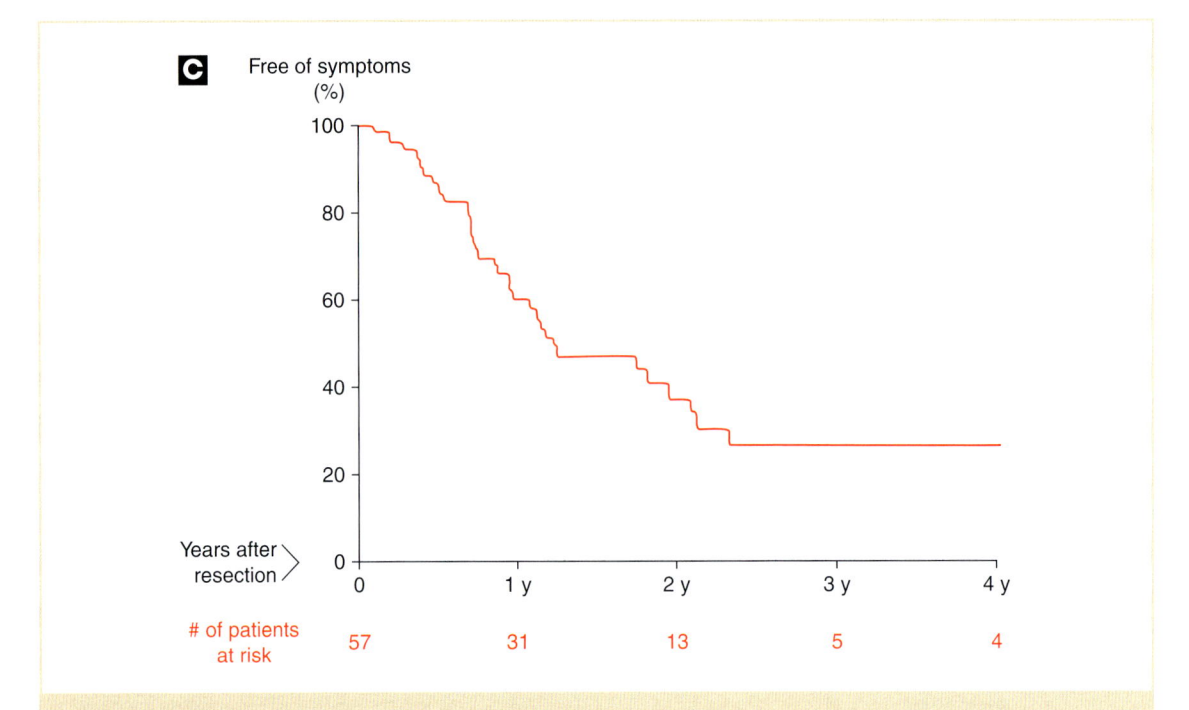

Figure 7-1: (A) Overall survival was approximately 75% at four years in 75 patients with neuroendocrine metastases to the liver after hepatic resection. (B) There was no significant difference in survival between patients undergoing complete margin-negative (R_0) resection or incomplete conventional resection or resection including extended lymph node dissection (R_{1-2}). (C) Mean duration of symptom response was nearly two years. Reprinted from Que FG, Nagorney DM, Batts KP, et al. *Amer J Surg.* 1995;169:36–42 with permission from Elsevier.[41]

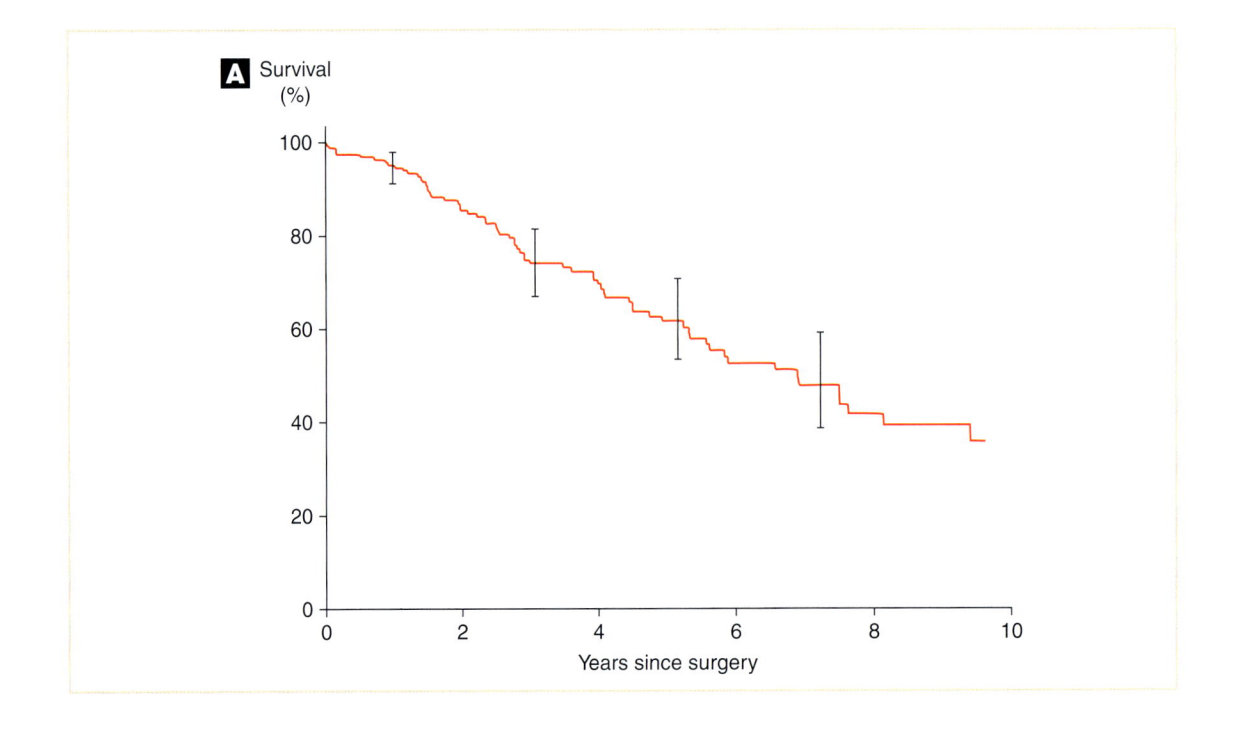

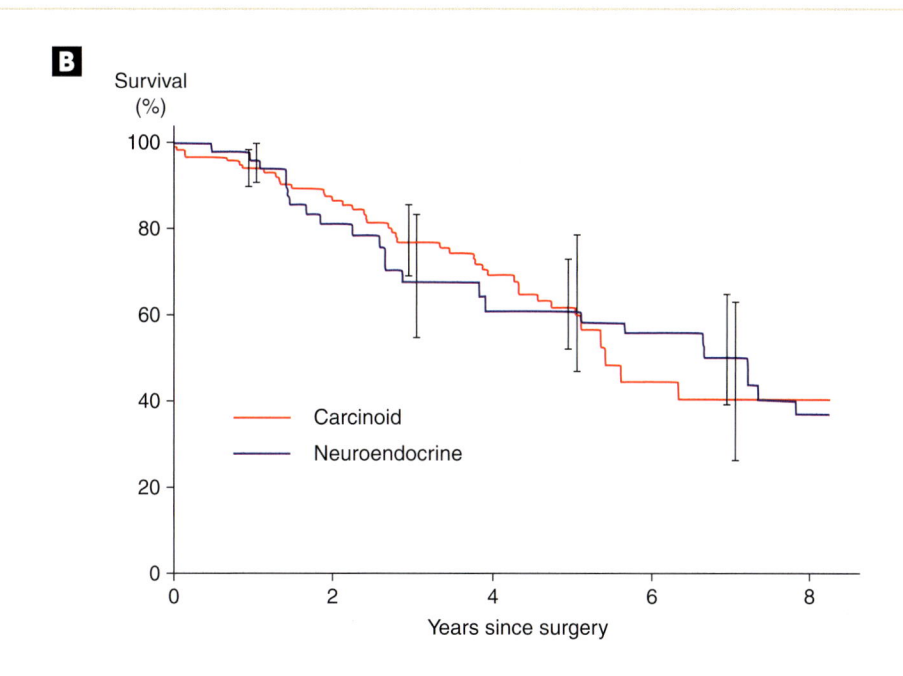

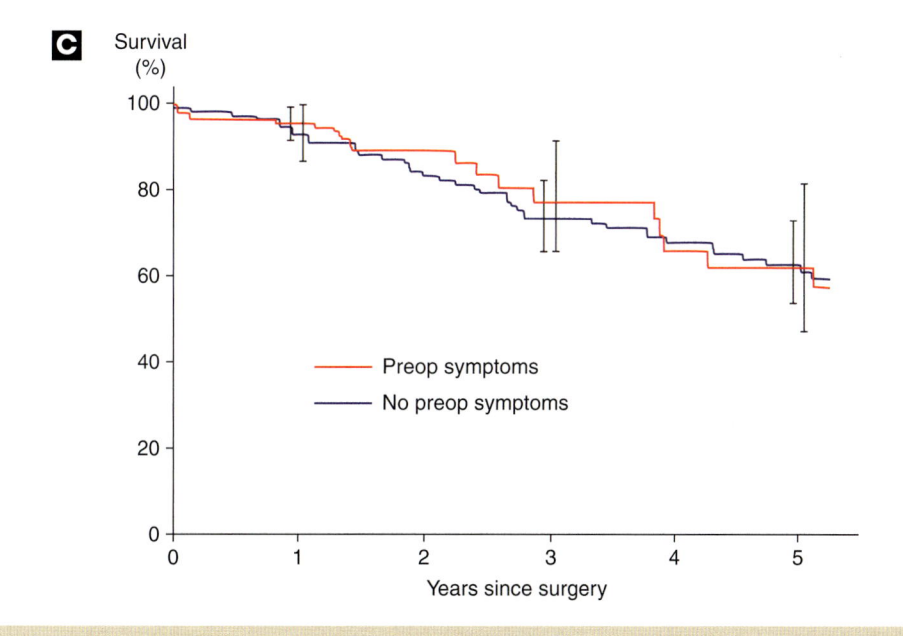

Figure 7-2: (A) In a study of 170 patients with both functioning and nonfunctioning tumors who underwent hepatic resection, symptoms resolved in 98% of patients. Median time to symptom recurrence was 45 months; 59% of patients experienced recurrent symptoms at five years. Overall survival was 61% at 5 years and 35% at 10 years. (B) There was no significant difference in recurrence of symptoms for patients with carcinoid (red) versus pancreatic neuroendocrine (blue). (C) There was no significant difference in survival between patients who were preoperatively symptomatic (red) or those who were not (blue). Reprinted from Sarmiento JM, Heywood G, Rubin J, et al. *J Amer Coll Surg.* 2003;197:29–37 with permission from Elsevier.[42]

absence of other distant metastases, and adequate hepatic and cardiac reserve.[46] It is imperative that operative candidates with NETs are optimized. The likely risk factors that require careful attention including clinical endocrinopathy, carcinoid heart disease, other significant comorbidity such as diabetes and finally anticipate occult non-NETs. Somatostatin (or its analogs) should be utilized preoperatively in carcinoid patients to prevent an intraoperative crisis related to excess release of hormonally active agents.

The technical caveats for resection of hepatic metastases include addressing the planned remnant metastases first, accepting a grossly negative resection margin especially near major ducts and vessels, ablating deep remnant metastases, employing ischemic preconditioning, and for staged resection where appropriate.

A review of the current literature on hepatic resection for metastatic NET with studies reporting on >30 patients is summarized in Table 7-2.[19,40,46,104–107] The cumulative findings from these reports support an aggressive operative approach for metastatic NETs. Overall five-year survival has ranged from 41% to 82%, with a median five-year survival of 74%. Resolution of endocrine symptoms, when addressed, exceeded 90% in most series. The duration was not routinely reported. Survival was not markedly different between carcinoid and noncarcinoid patients. The presence of endocrinopathy has not shown adverse outcome to date. Interestingly, although complete resection of hepatic metastases has been undertaken more frequently, survival has not significantly differed between patients with complete or incomplete hepatic resection of metastatic NET provided that cytoreduction exceeds 90% of the estimated hepatic cancer volume, and is associated with improvement in quality of life.[41,47,48] These data suggest that hepatic resection of metastatic NET is safe and clinically effective, and overall operative survival is nearly double to that of patients with unresected metastases. Few other factors related to the primary NET, metastatic disease, or patients have been correlated with survival.

The cytoreductive concept requires further discussion because of important patient implication. Resection of >90% of the volume of hepatic metastases resulting in varying residual disease can lead to significantly different residual cancer volumes based on variations of the incident metastatic volume, thus affecting both the time to recurrence of symptoms and survival. The clinical implication of cytoreductive hepatic resection is not only >90% resection of metastatic NET in the liver but striving to minimize residual metastatic volume that is not resected. It is the latter that determines disease recurrence and any contingent endocrinopathy. Excellent outcomes are possible for prolonged periods with a rigorous operative strategy as can be seen in Figure 7-3.

The overall frequency of recurrence or progression after hepatic resection is approximately 80% at five years. Intrahepatic progression of residual

TABLE 7-2: Hepatic Resection for Metastatic Neuroendocrine Tumor

Study	Patients (N)	Perioperative Mortality (N)	Postoperative Symptom Control (%)	5-y Survival (%)
Chamberlain, 2000[19]	34	2	90	76
Nave, 2001[104]	31	0	–	47
Ringe, 2001[105]	31	0	–	47
Sarmiento, 2003[46]	170	2	96	61
Chambers, 2008[a, 40]	30	0	75	74
Kianmanesh, 2008[106]	41	0	–	79
Eriksson, 2008[a, 54]	42	0	70	80 disease free survival
Scigliano, 2009[b, 107]	38	0	–	79

[a]Cytoreductive.
[b]Curative.

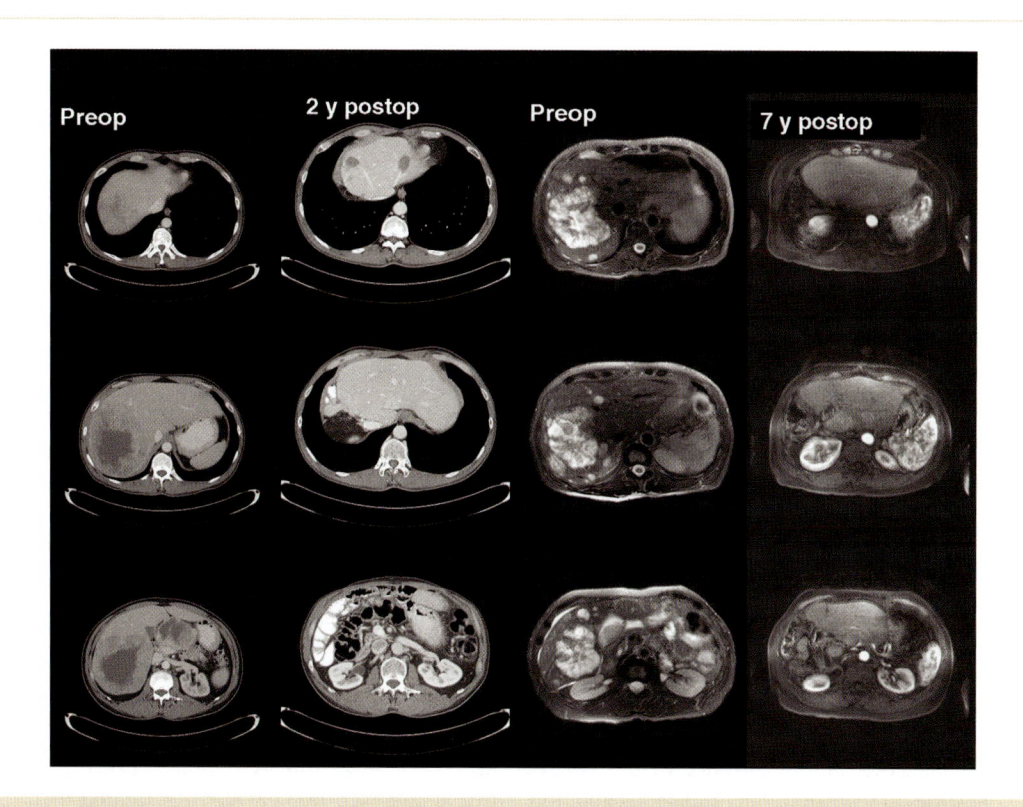

Figure 7-3: Preoperative and postoperative results of operative cytoreduction of hepatic neuroendocrine metastases in two cases: at two years and seven years postoperative. Reprinted from Maithel SK, Fong Y. *J Surg Oncol.* 2009;100:635–638 with permission from John Wiley and Sons.[50]

metastases after R_{1-2} resection or recurrence after R_0 resection dictates subsequent liver-directed therapy unless such therapy risks liver failure or extrahepatic metastases become dominant.

Although cure of patients with metastatic NET to the liver is infrequent, prolonged palliation is possible. Patterns of intrahepatic recurrence have not been well studied. Intrahepatic recurrence is typically multicentric in our experience. The extent and distribution of hepatic recurrence dictates the choice of therapy. For solitary recurrences, either resection or ablation is appropriate. Given that serial imaging usually identifies small recurrences after hepatic resection, percutaneous ablative approaches are preferable because morbidity associated with percutaneous radiofrequency ablation (RFA) is less than that after repeat resection. Repeat hepatic resection is advised for lesions in sites that preclude safe RFA. Sequential ablation or resection is undertaken as recurrence is recognized until precluded by the extent of recurrence within the liver. Metastatic NET precluding ablation or resection is treated by other therapies, as outlined below and in the diagrammatic schema.

Ablative Therapies

Multiple minimally invasive ablative modalities exist for the treatment of liver tumors, including cryotherapy, percutaneous ethanol injection (PEI), and thermal techniques such as RFA, microwave ablation (MW), and interstitial laser thermotherapy.[49]

Indeed, because reports of surgical experience have shown that cytoreduction of NETs can considerably improve patient survival and symptoms, the corollary of an aggressive ablation of progressive hepatic NE metastases should provide similar patient benefit. There are three clinical scenarios for ablation of NE hepatic metastases[50]: (1) adjunct to concurrent surgical resection of hepatic metastases; (2) treatment of limited hepatic metastases in patients unfit for operation; and (3) the primary hepatic therapy when clinical expertise or intraoperative circumstances preclude safe resection. Palliation of symptoms is an inherent aim for all patients with functional NE symptoms.

In contrast to non-NE metastases, there is justification based on surgical experience for subtotal debulking of significant hepatic tumor by the ablation of multiple metastases. Generally speaking, if the metastasis is visible with imaging, it can be treated in some manner with percutaneous ablation, provided there is sufficient preserved liver parenchyma to prevent hepatic decompensation.

This large volume ablation contrasts with the ablation of limited disease. Such a patient might have one or two very small hepatic metastases such that surgical resection might be considered overly aggressive given the effectiveness of percutaneous RFA in treating such tumors. Percutaneous treatment may be performed on an outpatient basis and obviates the longer hospitalization after resection. Moreover, given the invariable recurrence of metastases following surgical resection,[42] percutaneous ablation is well suited for the patient who has undergone prior liver surgery. Unlike surgical resection, ablation can easily be performed on multiple occasions based on occurrence of new metastases.

Radiofrequency Ablation

Currently, RFA is likely the most widely used ablative technique due to its effectiveness in treating larger tumors, versatility, ease of use, and relatively low risk of complications.[51-55] RFA has largely become the dominant modality used for ablation of NE metastases to the liver. Technologic advances, such as internally water-cooled electrode tips and expandable electrode tines, have made delivery of the thermal energy to the tumor more efficient and effective. The increasing expertise with percutaneous and laparoscopic approaches has made this technique more attractive by reducing its associated morbidity by treating patients in a minimally invasive way.[56,57]

RFA complements intraoperative resection of hepatic NE metastases. Given the extensive hepatic tumor burden typically encountered, ablation affords selective treatment of metastases located deep in the liver or in sites not further resectable after partial hepatectomy. Adjunctive RFA optimizes debulking of hepatic metastases, reduces the extent of resection, and increases overall candidacy for surgical treatment.

Resection is precluded in many patients with NE metastases to the liver because of the extent of tumor burden, comorbid disease, or prior hepatic resection. In such patients, percutaneous ablation allows less invasive tumor debulking and may have some advantage over chemotherapy alone, as shown by Ruers and colleagues.[58]

Published experience with RFA for NE hepatic metastases has been limited. RFA has been employed both primarily and as an adjunct to resection. Objective tumor destruction has been well documented and has been shown highly effective in local tumor control, with local recurrence in 3%–5% of treated metastases.[59,60] Duration of follow-up is insufficient to determine actual durability of local control given the protracted natural history of NE cancers. Progression of hepatic metastases has occurred in approximately 30% of patients within two years. Specific factors of the hepatic metastases such as site, degree of necrosis or fibrosis, and hormonal markers have not yet been correlated to RFA response. Local tumor control is achieved in 82%–98% of treated metastases, though duration of follow-up varied.[54,56,59,61-63] Local recurrence rates were greater in patients with colorectal metastases and fewer in those patients with NE hepatic metastases,[64] which may relate to different morphological characteristics of these tumors. Successful ablation typically occurred in the treatment of small metastases (<3 cm).[64-66] Only 50% of large tumors (>5 cm) were ablated completely, even with repeated ablation.

RFA has effectively relieved clinical endocrinopathies related to NE hepatic metastases. Nearly 90% of patients have experienced some degree of symptom relief following ablation of metastases.[59,60,63] Duration of relief from symptoms usually was 10 months or longer. These findings approach those reported after hepatic resection of metastatic NET. For limited hepatic metastases, RFA can achieve similar results percutaneously. In the setting of extrahepatic disease, isolated hepatic ablation will have a limited effect on symptoms.[63] However, clinical efficacy will depend upon the volume and site of extrahepatic tumor and the specific hormone expression.

Serum and urine NE tumor markers are generally proportional to tumor burden.[67] The response of such markers to RFA has been variable. In a study of 34 patients treated with intraoperative RFA, only 65% of patients had a decrease in serum tumor markers following ablation.[59] Persistently elevated tumor markers after RFA likely reflect patient selection, completeness of ablation, and occult or overt NE cancer within the abdomen or elsewhere. A favorable response in reduction of serum tumor markers following ablation may predict the durability of symptomatic response and be associated with improved survival and decreased incidence of disease progression.[59]

Microwave Ablation

MW therapy is a local treatment by which tumors are destroyed by coagulation from the passage of MWs into tissue. Microwave therapy is emerging as a reliable technique under a variety of clinical situations. Two main zones are described after ablative therapy (central and transitional). No viable cells even up to 6 cm in diameter were demonstrated in 93% of lesions after treatment.[68] Although data comparing RFA with MW are awaited, the results reported in observational studies indicate that MW may have a role when larger ablation zones are required in peripheral NETs.[69]

Ethanol Ablation

Ethanol ablation has also been incorporated into the treatment of primary and secondary hepatic neoplasms, including metastases from NE malignancies in selected patients.[49,61,70] Several studies have documented a complete intrahepatic response in patients with hepatic NE metastases treated with PEI. PEI permits ablation of metastases located adjacent to structures at risk of damage by RFA.

Highly selective ethanol ablation can be performed on metastases located adjacent to vital structures (such as the hepatic flexure of the colon), metastases adjacent to large vessels vulnerable to the heat-sink effect, and metastases adjacent to central bile ducts, where subsequent biliary stricture may occur. Moreover, metastases of very small size can also be ablated successfully with ethanol, with limited collateral injury to adjacent liver.

Cryoablation

Intraoperative cryoablation is effective in the treatment of primary and secondary tumors of the liver.[71–74] Cryoablation has predominantly been replaced by RFA because of the possibility of potentially devastating complications, increased time for use, and difficulty in monitoring disease recurrence.

Hepatic Transplantation

Orthotopic liver transplantation (OLT) has been employed increasingly for the treatment of metastatic NET. The rationale for OLT is similar to that for resection with the caveat that adequate cytoreduction by resection is precluded by the extent of intrahepatic disease and the absence of extrahepatic metastases. OLT during the time period of intrahepatic disease may be curative or, at least, significantly palliative. Unlike resection, OLT addresses all hepatic metastases and should at least provide similar, if not greater, duration of palliation of symptoms and survival. The attractiveness of R_0 resection afforded by OLT and the high recurrence rate of NETs associated with resection have fostered ongoing evaluation of OLT for metastatic NET.[75]

A current literature review of OLT, with series reporting >10 patients for NETs, is summarized in Table 7-3.[10,108–114] As with resection, OLT was undertaken if the primary and regional NET had been resected and distal metastases were excluded by octreotide scintigraphy and dynamic CT or MR imaging. Results and selection criteria have varied, and actual duration of follow-up has been limited. One-year survival has ranged from 50% to 100% (mean 82%) and five-year survival from 36% to 89% (mean 57%) with a mean overall follow-up of 36 months. Symptomatic relief from clinical endocrinopathies, when present, has been uniformly complete, but duration of symptomatic relief after OLT has not been clearly documented. The rate of recurrence is similar to that after resection and the criteria of patient selection for OLT likely account for this finding.

Current data do not support OLT as a primary treatment modality for metastatic NET[25,76] and should probably be considered only in patients with resected primary NET after a period of disease stability with exclusion of any extrahepatic disease; the parameters that predict reasonable outcome posttransplant include age <50 years, "limited" liver disease, low Ki 67 index, regular E-cadherin staining, and complete local-regional primary control ≥1 year.[25]

TABLE 7-3: Hepatic Transplantation for Metastatic Neuroendocrine Cancer

Study	Patients (N)	Median Follow-Up (mo)	1-y Survival (%)	5-y Survival (%)
Lehnert, 1998[103]	103	–	70	47
Rosenau, 2002[109]	19	38	89	80
Florman, 2004[110]	11	30	73	36
van Vilsteren, 2006[111]	19	18	87	–
Marin, 2007[112]	10	34	86	57 (3 y)
Olausson, 2007[113]	15	55	90	90
Frilling, 2006 & 2009[10,114] (4 perioperative deaths)	17	60	–	67

Chemoembolization/Radioembolization

NE metastases are intensely hypervascular. Embolization of the hepatic arteries results in ischemia of the metastases and causes variable degrees of tumor necrosis, which can alleviate symptoms or endocrinopathies.[77] Embolization alone or in combination with intra-arterial chemotherapy (chemoembolization) has been employed for relief of symptoms.[78] Repeated embolization is possible depending upon the interventional vascular technique employed (selective or nonselective). Objective tumor responses to embolization alone have ranged from 30% to 70% with similar symptomatic response rates.[79–81] Chemotherapy following embolization has prolonged duration of response.[82] These findings coupled with the theoretical advantages of high intrahepatic concentration afforded by arterial infusion of chemotherapeutic agents prompted evaluation of chemoembolization. Although chemoembolization has been employed for metastatic NETs, range and duration of response has been similar to embolization alone.[83,84] To date, no randomized trial comparing embolization with and without chemotherapy has confirmed a significant difference in outcomes or response; observational data have shown no statistical difference between the two groups.[78]

Complications are generally tolerable, though not insignificant. The postembolization syndrome consisting of nausea, right upper quadrant abdominal pain, fever, and elevation of serum transaminases usually lasting for three to seven days is common. Parenteral analgesics, intravenous hydration, and antipyretics are often necessary. Antibiotic prophylaxis is recommended for embolization. Other side effects include gallbladder necrosis, hepatic abscess, and renal failure. Patients with large (>5–10 cm) metastases and those with >50%–70% hepatic replacement are at greater risk of complications. Sequential lobar embolization may reduce the severity of the postembolization syndrome and risk of complications. Mortality after embolization has ranged from 2% to 7%.[77,85]

Radioembolization through the use of Yttrium-90 TheraSpheres® (MDS Nordion Inc., Ottawa, ON, Canada) has recently shown promise in the management of patients with other solid tumors; data with regard to its use in hepatic NETs are awaited.[86,87]

Medical (systemic) and Radiopharmaceutical Treatments

There are several approaches for the medical treatment of metastatic NET. These approaches include somatostatin analogs, chemotherapy, immunotherapy, targeted somatostatin analogs, and internal irradiation with I^{131} conjugates, and newer drugs.[88]

Somatostatin Analogs

Octreotide is a synthetic somatostatin analog with a significantly longer half-life and duration of action than native somatostatin.[89] It is primarily cytostatic but can also be cytotoxic. The effect of somatostatin analogs is mediated through type 2 and type 5 SSTR, inhibiting the cellular release of hormone. Response may correlate to SSTR scintigraphy.[90] The analogs also can affect cell cycle arrest in G1 phase, induce apoptosis, and inhibit angiogenesis. Lanreotide is currently the longest acting or slow release analog. Octreotide dose ranges from 100 to 500 μg three times daily and Lanreotide for 60–120 mg every four weeks.

Somatostatin analogs have been associated with a biochemical response in approximately 70% of patients, and symptomatic relief in 60%–90% of patients.[91] Objective reduction in tumor size (>50% of largest diameter) has occurred in <10% of patients. Stabilization of NET has been observed in 36%–70% of patients for a median duration of 12 months.[91] As expected, symptomatic response has been correlated with improved quality of life. Response to somatostatin analog therapy varies by type of NET. Only one prospective, multicenter, placebo-controlled, randomized study exists that evaluated the effect of "long-acting" octreotide on tumor control and deprogression. In midgut NET ($n = 85$), Rinke et al demonstrated a 14.3-month versus a 6-month tumor-to-tumor progression in patients receiving long-acting octreotide versus placebo ($P = 0.00072$). Overall, active treatment resulted in stable disease in 66.7% of patients versus 37.2% of those receiving placebo ($P = 0.0079$) over six months of treatment.

Chemotherapy

The crucial issue with rigorous assessment of medical treatment is that most studies are retrospective, assess heterogeneous tumors, commonly lack standardized entry criteria, reflect single-center experience, and are underpowered.

Systemic chemotherapy is generally reserved for patients with advanced or progressive disease where other treatment efforts have failed.[93] Carcinoid tumors may be less sensitive to cytotoxic agents due to the preponderance of low-grade malignant (well differentiated) histology and low proliferation index.[94] Dacarbazine, 5-FU, and epirubicin combination therapy has achieved objective tumor response in approximately 30% of patients with carcinoid tumors.[95] Median duration of response for carcinoid tumors is approximately six months.

Alpha Interferon

Systemic alpha interferon (αIFN) may be used to treat advanced NET. The mechanism of αIFN is mediated through direct inhibitors of cell cycle (G1/S phase), of protein and hormone production, antiangiogenesis, and indirectly by increased immune stimulation.[91] Although an objective tumor response is seen in only 10%–15%, both symptomatic and biochemical responses have been observed in approximately 40%–60% of patients.[91,96–97] Disease stabilization has occurred in 40%–60% of patients. Adverse reactions to αIFN are common and may dictate discontinuation of αIFN. Chronic fatigue and hematologic cytopenias are the most common side effects.

New Drugs and Targets

Traditional DNA-damaging cytotoxic drugs are of limited efficacy in GEP NETs because of reasons outlined above. Several proangiogenic molecules are overexpressed in NETs: for example, vascular endothelial growth factor and its receptors, and related signaling- pathway components such as epithelial growth factor receptor, insulin-like growth factor 1 receptor, phosphoinositide-3-kinase, RAC-alpha serine/threonine-protein kinase (AKT), and mammalian target of rapamycin (mTOR).[98] New drugs that target some of these molecules are under assessment in early clinical trials, such as Bevacizumab (monoclonal antibody against vascular endothelial growth factor), Sunitinib, Surafinib, Vetalinib, and so forth (tyrosine kinase inhibitors of vascular endothelial growth factor).[99] Angiogenesis and mTOR inhibitors might have potential (Temsirolimus, Everolimus), although <20% of patients have a radiological response.[99,100] Although strategies that use these biological agents might advance the management of GEP NETs, they were first developed for other tumor types. The development of more effective drugs for GEP NETs will need improved understanding of the biology and perhaps the discovery of a molecular target specific to all or some subtypes of GEP NETs. Use of SSTR to target the so-called passenger drugs (i.e., active cytotoxic drugs that are physically linked to agents that bind to SSTR) might hold potential.

Peptide Receptor Radionuclide Therapy

GEP NETs overexpress peptide receptors, mainly subtype 2, which become internalized after ligand binding. Therefore, they are targets for cytotoxic drugs coupled to somatostatin (e.g., radiolabeled somatostatin analogs). Diagnostic scintigraphy for these receptors (using Indium-111) can identify tumors that express SSTR.[101,102]

The most recent research studies involve the compound [177LuDOTA0Tyr3] octreotate. The somatostatin analog octreotate differs from octreotide in that the C-terminal threoninol is replaced with the amino acid threonine, resulting in a substantial increase in affinity for SSTR subtype 2. Recently published data on 131 patients treated demonstrated an objective response rate of 28% with favorable rates of nephrotoxicity and bone marrow suppression. Among the 103 patients who had stable disease or tumor regression, median time to progression was >36 months.[103]

Conclusions

It is clear that to optimize outcomes of these complex tumor types, treatment needs to be planned in the context of a multidisciplinary team preferably concentrated in centers that have developed expertise in this complex arena. We suggest an overall multimodal management plan (Figure 7-4), but one must also consider that there is a plethora of other often expensive treatments with poor evidence base that need only to be utilized in the context of a clinical trial.

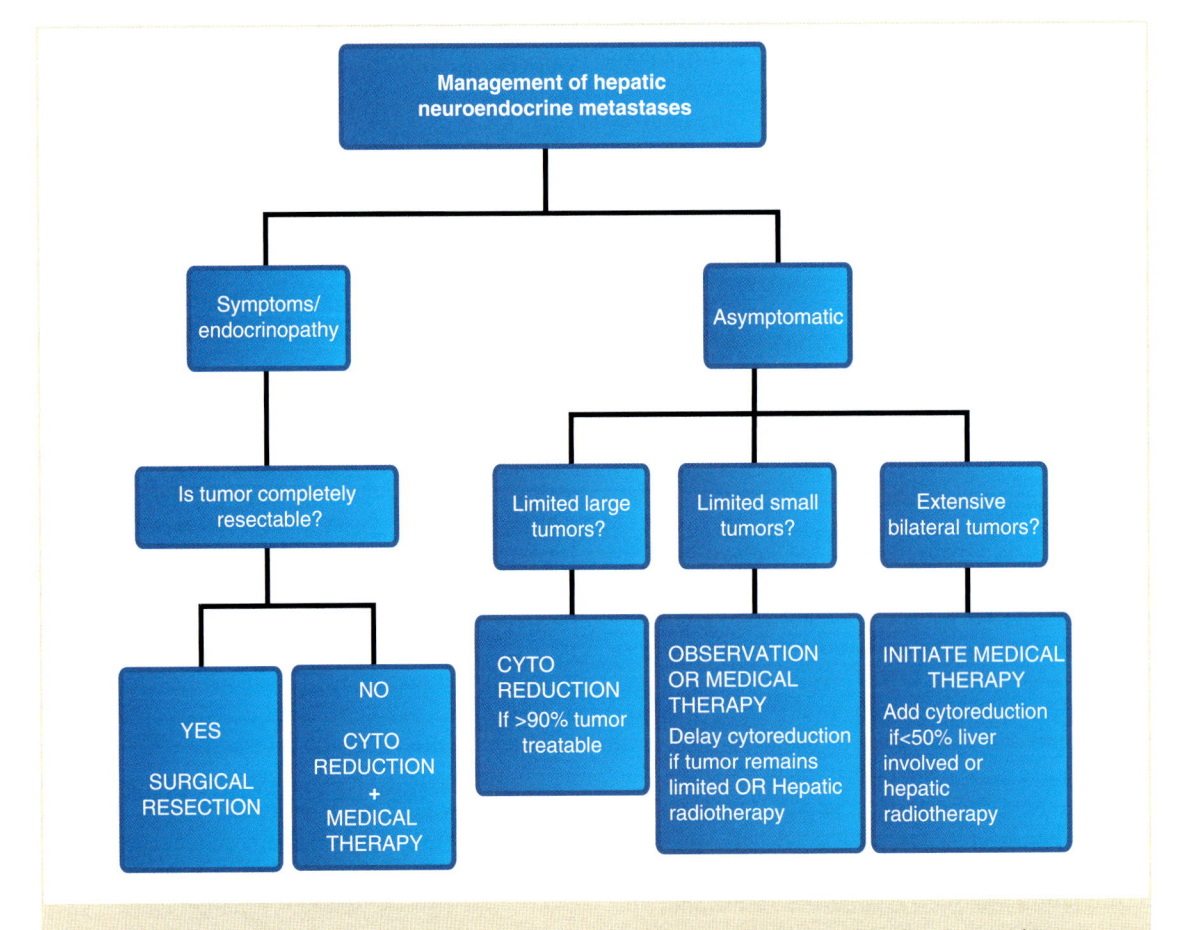

Figure 7-4: Management algorithm for neuroendocrine hepatic metastases, cytoreduction—either ablation or resection.[50]

References

1. Lubarsch O. Ueber dem primären Krebs des Ileum nebst Bemerkungen b¨ er das gleichzeitige Vorkommen von Krebs und Tuberculose. *Virchows Arch Pathol Anat* 1888;111:280–317.
2. Obendorfer S. Karzinoide tumoren des dunndarms. *Frankf Zschr Pathol* 1907;1:426–430.
3. Lembeck F. [Current status of carcinoid research; pharmacological report] [German]. *Krebsarzt*. 1958;13:196–202.
4. Kvols L, Brendtro K. The North American Neuroendrocine Tumor Society (NANETS) guidelines: mission, goals, and process. *Pancreas*. 2010;39:705–706.
5. Rindi G, Capella C, Solcia E. Introduction to a revised clinicopathological classification of neuroendocrine tumors of the gastroenteropancreatic tract. (Review). *Q J Nuc Med*. 2000;44:13–21.
6. Ong SL, Garcea G, Pollard CA, et al. A fuller understanding of pancreatic neuroendocrine tumours combined with aggressive management improves outcome. *Pancreatology*. 2009;9:583–600.
7. Rindi G, Kloppel G, Couvelard A, et al. TNM staging of midgut and hindgut (neuro) endocrine tumors: a consensus proposal including a grading system. *Virschows Arch*. 2007;451:757–762.
8. Fischer L, Kleeff J, Esposito I, et al. Clinical outcome and long-term survival in 118 consecutive patients with neuroendocrine tumours of the pancreas. *Br J Surg*. 2008;95:627–635.
9. Pape U, Berndt U, Muller-Nordhorn J, et al. Prognostic factors of long-term outcome in gastroenteropancreatic neuroendocrine tumours. *Endocr Relat Cancer*. 2008;15:1083–1097.
10. Frilling A, Li J, Malamutmann E, et al. Treatment of liver metastases from neuroendocrine tumours in relation to the extent of hepatic disease. *Brit J Surg*. 2009;96:175–184.
11. Klimstra D, Modlin I, Coppola D, et al. The Pathologic classification of neuroendocrine tumors: a review of nomenclature, grading, and staging systems. *Pancreas*. 2010;39:707–712.
12. Tsikitis VL, Wertheim BC, Guerrero MA. Trends of incidence and survival of gastrointestinal neuroendorine tumors in the United States: a seer analysis. *J Cancer* 2012;3:292–302.
13. Hauso O, Gustafsson B, Kidd M, et al. Neuroendocrine tumor epidemiology: contrasting Norway and North America. *Cancer*. 2008;113:2655–2664.
14. Yao J, Hassan M, Phan A, et al. One hundred years after "carcinoid": epidemiology of and prognostic factors for neuroendocrine tumors in 35,825 cases in the United States. *J Clin Oncol*. 2008;26:3063–3072.
15. Tomassetti P, Migliori M, Lalli S, et al. Epidemiology, clinical features, and diagnosis of gastroenteropancreatic endocrine tumours. *Ann Oncol*. 2001;12(suppl 2):S95–S99.
16. Proye C. Natural history of liver metastasis of gastroenteropancreatic neuroendocrine tumors: place for chemoembolization. *World J Surg*. 2001;25:685–688.
17. House M, Cameron J, Lillemoe K, et al. Differences in survival for patients with resectable versus unresctable metastases from pancreatic islet cell cancer. *J Gastrointestin Surg*. 2006;10:138–145.
18. Soreide J, van Heerden J, Thompson G, et al. Gastrointestinal carcinoid tumors: long- term prognosis for surgically treated patients. *World J Surg*. 2000;24:1431–1436.
19. Chamberlain R, Cames D, Brown K, et al. Hepatic neuroendocrine metastases: does intervention alter outcomes? *J Amer Coll Surg*. 2000;190:432–445.
20. Rindi G, D'Adda T, Proio E, et al. Prognostic factors in gastrointestinal endocrine tumors. *Endocr Pathol*. 2007;18:145–149.
21. Bernheim A, Connolly H, Pellikka P. Carcinoid heart disease. *Curr Treat Option Cardiovasc Med*. 2007;9:482–489.
22. Bernheim A, Connolly H, Rubin J, et al. Role of hepatic resection for patients with carcinoid heart disease. *Mayo Clinic Proc*. 2008;83:143–150.
23. Vinik A, Anthony L, Boudreaux J, et al. Neuroendocrine tumors: a critical appraisal of management strategies. *Pancreas*. 2010;39:801–818.
24. Ramage JK, Goretzki PE, Manfredi R, et al. Consensus guidelines for the management of patients with digestive neuroendocrine tumours: well-differentiated colon and rectum tumour/carcinoma. *Neuroendocrinology*. 2008;87:31–39.
25. Steinmuller T, Kianmanesh R, Falconi M, et al. Consensus guidelines for the management of patients with liver metastases from digestive (neuro)endocrine tumors: foregut, midgut, hindgut, and unknown primary. *Neuroendocrinology*. 2008;87:47–62.
26. Nikou GC, Marinou K, Thomakos P, et al. Chromogranin a levels in diagnosis, treatment and follow-up of 42 patients with non-functioning pancreatic endocrine tumours. *Pancreatology*. 2008;8:510–519.

27. Sondenaa K, Sen J, Heinle F, et al. Chromogranin A, a marker of the therapeutic success of resection of neuroendocrine liver metastases: preliminary report. *World J Surg*. 2004;28:890–895.
28. Zatelli MC, Torta M, Leon A, et al. Chromogranin A as a marker of neuroendocrine neoplasia: an Italian multicenter study. *Endo Relat Cancer*. 2007;14:473–482.
29. Reznek RH. CT/MRI of neuroendocrine tumours. *Cancer Imaging*. 2006;6:S163–S177.
30. Chatzipantelis P, Salla C, Konstantinou P, et al. Endoscopic ultrasound-guided fine- needle aspiration cytology of pancreatic neuroendocrine tumors: a study of 48 cases. *Cancer*. 2008;114:255–262.
31. Chiti A, van Graafeiland BJ, Savelli G, et al. Imaging of neuroendocrine gastro-entero- pancreatic tumours using radiolabelled somatostatin analogues. *Ital J Gastroenterol Hepatol*. 1999;31(suppl 2):S190–S194.
32. Ramage JK, Williams R, Buxton-Thomas M. Imaging secondary neuroendocrine tumours of the liver: comparison of I123 metaiodobenzylguanidine (MIBG) and In111-labelled octreotide (Octreoscan). *QJM*. 1996;89:539–542.
33. Garin E, Le Jeune F, Devillers A, et al. Predictive value of 18F-FDG PET and somatostatin receptor scintigraphy in patients with metastatic endocrine tumors. *J Nuc Med*. 2009;50:858–864.
34. Kauhanen S, Seppanen M, Ovaska J, et al. The clinical value of [18F]fluoro-dihydroxyphenylalanine positron emission tomography in primary diagnosis, staging, and restaging of neuroendocrine tumors [erratum appears in *Endocr Relat Cancer*. 2009 Jun;16(2):661]. *Endocr Relat Cancer*. 2009;16:255–265.
35. Binderup T, Knigge U, Loft A, et al. Functional imaging of neuroendocrine tumors: a head-to-head comparison of somatostatin receptor scintigraphy, 123I-MIBG scintigraphy, and 18F-FDG PET. *J Nuc Med*. Epub ahead of print 2010;N/A:N/A.
36. Namasivayam S, Martin DR, Saini S. Imaging of liver metastases: MRI. *Cancer Imaging*. 2007;7:2–9.
37. Rockall AG, Planche K, Power N, et al. Detection of neuroendocrine liver metastases with MnDPDP-enhanced MRI. *Neuroendocrinology*. 2009;89:288–295.
38. Anthony L, Strosberg J, Klimstra D, et al. The NANETS consensus guidelines for the diagnosis and management of gastrointestinal neuroendocrine tumors (NETs): well-differentiated NETs of the distal colon and rectum. *Pancreas*. 2010;39:767–774.
39. Kulke M, Anthony L, Bushnell D, et al. NANETS treatment guidelines: well-differentiated neuroendocrine tumors of the stomach and pancreas. *Pancreas*. 2010;39:735–752.
40. Chambers AJ, Pasieka JL, Dixon E, Rorstad O. The palliative benefit of aggressive surgical intervention for both hepatic and mesenteric metastases from neuroendocrine tumors. *Surgery*. 2008;144: 645–651; discussion 651–653.
41. Que FG, Nagorney DM, Batts KP, et al. Hepatic resection for metastatic neuroendocrine carcinomas. *Amer J Surg*. 1995;169:36–42; discussion 42–43.
42. Sarmiento JM, Heywood G, Rubin J, et al. Surgical treatment of neuroendocrine metastases to the liver: a plea for resection to increase survival. *J Amer Coll Surg*. 2003;197:29–37.
43. Sarmiento JM, Que FG, Grant CS, et al. Concurrent resections of pancreatic islet cell cancers with synchronous hepatic metastases: outcomes of an aggressive approach. *Surgery*. 2002;132:976–982; discussion 982–983.
44. Gaujoux S, Gonen M, Tang L, et al. Synchronous resection of primary and liver metastases for neuroendocrine tumors. *Ann Sug Oncol*. 2012;19(13): 4270–4277. Epub 2012 Jul 3.
45. Kandil E, Noureidine SI, Koffron A, et al. Outcomes of laparoscopic and open resection for neuroendocrine liver metastases. *Surgery*. 2012;152(6): 1225–1231. Epub 2012 Oct 13.
46. Sarmiento JM, Que FG. Hepatic surgery for metastases from neuroendocrine tumors. *Surg Oncol Clin N Amer*. 2003;12:231–242.
47. Knox CD, Feurer ID, Wise PE, et al. Survival and functional quality of life after resection for hepatic carcinoid metastasis. *J Gastrointestin Surg*. 2004;8:653–659.
48. Sartori P, Mussi C, Angelini C, et al. Palliative management strategies of advanced gastrointestinal carcinoid neoplasms. *Langenbecks Arch Surg*. 2005;390:391–396.
49. Siperstein AE, Berber E. Cryoablation, percutaneous alcohol injection, and radiofrequency ablation for treatment of neuroendocrine liver metastases. *World J Surgery*. 2001;25:693–696.
50. Maithel SK, Fong Y. Hepatic ablation for neuroendocrine tumor metastases. *J Surg Oncol*. 2009;100:635–638.

51. Choy PYG, Koea J, McCall J, et al. The role of radiofrequency ablation in the treatment of primary and metastatic tumours of the liver: initial lessons learned. *New Zealand Med J.* 2002;115:U128.
52. Crocetti L, de Baere T, Lencioni R. Quality improvement guidelines for radiofrequency ablation of liver tumours. *Cardiovasc Intervent Radiol.* 2010;33:11–17.
53. Elias D, Goere D, Leroux G, et al. Combined liver surgery and RFA for patients with gastroenteropancreatic endocrine tumors presenting with more than 15 metastases to the liver. *Euro J Surg Oncol.* 2009;35:1092–1097.
54. Eriksson J, Stalberg P, Nilsson A, et al. Surgery and radiofrequency ablation for treatment of liver metastases from midgut and foregut carcinoids and endocrine pancreatic tumors. *World J Surg.* 2008;32:930–938.
55. Livraghi T, Solbiati L, Meloni F, et al. Percutaneous radiofrequency ablation of liver metastases in potential candidates for resection: the "test-of-time approach." *Cancer.* 2003;97:3027–3035.
56. Berber E, Siperstein A. Local recurrence after laparoscopic radiofrequency ablation of liver tumors: an analysis of 1032 tumors. *Ann Surg Oncol.* 2008;15:2757–2764.
57. Mazzaglia PJ, Berber E, Siperstein AE. Radiofrequency thermal ablation of metastatic neuroendocrine tumors in the liver. *Curr Treat Options Oncol.* 2007;8:322–330.
58. Ruers TJM, Joosten JJ, Wiering B, et al. Comparison between local ablative therapy and chemotherapy for non-resectable colorectal liver metastases: a prospective study. *Annals of Surg Oncol.* 2007;14:1161–1169.
59. Berber E, Flesher N, Siperstein AE. Laparoscopic radiofrequency ablation of neuroendocrine liver metastases. *World J Surgery.* 2002;26:985–990.
60. Hellman P, Ladjevardi S, Skogseid B, et al. Radiofrequency tissue ablation using cooled tip for liver metastases of endocrine tumors. *World J Surg.* 2002;26:1052–1056.
61. Atwell TD, Charbonneau JW, Que FG, et al. Treatment of neuroendocrine cancer metastatic to the liver: the role of ablative techniques. *Cardiovasc Intervent Radiol.* 2005;28:409–421.
62. Gillams A, Cassoni A, Conway G, Lees W. Radiofrequency ablation of neuroendocrine liver metastases: the Middlesex experience. *Abdom Imaging.* 2005;30:435–441.
63. Henn AR, Levine EA, McNulty W, Zagoria RJ. Percutaneous radiofrequency ablation of hepatic metastases for symptomatic relief of neuroendocrine syndromes. *Amer J Roentgenol.* 2003;181:1005–1010.
64. Solbiati L, Ierace T, Tonolini M, et al. Radiofrequency thermal ablation of hepatic metastases. *Eur J Ultrasound.* 2001;13:149–158.
65. Kettenbach J, Muller SL, Schindl M. [Interventional therapy of neuroendokrine tumors of the gastrointestinal tract]. *Wien Klin Wochenschr.* 2003;115 (suppl 2):56–64.
66. Wood TF, Rose DM, Chung M, et al. Radiofrequency ablation of 231 unresectable hepatic tumors: indications, limitations, and complications. *Ann Surg Oncol.* 2000;7:593–600.
67. Jensen EH, Kvols L, McLoughlin JM, et al. Biomarkers predict outcomes following cytoreductive surgery for hepatic metastases from functional carcinoid tumors. *Ann Surg Oncol.* 2007;14:780–785.
68. Gravante G, Ong SL, Metcalfe MS, et al. Hepatic microwave ablation: a review of the histological changes following thermal damage. *Liver Int.* 2008;28:911–921.
69. Boutros C, Somasundar P, Garrean S, et al. Microwave coagulation therapy for hepatic tumors: review of the literature and critical analysis. *Surg Oncol.* 2010;19:e22–e32.
70. Garrean S, Hering J, Helton WS, Espat NJ. A primer on transarterial, chemical, and thermal ablative therapies for hepatic tumors. *Amer J Surg.* 2007;194:79–88.
71. Bhardwaj N, Strickland AD, Ahmad F, et al. Liver ablation techniques: a review. *Surg Endosc.* 2010;24:254–265.
72. Goering J, Mahvi D, Niederhuber J, et al. Cryoablation and liver resection for noncolorectal liver metastases. *Amer J Surg.* 2002;183:384–389.
73. Neeleman N, Wobbes T, Jager GJ, Ruers TJ. Cryosurgery as treatment modality for colorectal liver metastases. *Hepato-Gastroenterol.* 2001;48:325–329.
74. Sheen AJ, Poston GJ, Sherlock DJ. Cryotherapeutic ablation of liver tumours. *Brit J Surg.* 2002;89:1396–1401.
75. Mazzaferro V, Pulvirenti A, Coppa J. Neuroendocrine tumors metastatic to the liver: how to select patients for liver transplantation? *J Hepatol.* 2007;47:460–466.
76. Fernández J, Robles R, Marín C, et al. Role of liver transplantation in the management of

metastatic neuroendocrine tumors. *Transpl Proc.* 2003;35:1832–1833.

77. Christante D, Pommier S, Givi B, Pommier R. Hepatic artery chemoinfusion with chemoembolization for neuroendocrine cancer with progressive hepatic metastases despite octreotide therapy. *Surgery.* 2008;144:885–893; discussion 893–894.

78. Pitt S, Knuth J, Keily J, et al. Hepatic neuroendocrine metastases: chemo- or bland embolization? *J Gastrointestin Surg.* 2008;12:1951–1960.

79. Gupta S, Johnson MM, Murthy R, et al. Hepatic arterial embolization and chemoembolization for the treatment of patients with metastatic neuroendocrine tumors: variables affecting response rates and survival. *Cancer.* 2005;104:1590–1602.

80. Ho AS, Picus J, Darcy MD, et al. Long-term outcome after chemoembolization and embolization of hepatic metastatic lesions from neuroendocrine tumors. *Amer J Roentgenol.* 2007;188:1201–1207.

81. Perry LJ, Stuart K, Stokes KR, Clouse ME. Hepatic arterial chemoembolization for metastatic neuroendocrine tumors. *Surgery.* 1994;116:1111–1116; discussion 1116–1117.

82. Moertel CG, Johnson CM, McKusick MA, et al. The management of patients with advanced carcinoid tumors and islet cell carcinomas. *Ann Int Med.* 1994;120:302–309.

83. Fiorentini G, Rossi S, Bonechi F, et al. Intra-arterial hepatic chemoembolization in liver metastases from neuroendocrine tumors: a phase II study. *J Chemother.* 2004;16:293–297.

84. Ruutiainen AT, Soulen MC, Tuite CM, et al. Chemoembolization and bland embolization of neuroendocrine tumor metastases to the liver. *J Vascul Intervent Rad.* 2007;18:847–855.

85. Nakamura Y, Nakamura Y, Hori E, et al. Tumor lysis syndrome after transcatheter arterial infusion of cisplatin and embolization therapy for liver metastases of melanoma. *Int J Dermatol.* 2009;48:763–767.

86. Murthy R, Mutha P, Lee JH, Oh Y. Yttrium-90-labeled microsphere radioembolotherapy of liver-dominant metastases from thoracic malignancies. *J Vasc Intervent Radiol.* 2008;19:299–300.

87. Sato K, Lewandowski RJ, Bui JT, et al. Treatment of unresectable primary and metastatic liver cancer with yttrium-90 microspheres (TheraSphere): assessment of hepatic arterial embolization. *Cardiovasc Intervent Radiol.* 2006;29:522–529.

88. van Essen M, Krenning EP, Kam BLR, et al. Peptide-receptor radionuclide therapy for endocrine tumors. *Nate Rev Endocrinol.* 2009;5:382–393.

89. Williams G, Anderson JV, Williams SJ, Bloom SR. Clinical evaluation of SMS 201–995. Long-term treatment in gut neuroendocrine tumours, efficacy of oral administration, and possible use in non-tumoural inappropriate TSH hypersecretion. *Acta Endocrinol Suppl.* 1987;286:26–36.

90. Janson ET, Westlin JE, Eriksson B, et al. [111In-DTPA-D-Phe1]octreotide scintigraphy in patients with carcinoid tumours: the predictive value for somatostatin analogue treatment. *Eur J Endocrinol.* 1994;131:577–581.

91. Oberg K, Kvols L, Caplin M, et al. Consensus report on the use of somatostatin analogs for the management of neuroendocrine tumors of the gastroenteropancreatic system. *Ann Oncol.* 2004;15:966–973.

92. Rinke A, Muller H, Schade-Brittinger C, et al. Placebo-controlled, double-blind, prospective, randomized study on the effect of octreotide LAR in the control of tumor growth in patients with metastatic neuroendocrine midgut tumors: a report from the PROMID Study Group. *J Clin Oncol* 2009; 27(28):4656–4663.

93. Kaltsas GA, Besser GM, Grossman AB. The diagnosis and medical management of advanced neuroendocrine tumors. *Endocr Rev.* 2004;25:458–511.

94. Bajetta E, Procopio G, Buzzoni R, et al. Advances in diagnosis and therapy of neuroendocrine tumors. *Expert Rev Anticancer Ther.* 2001;1:371–381.

95. Strosberg JR, Kvols LK. A review of the current clinical trials for gastroenteropancreatic neuroendocrine tumours. *Expert Opin Investig Drugs.* 2007;16:219–224.

96. Moertel CG, Rubin J, Kvols LK. Therapy of metastatic carcinoid tumor and the malignant carcinoid syndrome with recombinant leukocyte A interferon. *J Clin Oncol.* 1989;7:865–868.

97. Oberg K. Neuroendocrine gastrointestinal tumours. *Ann Oncol.* 1996;7:453–463.

98. Phan AT, Yao JC. Neuroendocrine tumors: novel approaches in the age of targeted therapy. *Oncology.* 2008;22:1617–1623; discussion 1623–1624, 1629.

99. Dimou AT, Syrigos KN, Saif MW. Neuroendocrine tumors of the pancreas: what's new. Highlights from the "2010 ASCO Gastrointestinal Cancers Symposium." Orlando, FL, USA. January 22–24,

2010. *Jop: J Pancreas [Electronic Resource]*. 2010;11:135–138.

100. Yao JC, Phan A, Hoff PM, et al. Targeting vascular endothelial growth factor in advanced carcinoid tumor: a random assignment phase II study of depot octreotide with bevacizumab and pegylated interferon alpha-2b. *J Clin Oncol*. 2008;26:1316–1323.

101. de Jong M, Breeman WAP, Kwekkeboom DJ, et al. Tumor imaging and therapy using radiolabeled somatostatin analogues. *Acc Chem Res*. 2009; 42:873–880.

102. Nasir A, Stridsberg M, Strosberg J, et al. Somatostatin receptor profiling in hepatic metastases from small intestinal and pancreatic neuroendocrine neoplasms: immunohistochemical approach with potential clinical utility. *Cancer Control*. 2006;13:52–60.

103. Kwekkeboom DJ, de Herder WW, Kam BL, et al. Treatment with the radiolabeled somatostatin analog [177 Lu-DOTA 0,Tyr3]octreotate: toxicity, efficacy, and survival. *J Clin Oncol*. 2008;26:2124–2130.

104. Nave H, Mossinger E, Feist H, et al. Surgery as primary treatment in patients with liver metastases from carcinoid tumors: a retrospective, unicentric study over 13 years. *Surgery*. 2001;129:170–175.

105. Ringe B, Lorf T, Dopkens K, Canelo R. Treatment of hepatic metastases from gastroenteropancreatic neuroendocrine tumors: role of liver transplantation. *World J Surg*. 2001;25:697–699.

106. Kianmanesh R, Sauvanet A, Hentic O, et al. Two-step surgery for synchronous bilobar liver metastases from digestive endocrine tumors: a safe approach for radical resection. *Ann Surg*. 2008;247:659–665.

107. Scigliano S, Lebtahi R, Maire F, et al. Clinical and imaging follow-up after exhaustive liver resection of endocrine metastases: a 15-year monocentric experience. *Endo Relat Cancer*. 2009;16:977–990.

108. Lehnert T. Liver transplantation for metastatic neuroendocrine carcinoma: an analysis of 103 patients. *Transplantation*. 1998;66:1307–1312.

109. Rosenau J, Bahr MJ, von Wasielewski R, et al. Ki67, E-cadherin, and p53 as prognostic indicators of long-term outcome after liver transplantation for metastatic neuroendocrine tumors. Transplantation. 2002;73:386–394.

110. Florman S, Toure B, Kim L, et al. Liver transplantation for neuroendocrine tumors. J Gastrointest Surgery. 2004;8:208–212.

111. van Vilsteren FGI, Baskin-Bey ES, Nagorney DM, et al. Liver transplantation for gastroenteropancreatic neuroendocrine cancers: defining selection criteria to improve survival. Liver Transpl. 2006;12:448–456.

112. Marin C, Robles R, Fernandez JA, et al. Role of liver transplantation in the management of unresectable neuroendocrine liver metastases. Transplant Proc. 2007;39:2302–2303.

113. Olausson M, Friman S, Herlenius G, et al. Orthotopic liver or multivisceral transplantation as treatment of metastatic neuroendocrine tumors. Liver Transpl. 2007;13:327–333.

114. Frilling A, Malago M, Weber F, et al. Liver transplantation for patients with metastatic endocrine tumors: single-center experience with 15 patients. Liver Transpl. 2006;12:1089–1096.

CHAPTER 8

The Role of Liver-Directed Therapy for Noncolorectal, Non-neuroendocrine Liver Metastasis

Junaid Haroon & Ronald S. Chamberlain

Introduction

The liver is a commonly involved site in tumor metastases, with the mechanism of involvement varying depending on the site of the primary tumor. Colorectal, neuroendocrine tumors and other gastrointestinal tumors most often spread to the liver through the portal system or local lymphatic drainage. As a result, these diseases often present as localized hepatic disease allowing for a curative role for hepatic metastasectomy, which in the setting of colorectal cancer has yielded five-year survival rates[1-4] between 20% and 54%. Recent advances in anesthesia, surgical technique and perioperative management have further improved outcomes by limiting the postoperative mortality following hepatic resection to <5% in experienced hands.[5,6] Hepatic resection for neuroendocrine liver metastases has similarly proven effective for local control, demonstrating improvement of symptoms in up to 96% of patients and five-year survival rates up to 61% for this inherently indolent disease process.[7,8] Various other primary tumors also often spread to the liver through the systemic circulation and in these cases hepatic metastases typically a part of multiorgan involvement. In the rare scenario when the liver is the sole site of systemic involvement for noncolorectal, nonneuroendocrine (NCNN) metastases, they are usually multifocal and/or bilobar, making surgical resection prohibitive.

A precise algorithm for when hepatic resection for noncolorectal liver metastases (NCRLM) is indicated has proven difficult if not impossible. Most early reports included neuroendocrine tumors that typically have a substantially better prognosis[9,10] and have thus skewed survival rates to imply benefit that may not be true if only NCNN liver metastases are studied.[11-13] More recent rare studies have focused exclusively on the role of hepatic metastasectomy in highly selected patients with NCNN tumors, and though limited, these do suggest outcomes comparable to those achieved with hepatic resection for colorectal tumors in highly selected patients.[14-17] Unfortunately comparing these studies is impossible since most analysis is flawed clustering hepatic metastases from various malignancies into a single group, thus limiting the ability to form specific guidelines. Understanding the unique tumor biology of liver metastases (LM) from different primary sites however is the sine qua non for devising appropriate strategies and will be the focus of the remainder of this chapter.

Breast Cancer

More than one million cases of breast cancer are diagnosed each year, with approximately 40,000 women dying of metastatic breast cancer annually.[18] Approximately 50% of these patients develop hepatic metastases with a median survival of 2–14 months from detection, and isolated liver metastases occur in only 5%–25% of cases.[19-26] As such, the presence of breast cancer liver metastases implies a poor prognosis with a median survival of less than six months, and an overall survival of less than two years even when adjuvant chemotherapy or hormonal therapy is provided.[6,27,28] Although significant progress has been made in the multimodal treatment of systemic breast cancer, including new chemotherapeutic agents (anthracyclines and taxanes), antihormonal therapy (aromatase inhibitors and selective estrogen receptor modulators), and targeted biological agents (trastuzumab), the development of distant metastases continues to be associated with a dismal prognosis. In nearly all cases hepatic metastases are a manifestation of systemic dissemination of breast cancer in which case systemic chemotherapy remains the primary, if not the only available treatment. That said, neither chemotherapy nor radiation has been shown to improve survival in the setting of liver metastases,[26] a fact likely related to the reality that 70% of breast cancer liver metastases have no hormonal receptors and are nonresponsive to antiestrogen therapy.[29,30] Hepatic resection can be considered in isolated cases, although even among those considered for resection, only 13%–65% ultimately undergo resection since intraoperative findings often reveal undetected diffuse liver metastases or peritoneal carcinomatosis.[31] Patients who are not candidates for surgical resection have been treated with various other liver-directed modalities, including radiofrequency ablation (RFA), hepatic arterial infusion chemotherapy (HAIC), and other novel approaches, but only limited data related to efficacy are available.

Hepatic Metastasectomy Outcomes: Breast Cancer (Table 8-1)

At present, 19 different studies have reported on the outcomes of hepatic resection in patients with breast cancer liver metastases. Overall, these reports include a total of 973 highly selected breast cancer liver metastases patients and report a five-year survival between 9% and 61%.[6,11,14,16,17,32-45]

The largest cohort study included 454 patients and was reported by Adam et al. (2006) as part of a larger study analyzing the outcomes of hepatic metastasectomy for various different NCNN liver metastases. The authors reported a 45-month median survival and a five-year survival rate of 41% in patients with breast cancer liver metastases, and this was the only study to report 10-year survival rate that was 22%. The authors failed to report any tumor-specific morbidity or mortality rates.[11]

Only three additional studies with a cohort size of greater than 50 patients have been reported; the studies had sample sizes of 54, 85, and 86 patients, respectively.[38,41,45] Elias et al. (2003) reported on 54 breast cancer liver metastases (BCLM) patients. Criteria for selection included no extrahepatic metastases, good performance status, judged to pose limited resection risks, and achieved objective response or stabilization of liver metastases after three months of chemotherapy and hormonal therapy (where indicated). Nine patients did not fit these criteria; three presented with bone metastases and six showed progression after chemotherapy. Postoperative morbidity occurred in 12.9%; however, there was no postoperative mortality. Overall survival was 50% at three years and 34% at five years, whereas disease-free survival (DFS) was 42% at three years and 22% at five years. Median survival was 34.3 months. Hormone receptor negativity was a significant prognostic indicator for survival, increasing the risk of death by threefold.[38] In a separate study, Adam et al. (2006) identified 85 breast cancer patients with technically resectable breast cancer liver metastases. Among this group, 16 patients had extrahepatic metastases but were included since the disease was resectable or well controlled. Eleven patients had their additional metastases resected or were in remission following systemic therapy, whereas five had stable bone metastases. When an R0 resection was not achieved intraoperatively, residual disease was treated with postoperative hepatic arterial chemotherapy. Local morbidity was 22%, but there was no postoperative mortality. The median survival following first hepatic resection was 32 months, and the five-year survival rate was 37%. Lack of response to preoperative chemotherapy, inability to complete R0 resection and recurrence of metastases outside the

TABLE 8-1: Studies of Outcomes of Hepatic Metastasectomy in Patients with Breast Cancer

Study	Sample (N)	Median Survival (mo)	1 y	3 y	5 y	10 y
Elias (1991)[32]	12	37				
Elias (1995)[33]	21	26		50 (2-y)	9	
Harrison (1997)[14]	7				14	
Raab (1998)[34]	34	27			18	
Seifert (1999)[35]	15	57	100	54		
Yamada (2001)[36]	4				25	
Carilini (2002)[37]	17	53			46	
Elias (2003)[38]	54	34.3		50	34	
Vlastos (2004)[40]	31	63		86 (2-y)	61	
Arena (2004)[39]	17		92	52	41	
Ercolani (2005)[17]	21	40		54	25	
Weitz (2005)[16]	29	48				
Adam (2006)[41]	85	32			37	
Adam (2006)[11]	454	45			41	22
Reddy (2007)[6]	20	67				
Caralt (2008)[42]	12	35.9	100	79	33	
Hoffmann (2010)[43]	41	79		68	48	
Bresadola (2011)[44]	13	44				
Abbott (2012)[45]	86	57				

liver or in an unresectable location within the liver were associated with poor prognosis. Of note, bilateral liver metastases were predictive of a high recurrence rate.[41] Finally, in a recently published study, Abbott et al. (2012) reported on 86 breast cancer liver metastases patients who underwent hepatic resection in an effort to identify factors associated with prolonged survival. Patients with treated or stable extrahepatic disease were included. Patients deemed unresectable pre- or intraoperatively were excluded from the analysis, as were cases in which RFA was the only definitive hepatic therapy. No postoperative deaths were reported. The median follow-up period was 62 months, and the median disease-free survival and overall survival were 14 and 57 months, respectively. Estrogen receptor–negative primary tumor that failed to respond to preoperative chemotherapy were associated with worse outcomes.[45]

Additional smaller cohort studies have been reported and are useful to identify risks associated with hepatic resection as well as to further elucidate factors predictive of poor outcomes in such patients.[6,14,16,17,32–37,39,40,42–44] As a whole, these small cohort studies report morbidity rates ranging from 0% to 29%, and only one study reported a lone postoperative mortality.[34] Factors predictive of favorable outcomes following hepatic resection for breast cancer liver metastases patients included an oncologically complete resection[34,35,43,46] and a long disease-free interval (DFI) from primary breast surgery.[37,42,43,47] Although a longer disease-free interval was a prognostic indicator, there is currently no consensus on the ideal disease-free interval stimulating consideration of hepatic resection with different studies using cut-offs ranging from 12 to 36 months. In nearly all studies, an R0 resection was associated with a decreased risk of local recurrence,[35] whereas lymph node status did not demonstrate prognostic significance.[32]

Outcomes of Additional Liver-Directed Therapeutic Modalities: Breast Cancer (Table 8-2)

RFA is a well-established modality in the management of hepatic tumors. In comparison with surgery, it is less invasive, less expensive, associated with fewer contraindications and can be easily repeated if local tumor progression or new metastases are observed. Similar to surgical resection, RFA aims to ablate all visible metastases with a rim of normal tissue simulating an R0 "surgical margin." To date, seven studies have examined the efficacy of RFA in a total of 182 breast cancer liver metastases patients. Overall, these studies report a response rate of 92%–100% in a highly selected patient population. The average reported survival ranged from 11 to 60 months, and the five-year survival rate ranged from 27% to 64% when reported.[48–54] The only poor prognostic indicator identified in multiple studies was the presence of extrahepatic disease.[50,51]

The two largest studies evaluating the efficacy of RFA in patients with breast cancer liver metastases are composed of a total of 110 patients. Jakobs et al. (2009) reported on 43 patients with 111 breast cancer liver metastases to elaborate technical success, technical effectiveness, and survival following RFA. Primary technique effectiveness was achieved in 96%. Patients undergoing RFA under CT guidance had a median survival of 59 months from the date of RFA. Presence of extrahepatic disease was associated with a worse outcome; however, this was not true for skeletal metastases.[50] Meloni et al. (2009) identified 57 patients with breast cancer liver metastases and attempted to assess the local control rate and survival among patients undergoing percutaneous ultrasonography-guided RFA. Five patients were excluded from the study cohort, because they had more than five metastases or a single metastasis greater than 5 cm. Presence of extrahepatic metastases was considered a contraindication to RFA unless these metastases had been stable for at least six months following chemotherapy. There was no mortality reported and minor complications were reported in 4% of patients. Ninety-seven percent of the patients had their liver metastases completely treated. During follow-up, local tumor progression was seen in 25% of patients, whereas new intrahepatic metastases developed in 53%. Median survival from the date of diagnosis of liver metastases was 42 months, whereas the overall one-, three-, and five-year survival rates were 68%, 43%, and 27%, respectively. The only poor prognostic indicator identified was the diameter of the metastasis, either as a continuous variable or when using 2.5 cm as a cut-off.[53]

Although the efficacy of systemic chemotherapy in breast cancer liver metastases has been relatively limited, some institutions believe that regional chemotherapy is a promising therapy because higher drug concentrations can be achieved in the liver without significant systemic toxicity. In a study of multimodal treatments in 71 patients with breast cancer liver metastases, Peetz et al. (1982) demonstrated that a combination of HAIC, hormonal ablation, and systemic chemotherapy (median survival of 21 months) was superior to hormonal ablation and systemic chemotherapy alone (median survival of 15 months) both of which were better than systemic chemotherapy alone (3–9 months).[55] Four published studies have evaluated the outcomes among 118 patients treated with HAIC for breast cancer liver metastases. The overall response rate ranged from 45% to 59%, and the median survival ranged from 7 to 31 months. There was no procedure or chemotherapy-related mortality, and complications occurred in up to 22%.[56–59]

Stehlin et al. (1974) were not only the first to use HAIC for breast cancer liver metastases but have also reported the largest cohort. These authors treated 71 breast cancer liver metastases patients with HAIC, with 9 patients also undergoing hepatic resection. Forty-five percent of the patients responded to HAIC (median survival of 16 months), whereas 55% did not (median survival of three months).[59] Maes et al. (2008) published their experience with intrahepatic Mitomycin C (MMC) in 30 patients. Patients were selected if they had progressive, life-threatening liver disease as a major site of metastasis, and previous chemotherapy exposure was not taken into consideration. MMC (12 mg) was administered as a transcatheter bolus every four weeks. Thrombocytopenia, leukopenia, and allergic reaction were the most common side effects, occurring in 67%, 40%, and 13% of cases, respectively. No death or grade IV toxicity was recorded. A local response was obtained in 33% of patients, whereas 26% demonstrated a global response. The median progression-free survival was three months, whereas the overall survival was seven months.[56]

Transcatheter arterial chemoembolization (TACE) is an additional liver-directed therapeutic

TABLE 8-2: Studies of Outcomes of Nonresectional Therapy in Patients with Breast Cancer Metastases

Study	Modality	Sample (N)	Response (%)	Median (mo)	Survival 1 y (%)	3 y (%)	5 y (%)
Livraghi (2001)[52]	RFA	24	92				
Lawes (2006)[51]	RFA	19				42 (30 mo)	
Gunabushanam (2007)[49]	RFA	14	100		64		
Sofocleous (2007)[54]	RFA	12	93	60		70	30
Jakobs (2009)[50]	RFA	43	96	59			
Meloni (20009)[53]	RFA	57	97	42	68	43	27
Carrafiello (2011)[48]	RFA	13	100	11 (mean)			64
Stehlin (1974)[59]	HAIC	62	45	16 (responders)			
Schneebaum (1994)[58]	HAIC	18		28			
Melichar (2006)[57]	HAIC	8		31			
Li (2005)[63]	TACE	28	36		63	30	13
Cho (2010)[61]	TACE	10	20	24 (responders)			
Duan (2011)[62]	TACE	44	59		76	48	
Mack (2004)[64]	MR-guided thermotherapy	232		52	96	63	41

Abbreviations: RFA, radiofrequency ablation; HAIC, hepatic arterial infusion chemotherapy; TACE, transcatheter arterial chemoembolization; MR, magnetic resonance.

modality that utilizes a combination of regional chemotherapy and embolization of the hepatic vasculature to control liver metastases. Given the fact that liver metastases receives blood supply from the hepatic artery, this therapy is theoretically attractive.[60] Three studies have reported on the outcomes of TACE in breast cancer liver metastases patients, with a combined study population of 82 patients. Response rates ranged from 20% to 59%, and the overall three-year survival rates ranged from 30% to 48%.[61–63] When compared with systemic chemotherapy alone, these studies show an improved response rate (36% to 59% compared with 7% to 35%) as well as a much better one-year survival rate (63% to 76% vs. 34% to 48%); however, the patients were highly selected.[62,63] Postembolization syndrome was the most commonly reported complication. Li et al. (2005) compared the results of TACE and systemic chemotherapy among 48 patients. In this cohort, 28 patients were administered TACE (based on 5-Fluorouracil and cisplatin), and 20 patients were given anthracycline-based systemic chemotherapy. Response rates in the TACE group and the systemic chemotherapy group were 36% and 7%, respectively. The one-, three-, and five-year survival rates for the two groups were 63%, 30%, 13%; and 34%, 11%, 0%, respectively. Lymph node status of the primary tumor, clinical stage of liver metastases, the Child-Pugh score, estrogen receptor–negative primaries, disease-free survival of less than 24 months, treatment with chemotherapy only and weight loss were independent predictors of poor outcome.[62,63]

Occasional reports of magnetic resonance–guided thermotherapy using either laser or microwave for coagulation of breast cancer liver metastases have also been reported. One such study treated 232 patients with 578 liver metastases from breast cancer with magnetic resonance–guided laser thermotherapy. The indications for laser thermotherapy were less than five metastases, with no metastases greater than 5 cm. The authors reported a median survival of 4.3 years, and 1-, 2-, 3-, and 5-year survival rates of 96%, 80%, 63%, and 41%, respectively.[64] Two additional case reports on the use of magnetic resonance–guided microwave thermocoagulation have similarly demonstrated it to be a safe and potentially effective option for breast cancer liver metastases. A total of nine cases have been reported with a success rate of 100% and a median disease-free survival ranging from 15 to 26 months.[65,66]

Summary

Hepatic resection in highly selected patients with breast cancer liver metastases has achieved median survival in the range of 26 to 79 months and five-year survival rates of 9%–61%, which is significantly better than that expected for patients treated with systemic chemotherapy alone. Surgery should be considered only in patients in whom an R0 resection appears feasible as this is the most consistently reported factor associated with improved survival. Patient selection is improved by intraoperative ultrasonography that allows the identification of addition disease and the ability to achieve a negative margin.[67] Although extrahepatic disease is not an absolute contraindication to surgery, it should be well controlled or resectable at the time of surgery, and these cases should be extensively discussed at multidisciplinary tumor boards. Additional factors associated with improved survival following hepatic resection are numerous; however, response to preoperative chemotherapy and a longer disease-free interval after mastectomy appear to be most consistent in the published literature.

Hepatic resection for breast cancer liver metastases is feasible, and cure is possible in a limited number of patients. Additional liver-directed therapeutic options for patients who are not resection candidates include RFA, HAIC and TACE, with RFA being the most effective. Even when cure is not achieved, hepatectomy can effectively achieve local disease control in many cases and can prolong survival in highly selected patients.

Melanoma

Ocular melanoma is the most common primary intraocular malignancy in the Caucasian population. Uveal melanoma represents 6% of all melanoma diagnoses with a reported incidence of 4000 per annum in the United States.[68] The incidence of uveal melanoma has remained stable despite steady increase in cutaneous melanoma over the past few decades. Localized uveal melanoma is associated with a five-year survival rate of approximately 70% after treatment; however, approximately 50% of patients eventually develop metastases. Hematogenous dissemination is the most common mode of spread, and uveal melanoma demonstrate unique and selective oculo-hepatic tropism, with the liver being the only involved site in 70%–80% of cases and most often the cause of death.[69,70] The outcomes of patients with liver metastases from uveal melanoma are generally dismal, with a one-year survival rate of 10%.[71] Treatment options for uveal melanoma liver metastases (UMLM) include systemic- or hepatic-directed chemotherapy, hepatic resection, or hepatic artery embolization. Systemic chemotherapy is most often used although it is associated with a poor response rate and no demonstrable survival benefit.[72] Given a high frequency of solitary hepatic metastases, uveal melanoma patients have historically been considered good candidates for hepatic resection or other liver-directed therapies.[71] Hepatic arterial infusion of fotemustine or carboplatin has been shown to result in 22%–40% response rates with a median survival of 12–14 months.[73–75] Chemoembolization has demonstrated limited efficacy given UMLM are hypervascular with response rates of up to 36%; however, no survival benefit has been shown.[71] At present, the most promising survival rates are reported in patients with limited disease who are candidates for hepatic resection.[71,76,77]

Patients with cutaneous malignant melanoma differ significantly in their disease progression compared to uveal melanoma. Cutaneous malignant melanoma more typically spreads through lymphatic vessels, and major metastatic sites include regional lymph nodes, subcutaneous tissue, and lungs. The rate of hepatic metastases is 14%–20%, and the liver is rarely the only affected organ.[78] Five-year survival rates as low as 0%–3% have been reported in cases of cutaneous malignant melanoma with liver metastases.[79] In cases when disease is limited to the liver, R0 resection may offer a rare opportunity for long-term survival,[80] with five-year survival rates in the range of 20%–30%.[11,14,44] To date, nearly all the published literature on the treatment of melanoma liver metastases focuses primarily on UMLM rather than cutaneous malignant melanoma.

Hepatic Metastasectomy Outcomes: Melanoma (Table 8-3)

To date, seven studies have evaluated the outcomes of hepatic resection in UMLM patients. Cumulatively, the studies report on 472 UMLM patients. The reported median survival ranges from 14 to 38 months and five-year survival rates range from 7 to 53%. Remarkably, no study reported significant postoperative morbidity or mortality.[11,76,81–85] Almost universally all studies identified an R0 resection as the most important positive prognostic indicator.[76,83–85] Other consistently identified positive prognostic indicators were a limited number of metastases[82–85] and a long disease-free interval.[81,82,85]

The two largest studies evaluated 104 and 255 UMLM patients and were reported by Adam et al. (2006) and Mariani et al. (2009), respectively. Adam et al. (2006) studied the overall outcomes of a large cohort of patients with NCNN liver metastases undergoing hepatic resection, which included 104 patients with UMLM. In the UMLM group, the observed overall median survival was 19 months, with a five-year survival rate of 21%.[11] Mariani et al. (2009) reported the largest series of UMLM patients who underwent surgical management (N = 255). The overall survival rate was 57% at one year and 7% at five years. The median overall survival was 14 months, but increased to 27 months in cases in which an R0 resection was achieved. Positive prognostic factors included DFS greater than 24 months, R0 resection, four or less metastases, and absence of miliary liver disease.[85]

Outcomes of Additional Liver-Directed Therapeutic Modalities: Melanoma

HAIC as discussed earlier for the treatment of liver metastases achieves high intratumoral chemotherapy concentration while minimizing systemic toxicity.[86] In most studies, HAIC is combined with systemic chemotherapy,[75] hyperthermia,[87] or as a part of TACE[88–91] in an effort to achieve synergistic response. HAIC has also been shown to potentially improve outcomes when used in combination with hepatic resection in UMLM patients.[76] Eight studies have reported the outcomes associated with HAIC in 204 UMLM patients (see Table 8-4). Response rates ranged from 17% to 40% and median survival ranged from 8 to 24 months. Time to progression was 6–17 months in these studies. Severe procedure or catheter-related complications were seen in as many as 20% of patients, although no mortalities were reported.[73–75,87,92–95] A high baseline lactate dehydrogenase (LDH) level was the most significant poor prognostic indicator.[73,93] The use of fotemustine-based therapy was associated with improved outcomes when compared to other chemotherapy regimens.[75] Anecdotal reports have described UMLM patients surviving as long as 9 years after multimodal HAIC-based treatment with or without hepatic resection for UMLM.[96–98]

TABLE 8-3: Studies of Outcomes of Hepatic Metastasectomy in Patients with Ocular Melanoma

Study	Sample (N)	Median Survival (mo)	Survival (%) 1 y	3 y	5 y
Salmon (1998)[76]	17 (curative surgery)	22			
Aoyama (2000)[81]	10	27			53
Hsueh (2004)[82]	24	38			39
Rivoire (2005)[83]	28	15	59	29 (2 y)	13 (4 y)
Adam (2006)[11]	104	19			21
Frenkel (2009)[84]	34	23			
Mariani (2009)[85]	255	14	57		7

TABLE 8-4: Studies of Outcomes of Nonresectional Therapy in Patients with Hepatic Metastases from Melanoma

Study	Modality	Sample (N)	Response (%)	Median (mo)	Survival 1 yr (%)	Survival 3 yr (%)
Storm (1982)[87]	HAIC + hyperthermia	10	30	8.5		
Cantore (1994)[74]	HAIC	8	37.5	15		
Leyvraz (1997)[73]	HAIC	30	40	14		23 (2 y)
Egerer (2001)[92]	HAIC	7	29	24		47 (2 y)
Becker (2002)[75]	HAIC	48	22	16		
Peters (2006)[93]	HAIC	101	36	15	67	12
Melichar (2009)[94]	HAIC	10	20	10		
Farolfi (2011)[95]	HAIC	18	17	21		
Mavligit (1988)[99]	TACE	30	46	11		
Feun (1994)[100]	TACE	4	50	7		
Bedikian (1995)[71]	TACE	201	33			
Agarwala (2004)[88]	TACE	19	16			
Siegel (2007)[101]	TACE	30	30	14		
Vogl (2007)[91]	TACE	12	25	19.5		
Sharma (2008)[103]	TACE	20	35 (response + stabilization)	9	43	
Sato (2008)[102]	TAIE	39	32	14	62	
Yamamoto (2009)[105]	TACE/TAIE	53	24	10 (TACE) 20 (TAIE)		
Fiorentini (2009)[104]	TACE	10	100			
Huppert (2010)[106]	TACE	14	86	11.5	50	14 (2 y)
Schuster (2010)[107]	TACE	25	16	6	15	
Ahrar (2011)[108]	TACE	42	39	8		
Noter (2004)[109]	IHP	8	50	10	50	37.5 (2 y)
Rizell (2008)[110]	IHP	27	70	7.5		

Abbreviations: HAIC, hepatic arterial infusion chemotherapy; TACE, transcatheter arterial chemoembolization; TAIE, transcatheter arterial immune-embolization; IHP, isolated hepatic perfusion.

The largest HAIC study reported included 101 UMLM patients treated with fotemustine-based therapy and noted a response rate of 36% (15% showed complete response), leading to a median survival of 15 months and a one-, two-, and three-year survival rates of 67%, 29%, and 12%, respectively. Patients were included if they had good performance status, unresectable liver metastases, histologically confirmed uveal melanoma, minimal extrahepatic tumor burden, and adequate blood and renal tests. Hepatic dysfunction was not an exclusion criterion if it was felt to be related to tumor involvement. Severe drug-related complications occurred in 11% of patients and catheter-related complications in 21%. LDH levels greater than 1.5 times the upper limit of normal, male gender, and no hepatic resection of liver metastases were all associated with worse prognosis.[93] Becker et al. (2002) utilized sequential fotemustine, interferon-α, and interleukin-2 as in 48 UMLM patients in an effort to optimize treatment protocols for both isolated UMLM and disseminated disease. Patients with isolated liver metastases were treated with HAIC, whereas patients with systemic disease were treated with the same drugs systemically. Patients in the HAIC group showed a higher response rate (22% vs. 8%), although there was no significant difference in survival (12 vs. 11 months). Both groups had improved overall survival compared to patients not treated with fotemustine.[75]

Storm et al. (1982) combined dacarbazine-based HAIC with localized hyperthermia in an attempt to enhance response in patients with UMLM. Among 10 patients, response rates were 30%, and disease stabilization was achieved in 50%. The median time to progression was 6.5 months, and the median overall survival was 8.5 months. Minimal myelosuppression and hyperthermia-associated complications were observed. When patients with comparable disease were reviewed retrospectively, no responses were observed in cases treated with systemic dacarbazine or with systemic dacarbazine combined with hyperthermia.[87]

Fourteen studies involving 529 UMLM patients treated with TACE have been reported. Response rates have ranged from 16% to 100%, median survival varied from 7 to 22 months, and one-year survival rates were 15%–62%. Morbidity rates varied considerably, ranging from none to 100% of patients needing to discontinue therapy.[71,88,90,91,99–108] This wide variation is most likely attributable to variations in treatment protocols and chemotherapy doses. Various chemotherapeutic agents, including cisplatin and fotemustine, and different embolization agents were used in the 14 different study protocols. That said, differences in type of chemotherapy have not been correlated with the outcome.[107] The type of melanoma treated, cutaneous or uveal, also showed no correlation with the outcome.[101] However, a high LDH level (greater than 2 times the upper limit of normal) was strongly associated with a worse outcome.[101,108]

The largest TACE UMLM study was conducted by Bedikian et al. (1995) and involved 201 patients treated with systemic chemotherapy, HAIC, and TACE. Systemic chemotherapy generated a minimal response rate of 1%. Outcomes were most optimal in the TACE group, with a response rate of 33% and stabilization rate of 37%. The authors recommended TACE as the only effective modality among those evaluated. Serum alkaline phosphatase levels and short disease-free interval after treatment of the primary tumor were independently associated with poor prognosis.[71]

Melphalan-based isolated hepatic perfusion (IHP) has also been utilized as a novel treatment for liver metastases from malignant melanoma. The first study was performed to demonstrate the efficacy and potential safety of such a therapy in eight patients with UMLM treated with high-dose Melphalan (200 mg) for one hour. Grade III or IV hepatotoxicity was reported in 37.5% of patients but was typically transient and resolved in three months. The authors achieved a response rate of 50%, with median time to progression of 7 months and overall survival of 10 months. The one- and two-year survival rates were 50% and 37.5%, respectively.[109] A separate study by Rizell et al. (2008) aimed to clarify the ideal IHP protocol and included 27 patients, among whom 74% had uveal melanoma. Various treatment protocols were utilized with optimal results achieved in patients treated with IHP at a dose of 1.0 mg/kg, heated to a temperature of 40°C. The overall response rate for the entire study was 70%; however, 100% of patients in this subgroup achieved a complete response. No difference in outcomes was observed between ocular and cutaneous melanoma. Six patients (22%) died postoperatively due to multiorgan failure and hepatic insufficiency, and eight patients (30%) had severe complications. The authors recommended additional research to be completed to define a more clinically tolerable protocol and encouraged the simultaneous use of systemic chemotherapy to control systemic disease when targeted liver-directed perfusion therapy is utilized.[110]

Summary

Although uveal and cutaneous melanomas differ dramatically with regard to tumor biology, multiple studies have reported comparable outcomes following either hepatic resection or nonresectional liver-directed therapy of liver metastases from melanoma subtype in selected patients. Although surgery remains the only potentially curative option; five-year survival rates vary widely between 7% and 53%, and it is utilized far less often than alternate approaches primarily due to the biologic tendency of melanoma to widely disseminate. When liver surgery is feasible, an R0 resection and limited tumor burden are associated with improved outcomes.

In instances when surgery is not feasible, TACE should be considered as second-line treatment. TACE combines liver-directed chemotherapy with embolization techniques and can provide effective local control with few complications. Patients with a low LDH do significantly better following TACE compared to patients with high LDH. Although response rates range from 16% to 100%, considerable research is ongoing to optimize the effectiveness of TACE. Newer therapies based on fotemustine are at least as effective as traditional platinum-based chemotherapies while having considerably fewer side effects. Immunoembolization using granulocyte-macrophage colony-stimulating factor also appears to be a promising new approach.[102,105]

IHP although associated with a high regression rate and a demonstrable survival benefit may have a prohibitively high morbidity and mortality rate, making it a less favorable option until further research is conducted.

Soft-Tissue Sarcoma

Sarcomas are a rare and heterogeneous group of malignant tumors of mesenchymal origin that comprise approximately 1% of all adult malignancies. Approximately 80% of sarcomas originate from soft tissue, with 11,280 soft-tissue sarcomas (STS) diagnosed each year in the United States associated with 3900 deaths.[111] STS liver metastases (STSLM) develop in up to 25% of such patients. However isolated STSLM are rare and most likely occur as a result of hematogenous spread.[112] Histologic grade, histologic type, and primary site are all risk factors for the development of hepatic metastases but do not affect outcomes once metastases develop.[113] Patients with STSLM rarely respond to systemic chemotherapy or nonsurgical regional therapies.[91,132,133] Although R0 surgical resection is achievable in a minority of patients with completion rates up to 38%,[113] when achievable it can be curative or associated with prolonged survival similar to what has been demonstrated for pulmonary STS metastasectomy.[114]

Gastrointestinal stromal tumors (GISTs) report a biologically distinct STS that express the CD117 antigen and often exhibit a remarkable response to targeted chemotherapy and will be addressed in a separate section.[112]

Hepatic Metastasectomy Outcomes: Soft-Tissue Sarcoma (Table 8-5)

Twenty individual studies have studied the role of hepatic resection in patients with STSLM. Overall these studies have reported on 496 patients with a median survival ranging from 11 to 103 months and five-year survival rates ranging from 4% to 51%. No procedure-related mortalities were reported in any of the published studies.[6,10,11,14,17,24,44,113,115–126] The most consistently identified risk factor for recurrence and decreased survival was a disease-free interval less than 24 months between the resection of the primary tumor and identification of liver metastases.[24,124] Other poor prognostic indicators include larger size of metastases[126] and inability to achieve an R0 surgical resection. Although cytoreductive surgery did appear to offer a slight survival benefit over conservative therapy in most reports, it is important to consider that these were highly selected patient, and the inference cannot be generalized.[24,122] The presence of extrahepatic metastases did not confer a worse prognosis as long as they could be simultaneously resected.[122]

The three largest studies examining the role of hepatic resection for STSLM included a total of 247 patients. DeMatteo et al. (2001) analyzed 331 STSLM patients among whom 56 underwent complete metastasectomy. There was no perioperative mortality in the resection group. Postoperative survival rates of one, three, and five years were 88%, 50%, and 30%, respectively, with a median survival of 39 months. Five-year survival rate among those who did not undergo complete resection was 4%. A disease-free interval from the primary tumor to the development of liver metastases of greater than two years was a positive prognostic indicator.[24] Pawlik et al. (2006)

TABLE 8-5: Studies of Outcomes of Hepatic Metastasectomy in Patients with Soft-Tissue Sarcoma

Study	Sample (N)	Median Survival (mos)	1 y	3 y	5 y	10 y
Foster (1978)[116]	12	11			11	
Jaques (1995)[113]	14	30				
Harrison (1997)[14]	27	31			4	
Elias (1998)[10]	13			62	18	
Chen (1998)[115]	11	39		27		
Hemming (2000)[118]	7				29	
Lang (2000)[122]	26	32 (R0 resection)			20	
Van Ruth (2001)[121]	6	27		33		
DeMatteo (2001)[24]	56	39	88	50	30	
Goering (2002)[117]	14			44		
Ercolani (2005)[17]	10	44		64	36	
Pawlik (2006)[123]	66		91	65	27	
Teo (2006)[120]	7	28				
Adam (2006)[11]	125	32			31	
Lendoire (2007)[119]	23	19		18	9	
Reddy (2007)[6]	19	38				
Rehders (2009)[124]	27	44			49	
Bresadola (2011)[44]	3	32				
Chua (2011)[125]	15	103			51	37
Zacherl (2011)[126]	15	34			27	

evaluated the role of either hepatic resection or RFA in the treatment of selected STSLM patients. Sixty-six STSLM patients were selected that included 36 patients with GISTs. Fifty-three patients underwent hepatic resection with or without RFA and 13 underwent RFA alone. There was no mortality in the study cohort; however, major complications were seen in 15%. The overall one-, three-, and five-year survival rates were 91%, 65%, and 27%, respectively. Treatment with RFA and lack of adjuvant chemotherapy were associated with a shorter disease-free interval.[123] The largest cohort is drawn from a study by Adam et al. (2006) evaluating various NCNN liver metastases patients that included 125 patients with STSLM. Median survival after hepatic resection was 32 months. Long-term survival greater than five years was achieved in one-third of the STSLM group.[11]

Outcomes of Additional Liver-Directed Therapeutic Modalities: Soft-Tissue Sarcoma

Very limited reports on the use of nonsurgical alternatives for the treatment of STSLM have been published. Motsumoto et al. (1990) were among the first to successfully demonstrate the effectiveness of transcatheter arterial embolization in liver metastases arising from gastrointestinal leiomyosarcoma in three patients.[127] In a separate study, two cases of gastrointestinal leiomyosarcoma were treated with cisplatin-based TACE (150 mg), using polyvinyl sponge for embolization, followed by HAIC using vinblastine (10 mg/m² over two hours). Both patients achieved durable tumor regression after failing combination systemic chemotherapy.[128] These same authors expanded their initial study to include

14 additional STSLM patients. A partial response was demonstrated in 71% of patients, which lasted a median duration of 12 months. Transient complications included right upper quadrant pain, elevated liver enzymes, electrolyte abnormalities, and mild hematologic derangements.[89] Finally Melichar et al. (2005) evaluated the use of HAIC in six STSLM patients. Analysis was completed in five patients, and there was no response with all patients showing disease progression. The median survival was 20 months. The study was subsequently expanded to include 22 STSLM patients among whom a partial response was seen (48%). Responders had better overall survival than nonresponders (35 vs. 14 months).[129]

Summary

Metastatic sarcoma is generally associated with a poor prognosis and a dismal response to chemotherapy. Although anecdotal reports of dramatic response to TACE or regional chemotherapy have resulted in long-term survival, these are rare. An R0 resection remains the only treatment option with a reproducible survival benefit and an opportunity for cure.

Extrahepatic metastases are not an absolute contraindication to liver resection if they can be completely resected concurrently. Although cytoreductive surgery has shown a slight improvement in survival compared to conservative management, the benefit is not sufficient to justify surgical intervention when all disease cannot be removed. Curative resection for STSLM is associated with a median survival 19–103 months and a five-year survival rate of 4%–51%. Anecdotal reports of 10-year survival after surgery do exist.[125] Repeat hepatic resection of recurrences is feasible as long as an R0 resection is expected and in the absence of extrahepatic disease.

Gastrointestinal Stromal Tumors

Primary malignant tumors of the small intestine are rare in general. GISTs represent the third most common neoplasms among primary malignant small intestinal tumors[130] and account for 1%–3% of all tumors of the gastrointestinal tract and 5%–6% of all sarcomas.[131,132] GISTs express CD117 and CD34, with CD117 representing KIT (a tyrosine-kinase receptor). A mutation of KIT leads to constitutional activation of the tyrosine-kinase pathway, forming a base for tumor development, as well as a site for targeted therapy. Various novel therapeutic agents for GIST have been detected, specifically targeting inhibition of this pathway.[133,134]

Metastases from GIST usually occur locally or in the liver.[135] Up to 80% of patients with GIST develop local recurrence or metastasis after radical surgery, and the liver is the most common site (16% overall).[136] Surgical resection has historically been the standard of care for GIST liver metastases patients; however, recurrence rates after GIST liver metastases resection are high (70%–77%).[24] Survival with GIST liver metastases is generally poor, even after hepatic resection,[24] and until recently, GISTs were refractory to standard chemotherapy regimens. The recent development of targeted therapy using tyrosine kinase inhibitors such as imatinib has altered the survival outlook for advanced GIST. Very high response rate to iImatinib therapy are commonplace (complete response: 6%, partial response: 51%, and disease stabilization: 32%) and when combined with hepatic resection can result in macroscopically curative resections in 50%–80% of cases.[137] At present it is recommended that nearly all patients undergo a neoadjuvant course of imatinib and continue a postoperative course of imatinib, though the duration of such therapy is ill-defined.[138]

Hepatic Metastasectomy Outcomes: GIST

It is only in the past decade that GIST was identified as a separate entity from STS, and as such literature on the outcomes of hepatic resection for GIST liver metastases is limited.[130] Previous reports bundled GIST with other STSLM and likely skewed the outcomes toward more unfavorable results for this subgroup. Among those combinational studies, five-year survival rates have ranged from 27% to 49% and median survival was 39–76 months.[24,123,124]

Sato et al. (2004) reported a single case of a gastric GIST with synchronous hepatic metastases treated with gastrectomy and multiple hepatic metastasectomies for recurrent disease, resulting in a survival of over three years.[139] In an additional patient, imatinib therapy and embolization resulted in tumor shrinkage permitting surgical resection.[140] The largest study to date has reported on the outcomes of 14 GIST patients with multimodal therapy including hepatic resection, microwave coagulation, RFA, and imatinib. A median survival of 65 months and a five-year survival rate greater than 50% was achieved.[141]

Outcomes of Additional Liver-Directed Therapeutic Modalities: Gastrointestinal Stromal Tumors (GIST) (Table 8-6)

Since the identification of GIST as a unique biological entity with overexpression of KIT and the development of imatinib therapy, the prognosis of GIST of all stages has dramatically improved. Multiple studies have reported on the use of imatinib for the treatment of GIST-liver metastases with response rates ranging from 37% to 100% and median survival of 7–48 months.[136,142–144] These studies have further demonstrated that imatinib therapy far superior to alternatives such as Epirubicin-based HAIC in controlling GIST liver metastases.[142]

The largest study reported to date was conducted by Zhu et al. (2007). These authors treated 21 patients with solitary LM after primary GIST resection. Fifty-two percent of the patients responded to therapy. Grade III or IV toxicities were rare; however, one patient died in the course of the study. The two-year progression-free and overall survival rates were 86% and 95%, respectively.[136] All the 42 patients with recurrent GIST liver metastases or intra-abdominal spread were treated with long-term imatinib without any significant complications. The three-year survival rate was 67%, median time to progression was 37 months, and median overall survival time was 48 months.[144]

A limited number of anecdotal reports have also reported on the effectiveness of imatinib therapy for treatment naïve or treatment refractory GIST liver metastases and have noted high rates of stabilization and long-term remissions.[145–148] The combined use of neoadjuvant imatinib therapy to improve liver resectability rates as well as the use of long-term adjuvant therapy to prevent recurrences has been similarly documented.[143,149–151] Short-term use of imatinib or termination of adjuvant therapy after curative surgical resection is associated with a high risk of recurrence, and long-term low-dose imatinib has shown efficacy and gained favor.[152,153] Selected patients who are not candidates for surgical resection or imatinib therapy, or have failed therapy, may be candidates for multimodal treatment including RFA, transcatheter arterial embolization, and other novel approaches that independently or in combination with surgery and imatinib have shown effectiveness in sporadic GIST liver metastases cases.[154–156]

Summary

The introduction of imatinib targeted therapy for GIST has revolutionized the treatment of disseminated GIST. Surgery continues to play a significant supportive role to eradicate any limited systemic metastases. imatinib therapy may render unresectable patients resectable when used neoadjuvantly and its long-term low-dose use may substantially prevent recurrence with only minimal side effects. Although imatinib and surgery are the primary therapy for advanced GIST, other therapeutic modalities such as RFA and TACE have been effective in sporadic cases.

Other Gastrointestinal Tumors

Although the liver most likely acts as a filter for noncolorectal gastrointestinal (NCRGI) metastases as it does for colorectal metastases, the outcomes are not comparable.[157] In nearly all cases, liver metastases from NCRGI tumors are associated with a dismal outcome even if metastasectomy is attempted.[14,158,159] Moreover, the outcomes of NCRGI liver metastases are also substantially worse than those reported for hepatic resections for other non-GI liver metastases.[44] Five-year survivors are rare occurrences, with very few studies demonstrating five-year survival rates better than 30%.[11,25,160–162]

NCRGI tumors represent a diverse group with overall poor but variable outcomes. For example, small bowel tumors show a better outcome than gastro-esophageal junction tumors (five-year survivals of 49% and 12%, respectively).[11] Gastric cancer is the most common NCRGI tumor to spread to the liver, with small intestine tumors being exceedingly

TABLE 8-6: Studies of Outcomes of Nonresectional Therapy in Patients with Hepatic metastases from Gastrointestinal Stromal Tumors

Study	Modality	Sample (N)	Response (%)	Median (mo)	Survival (%) 1 y	3 y	5 y
Rutkowski (2003)[143]	Imatinib	32	37.5	7.5			
Fiorentini (2006)[142]	Imatinib	2	100	>16 (still alive)			
Zhu (2007)[136]	Imatinib	21	52			95 (2 y)	
Zhu (2010)[144]	Imatinib	42		48		67	

rare, and most often of neuroendocrine origin. As such the majority of the literature on the role of hepatic resection for NCRGI liver meatastases deals primarily (if not exclusively) with gastric cancer liver meatastases).

Gastric cancer is the fourth most common cancer worldwide and the eighth leading cause of cancer death in the United States.[163,164] The prognosis of gastric cancer is poor, with five-year survival rates approaching 30%.[163] The liver is a common site of metastasis from gastric cancer, being involved in approximately 10% of cases.[165] Once liver meatastases develop, reported five-year survival rates drop to below 10%. Although gastric adenocarcinoma is associated with long-term survivors after hepatic resection for liver meatastases in Japan,[166] western studies have failed to corroborate these data. Gastric cancer liver meatastases are frequently associated with peritoneal carcinomatosis and extensive local disease,[166] and attempts at curative hepatic resection are abandoned more often than not.[166,167] In cases with direct invasion of the liver by the primary gastric tumor, en-bloc resection, if technically possible, offers the potential for long-term survival.[167]

Hepatic Metastasectomy Outcomes: Gastrointestinal Tumors (Table 8-7)

Twenty-three different studies have reported on the use of hepatic resection for gastric cancer liver metastases. In total, these studies have treated 749 patients with NCNN liver meatastases of gastrointestinal origins. The reported overall median survival ranges from 8 to 54 months, with five-year survival rates ranging from 0% to 38%.[11,14,16,17,25,44,118,159–162,167–178] Only one study reports a median survival greater than 84 months, but this study included only two patients.[175] Synchronous en-bloc resection has been shown to be associated with a better than expected prognosis for discontinuous metachronous hepatic resection since the former is felt to be a manifestation of local progression rather than systemic disease.[167] In the case of liver meatastases, frequently identified poor prognostic indicators include a greater size and number of liver meatastases,[25,170,172,176] bilobar involvement,[161,176] and the presence of nodal disease.[171,177]

Despite a large number of published studies on the treatment of gastrointestinal NCNN liver meatastases, only three reports have a sample size greater than 50 patients. The largest of these studies was reported by Adam et al. (2006) and included 230 patients with gastrointestinal liver meatastases as a subset of a larger sample of NCNN liver meatastases patients. The median survival for GINCNN liver meatastases was 26 months, and the five-year survival rate was 37%.[11] Makino et al. (2010) reported on outcomes of 63 patients with gastric cancer liver metastases treated with gastrectomy with or without hepatic resection. None of the patients had additional factors rendering them noncurative. Overall one-, three-, and five-year survival rates for the entire group were 62%, 17%, and 10%, respectively. Survival was significantly improved for patients who underwent hepatic resection (82%,

TABLE 8-7: Studies of Outcomes of Hepatic Metastasectomy in Patients with Gastrointestinal Cancers

Study	Sample (N)	Median Survival (mos)	1 y	3 y	5 y	10 y
Bines (1993)[167]	12	8				
Hoshima (1995)[168]	6	22				
Miyazaki (1997)[169]	21	26				
Harrison (1997)[14]	7	21		0	0	
Hemming (2000)[118]	7			0	0	
Fujii (2001)[170]	10	16			10	
Laurent (2001)[159]	15			14	14	
Saiura (2002)[171]	10	25	50	30	20	
Sakamoto (2003)[25]	22		73	38	38	
Takada (2003)[173]	9	6	33			
Shirabe (2003)[172]	36		64	26	26	26
Weitz (2005)[16]	12	21				
Ercolani (2005)[17]	18	26		17	9	
Li (2006)[174]	44	19 (curative resection)				
Lim (2006)[175]	2	>84 (still alive)	100	100	100	
Adam (2006)[11]	230	26			31	
Sakamoto (2007)[176]	37	31			11	
O'Rourke (2008)[160]	27	54			37	
Manba (2009)[177]	49	22			20	
Makino (2010)[161]	63	31	82	46	37	
Schmelzle (2010)[178]	17	15			0	
Bresadola (2011)[44]	31	13	59	23	11	
Takemura (2012)[162]	64	34	84	50	37	

46%, and 37%, respectively). Hepatic resection and uni-lobar metastases were associated with a better outcome.[161] Takemura et al. (2012) sought to clarify which patients with gastric cancer liver metastases may derive the most benefit from hepatic resection. Sixty-four patients who had undergone macroscopically complete hepatic resection were retrospectively evaluated. The one-, three-, and five-year survival rates were 84%, 50%, and 37%, respectively, with a median survival of 34 months. Serosal invasion of gastric cancer and large tumor size (>5 cm) were independently associated with a poor prognosis.[162]

Outcomes of Additional liver-Directed Therapeutic Modalities: Gastrointestinal Tumors (Table 8-8)

The most well-studied nonresectional liver-directed therapeutic modality for gastrointestinal NCNN liver metastases is HAIC. Multiple protocols and multiple chemotherapeutic agents have been utilized by various authors. These include 5-fluorouracil (5-FU), MMC, and cis-diamminedichloroplatinum (CDDP) in various combinations as well as the use of some novel antineoplastic agents such as fluoropyrimi-

TABLE 8-8: Studies of Outcomes of Nonresectional Therapy in Patients with Hepatic Metastases from Gastrointestinal Cancers

Study	Modality	Sample (N)	Response (%)	Median (mo)	Survival 1 y	Survival 3 y	Survival 5 y
Denck (1980)[181]	HAIC (5-FU)	50	76				
Denck (1984)[182]	HAIC (5-FU)	181	58				
Nojiri (1988)[183]	HAIC (CDDP)	7 (3 GCLM)	29				
Hasegawa (1991)[184]	HAIC (CDDP)	3	100	6–11			
Paquet (1992)[185]	HAIC (5-FU)	11		13			
Hoshima (1995)[168]	HAIC (5-FU, carboplatin)	15		19			
Hashimoto (1997)[186]	HAIC (FEM)	7	33	14	51		
Takahashi (2001)[187]	HAIC (5-FU, CDDP)	9	67			44 (2 y)	
Saikawa (2002)[179]	HAIC (CDDP, S-1)	4	75				
Shizawa (2002)[188]	HAIC (5-FU, CDDP, MMC)	4	75				
Takada (2003)[173]	HAIC	67		5	22		
Tono (2004)[180]	HAIC (paclitaxel)	2	100				
Ojima (2007)[190]	HAIC	18	83				
Ota el at. (2009)[191]	HAIC (5-FU)	11	91	8–34			
Kitamura (1989)[194]	TACE (MMC)	12	50				
Kitamura (1990)[193]	Hypertensive HAIC (MMC)	14	38				
Arai (1994)[195]	Hypertensive HAIC (MMC)	8	62.5	26			
Iwasaki (1998)[196]	Hypertensive HAIC (MMC,5-FU)	10	70				
Ohashi (1999)[197]	Hypertensive HAIC (5-FU)	11	55	12			
Yamakado (2005)[198]	HAIC + RFA	7	100	16.5			
Hofer (2008)[199]	RFA	30		34			

Abbreviations: HAIC, hepatic arterial infusion chemotherapy; 5-FU, 5-fluorouracil; CDDP, cis-diamminedichloroplatinum; GCLM, gastric cancer liver metastases; FEM, 5-FU + epirubicin + mitomycin C; S-1, fluoropriminidine; MMC, mitomycin C; TACE: transcatheter arterial chemoembolization; RFA: radiofrequency ablation.

dine (S-1).[179,180] Comparing outcomes among the 14 published studies is impossible given significant variation in study design. Overall, 408 gastrointestinal NCNN liver metastases patients treated with HAIC have been reported, response rates ranging from 21% to 100%, and median survival ranging from 5 to 34 months. Side effects varied from negligible to severe in as many as half the patients treated.[168,173,179–191] Overall, CDDP was the chemotherapeutic agent associated with the most significant improvement in outcomes,[184] and the combined use of HAIC and systemic chemotherapy was slightly better than either alone.[189] It is important to note that none of the studies were conducted using modern chemotherapy regimens; hence, they cannot be endorsed.

The two largest studies on the use of HAIC included 181 and 21 patients, respectively. The first study was conducted by Denck et al. (1984) for the treatment of gastric cancer liver metastases patients with 5-FU-based therapy using a loading dose of 6 g over three to six days interrupted by intervals of six to eight weeks. These authors recorded regression rates of 58%, with time to progression up to 50 months.[182] The second study used 5-FU, epirubicin, and MMC (FEM) therapy and reported a median survival of five months and a one-year survival rate of only 22% in a cohort of 21 patients treated with resection of the primary and FEM-based HAIC.[173]

Multiple additional studies have utilized HAIC with various agents as part of a multimodal therapy in gastric cancer liver metastases patients. Such studies have consistently shown optimal outcomes following resection of the primary (as well as LM), using both systemic and intra-arterial chemotherapy adjuncts.[165,168,173,192]

Only one study has reported on the use of TACE for gastrointestinal NCNN liver metastases. This study performed TACE using MMC and degradable starch molecules in 12 patients and achieved a 50% response rate but demonstrated no survival benefit.[193] The authors expanded their cohort by adding HAIC of various combinations in an additional 55 gastric cancer liver metastases patients (hepatic arterial infusion in 14 cases with isolated liver metastases, and intra-aortic infusion in 41 who also had extrahepatic disease). The patients who received MMC–5-FU combination along with angiotensin II (38% response rate, with one complete response) showed the most promising outcomes.[194]

A similar approach using HAIC in combination with intra-arterial hypertensive agents such as angiotensin II and noradrenaline to treat 43 GCLM patients has been reported. Response rates ranged from 38% to 70% although no survival benefit was noted. The author speculated that the addition of systemic chemotherapy to control distant metastases may improve the overall efficacy of the approach.[193,195–197]

A handful of studies have also looked at the efficacy of RFA in the treatment of gastric cancer liver metastases either alone, following neoadjuvant HAIC or palliatively to allow unresectable patients to become resectable.[198,199] Additional reports have also described novel approaches such as hyperthermo-radio-chemotherapy, stereotactic radiation therapy, and other less frequently used approaches.[200–204]

Given the dismal prognosis, once gastric cancer liver metastases develop, several authors have sought strategies to prevent them. Takahashi et al. (1989) were among the first to experiment with HAIC using MMC (20 mg) and 5-FU (500 mg) as a one-time dose and demonstrated a decrease in the subsequent incidence of gastric cancer liver metastases when compared to controls. Unfortunately this approach did not improve survival and was subsequently abandoned.[205]

Summary

Current consensus regarding the appropriate management of gastric cancer liver metastases is that it should be treated with systemic chemotherapy alone. Locally advanced primaries with serosal or vascular invasion, bi-lobar liver metastases, and large metastases (>5 cm) are associated with such a poor survival that major hepatic surgery is often limited to palliative value. Adam et al. (2006) have suggested that some patients with gastric cancer liver metastases may be surgical candidates and that initial response to chemotherapy can serve as a marker for those who may benefit and achieve long-term survival.[11] Patients who have direct extension of their gastric tumor to the liver represent a unique group in whom en-bloc resection should always be offered as it has consistently been associated with long-term survival.[167]

Genitourinary Tumors

Genitourinary cancers represent heterogeneous group of tumors; however given their rarity, particularly those with liver metastases amenable to therapy, they will be discussed as a group.

Renal cell carcinoma (RCC) is the most common malignancy of the kidney, accounting for approximately 90% of all renal cancers. RCC accounts for 3% of adult cancers in the United States and is the cause of 13,000 deaths annually. The five-year survival rate is estimated at 70%, primarily due to early detection.[206] However as many as 50% of RCC patients eventually develop distant metastases, even after treatment, and of these 20%–40% have liver involvement.[207] Once metastases develop, the survival rate drops significantly, with five-year rates reported to be less than 20%. Once liver metastases develop, the median survival drops to a mere seven months.[208] As RCC is generally highly resistant to virtually all standard chemotherapeutic agents, surgical resection has become the backbone of treatment for local as well as systemic disease.[209] Although there is consensus on the benefit of metastasectomy for pulmonary metastasis, similar agreement does not exist for liver metastases.[210] The treatment of metastatic RCC has changed dramatically after the introduction of biological therapy; however, the treatment of hepatic metastases remains a substantial clinical challenge.

Testicular cancers are the most common solid malignancies in young, adult males, making up 1% of all cancers in men. Nonseminomatous germ cell tumors (NSGCTs) constitute the vast majority of testicular cancers. NSGCT is one of the most curable malignancies, with a five-year survival rate better than 95%.[111] The principle therapy for NSGCT is chemotherapy till serum markers normalize.[211] Systemic chemotherapy is universally effective at all visceral sites of germ cell metastases and is the primary treatment of NSGCT hepatic metastases. Although additional options are available to treat hepatic metastases in instances when chemotherapy fails such as thermal ablation, HAIC, and TACE,[212,213] the effectiveness of chemotherapy has left liver-directed therapy a largely neglected topic.

Hepatic Metastasectomy Outcomes: Genitourinary Tumors (Table 8-9)

Seventeen different studies have reviewed the clinical outcomes of hepatic resection in patients with RCC liver metastases. These studies include a total of 635 patients and report a median survival ranging from 12 to 142 months, and five-year survival rates between 27% and 62%. Morbidity rates ranged from 0% to 15%, and only a single study reported an operative mortality.[6,11,14,16,17,159,160,210,214–222] Metachronous liver disease,[210,221,222] an R0 resection,[220,221] and a disease-free interval greater than 24 months have been recognized as positive prognostic factors.[214,219,223] Fewer and smaller size of RCC liver metastases and the primary tumor biology may also result in more favorable outcomes.[210,216,217,219–221,223]

Most studies on hepatic resection of RCC liver metastases have been reported as subsets of a larger cohort of NCNN liver metastases.[6,11,14,16,17,159,160] In these reports, median survival in the RCC liver metastases subgroups have ranged from 30 to 50 months and consistently boasted five-year survival of 27% or greater.[6,11,14,16,17,159,160] Adam et al. (2006) analyzed 332 patients with RCC liver metastases undergoing hepatic resection and identified a 48% five-year survival.[11] Interestingly, the immunobiology of RCC has been well documented and anecdotal reports of spontaneous remission of liver metastases following radical nephrectomy leading to long-term survival have been demonstrated.[224,225] The largest study focusing solely on the outcomes of hepatic resection for RCC liver metastases analyzed 88 patients and was reported by Staehler et al. (2010). Sixty-eight patients underwent surgery, whereas 20 who refused surgery were used as a comparison group. Patients who underwent surgery had a five-year survival rate of 62% and a median survival of 142 months compared to patients who did not undergo hepatic resection who experienced a five-year survival rate of 29% and median survival of 27 months. Patients with metachronous metastases and low-grade primary RCC each had a median survival of 155 months. Patients with synchronous metastases or high-grade RCC did not benefit from surgery.[210]

Owing to the availability of highly effective systemic chemotherapy for NSGCT, there are very few reports on the outcomes of hepatic resection for such patients. That said, all anecdotal reports have demonstrated a survival benefit after hepatic resection in NSGCT patients, irrespective of response to chemotherapy. The response has been most pronounced in patients who had low tumors marker levels. Some authors have recommended hepatic surgery as a regular part of the therapeutic approach to disseminated NSGCT, whereas others still promote surgery for refractory disease only. Either way, all clinicians agree that there is a survival benefit of hepatic resection in NSGCT, and it should not be denied to any patient who is a candidate.[212,213,226–228]

TABLE 8-9: Studies of Outcomes of Hepatic Metastasectomy in Patients with Renal Cell Carcinoma

Study	Sample (N)	Median Survival (mo)	1 y	3 y	5 y
Tanaka (1989)[214]	7 (DFS > 6 mo)	21			
Antoniewicz (1994)[215]	2			50 (2 y)	
Fujisaka (1997)[216]	3	12	67		
Stief (1997)[217]	13	16			
Harrison (1997)[14]	34				60
Kawata (2000)[218]	4		66	33	
Laurent (2001)[159]	12			49	49
Alves (2003)[219]	14	26	69	26	
Ercolani (2005)[17]	15	53		50	42
Weitz (2005)[16]	11			18 (2 y)	
Adam (2006)[11]	332				48
Thelen (2007)[220]	31		82	54	39
Reddy (2007)[6]	18	37			
O'Rourke (2008)[160]	32	46			39
Staehler (2010)[210]	60	142			62
Ruys (2011)[221]	29		79	47	43
Langan (2012)[222]	18	24 (resection group)	89	40	27

Abbreviation: DFS, Disease-free survival.

Outcomes of Additional Liver-Directed Therapeutic Modalities: Genitourinary Tumors (Table 8-10)

Lipoidol has been demonstrated to be an effective means to target therapy to RCC liver metastases without any adverse events, and in some centers, it has been combined with HAIC.[229] Pomer et al. (1996) treated five patients with RCC liver metastases with HAIC using a combination of interleukin-2 (3 mg/d) and lipoidol (2–5 mL/d) noting only minimal grade I and II toxicities. One patient experienced a partial response, whereas four showed disease stabilization for a median of 32 months.[230] A separate study by Umeda et al. (2010) employed lipoidol-based HAIC using stylene-maleic acid neocarzinostatin to treat four patients with RCC liver metastases and demonstrated a median survival longer than 18 months, despite a response rate of only 17%.[231] In a case report by Kobayashi et al. (2011), one patient survived for five years after initial identification of renal pelvic cancer and failing systemic chemotherapy by using multiple administrations of HAIC as well as radiation therapy and transurethral resection of bladder tumors.[232] Additional novel immunotherapies including interferon-α and zoledronic acid have also been used to effectively treat RCC liver metastases inducing remission not only in the liver but also in other distant sites, including lung and bone.[233,234]

As in other tumor subtypes, TACE also has a limited role in the treatment of RCC liver metastases. Nabil et al. (2008) treated 31 patients with lipoidol-based TACE (using MMC) with starch microspheres and achieved responses rate of 59%, and a one-year survival rate of 31%.[235] Additional and more contemporary therapies include Yttrium-90 radioembolization and donor-lymphocyte infusions.[236,237]

TABLE 8-10: Studies of Outcomes of Nonresectional Therapy for Hepatic Metastases in Patients with Renal Cell Carcinoma

Study	Modality	Sample (N)	Response (%)	Median (mo)	Survival (%) 1 y	3 y	5 y
Pomer (1996)[230]	HAIC	5	20	32			
Umeda (2010)[231]	HAIC	6	17	>18			
Nabil (2008)[235]	TACE (MMC)	31	14	8	31	6 (2 y)	
Abdelmaksoud (2012)[237]	Radioembolization	6	67	7–64			

Abbreviations: HAIC, hepatic arterial infusion chemotherapy; TACE, transcatheter arterial chemoembolization; MMC, mitomycin C.

Summary

RCC liver metastases are often associated with excellent long-term survival compared to other solid tumor metastases. Five-year survival rates greater than 50% are documented following hepatic resection for RCC liver metastases. As such, all patients with RCC liver metastases should undergo evaluation for surgical resection. Operative criteria associated with improved outcomes include an R0 resection, a long disease-free interval before development of liver metastases and possibly the stage of the primary tumor. Rarely, resection of the primary tumor may lead to spontaneous regression of RCC liver metastases. For patients whose liver metastases do not regress and who are not candidates for surgical resection, HAIC with biological agents such as interleukin-2 and interferon-α represent novel therapeutic approaches with variable outcomes.

Current literature supporting hepatic resection of testicular cancer is scant, although occasional reports have shown improved survival. Hepatic resection is primarily a secondary modality for the treatment of NSGCT, as an adjunct to systemic chemotherapy in nonresponders. The use of other approaches in patients who fail systemic chemotherapy and are not candidates for surgical resection that may be considered include HAIC and TACE.

Ovarian/Gynecological Tumors

Ovarian cancer accounts for 3% of all cancers in women and causes approximately 15,000 deaths per annum in the United States. The overall five-year survival rate of women in the United States with ovarian cancer is 44%, which decreases to 27% once distant metastases develop.[206] Autopsy reports indicate that liver metastases are the second most common site of distant metastasis for epithelial ovarian cancers[238] and are associated with a median survival of 10–20 months.[239] Although the ideal treatment of advanced ovarian cancer is curative surgery, cytoreductive surgery is more commonly the primary approach because R0 surgery is often not practical. Following or before cytoreductive surgery, chemotherapy and less often radiation are used to consolidate surgical therapy. The role of cytoreduction for recurrent disease and for hepatic metastases, while feasible, remains controversial.[240] Theoretically cytoreduction should be effective whether it involves hepatectomy or in cases with no liver involvement,[241] but whether those with hematogenous hepatic spread represent a high-risk group is undetermined.

Additional gynecological malignancies include uterine, cervical, and fallopian tube malignancies; however, the current literature related to hepatic resection is dominated by ovarian cancer. For the purpose of this section, all tumors are considered gynecological malignancies and grouped as one.

Hepatic Metastasectomy Outcomes: Gynecological Malignancies (Table 8-11)

Very few reports involving small sample sizes have been published regarding the role of hepatic metastasectomy for gynecologic malignancies. In total,

TABLE 8-11: Studies of Outcomes of Hepatic Metastasectomy in Patients with Gynecological Cancer

Study	Sample (N)	Median Survival (mos)	Survival (%) 1 y	3 y	5 y
Chi (1997)[243]	12	27			
Hamy (2000)[245]	5	27			
Yoon (2003)[250]	24	62			
Merideth (2003)[247]	26	26			
Weitz (2005)[16]	12			86	
Ercolani (2005)[17]	15	52.5			
Bosquet (2006)[242]	35	27			
Lim (2009)[246]	14				51
Pekmezci (2010)[248]	4	39			
Yan (2011)[249]	10	26		60	

these studies have involved 265 patients. The overall median survival rate ranges from 26 to 62 months, with nearly all studies documenting a significant rate of postoperative morbidity,[247,249] but no perioperative mortality.[16,241–250] Factors predictive of improved survival were optimal cytoreduction[241,242,247] and a disease-free interval greater than 12 months.[242,247] Tumor deposits less than 2 cm was also predictive of improved outcomes.[241]

The largest series of ovarian cancer patients undergoing hepatic resection was reported by Bosquet et al. (2006). This series elaborated the outcomes of cytoreductive surgery including hepatic resection in 35 patients with metastatic ovarian cancer. Median overall disease-specific survival was 27 months. Optimal cytoreduction and disease-free interval greater than 12 months were the most significant prognostic indicators.[242]

Additional other studies with much smaller sample sizes have reported similar or higher survival rates among ovarian cancer patients undergoing hepatic metastasectomy. Published reports included patients with advanced epithelial ovarian cancers, recurrent ovarian or fallopian tube cancers, pure immature ovarian teratoma,[251] and lipoidal cell ovarian cancer.[244] Across the spectrum of pathologies, the median survival was more than two years.

Among those studies with significant patient follow-up, Lim et al. (2009) and Fan et al. (2001) followed patients for 5 and 10 years, respectively and reported five-year survival rates of 51% and 56% and 10-year survival rates of 39%.[246]

Outcomes of Additional Liver-Directed Therapeutic Modalities: Genitourinary Tumors

Insufficient data regarding the role of nonsurgical modalities in the treatment of liver metastases due to gynecologic malignancies currently exists. Modalities that have been reported include HAIC,[252–254] TACE,[255,256] and RFA.[257,258] Although limited reports have demonstrated response to nonsurgical liver-directed therapy,[254,255,257] these response rates are inferior to those achieved by hepatic resection.[249,256,258]

Vogl et al. (2012) reported the largest series involving the use of TACE as a palliative therapy in 65 patients with unresectable liver metastases due to ovarian cancer. These patients had failed chemotherapy and were selected to undergo different combinations of MMC-based TACE, using lipoidol and degradable starch molecules for embolization. Partial response was achieved in 17% and disease stabilization occurred in another 58.5% of patients. The overall survival rates at one, two, and three years were 58%, 19%, and 13%. The median survival time was 14 months.[256]

Interestingly, brachytherapy may represent a promising nonsurgical alternative for ovarian cancer liver metastases. Collettini et al. (2011) conducted a pilot study to evaluate the outcomes of CT-guided high-dose brachytherapy for cytoreduction of metachronous isolated liver metastases from ovarian cancer. Seven patients were recruited into this study, and all achieved complete disease remission. No post-procedure complications were noted. The one- and two-year survival rates were 100% and 86%, respectively.[259] Further studies with larger sample size should better inform us about the utility of this novel modality.

More recently Chao et al. (2001) tested the efficacy of percutaneous ethanol or acetic acid as curative therapy for isolated liver metastases from cervical cancer in two patients. Both patients were rendered free of disease after completion of treatment and remained disease free at one- and two-year follow-up.[260]

Summary

Despite the ongoing controversy in the gynecological community regarding the use of hepatic resection as a cytoreductive technique for disseminated ovarian cancer, current literature suggests a survival benefit in patients who are treated with optimal cytoreduction with median survival ranging from 26 to 62 months. The benefit is even greater when a curative R0 hepatic resection can be completed. Patients with a long disease-free survival before the development of liver metastases have a more significant survival benefit than do patients with synchronous liver disease, but both groups derive benefits.

Locoregional therapies like HAIC and RFA may have anecdotal roles, but survival benefit has not been documented.

Conclusion

Only a very small proportion of patients with NCNN liver metastases will be considered for hepatic resection. It is incumbent upon the treating surgeon and oncologist to identify those cases in which a survival benefit is most likely to accrue. Selection criteria for hepatic resection for NCNN metastases, like colorectal metastases, include control of the primary disease process, the potential for complete resection of all hepatic metastases and either the absence of extrahepatic metastases or completely resectable disease, if present.[14] Perhaps most importantly, the decision to resect hepatic metastases needs to be based on a firm understanding of the tumor biology of the primary malignancy.

Hepatic resection for BCLM is recommended in all cases with a disease-free interval longer than 24 months and if an R0 resection is technically possible. Lymph node involvement should not be considered a contraindication to surgery. In patients who are not candidates for surgery, RFA appears to be the most effective alternative modality and should be considered for all unresectable lesions smaller than 2.5 cm.

Liver metastases from melanoma may be resected in rare cases in which disease spread is limited to the liver, liver involvement is small (less than five lesions), and the DFI is longer than 24 months. Once again as R0 resection must be technically possible if a survival benefit is to be anticipated. TACE appears to be the most effective nonsurgical therapeutic modality for melanoma liver metastases and should be used in patients with a baseline LDH level less than two times the upper limit of normal. TACE appears beneficial for the treatment of liver metastases irrespective of whether the melanoma is ocular or cutaneous.

Sarcomatous liver metastases should be resected with curative intent if the DFI is longer than 24 months. This holds true even in the presence of extrahepatic disease, as long as this disease burden can be resected simultaneously. Surgical resection is recommended even in cases of local recurrence as a life-prolonging procedure. There is no indication for the use of nonsurgical therapies in patients who have unresectable liver metastases, and palliation should be the goal in such cases.

GIST represents a novel sarcomatous neoplasm expressing c-KIT that has resulted in a dramatic paradigm shift in management. Imatinib is first-line treatment for patients with systemic disease, and surgery is used supportively when imatinib is not effective, or the lesions are too large.

Although most advanced gastrointestinal malignancies are associated with a dismal prognosis once liver metastases develop, very rare selected patients may derive benefit from hepatic resection. Such patients must have uni-lobar disease with a few metastases, and no tumor greater than 5 cm. Patients who demonstrate nodal metastases or have serosal or lymphovascular invasion by the primary tumor should not be considered candidates for hepatic resection. Exception to this dogma exists in the setting of direct tumor extension into the liver, which should be resected en-bloc, allowing outcomes significantly better than metastatic disease. Nonsurgical options may be rarely utilized in patients who do not fulfill the above criteria, but the expectation should be to improve local disease control and not to offer long-term survival.

Hepatic metastasectomy for genitourinary cancers is associated with the highest survival rates, and metastasectomy should be considered in all patients with isolated liver disease. The best survival statistics are achieved in patients with metachronous disease and low-grade primary lesion. Repeat metastasectomy is also a feasible option in patients who develop local recurrence.

Gynecological malignancies constitute the only group that offers a survival benefit even after cytoreductive hepatic resection. In such patients, hepatic resection is indicated in all surgical candidates, understanding that the most pronounced survival benefit is achieved when curative resection can be performed.

Irrespective of the decision to perform a hepatic metastasectomy or not, all patients with liver metastases should be managed by a multidisciplinary team involving surgeons, medical oncologists, radiation oncologists, and interventional radiologists. Preoperative chemotherapy response is generally an independent predictor of improved outcomes, and all modalities of treatment should be considered when devising an individualized treatment plan.[11]

Although up to date, the recommendations made in this review are based on very small data sets when looked at from the perspective of individual cancer types. Further research focusing on a more detailed evaluation of when hepatic metastasectomy or other liver-directed therapies should be performed in NCNN tumor metastases remains essential.

References

1. Fong Y, Blumgart LH, Cohen AM. Surgical treatment of colorectal metastases to the liver. *CA Cancer J Clin*. 1995;45:50–62.
2. Gayowski TJ, Iwatsuki S, Madariaga JR, et al. Experience in hepatic resection for metastatic colorectal cancer: analysis of clinical and pathologic risk factors. *Surgery*. 1994;116:703–710; discussion 710–711.
3. Scheele J, Stang R, Altendorf-Hofmann A, Paul M. Resection of colorectal liver metastases. *World J Surg*. 1995;19:59–71.
4. Jaeck D, Nakano H, Bachellier P, et al. Significance of hepatic pedicle lymph node involvement in patients with colorectal liver metastases: a prospective study. *Ann Surg Oncol*. 2002;9:430–438.
5. Jarnagin WR, Gonen M, Fong Y, et al. Improvement in perioperative outcome after hepatic resection: analysis of 1,803 consecutive cases over the past decade. *Ann Surg*. 2002;236:397–406.
6. Reddy SK, Barbas AS, Marroquin CE, et al. Resection of noncolorectal nonneuroendocrine liver metastases: a comparative analysis. *J Am Coll Surg*. 2007;204:372–382.
7. Sarmiento JM, Heywood G, Rubin J, et al. Surgical treatment of neuroendocrine metastases to the liver: a plea for resection to increase survival. *J Am Coll Surg*. 2003;197:29–37.
8. Lang H, Nussbaum KT, Weimann A, Raab R. Liver resection for non-colorectal, non-neuroendocrine hepatic metastases. *Chirurg*. 1999;70:439–446.
9. Lindell G, Ohlsson B, Saarela A, et al. Liver resection of noncolorectal secondaries. *J Surg Oncol*. 1998;69:66–70.
10. Elias D, Cavalcanti de Albuquerque A, Eggenspieler P, et al. Resection of liver metastases from a noncolorectal primary: indications and results based on 147 monocentric patients. *J Am Coll Surg*. 1998;187:487–493.
11. Adam R, Chiche L, Aloia T, et al. Hepatic resection for noncolorectal nonendocrine liver metastases: analysis of 1,452 patients and development of a prognostic model. *Ann Surg*. 2006;244:524–535.
12. Savage AP, Malt RA. Survival after hepatic resection for malignant tumours. *Br J Surg*. 1992;79:1095–1101.
13. Iwatsuki S, Starzl TE. Personal experience with 411 hepatic resections. *Ann Surg*. 1988;208:421–434.
14. Harrison LE, Brennan MF, Newman E, et al. Hepatic resection for noncolorectal, non-neuroendocrine metastases: a fifteen-year experience with ninety-six patients. *Surgery*. 1997;121:625–632.
15. Karavias DD, Tepetes K, Karatzas T, et al. Liver resection for metastatic non-colorectal non-neuroendocrine hepatic neoplasms. *Eur J Surg Oncol*. 2002;28:135–139.
16. Weitz J, Blumgart LH, Fong Y, et al. Partial hepatectomy for metastases from noncolorectal, nonneuroendocrine carcinoma. *Ann Surg*. 2005;241:269–276.

17. Ercolani G, Grazi GL, Ravaioli M, et al. The role of liver resections for noncolorectal, non-neuroendocrine metastases: experience with 142 observed cases. *Ann Surg Oncol.* 2005;12: 459–466.

18. Takada T, Yasuda H, Amano H, et al. Simultaneous hepatic resection with pancreato-duodenectomy for metastatic pancreatic head carcinoma: does it improve survival? *Hepatogastroenterology.* 1997; 44:567–573.

19. Takada Y, Otsuka M, Seino K, et al. Hepatic resection for metastatic tumors from noncolorectal carcinoma. *Hepatogastroenterology.* 2001;48:83–86.

20. Musunuru S, Chen H, Rajpal S, et al. Metastatic neuroendocrine hepatic tumors: resection improves survival. *Arch Surg.* 2006;141:1000–1004; discussion 5.

21. Jardines L, Callans LS, Torosian MH. Recurrent breast cancer: presentation, diagnosis, and treatment. *Semin Oncol.* 1993;20:538–547.

22. Insa A, Lluch A, Prosper F, et al. Prognostic factors predicting survival from first recurrence in patients with metastatic breast cancer: analysis of 439 patients. *Breast Cancer Res Treat.* 1999;56:67–78.

23. Eichbaum MH, Kaltwasser M, Bruckner T, et al. Prognostic factors for patients with liver metastases from breast cancer. *Breast Cancer Res Treat.* 2006;96:53–62.

24. DeMatteo RP, Shah A, Fong Y, et al. Results of hepatic resection for sarcoma metastatic to liver. *Ann Surg.* 2001;234:540–547; discussion 7–8.

25. Sakamoto Y, Ohyama S, Yamamoto J, et al. Surgical resection of liver metastases of gastric cancer: an analysis of a 17-year experience with 22 patients. *Surgery.* 2003;133: 507–511.

26. Lee YT. Breast carcinoma: pattern of recurrence and metastasis after mastectomy. *Am J Clin Oncol.* 1984;7:443–449.

27. Cutler SJ, Ardyce JA, Taylor SG 3rd. Classification of patients with disseminated cancer of the breast. *Cancer.* 1969;24:861–869.

28. Metcalfe MS, Mullin EJ, Maddern GJ. Hepatectomy for metastatic noncolorectal gastrointestinal, breast and testicular tumours. *ANZ J Surg.* 2006;76: 246–250.

29. Elias D, Di Pietroantonio D. Surgery for liver metastases from breast cancer. *HPB (Oxford).* 2006;8: 97–99.

30. Samaan NA, Buzdar AU, Aldinger KA, et al. Estrogen receptor: a prognostic factor in breast cancer. *Cancer.* 1981;47:554–560.

31. Maksan SM, Lehnert T, Bastert G, Herfarth C. Curative liver resection for metastatic breast cancer. *Eur J Surg Oncol.* 2000;26:209–212.

32. Elias D, Lasser P, Spielmann M, et al. Surgical and chemotherapeutic treatment of hepatic metastases from carcinoma of the breast. *Surg Gynecol Obstet.* 1991;172:461–464.

33. Elias D, Lasser PH, Montrucolli D, et al. Hepatectomy for liver metastases from breast cancer. *Eur J Surg Oncol.* 1995;21:510–513.

34. Raab R, Nussbaum KT, Behrend M, Weimann A. Liver metastases of breast cancer: results of liver resection. *Anticancer Res.* 1998;18:2231–2233.

35. Seifert JK, Weigel TF, Gonner U, et al. Liver resection for breast cancer metastases. *Hepatogastroenterology.* 1999;46:2935–2940.

36. Yamada H, Katoh H, Kondo S, et al. Hepatectomy for metastases from non-colorectal and non-neuroendocrine tumor. *Anticancer Res.* 2001;21: 4159–4162.

37. Carlini M, Lonardo MT, Carboni F, et al. Liver metastases from breast cancer. Results of surgical resection. *Hepatogastroenterology.* 2002;49: 1597–1601.

38. Elias D, Maisonnette F, Druet-Cabanac M, et al. An attempt to clarify indications for hepatectomy for liver metastases from breast cancer. *Am J Surg.* 2003;185:158–164.

39. Arena E, Ferrero S. Surgical treatment of liver metastases from breast cancer. *Minerva Chir.* 2004;59:7–15.

40. Vlastos G, Smith DL, Singletary SE, et al. Long-term survival after an aggressive surgical approach in patients with breast cancer hepatic metastases. *Ann Surg Oncol.* 2004;11:869–874.

41. Adam R, Aloia T, Krissat J, et al. Is liver resection justified for patients with hepatic metastases from breast cancer? *Ann Surg.* 2006;244:897–907.

42. Caralt M, Bilbao I, Cortes J, et al. Hepatic resection for liver metastases as part of the "oncosurgical" treatment of metastatic breast cancer. *Ann Surg Oncol.* 2008;15:2804–2810.

43. Hoffmann K, Franz C, Hinz U, et al. Liver resection for multimodal treatment of breast cancer metastases: identification of prognostic factors. *Ann Surg Oncol.* 2010;17: 1546–1554.

44. Bresadola V, Rossetto A, Adani GL, et al. Liver resection for noncolorectal and nonneuroendocrine metastases: results of a study on 56 patients at a single institution. *Tumori*. 2011;97:316–322.
45. Abbott DE, Brouquet A, Mittendorf EA, et al. Resection of liver metastases from breast cancer: estrogen receptor status and response to chemotherapy before metastasectomy define outcome. *Surgery*. 2012;151:710–716.
46. Furka A, Halasz L, Szentkereszty Z, et al. Surgical treatment of liver metastases from breast cancer. *Hepatogastroenterology*. 2008; 55:1416–1418.
47. d'Annibale M, Piovanello P, Cerasoli V, Campioni N. Liver metastases from breast cancer: the role of surgical treatment. *Hepatogastroenterology*. 2005;52:1858–1862.
48. Carrafiello G, Fontana F, Cotta E, et al. Ultrasound-guided thermal radiofrequency ablation (RFA) as an adjunct to systemic chemotherapy for breast cancer liver metastases. *Radiol Med*. 2011;116:1059–1066.
49. Gunabushanam G, Sharma S, Thulkar S, et al. Radiofrequency ablation of liver metastases from breast cancer: results in 14 patients. *J Vasc Interv Radiol*. 2007;18:67–72.
50. Jakobs TF, Hoffmann RT, Schrader A, et al. CT-guided radiofrequency ablation in patients with hepatic metastases from breast cancer. *Cardiovasc Intervent Radiol*. 2009;32:38–46.
51. Lawes D, Chopada A, Gillams A, et al. Radiofrequency ablation (RFA) as a cytoreductive strategy for hepatic metastasis from breast cancer. *Ann R Coll Surg Engl*. 2006;88:639–642.
52. Livraghi T, Goldberg SN, Solbiati L, et al. Percutaneous radio-frequency ablation of liver metastases from breast cancer: initial experience in 24 patients. *Radiology*. 2001;220: 145–149.
53. Meloni MF, Andreano A, Laeseke PF, et al. Breast cancer liver metastases: US-guided percutaneous radiofrequency ablation--intermediate and long-term survival rates. *Radiology*. 2009;253:861–869.
54. Sofocleous CT, Nascimento RG, Gonen M, et al. Radiofrequency ablation in the management of liver metastases from breast cancer. *AJR Am J Roentgenol*. 2007;189:883–889.
55. Peetz M, Swanson J, Moseley HS, Fletcher WS. Endocrine ablation and hepatic artery infusion in the treatment of metastases to the liver from carcinoma of the breast. *Surg Gynecol Obstet*. 1982;155: 395–400.
56. Maes T, Wildiers H, Heye S, et al. Intra-hepatic Mitomycin C bolus infusion in the treatment of extensive liver metastases of breast cancer. *Breast Cancer Res Treat*. 2008;110:135–142.
57. Melichar B, Voboril Z, Cerman J Jr, et al. Regional chemotherapy in patients with breast carcinoma liver metastases. *Hepatogastroenterology*. 2006;53:100–105.
58. Schneebaum S, Walker MJ, Young D, et al. The regional treatment of liver metastases from breast cancer. *J Surg Oncol*. 1994;55:26–31; discussion 2.
59. Stehlin JS Jr, Hafstrom L, Greeff PJ. Experience with infusion and resection in cancer of the liver. *Surg Gynecol Obstet*. 1974;138:855–863.
60. Gelin LE, Lewis DH, Nilsson L. Liver blood flow in man during abdominal surgery. II. The effect of hepatic artery occlusion on the blood flow through metastatic tumor nodules. *Acta Hepatosplenol*. 1968;15:21–24.
61. Cho SW, Kitisin K, Buck D, et al. Transcatheter arterial chemoembolization is a feasible palliative locoregional therapy for breast cancer liver metastases. *Int J Surg Oncol*. 2010;2010:251621.
62. Duan XF, Dong NN, Zhang T, Li Q. Treatment outcome of patients with liver-only metastases from breast cancer after mastectomy: a retrospective analysis. *J Cancer Res Clin Oncol*. 2011;137:1363–1370.
63. Li XP, Meng ZQ, Guo WJ, Li J. Treatment for liver metastases from breast cancer: results and prognostic factors. *World J Gastroenterol*. 2005;11:3782–3787.
64. Mack MG, Straub R, Eichler K, et al. Breast cancer metastases in liver: laser-induced interstitial thermotherapy—local tumor control rate and survival data. *Radiology*. 2004;233:400–409.
65. Umeda T, Abe H, Kurumi Y, et al. Magnetic resonance-guided percutaneous microwave coagulation therapy for liver metastases of breast cancer in a case. *Breast Cancer*. 2005;12:317–321.
66. Abe H, Kurumi Y, Naka S, et al. Open-configuration MR-guided microwave thermocoagulation therapy for metastatic liver tumors from breast cancer. *Breast Cancer*. 2005;12:26–31.
67. Cassera MA, Hammill CW, Ujiki MB, et al. Surgical management of breast cancer liver metastases. *HPB (Oxford)*. 2011;13:272–278.
68. Singh AD, Topham A. Incidence of uveal melanoma in the United States: 1973–1997. *Ophthalmology*. 2003;110:956–961.

69. Rajpal S, Moore R, Karakousis CP. Survival in metastatic ocular melanoma. *Cancer*. 1983;52:334–336.

70. Seregard S, Kock E. Prognostic indicators following enucleation for posterior uveal melanoma. A multivariate analysis of long-term survival with minimized loss to follow-up. *Acta Ophthalmol Scand*. 1995;73:340–344.

71. Bedikian AY, Legha SS, Mavligit G, et al. Treatment of uveal melanoma metastatic to the liver: a review of the M. D. Anderson Cancer Center experience and prognostic factors. *Cancer*. 1995;76:1665–1670.

72. Albert DM, Niffenegger AS, Willson JK. Treatment of metastatic uveal melanoma: review and recommendations. *Surv Ophthalmol*. 1992;36:429–438.

73. Leyvraz S, Spataro V, Bauer J, et al. Treatment of ocular melanoma metastatic to the liver by hepatic arterial chemotherapy. *J Clin Oncol*. 1997;15:2589–2595.

74. Cantore M, Fiorentini G, Aitini E, et al. Intra-arterial hepatic carboplatin-based chemotherapy for ocular melanoma metastatic to the liver. Report of a phase II study. *Tumori*. 1994;80:37–39.

75. Becker JC, Terheyden P, Kampgen E, et al. Treatment of disseminated ocular melanoma with sequential fotemustine, interferon alpha, and interleukin 2. *Br J Cancer*. 2002;87:840–845.

76. Salmon RJ, Levy C, Plancher C, et al. Treatment of liver metastases from uveal melanoma by combined surgery-chemotherapy. *Eur J Surg Oncol*. 1998;24:127–130.

77. Einhorn LH, Burgess MA, Vallejos C, et al. Prognostic correlations and response to treatment in advanced metastatic malignant melanoma. *Cancer Res*. 1974;34:1995–2004.

78. Leiter U, Meier F, Schittek B, Garbe C. The natural course of cutaneous melanoma. *J Surg Oncol*. 2004;86:172–178.

79. Barth A, Wanek LA, Morton DL. Prognostic factors in 1,521 melanoma patients with distant metastases. *J Am Coll Surg*. 1995;181:193–201.

80. Rose DM, Essner R, Hughes TM, et al. Surgical resection for metastatic melanoma to the liver: the John Wayne Cancer Institute and Sydney Melanoma Unit experience. *Arch Surg*. 2001;136:950–955.

81. Aoyama T, Mastrangelo MJ, Berd D, et al. Protracted survival after resection of metastatic uveal melanoma. *Cancer*. 2000;89:1561–1568.

82. Hsueh EC, Essner R, Foshag LJ, et al. Prolonged survival after complete resection of metastases from intraocular melanoma. *Cancer*. 2004;100:122–129.

83. Rivoire M, Kodjikian L, Baldo S, et al. Treatment of liver metastases from uveal melanoma. *Ann Surg Oncol*. 2005;12:422–428.

84. Frenkel S, Nir I, Hendler K, et al. Long-term survival of uveal melanoma patients after surgery for liver metastases. *Br J Ophthalmol*. 2009;93:1042–1046.

85. Mariani P, Piperno-Neumann S, Servois V, et al. Surgical management of liver metastases from uveal melanoma: 16 years' experience at the Institut Curie. *Eur J Surg Oncol*. 2009;35:1192–1197.

86. Venook AP, Warren RS. Regional chemotherapy approaches for primary and metastatic liver tumors. *Surg Oncol Clin N Am*. 1996;5:411–427.

87. Storm FK, Kaiser LR, Goodnight JE, et al. Thermochemotherapy for melanoma metastasis in liver. *Cancer*. 1982;49:1243–1248.

88. Agarwala SS, Panikkar R, Kirkwood JM. Phase I/II randomized trial of intrahepatic arterial infusion chemotherapy with cisplatin and chemoembolization with cisplatin and polyvinyl sponge in patients with ocular melanoma metastatic to the liver. *Melanoma Res*. 2004;14:217–222.

89. Mavligit GM, Zukwiski AA, Ellis LM, et al. Gastrointestinal leiomyosarcoma metastatic to the liver. Durable tumor regression by hepatic chemoembolization infusion with cisplatin and vinblastine. *Cancer*. 1995;75:2083–2088.

90. Patel K, Sullivan K, Berd D, et al. Chemoembolization of the hepatic artery with BCNU for metastatic uveal melanoma: results of a phase II study. *Melanoma Res*. 2005;15:297–304.

91. Vogl T, Eichler K, Zangos S, et al. Preliminary experience with transarterial chemoembolization (TACE) in liver metastases of uveal malignant melanoma: local tumor control and survival. *J Cancer Res Clin Oncol*. 2007;133:177–184.

92. Egerer G, Lehnert T, Max R, et al. Pilot study of hepatic intraarterial fotemustine chemotherapy for liver metastases from uveal melanoma: a single-center experience with seven patients. *Int J Clin Oncol*. 2001;6:25–28.

93. Peters S, Voelter V, Zografos L, et al. Intra-arterial hepatic fotemustine for the treatment of liver

metastases from uveal melanoma: experience in 101 patients. *Ann Oncol.* 2006;17:578–583.
94. Melichar B, Voboril Z, Lojik M, Krajina A. Liver metastases from uveal melanoma: clinical experience of hepatic arterial infusion of cisplatin, vinblastine and dacarbazine. *Hepatogastroenterology.* 2009;56:1157–1162.
95. Farolfi A, Ridolfi L, Guidoboni M, et al. Liver metastases from melanoma: hepatic intra-arterial chemotherapy. A retrospective study. *J Chemother.* 2011;23:300–305.
96. Kodjikian L, Grange JD, Rivoire M. Prolonged survival after resection of liver metastases from uveal melanoma and intra-arterial chemotherapy. *Graefes Arch Clin Exp Ophthalmol.* 2005;243:622–624.
97. Brasiuniene B, Sokolovas V, Brasiunas V, et al. Combined treatment of uveal melanoma liver metastases. *Eur J Med Res.* 2011;16:71–75.
98. Metzger U, Rothlin M, Burger HR, Largiader F. Long-term complete remission of melanoma liver metastases after intermittent intra-arterial cisplatin chemotherapy and surgery. *Eur J Surg Oncol.* 1997;23:270–274.
99. Mavligit GM, Charnsangavej C, Carrasco CH, et al. Regression of ocular melanoma metastatic to the liver after hepatic arterial chemoembolization with cisplatin and polyvinyl sponge. *JAMA.* 1988;260:974–976.
100. Feun LG, Reddy KR, Yrizarry JM, et al. A phase I study of chemoembolization with cisplatin and lipiodol for primary and metastatic liver cancer. *Am J Clin Oncol.* 1994;17:405–410.
101. Siegel R, Hauschild A, Kettelhack C, et al. Hepatic arterial Fotemustine chemotherapy in patients with liver metastases from cutaneous melanoma is as effective as in ocular melanoma. *Eur J Surg Oncol.* 2007;33:627–632.
102. Sato T, Eschelman DJ, Gonsalves CF, et al. Immunoembolization of malignant liver tumors, including uveal melanoma, using granulocyte-macrophage colony-stimulating factor. *J Clin Oncol.* 2008;26:5436–5442.
103. Sharma KV, Gould JE, Harbour JW, et al. Hepatic arterial chemoembolization for management of metastatic melanoma. *AJR Am J Roentgenol.* 2008;190:99–104.
104. Fiorentini G, Aliberti C, Del Conte A, et al. Intra-arterial hepatic chemoembolization (TACE) of liver metastases from ocular melanoma with slow-release irinotecan-eluting beads. Early results of a phase II clinical study. *In Vivo.* 2009;23:131–137.
105. Yamamoto A, Chervoneva I, Sullivan KL, et al. High-dose immunoembolization: survival benefit in patients with hepatic metastases from uveal melanoma. *Radiology.* 2009;252:290–298.
106. Huppert PE, Fierlbeck G, Pereira P, et al. Transarterial chemoembolization of liver metastases in patients with uveal melanoma. *Eur J Radiol.* 2010;74:e38–e44.
107. Schuster R, Lindner M, Wacker F, et al. Transarterial chemoembolization of liver metastases from uveal melanoma after failure of systemic therapy: toxicity and outcome. *Melanoma Res.* 2010;20:191–196.
108. Ahrar J, Gupta S, Ensor J, et al. Response, survival, and prognostic factors after hepatic arterial chemoembolization in patients with liver metastases from cutaneous melanoma. *Cancer Invest.* 2011;29:49–55.
109. Noter SL, Rothbarth J, Pijl ME, et al. Isolated hepatic perfusion with high-dose melphalan for the treatment of uveal melanoma metastases confined to the liver. *Melanoma Res.* 2004;14:67–72.
110. Rizell M, Mattson J, Cahlin C, et al. Isolated hepatic perfusion for liver metastases of malignant melanoma. *Melanoma Res.* 2008;18:120–126.
111. Siegel R, Naishadham D, Jemal A. Cancer statistics, 2012. *CA Cancer J Clin.* 2012;62:10–29.
112. Van Glabbeke M, van Oosterom AT, Oosterhuis JW, et al. Prognostic factors for the outcome of chemotherapy in advanced soft tissue sarcoma: an analysis of 2,185 patients treated with anthracycline-containing first-line regimens—a European Organization for Research and Treatment of Cancer Soft Tissue and Bone Sarcoma Group Study. *J Clin Oncol.* 1999;17:150–157.
113. Jaques DP, Coit DG, Casper ES, Brennan MF. Hepatic metastases from soft-tissue sarcoma. *Ann Surg.* 1995;221:392–397.
114. Billingsley KG, Burt ME, Jara E, et al. Pulmonary metastases from soft tissue sarcoma: analysis of patterns of diseases and postmetastasis survival. *Ann Surg.* 1999;229:602–610; discussion 10–12.
115. Chen H, Pruitt A, Nicol TL, et al. Complete hepatic resection of metastases from leiomyosarcoma prolongs survival. *J Gastrointest Surg.* 1998;2:151–155.
116. Foster JH. Survival after liver resection for secondary tumors. *Am J Surg.* 1978;135:389–394.

117. Goering JD, Mahvi DM, Niederhuber JE, et al. Cryoablation and liver resection for noncolorectal liver metastases. *Am J Surg*. 2002;183:384–389.
118. Hemming AW, Sielaff TD, Gallinger S, et al. Hepatic resection of noncolorectal nonneuroendocrine metastases. *Liver Transpl*. 2000;6:97–101.
119. Lendoire J, Moro M, Andriani O, et al. Liver resection for non-colorectal,non-neuroendocrine metastases: analysis of a multicenter study from Argentina. *HPB (Oxford)*. 2007;9:435–439.
120. Teo MC, Tan YM, Chung AY, et al. Metastectomy for non-colorectal, non-neuroendocrine liver secondaries. *ANZ J Surg*. 2006;76:575–578.
121. van Ruth S, Mutsaerts E, Zoetmulder FA, van Coevorden F. Metastasectomy for liver metastases of non-colorectal primaries. *Eur J Surg Oncol*. 2001;27:662–667.
122. Lang H, Nussbaum KT, Kaudel P, et al. Hepatic metastases from leiomyosarcoma: a single-center experience with 34 liver resections during a 15-year period. *Ann Surg*. 2000;231:500–505.
123. Pawlik TM, Vauthey JN, Abdalla EK, et al. Results of a single-center experience with resection and ablation for sarcoma metastatic to the liver. *Arch Surg*. 2006;141:537–543; discussion 43–44.
124. Rehders A, Peiper M, Stoecklein NH, et al. Hepatic metastasectomy for soft-tissue sarcomas: is it justified? *World J Surg*. 2009;33:111–117.
125. Chua TC, Chu F, Morris DL. Outcomes of single-centre experience of hepatic resection and cryoablation of sarcoma liver metastases. *Am J Clin Oncol*. 2011;34:317–320.
126. Zacherl M, Bernhardt GA, Zacherl J, et al. Surgery for liver metastases originating from sarcoma-case series. *Langenbecks Arch Surg*. 2011;396:1083–1091.
127. Matsumoto S, Takeuchi T, Morita S. Transcatheter arterial embolization for cystic hepatic metastases from leiomyosarcoma of gastrointestinal tract. *Rinsho Hoshasen*. 1990;35:453–458.
128. Mavligit GM, Zukiwski AA, Salem PA, et al. Regression of hepatic metastases from gastrointestinal leiomyosarcoma after hepatic arterial chemoembolization. *Cancer*. 1991;68:321–323.
129. Melichar B, Voboril Z, Nozicka J, et al. Hepatic arterial infusion chemotherapy in sarcoma liver metastases: a report of 6 cases. *Tumori*. 2005;91:19–23.
130. Kamoshita N, Yokomori T, Iesato H, et al. Malignant gastrointestinal stromal tumor of the jejunum with liver metastasis. *Hepatogastroenterology*. 2002;49:1311–1314.
131. Lewis JJ, Brennan MF. Soft tissue sarcomas. *Curr Probl Surg*. 1996;33:817–872.
132. Nishida T, Hirota S. Biological and clinical review of stromal tumors in the gastrointestinal tract. *Histol Histopathol*. 2000;15:1293–1301.
133. Hirota S, Isozaki K, Moriyama Y, et al. Gain-of-function mutations of c-kit in human gastrointestinal stromal tumors. *Science*. 1998;279:577–580.
134. Corless CL, McGreevey L, Haley A, et al. KIT mutations are common in incidental gastrointestinal stromal tumors one centimeter or less in size. *Am J Pathol*. 2002;160:1567–1572.
135. Sawai H, Okada Y, Funahashi H, et al. Gastrointestinal stromal tumor of the rectum with liver metastasis: report of a case. *Hepatogastroenterology*. 2007;54:1113–1115.
136. Zhu J, Wang Y, Hou M, et al. Imatinib mesylate treatment for advanced gastrointestinal stromal tumor: a pilot study focusing on patients experiencing sole liver metastasis after a prior radical resection. *Oncology*. 2007;73:324–327.
137. Ye YJ, Gao ZD, Poston GJ, Wang S. Diagnosis and multi-disciplinary management of hepatic metastases from gastrointestinal stromal tumour (GIST). *Eur J Surg Oncol*. 2009;35:787–792.
138. Zalinski S, Palavecino M, Abdalla EK. Hepatic resection for gastrointestinal stromal tumor liver metastases. *Hematol Oncol Clin North Am*. 2009;23:115–127, ix.
139. Sato T, Ohyama S, Kokudo N, et al. The repeated hepatectomy for frequent recurrence of hepatic metastasis from gastrointestinal stromal tumor of the stomach. *Hepatogastroenterology*. 2004;51:181–183.
140. Radkani P, Ghersi MM, Paramo JC, Mesko TW. A multidisciplinary approach for the treatment of GIST liver metastasis. *World J Surg Oncol*. 2008;6:46.
141. Maehara N, Chijiiwa K, Eto T, et al. Surgical treatment for gastric GIST with special reference to liver metastases. *Hepatogastroenterology*. 2008;55:512–516.
142. Fiorentini G, Bernardeschi P, Rossi S, et al. Imatinib mesylate induces responses in patients with liver metastases from gastrointestinal

stromal tumor failing intra-arterial hepatic chemotherapy. *J Cancer Res Ther*. 2006;2:68–71.

143. Rutkowski P, Nyckowski P, Grzesiakowska U, et al. The clinical characteristics and the role of surgery and imatinib treatment in patients with liver metastases from c-Kit positive gastrointestinal stromal tumors (GIST). *Neoplasma*. 2003;50:438–442.

144. Zhu J, Yang Y, Zhou L, et al. A long-term follow-up of the imatinib mesylate treatment for the patients with recurrent gastrointestinal stromal tumor (GIST): the liver metastasis and the outcome. *BMC Cancer*. 2010;10:199.

145. Itoh G, Ogawa M, Osaka H, et al. A case of long survival after resection and treatment with imatinib mesylate against metachronous liver metastases and a lung metastasis of a small intestine gastrointestinal stromal tumor. *Gan To Kagaku Ryoho: Japanese Journal of Cancer and Chemotherapy*. 2012;39:835–837.

146. Kimura O, Yamamoto O, Hisamitsu K, et al. Usefulness of low-dose and long-term administration of imatinib in patients with liver metastases of rectal GIST and GIST of stomach. *Gan To Kagaku Ryoho: Japanese Journal of Cancer and Chemotherapy*. 2010;37:2285–2287.

147. Suzuki S, Sasajima K, Miyamoto M, et al. Pathologic complete response confirmed by surgical resection for liver metastases of gastrointestinal stromal tumor after treatment with imatinib mesylate. *World J Gastroenterol*. 2008;14:3763–3767.

148. Yamamoto S, Kubo S, Shuto T, et al. Treatment with STI571, a tyrosine kinase inhibitor, for gastrointestinal stromal tumor with peritoneal dissemination and multiple liver metastases. *J Gastroenterol*. 2003;38:896–899.

149. Kittaka H, Yamada T, Goto K, et al. Hepatic metastasis from gastric GIST radically resected after imatinib mesylate therapy—a case report. *Gan To Kagaku Ryoho: Japanese Journal of Cancer and Chemotherapy*. 2011;38:2508–2510.

150. Onoe S, Sakamoto Y. A case of hepatic metastasis from gastric GIST successfully resected following neoadjuvant targeted therapy. *Jpn J Clin Oncol*. 2011;41:590.

151. Sakakura C, Hagiwara A, Soga K, et al. Long-term survival of a case with multiple liver metastases from duodenal gastrointestinal stromal tumor drastically reduced by the treatment with imatinib and hepatectomy. *World J Gastroenterol*. 2006;12:2793–2797.

152. Tsutsui M, Yoshino S, Sakamoto K, Oka M. Long-term survival after surgery and adjuvant imatinib in a patient with rectal GIST, local recurrence, liver metastases and mediastinal pleural metastasis. *Gan To Kagaku Ryoho: Japanese Journal of Cancer and Chemotherapy*. 2009;36:2351–2353.

153. Yamamura M, Hirai T, Higashida M, et al. A resected case of postoperative liver metastasis of a gastrointestinal stromal tumor showing complete response after imatinib treatment. *Gan To Kagaku Ryoho: Japanese Journal of Cancer and Chemotherapy*. 2008;35:1945–1949.

154. Ishikawa A, Teratani T, Ono S, et al. A case of gastrointestinal stromal tumor with liver and bone metastases effectively treated with radiofrequency ablation and imatinib mesylate. *Nihon Shokakibyo Gakai Zasshi: Japanese Journal of Gastroenterology*. 2006;103:1274–1279.

155. Minami T, Sato S, Watanabe Y, et al. Successful treatment of a gastrointestinal stromal tumor with liver metastases in a case that tolerated imatinib administration, by radiofrequency ablation using contrast-enhanced ultrasonography. *Nihon Shokakibyo Gakai Zasshi: Japanese Journal of Gastroenterology*. 2010;107:442–448.

156. Tamura J, Nakayama Y, Kitaguchi K, et al. A successfully resected case of liver metastasis of gastrointestinal stromal tumor responding to neoadjuvant chemotherapy with imatinib mesylate and interventional radiology. *Gan To Kagaku Ryoho: Japanese Journal of Cancer and Chemotherapy*. 2009;36:1769–1772.

157. Koch M, Weitz J, Kienle P, et al. Comparative analysis of tumor cell dissemination in mesenteric, central, and peripheral venous blood in patients with colorectal cancer. *Arch Surg*. 2001;136:85–89.

158. Berney T, Mentha G, Roth AD, Morel P. Results of surgical resection of liver metastases from non-colorectal primaries. *Br J Surg*. 1998;85:1423–1427.

159. Laurent C, Rullier E, Feyler A, et al. Resection of noncolorectal and nonneuroendocrine liver metastases: late metastases are the only chance of cure. *World J Surg*. 2001;25:1532–1536.

160. O'Rourke TR, Tekkis P, Yeung S, et al. Long-term results of liver resection for non-colorectal, non-neuroendocrine metastases. *Ann Surg Oncol*. 2008;15:207–218.

161. Makino H, Kunisaki C, Izumisawa Y, et al. Indication for hepatic resection in the treatment of

162. Takemura N, Saiura A, Koga R, et al. Long-term outcomes after surgical resection for gastric cancerliver metastasis: an analysis of 64 macroscopically complete resections. *Langenbecks Arch Surg*. 2012;397:6, 951–957.

163. Thun MJ, DeLancey JO, Center MM, et al. The global burden of cancer: priorities for prevention. *Carcinogenesis*. 2010;31:100–110.

164. Jemal A, Murray T, Ward E, et al. Cancer statistics, 2005. *CA Cancer J Clin*. 2005;55:10–30.

165. Okuyama K, Isono K, Juan IK, et al. Evaluation of treatment for gastric cancer with liver metastasis. *Cancer*. 1985;55:2498–2505.

166. Ochiai T, Sasako M, Mizuno S, et al. Hepatic resection for metastatic tumours from gastric cancer: analysis of prognostic factors. *Br J Surg*. 1994;81:1175–1178.

167. Bines SD, England G, Deziel DJ, et al. Synchronous, metachronous, and multiple hepatic resections of liver tumors originating from primary gastric tumors. *Surgery*. 1993;114:799–805; discussion 4–5.

168. Hoshima M, Taniguchi H, Mugitani T, et al. Hepatic arterial infusion therapy for gastric liver metastasis using implanted reservoir. *Gan To Kagaku Ryoho: Japanese Journal of Cancer and Chemotherapy*. 1995;22:1515–1518.

169. Miyazaki M, Itoh H, Nakagawa K, et al. Hepatic resection of liver metastases from gastric carcinoma. *Am J Gastroenterol*. 1997;92:490–493.

170. Fujii K, Fujioka S, Kato K, et al. Resection of liver metastasis from gastric adenocarcinoma. *Hepatogastroenterology*. 2001;48:368–371.

171. Saiura A, Umekita N, Inoue S, et al. Clinicopathological features and outcome of hepatic resection for liver metastasis from gastric cancer. *Hepatogastroenterology*. 2002;49:1062–1065.

172. Shirabe K, Shimada M, Matsumata T, et al. Analysis of the prognostic factors for liver metastasis of gastric cancer after hepatic resection: a multi-institutional study of the indications for resection. *Hepatogastroenterology*. 2003;50:1560–1563.

173. Takada J, Katsuki Y, Hamada H, Tsuji Y. Evaluation of intraarterial infusion chemotherapy for liver metastasis from gastric cancer FEM: combination therapy of 5-FU, epirubicin and MMC. *Gan To Kagaku Ryoho: Japanese Journal of Cancer and Chemotherapy*. 2003;30:1627–1630.

174. Li YM, Zhan WH, Han FH, et al. Clinicopathological analysis of synchronous liver metastasis in gastric cancer and evaluation of surgical outcomes. *Zhonghua Wei Chang Wai Ke Za Zhi: Chinese Journal of Gastrointestinal Surgery*. 2006;9:127–130.

175. Lim JK, Ahn JB, Cheon SH, et al. Long-term survival after surgical resection for liver metastasis from gastric cancer: two case reports. *Cancer Res Treat*. 2006;38:184–188.

176. Sakamoto Y, Sano T, Shimada K, et al. Favorable indications for hepatectomy in patients with liver metastasis from gastric cancer. *J Surg Oncol*. 2007;95:534–539.

177. Manba N, Nashimoto A, Yabusaki H, et al. Evaluation of hepatic resection for synchronous liver metastasis from gastric cancer. *Gan To Kagaku Ryoho: Japanese Journal of Cancer and Chemotherapy*. 2009;36:2016–2018.

178. Schmelzle M, Eisenberger CF, am Esch JS 2nd, et al. Non-colorectal, non-neuroendocrine, and non-sarcoma metastases of the liver: resection as a promising tool in the palliative management. *Langenbecks Arch Surg*. 2010;395:227–234.

179. Saikawa Y, Kanai T, Kawano Y, et al. A novel combined chemotherapy using TS-1 and low-dose cisplatin against liver metastasis of gastric cancer. *Gan To Kagaku Ryoho: Japanese Journal of Cancer and Chemotherapy*. 2002;29:1241–1245.

180. Tono T, Iwazawa T, Matsui S, et al. Hepatic arterial infusion of paclitaxel for liver metastasis from gastric cancer. *Cancer Invest*. 2004;22:550–554.

181. Denck H. Regional cytostatic infusion therapy in patients with inoperable gastrointestinal carcinomas and metastases in the liver (author's translation). *Wien Med Wochenschr: Wiener Medizinische Wochenschr (Vienna Medical Journal)*. 1980;130:36–39.

182. Denck H. Results of intermittent intra-arterial chemotherapy with 5-FU in liver metastases and inoperable tumors of the gastrointestinal and urogenital tracts. *Onkologie: Onkologie International Journal for Cancer Research and Treatment*. 1984;7:167–176.

183. Nojiri O, Nakamura M, Tanaka Y, Banno T. Two-route chemotherapy by CDDP and STS in liver metastasis of gastrointestinal adenocarcinoma. *Gan To Kagaku Ryoho: Japanese Journal of Cancer and Chemotherapy*. 1988;15:47–51.

184. Hasegawa Y, Honnma S, Takanashi K, et al. CDDP-ip PMUE therapy in gastric cancer

185. Paquet KJ, Kalk JF, Cuan-Orozco F, et al. Hepatic chemoinfusion of 5-FU in metastasis of gastrointestinal cancer and advanced primary hepatocellular carcinoma. *Eur J Surg Oncol.* 1992;18:156–161.
186. Hashimoto M, Tsuji Y, Tomita I, et al. Evaluation of intra-arterial infusion chemotherapy for liver metastasis from gastric cancer. *Gan To Kagaku Ryoho: Japanese Journal of Cancer and Chemotherapy.* 1997;24:1715–1718.
187. Takahashi H, Tono T, Tamagaki S, et al. Usefulness of hepatic arterial infusion chemotherapy for liver metastasis in gastric cancer. *Gan To Kagaku Ryoho: Japanese Journal of Cancer and Chemotherapy.* 2001;28:1724–1727.
188. Shizawa R, Nagahori Y, Kumamoto N, et al. Effect of hepatic arterial infusion chemotherapy for liver metastasis from gastric cancer. *Gan To Kagaku Ryoho: Japanese Journal of Cancer and Chemotherapy.* 2002;29:2092–2095.
189. Takeno A, Fujitani K, Tsujinaka T, et al. Evaluation of arterial infusion chemotherapy for liver metastasis from gastric cancer. *Gan To Kagaku Ryoho: Japanese Journal of Cancer and Chemotherapy.* 2003;30:1631–1634.
190. Ojima H, Ootake S, Yokobori T, et al. Treatment of multiple liver metastasis from gastric carcinoma. *World J Surg Oncol.* 2007;5:70.
191. Ota T, Shuto K, Ohira G, et al. Evaluation of hepatic arterial infusion chemotherapy for liver metastasis from gastric cancer. *Gan To Kagaku Ryoho: Japanese Journal of Cancer and Chemotherapy.* 2009;36:2019–2021.
192. Takada J, Katsuki Y, Hamada H, Tsuji Y. Evaluation of intra-arterial infusion chemotherapy for liver metastasis from gastric cancer FEM--combination therapy of 5 FU, epirubicin and MMC. *Gan To Kagaku Ryoho: Japanese Journal of Cancer and Chemotherapy.* 2002;29:2089–2091.
193. Kitamura M, Arai K, Miyashita K. Evaluation of the liver and peritoneal metastasis in the treatment of gastric carcinoma with intra-arterial injection in terms of survival period. *Gan To Kagaku Ryoho: Japanese Journal of Cancer and Chemotherapy.* 1990;17:1657–1660.
194. Kitamura M, Arai K, Miyashita K, Kosaki G. Arterial infusion chemotherapy in patients with gastric cancer in liver metastasis and long-term survival after treatment. *Gan To Kagaku Ryoho: Japanese Journal of Cancer and Chemotherapy.* 1989;16:2936–2639.
195. Arai K, Kitamura M, Iwasaki Y. Effects and problems of intraarterial noradrenaline-induced hypertensive chemotherapy for liver metastasis of gastric cancer. *Gan To Kagaku Ryoho: Japanese Journal of Cancer and Chemotherapy.* 1994;21:2132–2135.
196. Iwasaki Y, Kitamura M, Arai K. Intrahepatic arterial infusion chemotherapy with angiotensin II for liver metastasis from gastric cancer. *Gan To Kagaku Ryoho: Japanese Journal of Cancer and Chemotherapy.* 1998;25:1412–1415.
197. Ohashi M, Arai K, Iwasaki Y, Takahashi T. Efficacy and problems of hepatic arterial chemotherapy with angiotensin II for liver metastasis from gastric cancer. *Gan To Kagaku Ryoho: Japanese Journal of Cancer and Chemotherapy.* 1999;26:1777–1780.
198. Yamakado K, Nakatsuka A, Takaki H, et al. Prospective study of arterial infusion chemotherapy followed by radiofrequency ablation for the treatment of liver metastasis of gastric cancer. *J Vasc Interv Radiol.* 2005;16:1747–1751.
199. Hofer S, Oberholzer C, Beck S, et al. Ultrasound-guided radiofrequency ablation (RFA) for inoperable gastrointestinal liver metastases. *Ultraschall Med.* 2008;29:388–392.
200. Ito G, Kubo N, Tanaka H, et al. A case of long-term survival after undergoing S-1 based multidisciplinary therapy for liver metastasis of gastric cancer. *Gan To Kagaku Ryoho: Japanese Journal of Cancer and Chemotherapy.* 2011;38:2348–2350.
201. Urade M, Yonemura Y, Fujimura T, et al. A case of liver metastasis of gastric cancer which was made resectable by hypertheromo-chemo-radiotherapy. *Nihon Geka Gakkai Zasshi: Journal of the Japan Surgical Society.* 1989;90:446–449.
202. Fukuda Y, Takeshima F, Ogihara K, et al. Successful management of liver metastasis from gastric adenosquamous carcinoma with adjuvant chemotherapy and radiofrequency ablation. *Nihon Shokakibyo Gakai Zasshi: Japanese Journal of Gastroenterology.* 2012;109:606–614.
203. Kimura Y, Taniguchi H, Yano H, et al. A case of liver metastasis from gastric cancer treated with stereotactic radiation therapy. *Gan To Kagaku Ryoho: Japanese Journal of Cancer and Chemotherapy.* 2010;37:2499–2501.
204. Kushibiki K, Shimada M, Matsuoka H, et al. Successful UFT-E granule and 5-FUCDDP combination therapy for an unresectable advanced gastric cancer complicated with liver metastasis.

Gan To Kagaku Ryoho: Japanese Journal of Cancer and Chemotherapy. 1996;23:1313–1315.

205. Takahashi Y, Mai M, Fujimoto T, et al. Preventive hepatic arterial infusion in high risk cases of liver metastasis from gastric cancer. *Gan To Kagaku Ryoho: Japanese Journal of Cancer and Chemotherapy.* 1989;16:2756–2759.

206. Cancer Facts and Figures 2012. American Cancer Society, 2012. http://www.cancer.org/Research/CancerFactsFigures/CancerFactsFigures/cancer-facts-figures-2012.

207. Aloia TA, Adam R, Azoulay D, et al. Outcome following hepatic resection of metastatic renal tumors: the Paul Brousse Hospital experience. *HPB (Oxford).* 2006;8:100–105.

208. Motzer RJ, Mazumdar M, Bacik J, et al. Survival and prognostic stratification of 670 patients with advanced renal cell carcinoma. *J Clin Oncol.* 1999;17:2530–2540.

209. Yagoda A, Petrylak D, Thompson S. Cytotoxic chemotherapy for advanced renal cell carcinoma. *Urol Clin North Am.* 1993;20:303–321.

210. Staehler MD, Kruse J, Haseke N, et al. Liver resection for metastatic disease prolongs survival in renal cell carcinoma: 12-year results from a retrospective comparative analysis. *World J Urol.* 2010;28:543–547.

211. Einhorn LH. Treatment of testicular cancer: a new and improved model. *J Clin Oncol.* 1990;8:1777–1781.

212. Goulet RJ Jr, Hardacre JM, Einhorn LH, et al. Hepatic resection for disseminated germ cell carcinoma. *Ann Surg.* 1990;212:290–293; discussion 3–4.

213. Eastham JA, Wilson TG, Russell C, et al. Surgical resection in patients with nonseminomatous germ cell tumor who fail to normalize serum tumor markers after chemotherapy. *Urology.* 1994;43:74–80.

214. Tanaka Y, Kakizoe T, Tobisu K, Takai K. Analysis of renal cell carcinoma with tumorous legion in the liver. *Nihon Hinyokika Gakkai Zasshi: The Japanese Journal of Urology.* 1989;80:229–235.

215. Antoniewicz AA, Krawczyk M, Polanski JA, et al. Resection of the liver in a metastatic disease caused by renal carcinoma. *Mater Med Pol.* 1994;26:143–144.

216. Fujisaki S, Takayama T, Shimada K, et al. Hepatectomy for metastatic renal cell carcinoma. *Hepatogastroenterology.* 1997;44:817–819.

217. Stief CG, Jahne J, Hagemann JH, et al. Surgery for metachronous solitary liver metastases of renal cell carcinoma. *J Urol.* 1997;158:375–377.

218. Kawata N, Hirakata H, Yuge H, et al. Cytoreductive surgery with liver-involved renal cell carcinoma. *Int J Urol.* 2000;7:382–385.

219. Alves A, Adam R, Majno P, et al. Hepatic resection for metastatic renal tumors: is it worthwhile? *Ann Surg Oncol.* 2003;10:705–710.

220. Thelen A, Jonas S, Benckert C, et al. Liver resection for metastases from renal cell carcinoma. *World J Surg.* 2007;31:802–807.

221. Ruys AT, Tanis PJ, Iris ND, et al. Surgical treatment of renal cell cancer liver metastases: a population-based study. *Ann Surg Oncol.* 2011;18:1932–1938.

222. Langan RC, Ripley RT, Davis JL, et al. Liver directed therapy for renal cell carcinoma. *J Cancer.* 2012;3:184–190.

223. Tongaonkar HB, Kulkarni JN, Kamat MR. Solitary metastases from renal cell carcinoma: a review. *J Surg Oncol.* 1992;49:45–48.

224. Ritchie AW, Layfield LJ, deKernion JB. Spontaneous regression of liver metastasis from renal carcinoma. *J Urol.* 1988;140:596–597.

225. Wyczolkowski M, Klima W, Bieda W, Walas K. Spontaneous regression of hepatic metastases after nephrectomy and metastasectomy of renal cell carcinoma. *Urol Int.* 2001;66:119–120.

226. Hahn TL, Jacobson L, Einhorn LH, et al. Hepatic resection of metastatic testicular carcinoma: a further update. *Ann Surg Oncol.* 1999;6:640–644.

227. Maluccio M, Einhorn LH, Goulet RJ. Surgical therapy for testicular cancer metastatic to the liver. *HPB (Oxford).* 2007;9:199–200.

228. You YN, Leibovitch BC, Que FG. Hepatic metastasectomy for testicular germ cell tumors: is it worth it? *J Gastrointest Surg.* 2009;13:595–601.

229. Stansby G, Bhattacharya S, Hilson AJ, et al. Case report: localization of lipiodol-radioiodine in hepatic metastases from renal cell carcinoma. *Br J Radiol.* 1994;67:822–824.

230. Pomer S, Brado M, Roeren T, et al. Repetitive immuno-embolization of inoperative liver metastases of renal cell carcinoma. Method characterization and preliminary results. *Urologe A.* 1996;35:310–314.

231. Umeda S, Ito K, Takahashi E, et al. Clinical experience of treatment of liver metastasis of renal cell carcinoma treated with SMANCS/lipiodol therapy. *Hinyokika Kiyo: Acta Urologica Japonica.* 2010;56:543–549.

232. Kobayashi M, Kinouchi T, Kinoshita T, et al. A case of renal pelvic cancer with hepatic metastasis where hepatic arterial infusion chemotherapy (HAIC) proved effective: a case report. *Hinyokika Kiyo: Acta Urologica Japonica*. 2011;57:627–631.

233. Miwa S, Mizokami A, Konaka H, et al. A case of bone, lung, pleural and liver metastases from renal cell carcinoma which responded remarkably well to zoledronic acid monotherapy. *Jpn J Clin Oncol*. 2009;39:745–750.

234. Okaneya T, Murata Y, Kinebuchi Y. Complete remission of lung and hepatic metastases from renal cell carcinoma by interferon alpha-2b therapy: a case report. *Hinyokika Kiyo: Acta Urologica Japonica*. 1999;45:617–619.

235. Nabil M, Gruber T, Yakoub D, et al. Repetitive transarterial chemoembolization (TACE) of liver metastases from renal cell carcinoma: local control and survival results. *Eur Radiol*. 2008;18:1456–1463.

236. Barkholt L, Danielsson R, Calissendorff B, et al. Indium-111-labelled donor-lymphocyte infusion by way of hepatic artery and radio-frequency ablation against liver metastases of renal and colon carcinoma after allogeneic hematopoietic stem-cell transplantation. *Transplantation*. 2004;78:697–703.

237. Abdelmaksoud MH, Louie JD, Hwang GL, et al. Yttrium-90 radioembolization of renal cell carcinoma metastatic to the liver. *J Vasc Interv Radiol*. 2012;23:323–330 e1.

238. Lyass O, Brufman G, Edelmann DZ, et al. Multiple parenchymal liver metastases as the first site of recurrent ovarian carcinoma: a case report and review of the literature. *Eur J Gynaecol Oncol*. 1997;18:68–70.

239. Loizzi V, Rossi C, Cormio G, et al. Clinical features of hepatic metastasis in patients with ovarian cancer. *Int J Gynecol Cancer*. 2005;15:26–31.

240. Chi DS, McCaughty K, Diaz JP, et al. Guidelines and selection criteria for secondary cytoreductive surgery in patients with recurrent, platinum-sensitive epithelial ovarian carcinoma. *Cancer*. 2006;106:1933–1939.

241. Naik R, Nordin A, Cross PA, et al. Optimal cytoreductive surgery is an independent prognostic indicator in stage IV epithelial ovarian cancer with hepatic metastases. *Gynecol Oncol*. 2000;78:171–175.

242. Bosquet JG, Merideth MA, Podratz KC, Nagorney DM. Hepatic resection for metachronous metastases from ovarian carcinoma. *HPB (Oxford)*. 2006;8:93–96.

243. Chi DS, Fong Y, Venkatraman ES, Barakat RR. Hepatic resection for metastatic gynecologic carcinomas. *Gynecol Oncol*. 1997;66:45–51.

244. Garduno-Lopez AL, Mondragon-Sanchez R, Herrera-Goepfert R, Bernal-Maldonado R. Resection of liver metastases from a virilizing steroid (lipoid) cell ovarian tumor. *Hepatogastroenterology*. 2002;49:657–659.

245. Hamy AP, Paineau JR, Mirallie EC, et al. Hepatic resections for non-colorectal metastases: forty resections in 35 patients. *Hepatogastroenterology*. 2000;47:1090–1094.

246. Lim MC, Kang S, Lee KS, et al. The clinical significance of hepatic parenchymal metastasis in patients with primary epithelial ovarian cancer. *Gynecol Oncol*. 2009;112:28–34.

247. Merideth MA, Cliby WA, Keeney GL, et al. Hepatic resection for metachronous metastases from ovarian carcinoma. *Gynecol Oncol*. 2003;89:16–21.

248. Pekmezci S, Saribeyoglu K, Aytac E, et al. Surgery for isolated liver metastasis of ovarian cancer. *Asian J Surg*. 2010;33:83–88.

249. Yan X, Bao Q, An N, et al. Significance of hepatic resection in the treatment of hepatic parenchymal metastasis of recurrent epithelial ovarian carcinoma. *Zhonghua Zhong Liu Za Zhi: Chinese Journal of Oncology*. 2011;33:132–137.

250. Yoon SS, Jarnagin WR, Fong Y, et al. Resection of recurrent ovarian or fallopian tube carcinoma involving the liver. *Gynecol Oncol*. 2003;91:383–388.

251. Fan Q, Huang H, Lian L, Lang J. Characteristics, diagnosis and treatment of hepatic metastasis of pure immature ovarian teratoma. *Chin Med J (Engl)*. 2001;114:506–509.

252. Scarabelli C, Campagnutta E. Intraarterial infusion chemotherapy in the treatment of liver metastases from ovarian cancer. *Eur J Gynaecol Oncol*. 1981;2:121–126.

253. Yokoyama H, Murakami T, Akagi T, et al. A case of ovarian cancer with liver metastasis successfully treated by PAC therapy. *Gan To Kagaku Ryoho: Japanese Journal of Cancer and Chemotherapy*. 1991;18:1203–1207.

254. Tohya T, Shimajiri S, Onoda C, Yoshimura T. Complete remission of ovarian endometrioid adenocarcinoma associated with hyperamylasemia

and liver metastasis treated by paclitaxel and carboplatin chemotherapy: a case report. *Int J Gynecol Cancer*. 2004;14:378–380.
255. Hayashi S, Kohlita Y, Fujii I. Arterial chemoembolization for multiple liver metastases of uterine cancer. Two case reports. *Eur J Gynaecol Oncol*. 1990;11:439–445.
256. Vogl TJ, Naguib NN, Lehnert T, et al. Initial experience with repetitive transarterial chemoembolization (TACE) as a third line treatment of ovarian cancer metastasis to the liver: indications, outcomes and role in patient's management. *Gynecol Oncol*. 2012;124:225–229.
257. Bojalian MO, Machado GR, Swensen R, Reeves ME. Radiofrequency ablation of liver metastasis from ovarian adenocarcinoma: case report and literature review. *Gynecol Oncol*. 2004;93:557–560.
258. Mateo R, Singh G, Jabbour N, et al. Optimal cytoreduction after combined resection and radiofrequency ablation of hepatic metastases from recurrent malignant ovarian tumors. *Gynecol Oncol*. 2005;97:266–270.
259. Collettini F, Poellinger A, Schnapauff D, et al. CT-guided high-dose-rate brachytherapy of metachronous ovarian cancer metastasis to the liver: initial experience. *Anticancer Res*. 2011;31:2597–2602.
260. Chao A, Lai CH, Hsueh S, et al. Intralesional injection for hepatic metastasis from cervical carcinoma. A report of two cases. *J Reprod Med*. 2001;46:1008–1012.

CHAPTER 9

Surgical Resection for Non-colorectal, Non-neuroendocrine Liver Metastases

Christoph Kahlert & Jergen Weitz

The sole curative approach for malignant liver tumors is surgical resection. Only 10% of malignant liver tumors derive from primary liver or bile duct cancer, whereas the vast majority of cancerous hepatic lesions originate from extrahepatic primary tumors. Resection of hepatic tumors can be accomplished safely with an appropriate risk of perioperative mortality and morbidity.[1]

The survival rate of patients with colorectal liver metastases, who have undergone partial hepatectomy, amounts to 30%–61% after three years, and still reaches 16%–51% after five years.[2-4] For patients with hepatic metastasized neuroendocrine tumors, surgical resection even results in five-year survival rates of 76%.[5] Nevertheless, a surgical intervention with a curative intent remains highly controversial for noncolorectal, nonneuroendocrine metastases. First, noncolorectal, nonneuroendocrine liver metastases often arise from very aggressive types of cancer. Even if the resection of the hepatic lesions is feasible from a technical point of view, the postoperative clinical course is still associated with a dismal prognosis. Moreover, many noncolorectal, nonneuroendocrine liver metastases originate from extraabdominal primary tumors. In contrast to intra-abdominal tumors, which disseminate through the portal vein with the liver theoretically being the first filter organ, liver metastases of extraabdominal primary tumors imply a simultaneous, extrahepatic tumor metastasization.

However, certain patients with noncolorectal, nonneuroendocrine liver metastases might benefit from a surgical approach due to a more favorable tumor biology. To select these patients, a careful assessment of each individual patient is required. Prior to the decision regarding a surgical approach, three prerequisites have to be accomplished: (1) the feasibility of a complete excision of all intrahepatic disease, (2) reliable control of the primary tumor by means of complete resection, and (3) absence of extrahepatic lesions at time of partial hepatectomy. Furthermore, the decision-making criteria should include length of disease-free interval, response to chemotherapy before surgery, and the origin and histological type of the primary tumor.[6]

Breast Cancer

Breast cancer is the second most common malignant tumor of women in the western world. In fact, 40,170 deaths were anticipated in the United States[7] in 2009.

The incidence of breast cancer metastases confined to the liver amounts to 10%–20% at the stage of disseminated tumor disease[8,9] (Figure 9-1). Resection of liver metastases without the presence of extrahepatic dissemination resulted in a median overall survival between 36 and 63 months[6,10,11] (Figure 9-2), when patients underwent surgical treatment in addition to systemic chemotherapy. These numbers exceed the outcome of patients having merely received systemic chemotherapy.[12] However, before offering an operation to the individual patient, certain selection criteria should be taken into account. Negative predictive risk factors advising against a surgical approach are positive lymph node status of the initial breast cancer, recurrence of liver metastases within one year after resection of the primary tumor,[13] extensive hepatic lesions requiring a major resection[14] and failure to respond to preoperative chemotherapy[6] (Table 9-1). Patients, who are not amendable to surgery, might be offered ultrasound (US)-guided percutaneous, radiofrequency ablation. Treatment by this intervention has resulted in a median overall survival of 30 months and a five-year survival rate of 27%.[15] However, US-guided, percutaneous radiofrequency ablation requires highly selective inclusion criteria such as less than five hepatic lesions, tumor diameter < 2.5 cm and exclusion of extrahepatic tumor masses.

In summary, patients with breast cancer metastases confined solely to the liver may profit by a surgical intervention, if certain negative predictive risk factors can be excluded (Figure 9-2A and B). If these patients are not amendable to surgery, radiofrequency ablation should be taken into consideration as second-best alternative compared to systemic chemotherapy alone.

Gynecological Tumors

Gynecological tumors spreading to the liver mainly originate from ovarian cancer.

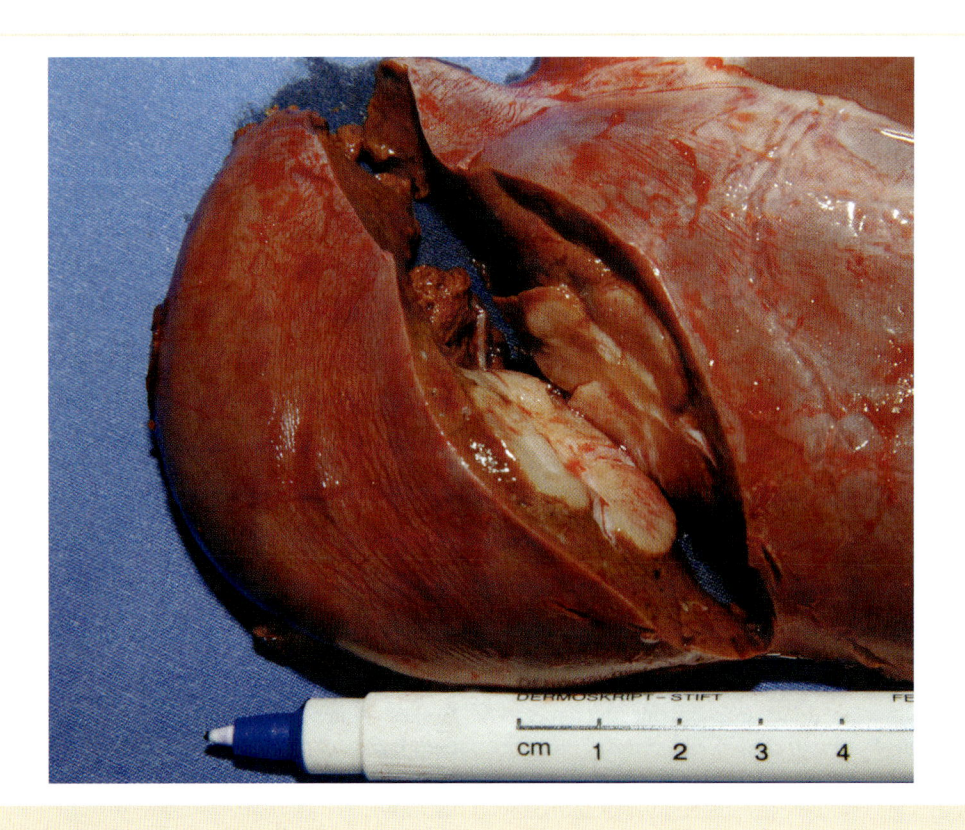

Figure 9-1: Solitary liver metastases originating from breast cancer.

TABLE 9-1: Assessment of Predictive Risk Factors Determining the Prognosis of Patients with Breast Cancer Metastases to the Liver

Positive predictive risk factors associated with a favorable prognosis	Negative risk factors associated with a dismal prognosis	Study
Interval between primary tumor and hepatic metastasis >1 y	Interval between primary tumor and hepatic metastasis <1 y	Hoffmann et al.[60] Selzner et al.[13]
Resection margin	Resection margin	Hoffmann et al.[60]
R0	R1/2	Selzner et al.[13]
Minor liver resection	Major liver resection	Pocard et al.[14]
N0 or N1 lymph node status of the initial breast cancer	N1b or N2 lymph node status of the initial breast cancer	Selzner et al.[13]
Response to chemotherapy	Failure to respond to preoperative chemotherapy	Adam et al.[6]

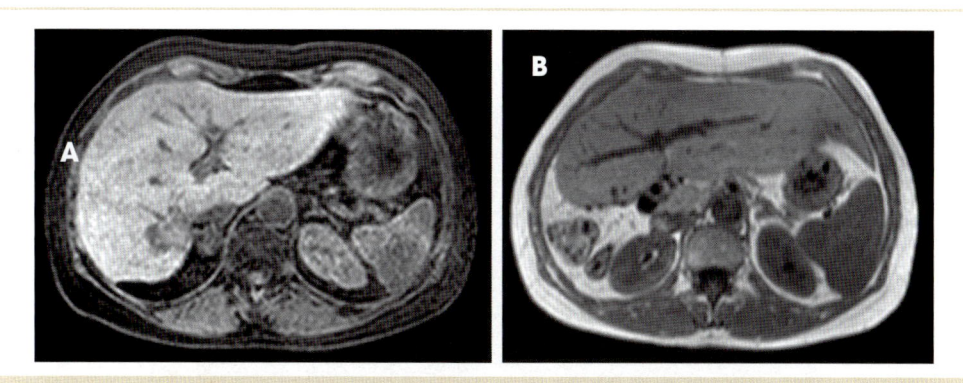

Figure 9-2: Abdominal MRI of a patient with a single breast cancer liver metastases one month before surgical resection (A) and 18 months postoperative (B).

Epithelial ovarian cancer is the fifth leading cause of tumor-related death in women in western countries and is the leading cause of gynecological cancer death.[7] Less frequent histological types of ovarian cancer encompass sarcomas, germ cell, and stromal tumors.[16] In approximately 50% of patients with ovarian cancer, liver metastases are diagnosed.[16] As there is an inverse correlation between the volume of the residual tumor and the patient overall survival, resection of liver metastases should be performed with optimal cytoreduction of extrahepatic lesions.[17,18] By this, median overall survival can be prolonged significantly.[17]

Uterine and cervical cancers metastasize most frequently through the lymphatic system, whereas hematogenous dissemination is a rare and rather late-stage event. Therefore, isolated uterine or cervical cancer liver metastases develop only in a minority of patients.[19,20] However, if extrahepatic metastatic sites can be excluded, partial hepatectomy should be evaluated as therapeutical option. Retrospective studies reported about a median overall survival of 35% and a five-year survival rate of 35% for uterine cancer[6,21] and also approved the feasibility of partial hepatectomy in the presence of cervical cancer liver metastases.[22–24]

In conclusion, surgical resection of liver metastases arising from gynecological tumors offers the only curative approach. Although ovarian cancer frequently disseminates into the liver, liver metastases originating from uterine and cervical cancer are a rare event. Before a surgical intervention, a diligent diagnostic investigation should warrant the absence of extrahepatic metastases. These patients will most likely benefit from a surgical approach, if all disease can be resected.

Pancreatic Cancer

Although the incidence of pancreatic cancer amounts only to 3% of all tumors, it contributes to one of the most major causes of cancer-related death in the United States.[7,25] Surgical resection remains the only potential curative therapeutic option. But at time of initial diagnosis, approximately only 25% of the patients with pancreatic cancer are still eligible for a curative surgical intervention. According to the established standard criteria, liver metastases represent a late stage of the disease, which disqualifies the patient for a curative surgical approach. Instead, the standard guidelines for hepatic metastatic pancreatic cancer recommend palliative systemic chemotherapy as best therapeutical option. But this palliative treatment only reaches a median overall survival of approximately six months.[26-29] Therefore, resection of pancreatic cancer liver metastases is occasionally performed as an individual curative attempt (Figure 9-3). This may extend the median overall survival from 6 to 20 months[6,23,30-39] and in single cases even longer than five years.[32] However, resection of pancreatic liver

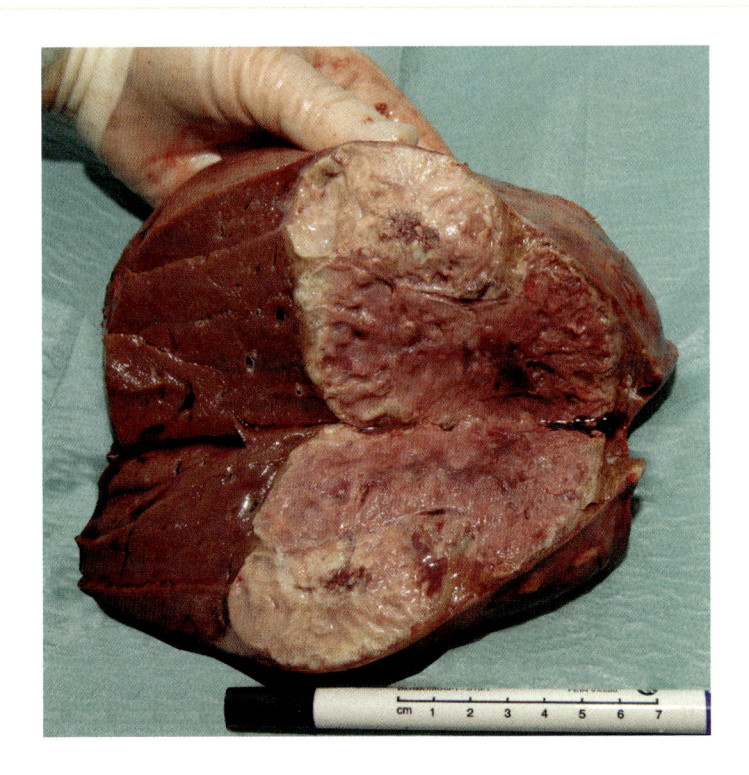

Figure 9-3: Solitary liver metastases of an pancreatic acinar cell carcinoma, resection with a R0 margin in a curative attempt.

metastases bears also a high risk of complications, if it is performed simultaneously with resection of the primary tumor in order to warrant a local control of the disease. Thus, the decision for the resection of pancreatic cancer liver metastases should be made on an individual basis where the patient is aware of a nonstandard treatment approach.

Gastric Cancer

The efficacy of a curative surgical approach for locally advanced gastric cancer has significantly been improved by multimodal therapeutic regimens including perioperative chemotherapy.[40] In contrast, the diagnosis of gastric cancer metastatic to the liver is still considered to be an indication for a palliative treatment. Systemic chemotherapy results in a median overall survival of 9–10 months.[40,41] This dismal prognosis has led to resection of gastric cancer liver metastases in a few cases as an individual curative attempt. Although median overall survival of 19–34 months has been achieved in patients undergoing complete resection of metastatic gastric cancer disease in the liver,[42–46] these data are certainly influenced by a selection bias. However, bearing in mind that surgical resection is the only hope for cure, patients should not be categorically excluded, but carefully evaluated for a surgical approach as an individual curative attempt. Positive prognostic factors are the presence of metachronous or solitary metastases[47] (Table 9-2). These parameters have been associated with a more favorable clinical outcome and may be useful as decision criteria to select appropriate patients eligible for partial hepatectomy.

Gastrointestinal Stromal Tumors

Gastrointestinal stromal tumors (GIST) account for most of the mesenchymal tumors emerging in the gastrointestinal wall.[48] In approximately 25%, GIST develop metastases isolated to the liver.[49] Partial hepatectomy is the preferred treatment of GIST liver metastases, when complete resection can be achieved. The clinical outcome of patients with GIST liver metastases has significantly been improved by the introduction of imatinib mesylate.[50,51] In the pre-tyrosine kinase inhibitor era, postoperative life expectancy after partial hepatectomy was estimated to reach 39 months and a five-year survival of 30% in a retrospective study.[52] By treating patients with imatinib in addition to surgical resection of liver metastases, the five-year survival rate increased[6] to 70% and median overall survival was not reached despite long periods of follow-up.[53] The observations by DeMatteo et al. and Gronchi et al. have been a fundamental impact on the therapy of hepatic metastases deriving from GIST. They demonstrated in two retrospective studies that mainly patients with metastatic GIST responding to a preoperative tyrosine kinase inhibitor therapy profit by a surgical approach, whereas nonresponder do not seem to benefit by tumor resection.[54,55] These findings should be included as major selection criteria before offering surgery to patients with liver metastases of GIST.

In conclusion, by introducing a multimodality approach based on molecular targeted therapy and surgery, the treatment of liver metastases arising from GIST has significantly improved. The indication for liver resection should be based on the response to chemotherapy by imatinib (Table 9-3). Patients with

TABLE 9-2: Assessment of Predictive Risk Factors Determining the Prognosis of Patients with Sarcoma Metastatic to the Liver

Positive predictive risk factors associated with a favorable prognosis	Negative risk factors associated with a dismal prognosis	Study
Time to liver metastases >2 y	Time to liver metastases <2 y	DeMatteo et al.[52]
Response to treatment with imatinib[a]	Nonresponse to imatinib[a]	DeMatteo et al.[54]
		Gronchi et al.[55]

[a]For gastrointestinal stromal tumors.

TABLE 9-3: Selection Criteria for Resection and Determining Clinical Outcome in Patients with Noncolorectal, Non-neuroendocrine Liver Metastases by Weitz et al.[23] and Adam et al.[6]

Independent prognostic factors determined by Weitz et al.[23]

- Disease-free interval
- Primary tumor Length of type
- Completeness of resection

Independent prognostic factors determined by Adam et al.[6]

- Patient age over 60 yrs
- Cancer of nonbreast origin
- Melanoma or squamous histology
- Disease-free interval of <12 mo
- Extrahepatic disease
- Incomplete macroscopic resection
- Major hepatectomy

a response will very likely profit by an operation, whereas nonresponders disqualify for surgery and should be treated by palliative therapy.

Sarcoma

Depending on the primary site, sarcomas display a different pattern of dissemination: extremity and trunk soft tissue sarcomas develop lung metastases, whereas primary visceral and retroperitoneal sarcomas often spread to the liver[49] (Figure 9-4). The median survival for patients receiving merely chemotherapy is poor, and fewer than 20% remain alive at two years.[56,57] In contrast, patients with resection of liver metastases survived 32–37 months on average and had a five-year survival rate of 27%–32%,[6,53] (Figure 9-5A and B). These data are probably affected by a selection bias, but they also demonstrate that surgical intervention can improve progression-free and overall survival in a selected subgroup of patients. Hence, the careful assessment of prognostic factors such as performance status, disease-free interval, histology, and tumor grade[52,56,58] (Table 9-3)

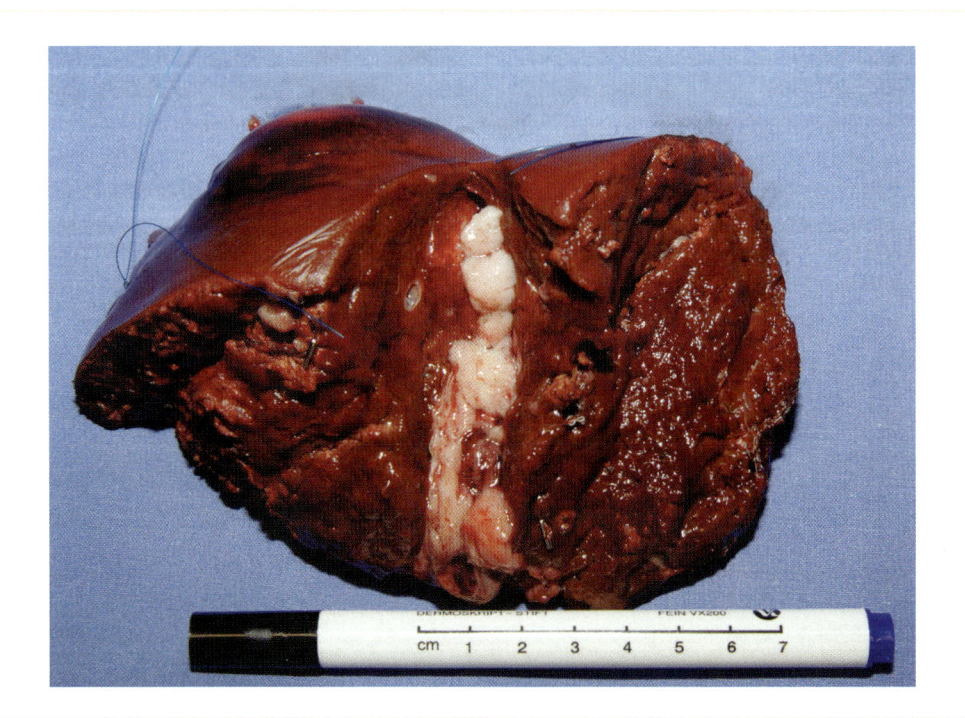

Figure 9-4: Liver metastases deriving from an extra-skeletal Ewing sarcoma.

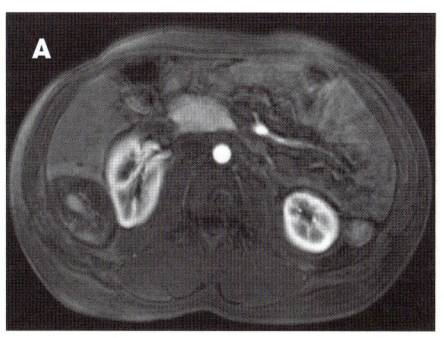

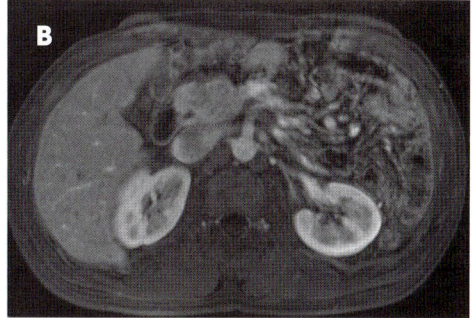

Figure 9-5: Corresponding MRI of the patient with an Ewing sarcoma metastatic to the liver four weeks before partial hepatectomy (A) and six months after (B).

can offer a guideline to select appropriate patients, who most likely will profit from a surgical approach.

Selection Criteria for Resection and Determining Clinical Outcome

The application of valid predictive factors is an essential prerequisite to select appropriate patients with noncolorectal, nonneuroendocrine liver metastases, who would benefit by partial hepatectomy. Weitz et al.[23] described length of disease-free interval, primary tumor type, and completeness of resection as independent prognostic factors in 141 patients undergoing hepatic resection between April 1981 and April 2002 (Table 9-3). A second large retrospective study by Adam et al. analyzed the outcome of 1452 patients from 41 centers undergoing hepatectomy between 1983 and 2004.[6] As independent adverse prognostic factors, they identified patient age over 60 years, nonbreast origin, melanoma or squamous histology, disease-free interval of less than 12 months, extrahepatic disease, incomplete macroscopic resection, and major hepatectomy (Table 9-3). On the basis of these prognostic factors, Adam et al. developed a prognostic scoring system to stratify patients into three risk groups. This risk model proved to distinguish low-risk patient with a five-year survival of 46% from mid-risk patients with a five-year survival rate of 33% and high-risk patients with a five-year survival of only 2%.

In future, these risk models might be used as decision-making device to determine patients with noncolorectal, nonneuroendocrine liver metastases, who will benefit by a surgical approach.

Summary

Hepatic resection for noncolorectal, nonneuroendocrine metastases is an effective curative treatment option in a selected subgroup of patients. A careful preoperative assessment is required to determine those patients, who will likely benefit by a surgical approach. This preoperative evaluation should be based on risk models accounting for a wide panel of prognostic and predictive risk factors. However, up to date, no randomized prospective study has evaluated a potential benefit of partial hepatectomy in the presence of noncolorectal, nonneuroendocrine liver metastases. Therefore, the data, which have been obtained by retrospective studies, are limited regarding a direct comparison to nonsurgical approaches. In conclusion, the decision to offer a surgical approach to a patient should be made on an individual basis. Furthermore, to reduce the risks of postoperative morbidity and mortality, it is recommendable to perform the surgical intervention on the liver at high-volume centers.[59]

References

1. Fortner JG, Fong Y. Twenty-five-year follow-up for liver resection: the personal series of Dr. Joseph G. Fortner. *Ann Surg.* 2009;250: 908–913.
2. Fong Y, Cohen AM, Fortner JG, et al. Liver resection for colorectal metastases. *J Clin Oncol.* 1997;15:938–946.

3. Scheele J, Stang R, Altendorf-Hofmann A, Paul M. Resection of colorectal liver metastases. *World J Surg*. 1995;19:59–71.
4. Schlag P, Hohenberger P, Herfarth C. Resection of liver metastases in colorectal cancer—competitive analysis of treatment results in synchronous versus metachronous metastases. *Eur J Surg Oncol*. 1990;16:360–365.
5. Chamberlain RS, Canes D, Brown KT, et al. Hepatic neuroendocrine metastases: does intervention alter outcomes? *J Am Coll Surg*. 2000;190:432–445.
6. Adam R, Chiche L, Aloia T, et al. Hepatic resection for noncolorectal nonendocrine liver metastases: analysis of 1,452 patients and development of a prognostic model. *Ann Surg*. 2006;244:524–535.
7. Jemal A, Siegel R, Ward E, et al. Cancer statistics, 2009. *CA Cancer J Clin*. 2009;59:225–249.
8. Atalay G, Biganzoli L, Renard F, et al. Clinical outcome of breast cancer patients with liver metastases alone in the anthracycline-taxane era: a retrospective analysis of two prospective, randomised metastatic breast cancer trials. *Eur J Cancer*. 2003;39:2439–2449.
9. Er O, Frye DK, Kau SW, et al. Clinical course of breast cancer patients with metastases limited to the liver treated with chemotherapy. *Cancer J*. 2008;14:62–68.
10. Caralt M, Bilbao I, Cortes J, et al. Hepatic resection for liver metastases as part of the "oncosurgical" treatment of metastatic breast cancer. *Ann Surg Oncol*. 2008;15:2804–2810.
11. Vlastos G, Smith DL, Singletary SE, et al. Long-term survival after an aggressive surgical approach in patients with breast cancer hepatic metastases. *Ann Surg Oncol*. 2004;11:869–874.
12. Alba E, Martin M, Ramos M, et al. Multicenter randomized trial comparing sequential with concomitant administration of Doxorubicin and Docetaxel as first-line treatment of metastatic breast cancer: a Spanish Breast Cancer Research Group (GEICAM-9903) phase III study. *J Clin Oncol*. 2004;22:2587–2593.
13. Selzner M, Morse MA, Vredenburgh JJ, et al. Liver metastases from breast cancer: long-term survival after curative resection. *Surgery*. 2000;127:383–389.
14. Pocard M, Pouillart P, Asselain B, et al. Hepatic resection for breast cancer metastases: results and prognosis (65 cases). *Ann Chir*. 2001;126:413–420.
15. Meloni MF, Andreano A, Laeseke PF, et al. Breast cancer liver metastases: US-guided percutaneous radiofrequency ablation—intermediate and long-term survival rates. *Radiology*. 2009;253:861–869.
16. Rose PG, Piver MS, Tsukada Y, Lau TS. Metastatic patterns in histologic variants of ovarian cancer. An autopsy study. *Cancer*. 1989;64:1508–1513.
17. Bristow RE, Montz FJ, Lagasse LD, et al. Survival impact of surgical cytoreduction in stage IV epithelial ovarian cancer. *Gynecol Oncol*. 1999;72:278–287.
18. Lim MC, Kang S, Lee KS, et al. The clinical significance of hepatic parenchymal metastasis in patients with primary epithelial ovarian cancer. *Gynecol Oncol*. 2009;112:28–34.
19. Carlson V, Delclos L, Fletcher GH. Distant metastases in squamous-cell carcinoma of the uterine cervix. *Radiology*. 1967;88:961–966.
20. Kim GE, Lee SW, Suh CO, et al. Hepatic metastases from carcinoma of the uterine cervix. *Gynecol Oncol*. 1998;70:56–60.
21. Kollmar O, Moussavian MR, Richter S, et al. Surgery of liver metastasis in gynecological cancer—indication and results. *Onkologie*. 2008;31:375–379.
22. Kaseki H, Yasui K, Niwa K, et al. Hepatic resection for metastatic squamous cell carcinoma from the uterine cervix. *Gynecol Oncol*. 1992;44:284–287.
23. Weitz J, Blumgart LH, Fong Y, et al. Partial hepatectomy for metastases from noncolorectal, nonneuroendocrine carcinoma. *Ann Surg*. 2005;241:269–276.
24. Wolf RF, Goodnight JE, Krag DE, Schneider PD. Results of resection and proposed guidelines for patient selection in instances of non-colorectal hepatic metastases. *Surg Gynecol Obstet*. 1991;173:454–460.
25. Jemal A, Siegel R, Ward E, et al. Cancer statistics, 2008. *CA Cancer J Clin*. 2008;58:71–96.
26. Moore MJ, Goldstein D, Hamm J, et al. Erlotinib plus gemcitabine compared with gemcitabine alone in patients with advanced pancreatic cancer: a phase III trial of the National Cancer Institute of Canada Clinical Trials Group. *J Clin Oncol*. 2007;25:1960–1966.
27. Heinemann V, Quietzsch D, Gieseler F, et al. Randomized phase III trial of gemcitabine plus cisplatin compared with gemcitabine alone in advanced pancreatic cancer. *J Clin Oncol*. 2006;24:3946–3952.
28. Louvet C, Labianca R, Hammel P, et al. Gemcitabine in combination with oxaliplatin compared with gemcitabine alone in locally

29. Michalski CW, Erkan M, Huser N, et al. Resection of primary pancreatic cancer and liver metastasis: a systematic review. *Dig Surg*. 2008;25: 473–480.
30. Shrikhande SV, Kleeff J, Reiser C, et al. Pancreatic resection for M1 pancreatic ductal adenocarcinoma. *Ann Surg Oncol*. 2007;14:118–127.
31. Gleisner AL, Assumpcao L, Cameron JL, et al. Is resection of periampullary or pancreatic adenocarcinoma with synchronous hepatic metastasis justified? *Cancer*. 2007;110:2484–2492.
32. Yamada H, Hirano S, Tanaka E, et al. Surgical treatment of liver metastases from pancreatic cancer. *HPB (Oxford)*. 2006;8:85–88.
33. Karavias DD, Tepetes K, Karatzas T, et al. Liver resection for metastatic non-colorectal non-neuroendocrine hepatic neoplasms. *Eur J Surg Oncol*. 2002;28:135–139.
34. Laurent C, Rullier E, Feyler A, et al. Resection of noncolorectal and nonneuroendocrine liver metastases: late metastases are the only chance of cure. *World J Surg*. 2001;25:1532–1536.
35. Benevento A, Boni L, Frediani L, et al. Result of liver resection as treatment for metastases from noncolorectal cancer. *J Surg Oncol*. 2000;74:24–29.
36. Lang H, Nussbaum K T, Weimann A, Raab R. Liver resection for non-colorectal, non-neuroendocrine hepatic metastases. *Chirurg*. 1999;70:439–446.
37. Takada T, Yasuda H, Amano H, et al. Simultaneous hepatic resection with pancreato-duodenectomy for metastatic pancreatic head carcinoma: does it improve survival? *Hepatogastroenterology*. 1997;44:567–573.
38. Howard JM. Pancreatoduodenectomy (Whipple resection) with resection of hepatic metastases for carcinoma of the exocrine pancreas. *Arch Surg*. 1997;132:1044.
39. Klempnauer J, Ridder GJ, Piso P, Pichlmayr R. Is liver resection in metastases of exocrine pancreatic-carcinoma justified? *Chirurg*. 1996;67:366–370.
40. Cunningham D, Allum WH, Stenning SP, et al. Perioperative chemotherapy versus surgery alone for resectable gastroesophageal cancer. *N Engl J Med*. 2006;355:11–20.
41. Van Cutsem E, Moiseyenko VM, Tjulandin S, et al. Phase III study of docetaxel and cisplatin plus fluorouracil compared with cisplatin and fluorouracil as first-line therapy for advanced gastric cancer: a report of the V325 Study Group. *J Clin Oncol*. 2006;24:4991–4997.
42. Koga R, Yamamoto J, Ohyama S, et al. Liver resection for metastatic gastric cancer: experience with 42 patients including eight long-term survivors. *Jpn J Clin Oncol*. 2007;37:836–842.
43. Morise Z, Sugioka A, Hoshimoto S, et al. The role of hepatectomy for patients with liver metastases of gastric cancer. *Hepatogastroenterology*. 2008;55:1238–1241.
44. Okano K, Maeba T, Ishimura K, et al. Hepatic resection for metastatic tumors from gastric cancer. *Ann Surg*. 2002;235:86–91.
45. Roh HR, Suh KS, Lee HJ, et al. Outcome of hepatic resection for metastatic gastric cancer. *Am Surg*. 2005;71:95–99.
46. Sakamoto Y, Ohyama S, Yamamoto J, et al. Surgical resection of liver metastases of gastric cancer: an analysis of a 17-year experience with 22 patients. *Surgery*. 2003;133:507–511.
47. Shirabe K, Shimada M, Matsumata T, et al. Analysis of the prognostic factors for liver metastasis of gastric cancer after hepatic resection: a multi-institutional study of the indications for resection. *Hepatogastroenterology*. 2003;50:1560–1563.
48. Connolly EM, Gaffney E, Reynolds JV. Gastrointestinal stromal tumours. *Br J Surg*. 2003; 90:1178–1186.
49. DeMatteo RP, Lewis JJ, Leung D, et al. Two hundred gastrointestinal stromal tumors: recurrence patterns and prognostic factors for survival. *Ann Surg*. 2000;231:51–58.
50. Demetri GD, von Mehren M, Blanke CD, et al. Efficacy and safety of imatinib mesylate in advanced gastrointestinal stromal tumors. *N Engl J Med*. 2002;347:472–480.
51. Schurr P, Kohrs D, Reichelt U, et al. Repeated surgery improves survival in recurrent gastrointestinal stromal tumors: a retrospective analysis of 144 patients. *Dig Surg*. 2009;26:229–235.
52. DeMatteo RP, Shah A, Fong Y, et al. Results of hepatic resection for sarcoma metastatic to liver. *Ann Surg*. 2001;234:540–547; discussion 547–548.
53. Pawlik TM, Vauthey JN, Abdalla EK, et al. Results of a single-center experience with resection and ablation for sarcoma metastatic to the liver. *Arch Surg*. 2006;141:537–543; discussion 543–534.
54. DeMatteo RP, Maki RG, Singer S, et al. Results of tyrosine kinase inhib-itor therapy followed by surgical resection for metastatic

gastrointestinal stromal tumor. *Ann Surg.* 2007; 245:347–352.

55. Gronchi A, Fiore M, Miselli F, et al. Surgery of residual disease following molecular-targeted therapy with imatinib mesylate in advanced/metastatic GIST. *Ann Surg.* 2007;245:341–346.

56. Maurel J, Lopez-Pousa A, de Las Penas R, et al. Efficacy of sequential high-dose doxorubicin and ifosfamide compared with standard-dose doxorubicin in patients with advanced soft tissue sarcoma: an open-label randomized phase II study of the Spanish group for research on sarcomas. *J Clin Oncol.* 2009;27:1893–1898.

57. Van Glabbeke M, van Oosterom AT, Oosterhuis JW, et al. Prognostic factors for the outcome of chemotherapy in advanced soft tissue sarcoma: an analysis of 2,185 patients treated with anthracycline-containing first-line regimens—a European Organization for Research and Treatment of Cancer Soft Tissue and Bone Sarcoma Group Study. *J Clin Oncol.* 1999;17:150–157.

58. Van Glabbeke M, Verweij J, Judson I, Nielsen OS. Progression-free rate asthe principal end-point for phase II trials in soft-tissue sarcomas. *Eur J Cancer.* 2002;38:543–549.

59. Weitz J, Koch M, Friess H, Buchler MW. Impact of volume and specialization for cancer surgery. *Dig Surg.* 2004;21:253–261.

60. Hoffmann K, Franz C, Hinz U, et al. Liver resection for multimodal treatment of breast cancer metastases: identification of prognostic factors. *Ann Surg Oncol.* 2010;17:1546–1554.

SECTION III

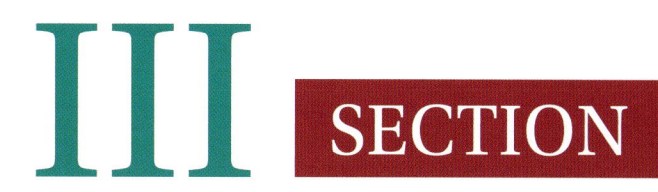

Diagnosis

Yuman Fong

CHAPTER 10

Imaging of Hepatobiliary Cancer: Ultrasonography, CT, PET-CT, and MRI

Thorsten Persigehl & Lawrence H. Schwartz

Introduction

Characterization of hepatobiliary lesions is an important objective of diagnostic imaging, more so because of the high prevalence of "incidental" detection of focal liver lesions in healthy adults and in patients with a known malignancy. Moreover, early diagnosis and differentiation of focal liver changes in liver cirrhosis is a special challenge as it is widely accepted that there is continuous carcinogenic progression of benign regenerating nodules to premalignant dysplastic nodules and then to malignant hepatocellular carcinoma (HCC).

Over the past few decades, substantial progresses has been made in developing and/or refining various radiological imaging methods, and these are now well established in the differential diagnosis of hepatobiliary masses. State-of-the-art imaging includes (1) (transabdominal) *ultrasonography* (US) partially performed with Doppler flow evaluation and usage of intravenous ultrasound contrast agents, (2) *computed tomography* (CT) including (dynamic) mechanical injection of intravenous nonionic iodinated contrast media, and (3) *magnetic resonance imaging* (MRI) with and without (dynamic) gadolinium-chelate-enhanced sequences. Nuclear medicine techniques, such as fluorodeoxyglucose–positron emission tomography (FDG-PET) or somatostatin receptor scintigraphy, appear to be indicated only for special cases.

General Indications

In the literature, a large number of varying imaging recommendations exists that take into account underlying disease (e.g., hepatitis B or C) and/or individual patient histories (e.g., previous cancer). The mentioned recommendations are based on the 2006 American College of Radiology (ACR) guidelines for liver imaging.[1] These general ACR guidelines assume that no prior diagnosis is available for comparison because no diagnostics have been done. For noninvasive HCC screening, differences exists between the guidelines of the Japanese Society of Hepatology,[2] the guidelines of the American Association for the Study of Liver Diseases,[3] and the European Association for the Study of the Liver.[4] However, after diagnosis of a hepatobiliary mass questions regarding further imaging or follow-up examination, or whether biopsy or surgery is required should be answered on a case-by-case basis.

Liver lesions with typical imaging features of a simple cyst, a hemangioma, or focal nodular hyperplasia (FNH) should be classified as benign. But, if there is any doubt that the hepatic mass is benign, especially in patients with suspected or known malignancy, follow-up imaging should be done to make sure that there is no change in lesion appearance. Alternatively, in the case of an unclear US or CT finding, additional MRI could be done to achieve a definitive diagnosis. Typical malignant hepatobiliary tumors on US, CT, or MRI do not require additional imaging for diagnosis but should be confirmed by serum tumor markers or percutaneous biopsy. However, further imaging for adequate tumor classification (e.g., TNM classification of malignant tumors) may be indicated. For indeterminate hepatobiliary masses at one imaging modality (e.g., US and CT), follow-up examination seems impractical due to the potential need of a rapid and appropriate treatment initiation, and additional imaging (e.g., MRI and FDG-PET-CT) may be required for precise tissue characterization. In case of prior indeterminate US and/or CT imaging, an additional procedure using MRI may be helpful. Nuclear medicine methods should be considered for special cases such as patients with suspected hepatic metastasis of colorectal cancer (FDG-PET) or neuroendocrine liver metastasis (somatostatin receptor scintigraphy). However, subcentimeter lesions might be difficult to characterize, and in patients with an extrahepatic primary malignancy, short-term follow-up imaging might be justified. For a highly suspicious liver lesion, the final diagnosis could be obtained by percutaneous biopsy, and, for masses of the bile duct, invasive ERCP diagnostic [supported by fluorescence in-situ hybridization (FISH)] should be discussed. For cirrhotic liver disease, diagnosis of suspicious liver lesions is best performed with dynamic contrast-enhanced (DCE) MRI followed by dynamic contrast-enhanced, multidetector CT (MDCT) and US. In recent studies, CE US showed similar sensitivities and specificities as dynamic CT and MRI. However, characterization is more accurate for larger lesions (>2 cm), and differentiation of small nodular inflammatory, benign dysplastic and malignant HCC lesions can be difficult. In cases of unclear (small) liver lesions, for final diagnostic correlation of serum tumor markers (e.g., alpha-fetoprotein [AFP]), percutaneous biopsy, and follow-up imaging might be necessary.

Imaging Methods

Ultrasonography

Conventional transabdominal US remains the most commonly used modality for screening healthy persons and patients at high risk of developing liver disease (e.g., liver cirrhosis) and/or a known malignancy (e.g., colon cancer), but US that is not CE is hampered by relative low sensitivity and specificity.[5,6] Additional US Doppler flow evaluation allows analysis of blood vessel flow characteristics and simplifies imaging of the biliary duct system. Recent studies demonstrated that CE US improves the detection and characterization of focal liver lesions compared to conventional grayscale US and shows similar sensitivity and specificity to dynamic CE CT and MRI.[7-9] US contrast agents (e.g., SonoVue® and Optison®) are approved in many countries for liver and/or cardiac indications and sometimes are used in an off-label fashion. In general, these contrast agents consist of microscopic bubbles of gas in an encapsulating shell, oscillating in response to a low-intensity ultrasound field and being disrupted in response to a high-intensity field.[10] CE US shows real-time arterial perfusion (5–25 seconds), portalvenous perfusion (25–60 seconds), and late perfusion (>120 seconds) visualization with a higher temporal resolution compared to CE CT and MR imaging.[11] In the case of multiple liver lesions, each lesion could be analyzed separately by a new bolus injection per lesion. These lung capillaries suitable microbubbles remain purely intravascular and show no extravasation into surrounding interstitial tissue. Thus, hepatobiliary tumors (e.g., cholangiocarcinomas), which usually show accumulation of permeable, low molecular weight CT and MR contrast agents, cause discordant CE US imaging patterns in late contrast phases.[12] However, CE US has limitations parallel to conventional non-CE US, such as dependency on the experience of the investigator, body shape of the patient, superimposition of bowel gas, and localization of the liver lesion (especially in hepatic steatosis).

Computed Tomography

CT of the abdomen is widely used for screening, staging, and follow-up in patients with known malignancy, but CT is hampered by the nephrotoxicity of iodine-containing contrast agents and ionization (especially for multi-phase imaging protocols in young patients).[13] MDCT, with substantially shorter acquisition times and reconstruction of thin slice sections in a single breathhold, allows multiphase imaging over one contrast bolus injection.[14] Postprocessing, three-dimensional multiplanar reformations (MPR) can not only improve the depiction of tumorous tissue regarding size, volume, and infiltration of surrounding structures but also provide information on secondary findings important for decisions regarding the adequacy of therapy (e.g., metastatic lymph nodes or liver cirrhosis). MDCT protocols may vary substantially for differing indications and between imaging centers depending on the used CT scanner (e.g., 4- to 256-detector rows), contrast power injector settings (e.g., flow rates between 3 and 5 mL/s), and contrast agent type (e.g., nonionic iodine concentrations between 300 and 400 mg/mL such as Ultravist® 300 or 370).[14] Moreover, determination of the circulation time is of great importance and could be achieved by a test bolus scan or care bolus technique. Thus, MDCT protocols have to be adapted for each specific clinical indication and imaging center to ensure optimal detection and characterization of hepatobiliary tumors.

For detection and characterization of hepatobiliary tumors, a dynamic enhancement pattern (e.g., centripetal/centrifugal "fill-in", homogeneous/heterogeneous enhancement, peripheral (discontinuous) nodular/ring enhancement, central scar, and "wash-out") after bolus injection of a nonionic iodine-containing contrast agent can help to achieve a more accurate diagnosis. Precontrast CT scans might be helpful in the characterization of an indeterminate mass by visualization of focal fat, hemorrhage, calcification, or Lipiodol retention after chemoembolization. Early arterial phase imaging 15–20 seconds after the start of the contrast injection with optimal enhancement of hepatic arteries might be useful for presurgical evaluation. During late arterial phase examinations, after 30–35 seconds, an optimal delineation of hypervascular lesions (e.g., capillary hemangioma, HCC, adenoma, FNH, or metastasis of neuroendocrine tumors (NETs) and clear cell renal carcinomas) seems to be most feasible. Hypovascular liver lesions (e.g., liver metastases) are best depicted using portal-venous phase imaging after 60–70 seconds. Delayed equilibrium phase imaging after 120–240 seconds helps diagnose lesions with pronounced "wash-out" compared to the surrounding liver tissue (e.g., diffuse HCC), delayed complete filling (e.g., cavernous hemangioma), or even on late imaging phases >5 minutes of delayed enhancement (e.g., cholangiocarcinoma). However, imaging of multiple phases seems to be unnecessary for a lot of screening and treatment follow-up examinations (e.g., screening and follow-up of liver metastasis at the portal-venous phase only).

Briefly, PET using [18F] FDG is widely established in oncologic imaging as it allows visualization and quantification of the metabolic activity of tumors in terms of their regional glucose uptake. Data regarding the applicability of FDG-PET imaging to hepatobiliary tumors are limited, but FDG-PET-CT might be used as a second-line modality in case of suspected metastasis of a hepatobiliary cancer (e.g., gallbladder carcinoma and cholangiocarcinoma), hepatic metastasis from a FDG-positive primary (e.g., from melanoma, breast, colon, and esophageal cancer), and lymphatic infiltration (e.g., non-Hodgkin lymphoma [NHL]).[15,16] Moreover, nuclear scintigraphy (e.g., somatostatin receptor scintigraphy) combined with single photon emission computed tomography (SPECT/CT) is an option for patients with suspected liver metastasis of NETs.[17]

Magnetic Resonance Imaging

MRI, with an excellent soft-tissue contrast, is a highly sensitive and specific method for evaluation of the liver and biliary system.[18,19] With recent technical advances in hardware (e.g., gradient field strengths), software (e.g., fast parallel imaging techniques), and intravenous contrast agents (e.g., hepatobiliary-specific contrast agents), MRI has been substantially improved. Combination of cross-sectional MRI and three-dimensional MR cholangiopancreatography (MRCP) allows a clear depiction of intra- and extra-hepatic biliary cancer by showing, noninvasively, the biliary duct system with associated strictures, the complete tumor with adjacent soft tissue and tumor infiltration into surrounding structures.[20] Thus, comprehensive MR protocols are widely established for detection, characterization, staging, and assessment of the resectability of hepatobiliary masses. Moreover, MRI's lack of ionizing radiation provides a significant advantage over MDCT in pediatrics and for patients with multiple follow-up examinations. MRI contraindications are, among others, cardiac pacemakers/defibrillators, brain neurostimulators, metal implants, a history of severe allergic reactions to MR contrast agents, and end-stage renal failure or perioperative liver transplantation with risk of nephrogenic systemic sclerosis (NSF).

MRI examinations are commonly performed at 1.5 Tesla using phased-array body coils in a parallel imaging technique and dynamic contrast application. Comprehensive MRI protocols include (1) axial T2-weighted two-dimensional spin-echo (with or without fat saturation), (2) unenhanced axial "in-phase/out-of-phase" T1-weighted two-dimensional gradient-echo or axial Dixon method, (3) dynamic CE

(DCE) T1-weighted three-dimensional gradient-echo (with fat suppression) sequences using a breath-hold technique and administration of a Gd-based MR contrast agent, and (4) optional additional axial diffusion-weighted imaging (DWI) with b-factors of 250 and 500 s/mm^2, and (5) heavily T2-weighted MRCP (or T1-weighted MR cholangiography after administration of hepatobiliary-specific contrast media).[18,19] Perfect bolus timing of dynamic CE MRI is more challenging compared to CT, predominantly because of the smaller amount of contrast agent, faster liver peak enhancement, and optimal data acquisition at the central k-space. For optimal enhancement of contrast at the lesion site, a mechanically administered bolus injection with flow rates of 2–3 mL/s and a test bolus scan or automated bolus detection technique is recommended. Commonly used dynamic CE MRI include scan phases (1) of 15–20 seconds for arterial, (2) of 45–60 seconds for portal-venous, and (3) of 3–5 minutes for delayed equilibrium imaging after injection of a nonspecific gadolinium chelate, and additional (4) late hepatobiliary phase imaging of 20 minutes after application of Gd-EOB-DTPA and 60 minutes after application of Gd-BOPTA in noncirrhotic patients.[19,21] However, MRI protocols show variations concerning optimized sequences for different tissues at differing field strengths and differing contrast media types. This makes image interpretation more complex for the reader as it combines information of the varying sequences (e.g., T2- and T1-weighted with or without fat suppression). Also, names of similar sequences may vary between differing vendors such as three-dimensional spoiled gradient echo sequence (1) LAVA (liver acquisition with volume acceleration) at GE, (2) THRIVE (T1 high resolution isotropic volume expansion) at Philips, and (3) VIBE (volume interpolated breathhold examination) at Siemens MR systems.

Contrast agents clinically used in hepatobiliary MR imaging can be divided into nonspecific extracellular gadolinium chelates, hepatobiliary-specific contrast agents, and reticuloendothelial specific (RES) contrast agents.

First, nonspecific extracellular gadolinium chelates (e.g., Gd-DTPA [Magnevist®], Gd-HP-DO3A [Prohance®], and Gd-DTPA-BMA [Omniscan®]) predominately shorten the T1 relaxation time with a resulting signal increase on T1-weighted images.[22] These low-molecular-weight contrast media, which are among the most widely clinical used MR contrast agents, are distributed initially within the intravascular compartment, and diffuse rapidly into the extravascular interstitial space, similar to iodinated contrast agents in CT. Thus, after bolus injection, dynamic information regarding tissue perfusion and permeability can be acquired.

Second, there are two principal classes of hepatobiliary-specific contrast agents, one based on manganese (Mn-DPDP [Teslascan®] and two are gadolinium based (Gd-BOPTA [MultiHance®] and Gd-EOB-DTPA [Eovist®/Primovist®]).[23] These agents are taken up by functioning hepatocytes, excreted in the bile, and mainly cause a shortening of the T1 relaxation period on T1-weighted sequences. However, these three MR contrast agents vary in form of administration (e.g., slow infusion of Mn-DPDP vs. bolus injection of Gd-EOB-DTPA), dose (e.g., 0.1 mmol/kg of Gd-BOPTA vs. 0.025 mmol/kg of Gd-EOB-DTPA), and degree of hepatocellular uptake and excretion through the biliary pathway (e.g., 3%–5% at Gd-BOPTA vs. 50% at Gd-EOB-DTPA). The two hepatobiliary-specific agents that are used most—Gd-EOB-DTPA and Gd-BOPTA—initially show an intra-vascular distribution. This is followed by a rapid extravasation of the agents into the extravascular interstitial compartment, and their subsequent uptake into functional hepatocytes. Hence, these two contrast agents provide dual benefits: (1) the capability of dynamic imaging with imaging characteristics that are similar to nonspecific extracellular gadolinium chelates and (2) delayed hepatobiliary phase imaging. This late hepatobiliary phase can be used to improve the detection and characterization of lesions of hepatocellular (e.g., hyperintense FNH) or nonhepatocellular origin (e.g., hypointense metastasis). However, the dependence of optimal hepatobiliary phase timing on the contrast agent and on liver function (e.g., 10–60 minute for Gd-EOB-DTPA and 60–120 minute for Gd-BOPTA) result in a prolongation of the total MR imaging time.[23] Moreover, hepatobiliary-specific contrast agents could be used for CE T1-weighted MR cholangiography[24,25] and assessment of liver function.[26]

Third, superparamagnetic iron oxides ("small particles of iron oxide"; SPIO) are reticuloendothelial-specific contrast agents that predominantly shorten T2 relaxation accompanied by a signal decrease on T2 (T2*)-weighted images (e.g., Resovist®, Feridex®/Endorem®).[27] SPIOs are taken up by the reticuloendothelial system (RES) in the liver (so-called Kupffer cells), spleen, and lymph nodes. Thus, normal liver parenchyma and lesions that contain Kupffer cells (e.g., hepatic adenoma, FNH, regenerating nodules, and well-differentiated HCC) show a signal loss at the accumulation phase (>10 minutes after injection), whereas other tissues remain unchanged and appear relatively more hyperintense. A combination of SPIO-enhanced MRI and DWI or dual-contrast MRI of SPIOs and Gd-based contrast media could improve diagnosis of liver lesions.[28,29] However, due to the recent decrease of the clinical availability of SPIOs, this MR technique is actually not routinely used.

Hepatobiliary Tumors

Benign Lesions

Fatty Infiltration

Fatty infiltration of liver parenchyma can be diffuse, patchy, or focal. The pattern could be lobar, segmental, or wedge-shaped and is partially related to regional perfusion differences. Diagnosis of focal fatty infiltration or even areas of spared infiltration in steatosis may be challenging. Such "pseudolesions" could be misinterpreted as true liver lesions. However, the presence of normal vessels within the lesion, and knowledge of typical locations of such "pseudolesions" could be helpful (e.g., adjacent to the gallbladder fossa).

At US, diffuse fatty infiltration results in an increased hepatic echogenicity that can hamper the visibility of the dorsal liver parenchyma.[30,31] Moreover, focal fatty infiltration appears hyperechogenic and focal fatty sparing hypoechogenic without suspicious abnormal perfusion characteristics on Doppler or CE US.

Noncontrast CT typically shows a decreased diffuse or focal density. Normally, liver shows a slightly higher density compared to spleen (of about 10 Hounsfield Units [HU]), and reversal of this relationship could be a first visible sign of hepatic steatosis.[31] Evaluation of fatty infiltration seems to be more accurate on noncontrast CT scans than on CE CT. But, in general, on delayed contrast phase images, the HU of steatotic liver should be lower than the HU in the spleen.

MRI allows, in most of cases, an accurate diagnosis due to differing signal characteristics.[31] On T2- and T1-weighted images, areas of fatty infiltration appear relatively hyperintense; in contrast, on fat suppressed images, these areas show low signal intensities. Moreover, "in-phase/out-of-phase" T1-weighted sequences allow to distinguish fat with high sensitivity. These specific "chemical shift" imaging technique rely on the different resonance frequencies of fat protons and water protons. In the presence of both components, and at "out-of-phase" echo times, the signals are opposite and will cancel each other out. Thus, tissue with relative equal quantities of fat and (normal) water appears dark on "out-of-phase" images, whereas tissue without fat remains similar bright to "in-phase" images. However, the presence of fat within other focal liver lesions (e.g., adenoma and HCC) should be taken into account before making the diagnosis of focal fatty infiltration. On postgadolinium T1-weighted images, fatty infiltration should not show a suspicious enhancement compared to the surrounding liver parenchyma.

Cysts

Simple hepatic or bile duct cysts are sharply margined, can vary in size, and appear as a solitary mass or as multiple lesions (hepatic polycystic disease).

On US, simple cysts are typically anechogenic, with enhanced echos (hyperchogenicity) posterior to the lesion due to unaffected transmission (Figure 10-1A). US should show a smooth wall without (contrast enhancing) solid nodules.[32]

On CT, cysts typically appear as well-defined hypodense lesion with densities similar to that of water (<20 HU) and no detectable contrast-enhancement of solid components or wall calcifications (Figure 10-1B).[33] Small cysts (<1 cm) may be difficult to characterize on CT because of volume averaging and an artificially higher number of HU.

On MRI, simple cysts show a homogenous hyperintense signal on T2-weighted images and appear hypointense on T1-weighted images, without detectable enhancement after contrast administration (Figure 10-1C).[33,34] Cysts maintain their high signal on "heavy" T2-weighted spin-echo sequences with long TE values (e.g., >120 ms).[35] Rarely, thin septations within hepatic cysts can be observed, which might be also caused by cysts that are located close together (Figure 10-1D).

However, cysts can be complicated (e.g., after infection or trauma) with a high protein or hemorrhagic content and may appear hypoechogenic or

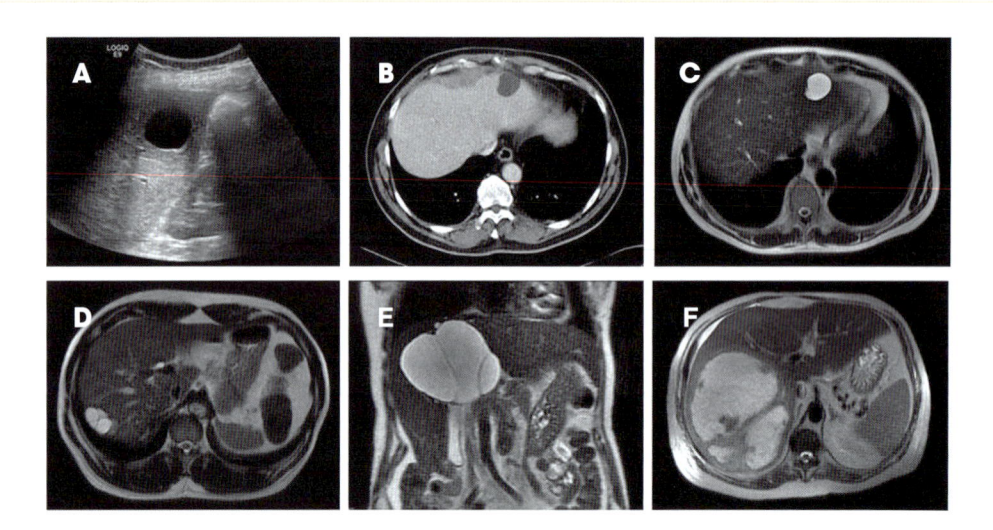

Figure 10-1: Hepatic cyst and cystic lesions. Hepatic cyst with a typical anechogenic appearance and hyperchogenicity posterior to the lesion on grayscale ultrasonography (A), a well-defined hypodense lesion on computed tomography (B), and a hyperintense signal on T2-weighted magnetic resonance imaging (C). Differential diagnosis include, among others, complicated cysts with fine septations (D), benign multicystic biliary cystadenoma (E), and hepatic abscess with contrast-enhancing wall and septations (F).

hyperechogenic on US, with increased HU on CT, or high signal on T1-weighted MR images. In case of an atypical imaging pattern (e.g., a multicystic mass, a thickened contrast-enhancing wall, and/or septations), one should consider in the differential diagnosis an infection or a super-infection (e.g., hepatic abscess [Figure 10-1F], amebic abscess, or echinococcal cyst), postoperative changes (e.g., biloma), metastasis (cystic or necrotic metastasis of, e.g., ovarian and pancreas cancer or GIST [Figure 10-6D]), a benign tumor (e.g., biliary cystadenoma [Figure 10-1E]), or a malignant tumor (e.g., biliary cystadenocarcinoma).

Hemangioma

Hemangiomas are usually well-defined, lobulated lesions and occur often as a set of multiple lesions. They can be divided into the more common cavernous hemangiomas and the less common (small) capillary hemangiomas. For large, cavernous hemangiomas, areas of central thrombosis, fibrosis, and/or calcification may be present.

On US, hemangiomas appear hyperechogenic with sharp borders (Figure 10-2A).[32] On additional color Doppler evaluation, peripheral feeding blood vessels may be detectable. Moreover, CE US usually allows real-time visualization of typical perfusion phenomena within the lesion, with early arterial peripheral nodular enhancement and progressive centripetal filling during following delayed phases (Figure 10-2B–E).[11]

On noncontrast CT, a hemangioma shows mostly a hypodense lesion, whereas large hemangiomas might be more heterogeneous in the presence of thrombotic or fibrotic changes, with possible calcifications. Classically, after contrast injection, initial peripheral (discontinuous) nodular enhancement with progressive centripetal complete filling on late phase imaging can be observed (Figure 10-2F–H).[33]

On MRI, hemangiomas are hyperintense on T2-weighted images (Figure 10-3A) and tend to retain their high signal on "heavy" T2-weighted sequences.[33,35] On T1-weighted images, hemangiomas are hypointense and generally show an initial peripheral (discontinuous) nodular enhancement with progressive centripetal complete filling, following the "blood pool" contrast over all imaging phases

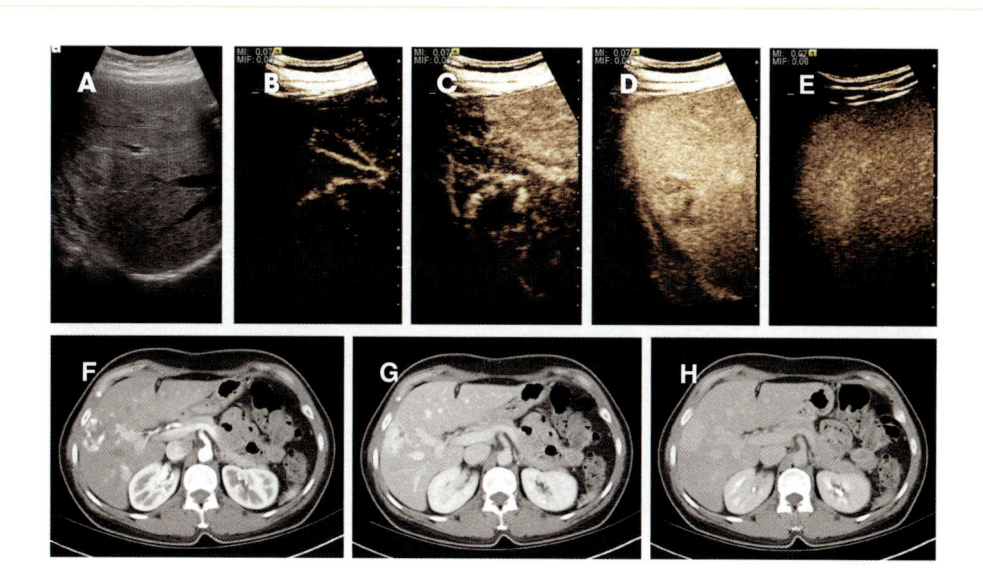

Imaging of Hepatobiliary Cancer: Ultrasonography, CT, PET-CT, and MRI   229

Figure 10-2: Hemangioma. Hemangioma with a typical hyperechogenic appearance and sharp borders on conventional ultrasonography (US) (A). Contrast-enhanced US demonstrates a real-time visualization of typical perfusion phenomena within the lesion, with early arterial peripheral nodular enhancement and progressive centripetal filling during following delayed phases (B–E). In line, dynamic contrast-enhanced computed tomography shows an initial arterial peripheral discontinuous nodular enhancement (F) with progressive centripetal complete filling in the portal-venous (G) and delayed equilibrium phase (H). Notice, contrast-enhancing parts of the hemangioma match the "blood pool" contrast at all imaging phases. (Courtesy of Dr. M. Palmowski, University Hospital Aachen, Germany.)

(Figure 10-3B–F). Using hepatobiliary-specific contrast agents, hemangiomas usually appear hypointense in the hepatobiliary phase, in line to the "blood pool" contrast. After injection of SPIOs, hemangiomas can initially show a signal loss on T2-weighted images in the perfusion phase due to "blood pool" effects but show no uptake in the delayed accumulation phase.[27]

However, accurate characterization of small capillary hemangiomas (<2 cm) with rapid "flash-filling" or large hemangiomas (5–10 cm) with incomplete filling (e.g., in the presence of a central thrombosis and/or fibrosis) can be difficult and might be best diagnosed using real-time CE US or MRI due to their typically strong T2 characteristics on "heavy" T2-weighted sequences.

Focal Nodular Hyperplasia

FNH usually appears as a well-defined liver lesion that contains all the elements of normal liver (e.g., hepatocytes, Kupffer cells, and small bile ducts) and that may show, even in larger tumors (>3 cm), a detectable central scar. FNH occurs predominantly as a solitary lesion but can also present as multiple lesions. At the time of diagnosis, the mean size is about 3 cm.

On conventional grayscale US, FNH is mostly slightly hypointense or isoechogenic, and only very rarely is it hyperechogenic compared to the surrounding liver parenchyma; or it may be detected only by a hypoechogenic central scar.[32,36] On color Doppler US, at the lesion center, one may find enlarged feeding vessels; at the periphery, draining vessels. However, CE US allows a more sophisticated analysis of the perfusion pattern. On CE US, a rapidly centrifugal ("spoke-wheel") enhancement of the lesion can usually be demonstrated, whereas the central scar typically remains hypoechogenic.[11,37]

On noncontrast CT scans, FNHs appear isodense or mildly hypodense and in some lesions there is a

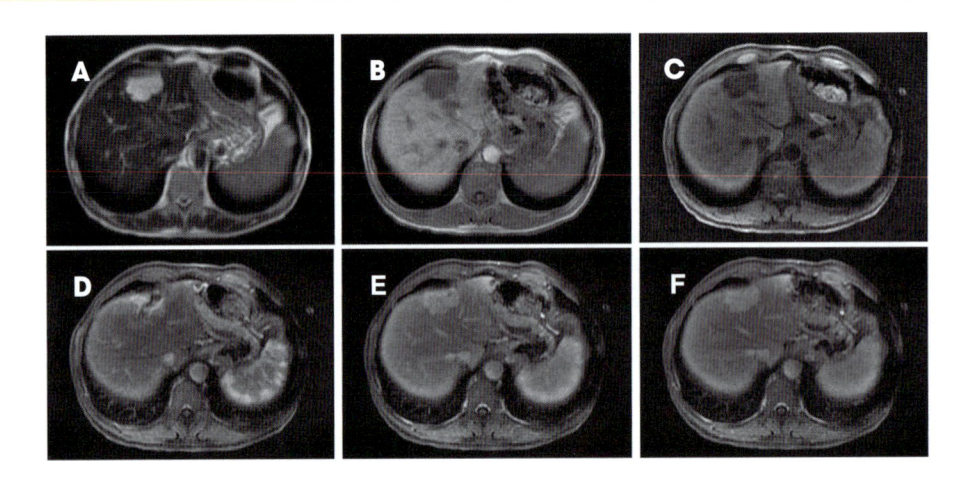

Figure 10-3: Hemangioma. Cavernous hemangiomas typically appear as well-defined, lobulated lesions with a hyperintense signal on T2-weighted (A) and hypointense signal on T1-weighted magnetic resonance images, without (B) and with fat suppression (C). Dynamic contrast-enhanced magnetic resonance imaging shows an initial arterial peripheral, discontinuous enhancement with successive centripetal complete filling, following the "blood pool" contrast over all imaging phases (D–F).

detectable central hypodensity.[36] Dynamic CE CT mostly shows a strong transient arterial hyperdense enhancement that becomes isodense in the portal-venous and delayed equilibrium phase. The central scar, if visible on CT, usually exhibits a mildly delayed enhancement.

On MRI examinations, FNH can appear minimally hyperintense to isointense on T2-weighted images (Figure 10-4A), and isointense to slightly hypointense on T1-weighted images (Figure 10-4B and C). After gadolinium injection, FNHs typically show an early strong arterial enhancement, which fades to an isointense appearance on delayed phase images (Figure 10-4D and E).[33,38] In contrast to HCC, FNH usually shows no relative hypodense "wash-out" in comparison with the surrounding liver parenchyma. The central scar appears mostly hyperintense on T2-weighted images and hypointense on T1-weighted images, with a delayed and prolonged contrast-enhancement on postgadolinium sequences. Using hepatobiliary-specific contrast agents, FNHs appear on the delayed hepatobiliary phase mostly isointense or even hyperintense compared to the surrounding normal liver parenchyma (Figure 10-4F).[23,39] This is due to contrast accumulation in functional hepatocytes and excretion into the (malformed) small bile ducts. As FNH normally contains Kupffer cells, it also shows uptake of SPIOs with a detectable signal loss on T2-weighted images, whereas the central scar typically remains hyperintense.[36,40]

Hepatic Adenoma

Hepatic adenomas (or hepatocellular adenoma [HCA]) are well-delineated lesions, possibly with a thin pseudocapsule. Hepatic adenomas are commonly solitary lesions (with a higher prevalence in the right lobe), but can occur, in some cases, as multiple lesions, with even more than 10 lesions (so-called adenomatosis). They can be large in size (>10 cm) and may contain fat, hemorrhages, calcifications, and/or a central, degenerative, scar-like fibrosis. Thus, the imaging pattern of HCAs can show extreme variations based on their histological appearance.

On conventional grayscale US, hepatic adenomas generally appear hypoechogenic, but can also be heterogeneous and hyperechogenic in the presence of fat, hemorrhage, or calcifications.[36] Color Doppler US may show a hypervascularization of the lesion with pronounced enlarged blood vessels at the

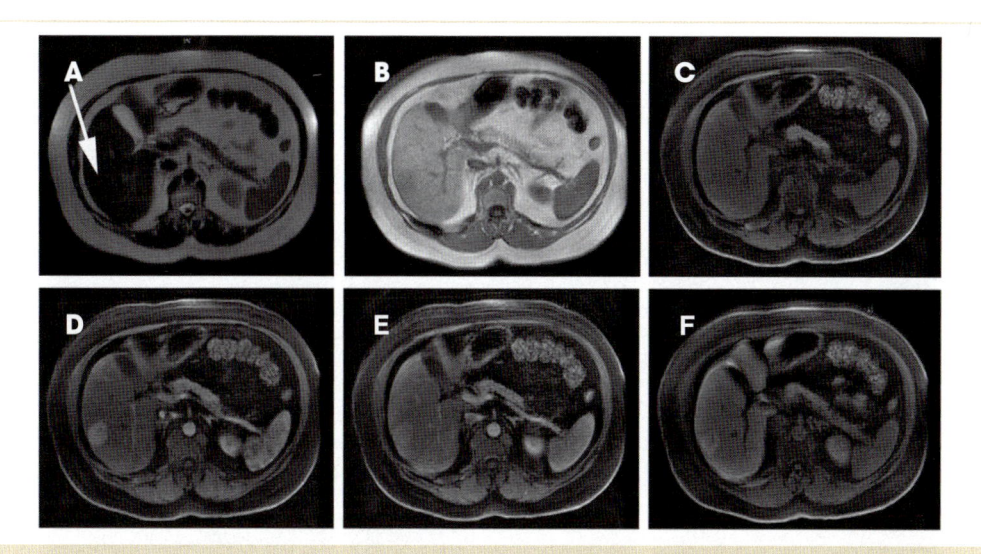

Figure 10-4: Focal nodular hyperplasia (FNH). FNH with an isointense signal on T2-weighted magnetic resonance imaging sequence, whereas the central (punctual) scar shows a typical hyperintensity (A). The well-defined FNH appears slightly hypointense on T1-weighted images (B) and isointense on fat suppressed T1-weigthed images before contrast injection (C). After injection of the hepatobiliary-specific contrast agent Gd-EOB-DTPA, the FNH shows a typically arterial enhancement (D), which fades to a more isointense appearance on delayed phase images (E). On the late hepatobiliary phase after 20 min, the FNH demonstrates a clear contrast uptake with a slightly hyperintense signal compared to the surrounding normal liver parenchyma.

periphery. CE US mostly shows a rapidly centripetal or diffuse perfusion in the real-time arterial phase with a homogeneous sustained "fill-in" and possible minor "wash-out" in the portal-venous phase.[10]

On noncontrast CT, hepatic adenomas appear as isodense to hypodense lesions, due to the amount of fat within the mass. On the contrary, hyperdense areas of hemorrhage or calcifications can also be observed in some cases. After contrast injection, small lesions may be associated with a strong homogeneous arterial enhancement, large lesions with a more inhomogeneous arterial enhancement. On portal-venous phase images, HCAs appear slightly hyperdense to isodense, and even on delayed-phase images, a mild "wash-out" may be detectable.[36] At the tumor periphery, enlarged vessels or a thin pseudocapsule may be visible.

On MRI, hepatic adenomas generally appear isointense or slightly hyperintense on T2-weighted images (Figure 10-5A). On T1-weighted images, HCAs may show a very varying appearance with heterogeneous hypodense, isointense, and slightly hyperintense regions (Figure 10-5B and C).[38] This variability is due to the amount of fat, haemosiderin, and/or calcification. However, the distribution of fat is usually more homogenous in HCAs compared with angiomyolipoma or HCC, which show more heterogeneous areas of fat. Infrequently, a surrounding pseudocapsule with a hyperintense signal on T2-weighted images, and a hypointense signal on T1-weighted images might be seen. HCAs may also show, rarely, a degenerative scar-like central area, which can mimic FNH. On dynamic CE MR sequences, hepatic adenomas usually show a strong homogeneous enhancement for small lesions and more heterogeneous enhancement for larger lesions (Figure 10-5D). This occurs in the arterial phase and fades to an isointense appearance in the late portal-venous and equilibrium phases (Figure 10-5E). In delayed phases, minor "wash-out" phenomena might be detectable, which could make a differentiation of HCA from HCC without clinical information impossible. Using hepatobiliary-specific contrast agents, HCAs mostly show, due to the absence of bile ducts and a portal tract system, no substantial contrast uptake and appear hypointense on hepatobiliary

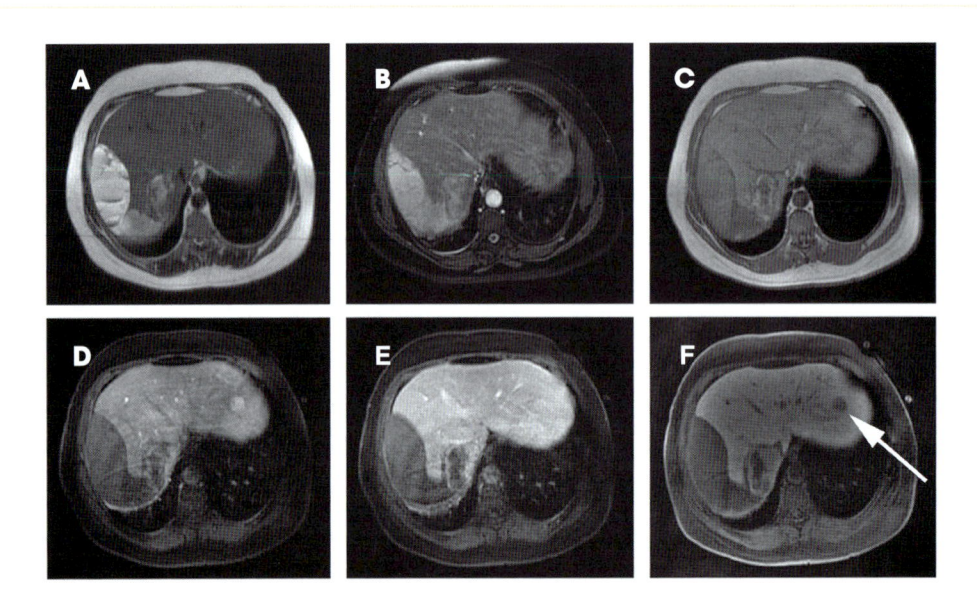

Figure 10-5: Hepatic adenoma. Hepatic adenoma in the dorsal right lobe of the liver with an acute subcapsular hematoma, whereas the hepatic adenoma itself appears widely isointense on T2-weighed (A), fat-suppressed T2-weighed (B), and T1-weighted images (C). Hepatic adenomas typically show a strong arterial enhancement (D), which normally fades to an isointense appearance in the delayed equilibrium phase (E). Using hepatobiliary-specific contrast agents, hepatic adenoma mostly show, due to the absence of bile ducts and a portal tract system, no substantial contrast uptake and appear hypointense on hepatobiliary phase imaging (F). Also notice the second hepatic adenoma in the left lobe of the liver (arrow), which could be clearly depicted on the arterial phase and hepatobiliary phase 20 min after injection of Gd-EOB-DTPA.

phase imaging, allowing a sensitive differentiation from FNH (Figure 10-5F).[23,36,39] After SPIO application, HCAs show, in a few cases, due to their presence Kupffer cells, a signal loss compared to the surrounding normal liver parenchyma, resulting in an unspecific hypointense, isointense, or relatively hyperintense appearance on T2-weighted images.[40]

Less Common Benign Tumors

Rare benign hepatobiliary tumors include cyst-like biliary hamartomas and biliary cystadenoma, as well as solid lesions such as angiomyolipoma of the liver.

Biliary Hamartoma

Biliary hamartomas (also known as von Meyenburg's complex) may appear as multiple or solitary masses and are usually small (< 1.5 cm), cyst-like, and well-delineated lesions.

On conventional grayscale US, biliary hamartomas appear as small hypoechogenic and hyperechogenic lesions or can even present as a heterogeneous liver texture with multiple subcentimeter lesions.[41] In a limited number of case reports, biliary hamartomas showed unspecific perfusion characteristics on CE US.[42]

Biliary hamartomas appear hypodense on noncontrast CT scans and, due to their cystic or fibrous content, show varying enhancement from hypodense to isodense after contrast application.[43]

On MRI, cyst-like lesions appear hyperintense and fibrous lesions more isointense on T2-weighted images.[38] On T1-weighted images, biliary hamartomas are generally hypointense. Cystic lesions may show a thin contrast-enhancing rim of compressed adjacent liver parenchyma, whereas solid fibrous lesions may exhibit an unspecific enhancement. Thus, the differential diagnosis from miliary metastasis (especially in patients with known breast cancer) can be very challenging. Normally, biliary hamartomas show no "central dot sign," as typically seen for Caroli disease. On MRCP images, usually no communication with the biliary duct system can be detected.

Biliary Cystadenoma

Biliary cystadenomas are rare and occur mostly in the liver. They can also occur, even more rarely, in the extrahepatic bile duct and gallbladder. They usually appear as well-defined, multiloculated cysts with possible calcifications and contrast enhancing septations or small nodules.

On US, large anechogenic lesions with septations, calcifications, and/or solid nodules are detectable. These cyst-like lesions, after internal hemorrhage, or mucinous lesions can exhibit hypoechogenic or hyperechogenic fluid content (levels).

Biliary cystadenomas appear on unenhanced CT as large hypodense cystic lesions with septations and possible cacifications. However, biliary cystadenoma with mucinous or hemorrhagic content can show increased HU. On postcontrast CT, solid parts may demonstrate a mild contrast enhancement.

On MRI, cystic biliary cystadenomas show a hyperintense signal on T2-weighted images and a hypointense signal on T1-weighted images (Figure 10-1E), whereas mucinous- filled cystadenomas could appear isointense to hyperintense on T1-weighted sequences.[44] A moderate contrast enhancement of solid components can be detected on postgadolinium, T1-weighted (fat suppressed) images.

However, all imaging patterns on US, CT, and MRI are unspecific and allow no reliable differentiation from biliary cystadenocarcinoma.

Angiomyolipoma

Hepatic angiomyolipoma is a well-defined tumor containing variable amounts of fat, smooth muscle, and blood vessels. Thus, a small angiomyolipoma with a high amount of fat can mimic a lipoma.

On conventional grayscale US, due to their divergent composition, angiomyolipomas normally show extensive heterogeneous hyperechogenic areas combined with hypoechogenic and anechogenic areas.[45] In most of the lesions, arterial flow signals can be detected by color Doppler imaging. CE US commonly shows an early high perfusion in the arterial phase, with slightly higher to similar perfusion characteristics on delayed phases.[46]

On noncontrast CT, hepatic angiomyolipomas appear, based on their composition, as well defined heterogeneous hypodense masses, typically containing areas of detectable fat with negative HU. After contrast injection, they may show an inhomogeneous hyperdense arterial enhancement of the non fatty parts, with a heterogeneous contrast enhancement on delayed phases.[33]

On MRI, angiomyolipomas frequently appear heterogeneous and hyperintense on T2-weighted images and on T1-weighted images, with accordingly hypointense signals on fat-suppressed sequences.[45] On "in-phase/out-of-phase" T1-weighted imaging, a clear signal loss on "out-of-phase" images can be seen for the fatty portions. On arterial phase MR imaging, angiomyolipomas show a strong contrast enhancement of the soft tissue parts, which fades to an isointense appearance on subsequent late equilibrium phase imaging.

Malignant Lesions

Hepatic Metastasis

Hepatic metastases occur as solitary or multiple lesions and tend to have less well-defined margins. Metastases show a very divergent appearance on US, CT, and MRI and may mimic other benign or malignant lesions. In addition, different types of focal hepatic lesions may coexist in the same patient, which could make diagnosis even more difficult. On the contrary, about half of small liver lesions (<1.5 cm) in cancer patients are benign but can be difficult to differentiate from small liver metastases. Metastases of the gall bladder are very rare and are predominately of melanotic origin.

On US, hepatic metastases exhibit varying imaging patterns from hyperechogenic, hypoechogenic to cystic anechogenic (Figure 10-6A). More- over, hepatic metastases could demonstrate on grayscale US a "target-sign" appearance with a hypoechogenic rim and isoechogenic center, and detectable blood vessels on color Doppler US (e.g., hepatic metastasis

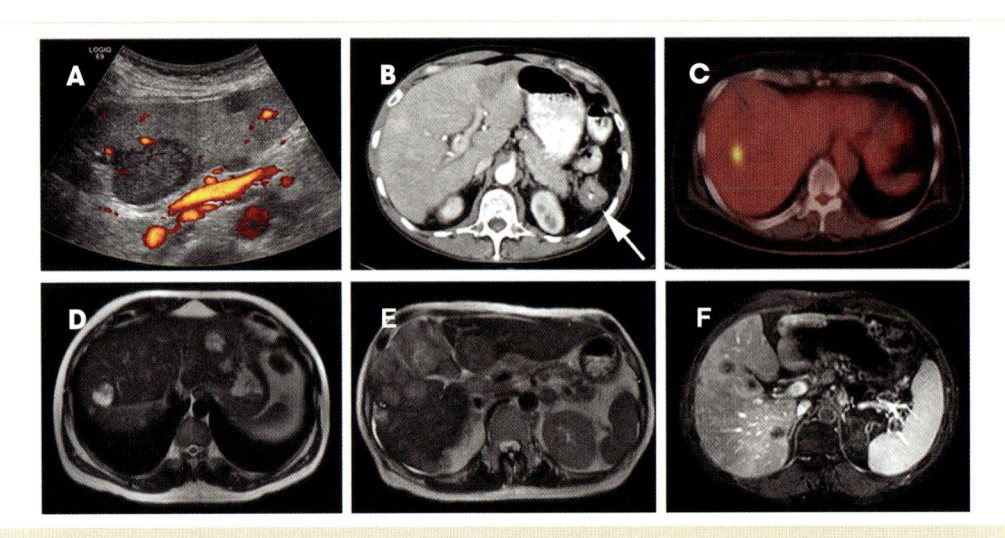

Figure 10-6: Hepatic metastasis. Hepatic metastasis of a breast cancer with a hypoechogenic appearance on grayscale ultrasonography (US) and few detectable blood vessels at the tumor rim on power Doppler US (A). Contrast-enhanced computed tomography (CT) with a hypovascularized, hypodense metastasis in the left hepatic lobe from a new diagnosed colon cancer (arrow) (B). Fluorodeoxyglucose (FDG)-positron emission tomography (PET)-CT of a small breast cancer metastasis, which shows a high FDG-uptake and was only hardly detectable on CT alone (C). Cystic hepatic metastasis of a pancreatic cancer with high, cyst-like signal on T2-weighted MR images, but irregular tumor margins (D). Multiple, diffuse infiltrating hepatic metastasis of a breast cancer with an intermediate hyperintense signal on a T2-weighted MR sequence (E). Multiple hepatic metastasis of a colon cancer with "target sign" appearance on postcontrast T1-weighed MRI with fat suppression (F).

of colorectal cancer). However, conventional US is hampered by low sensitivity and specificity, and additional CE US may be helpful to improve lesion detection and characterization. Based on their vascular pattern, hepatic metastases may exhibit, on real-time CE US, a suspici-ous early rim enhancement with central hypovascularization ("target-sign"), diffuse hypovascularization, or diffuse hypervascularization with "wash-out" phenomena.[10,11]

Hepatic metastases also show varying appearances on CT, which is widely performed for detection and follow-up of metastases in portal-venous phase "whole body" examinations. On noncontrast CT, metastasis mostly appear only slightly hypodense to isodense and can be invisible.[47,48] A minority of hepatic metastases contain hyperdense calcifications (e.g., from adenocarcinomas of the colon or ovary). Cystic metastases (e.g., from ovarian or pancreatic cancer) can demonstrate water-like densities (<20 HU) but normally show contrast-enhancing components (e.g., septations or thickened walls). On dynamic CE CT scans, hypovascularized metastases predominantly appear hypodense in the portal-venous phase (Figure 10-6B), with possible peripheral rim enhancement, representing angiogenic tissue, desmoplastic changes and/or compressed adjacent liver parenchyma. Hypervascularized metastases (e.g., from renal cell carcinoma, breast cancer, thyroid tumors, melanoma, endocrine pancreatic tumors, carcinoid tumors, or pheochromocytoma) can demonstrate strong enhancement in the arterial phase, fading to an isodense appearance in the portal-venous phase. Thus, for hypervascular tumors, it is critical to obtain arterial and portal-venous phase imaging. Moreover, hepatic metastases can show, in response to effective treatment, a heterogeneous enhancement with hypodense necrotic areas or, in the best-case scenario, complete necrosis without detectable contrast enhancement. A combination of CT with FDG-PET (e.g., FDG-PET-CT for metastases of colorectal cancer, melanoma, or breast cancer [Figure 10-6C]) or a combination of CT with SPECT (e.g., SPECT/CT) for metastasis of neuroendocrine colon and pancreas tumors (NETs) or thyroid carcinomas can be beneficial for detection, localization, characterization, and treatment monitoring in a "whole body" fashion.[16,17] However, data from FDG-PET-CT and SPECT/CT for imaging of hepatic metastases are limited and seem to be indicated as second-line modalities to be used on a case-by-case basis.

MRI has been shown to be highly sensitive and specific for imaging of hepatic metastases without exposure to ionizing radiation. Generally, on MRI, most metastases appear heterogeneous and moderate hyperintense on T2-weighted and moderately hypointense on T1-weighted images (Figure 10-6E).[38,48] Cystic metastases (e.g., from ovarian or pancreatic cancer) could demonstrate a cyst-like appearance with a high signal on T2-weighted sequences but normally show contrast-enhancing components (e.g., septations or thickened walls) (Figure 10-6D).[49] On optional DWI, metastases frequently appear hyperintense, and this characteristic might be helpful for improved lesion detection. Central calcification can result in a signal reduction on T2-weighted images. Metastases from melanomas can still appear hyperintense on precontrast T1-weighted sequences due to their melanin content. Nevertheless, metastases with a high protein (mucinous) content or calcification (e.g., from adenocarcinomas of the colon or ovary) can also appear hyperintense on these sequences. During dynamic CE MRI, hypovascular metastases (e.g., from colorectal cancer) usually show an early peripheral rim enhancement, with only minor to no contrast enhancement of the center in the delayed phases (Figure 10-6F). Hypervascularized metastases can show strong arterial enhancement, similar to FNH, HCA, or HCC. Hepatobiliary-specific contrast agents can improve detection and characterization, particularly for small liver lesions (<1 cm), due to their ability to be seen in both dynamic-phase and hepatobiliary-phase imaging.[23,50] Metastases usually appear hypointense in the hepatobiliary phase, which could be helpful for detection of small lesions, while information from early postcontrast and T2-weighted imaging can be helpful for characterization. Metastases typically show no uptake of SPIOs due to the absence of Kupffer cells, and appear hyperintense on T2-weighted sequences.[27]

Hepatocellular Carcinoma

The diagnosis of HCC on US, CT, and MRI is challenging due to the common association of these tumors with chronic liver disease, and micronodular or macronodular cirrhotic liver texture changes.[51,52] Besides the "de novo" HCC occurrence, it is widely accepted that there is a continuous carcinogenic progression (hepatocarcinogenesis) of benign regenerating nodules to premalignant dysplastic nodules, to well differentiated, and then to poorly differentiated malignant HCC, which makes a noninvasive HCC diagnosis even more difficult.[53] HCC lesions can be solitary, multifocal, and diffuse. Solitary large masses preferentially occur in noncirrhotic liver, multifocal small lesions in cirrhotic liver.

Conventional US has only a low sensitivity and specificity for the diagnosis of HCC, even in cirrhotic livers with regenerative nodular changes.[54] HCC may appear hypoechogenic, isoechogenic, or hyperechogenic, with a thin hypoechogenic capsule on grayscale US (Figure 10-7A). On color Doppler US, intramural flow signals may be detectable. CE US allows improved real-time perfusion imaging with sensitivity and specificity similar to CE CT and MRI. On CE US, HCC typically shows arterial hyperperfusion with "wash-out" phenomena in the delayed images.[10,11] However, in some HCCs, only areas of pronounced delayed hypoenhancement, or prolonged enhancement without detectable "wash-out," may be detectable, which could make it difficult to distinguish HCCs from regenerative changes and dysplastic nodules, and in a first further step, multimodality imaging (e.g., additional dynamic CE MRI) might be indicated.

On noncontrast CT, small HCC lesions appear mostly isodense to slightly hypodense and might be masked by fibrotic changes in cirrhotic livers.[55] Larger HCCs usually show up as moderately hypodense masses, possibly with a thin pseudocapsule, and with areas of necrosis, fat, and/or calcification (Figure 10-7B). After contrast injection, HCCs classically show a strong arterial enhancement that tends to fade to an isodense appearance in the portal-venous phase, with relatively hypodense "wash-out" characteristics in delayed phases. Although small HCC lesions mostly show a strong, homogenous, and hyperdense arterial enhancement, larger HCC lesions (>5 cm) more commonly demonstrate a moderately heterogeneous arterial enhancement with

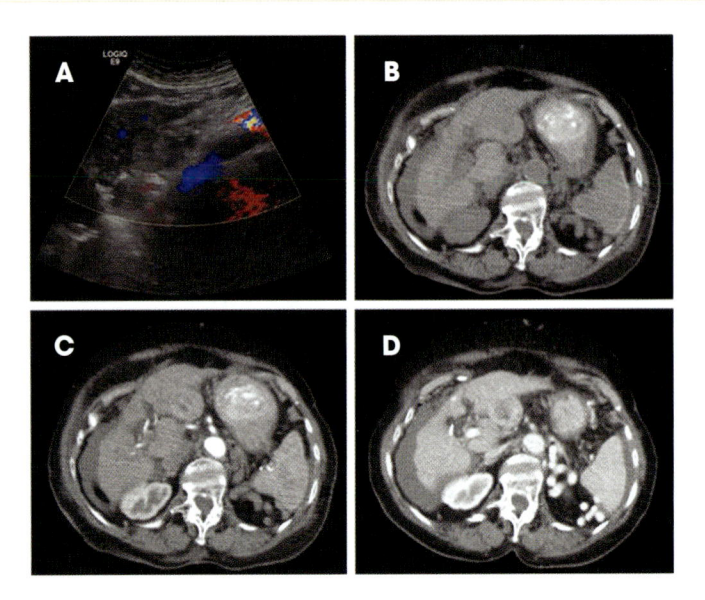

Figure 10-7: Hepatocellular carcinoma (HCC). HCC with a heterogeneous echogenicity and hypoechogenic rim to the adjacent cirrhotic liver parenchyma on ultrasonography (A). On the noncontrast computed tomography, the nodular HCC lesion demonstrate a slightly hypodense appearance with a small hypodense area at the tumor center, representing necrotic and/or fibrotic changes (B). After contrast injection, the HCC shows a moderate arterial enhancement (C) with central "wash-out" phenomena on the delayed contrast phase (D).

inhomogeneous "wash-out" in the delayed phases (Figure 10-7C and D).[52] In contrast, siderotic regenerative nodules may appear hyperdense on noncontrast CT scans, and dysplastic nodules can show arterial enhancement, but typically without detectable "wash-out" in the delayed phases. However, overlap of these imaging patterns with HCC has been reported. In HCC, an initial contrast-sparing vessel invasion with a delayed contrast-enhancing thrombus into the portal or hepatic veins could be seen.

On MRI, most HCCs appear slightly hyperintense on T2-weighted images and hypointense on T1-weighted images (Figure 10-8A–C), whereas small HCCs (<1–2 cm) may appear isointense on T2- and T1-weighted images and require dynamic CE MRI for detection.[56–58] In contrast, small siderotic regenerative nodules can show a moderately hypointense signal on T2-weighted images and dysplastic nodules can appear hyperintense on precontrast T1-weighted images (Figure 10-9A–C); but these imaging patterns do not allow accurate differentiation between early HCC and even small HCC lesions in dysplastic nodules ("nodule in nodule"). Within HCCs, areas of internal fat or hemorrhage can cause a high signal on precontrast T1-weighted images. Large HCCs frequently exhibit a heterogeneous texture on precontrast sequences, which is often, especially in diffuse HCC, poorly distinguishable from cirrhotic liver parenchyma, but sometimes best detectable at T2-weighted images. On CE MRI, HCC lesions show a variable pattern of enhancement owing to the histological and vascular nature of the lesions. HCCs classically show strong arterial enhancement with detectable "wash-out" in the late equilibrium phase, and a relative hypointense appearance compared with the surrounding liver parenchyma (Figure 10-8D–F). Large HCCs can show a moderately inhomogeneous arterial enhancement and even large diffuse HCC might be detectable only by "wash-out" phenomena in delayed contrast phases. In contrast, regenerative nodules

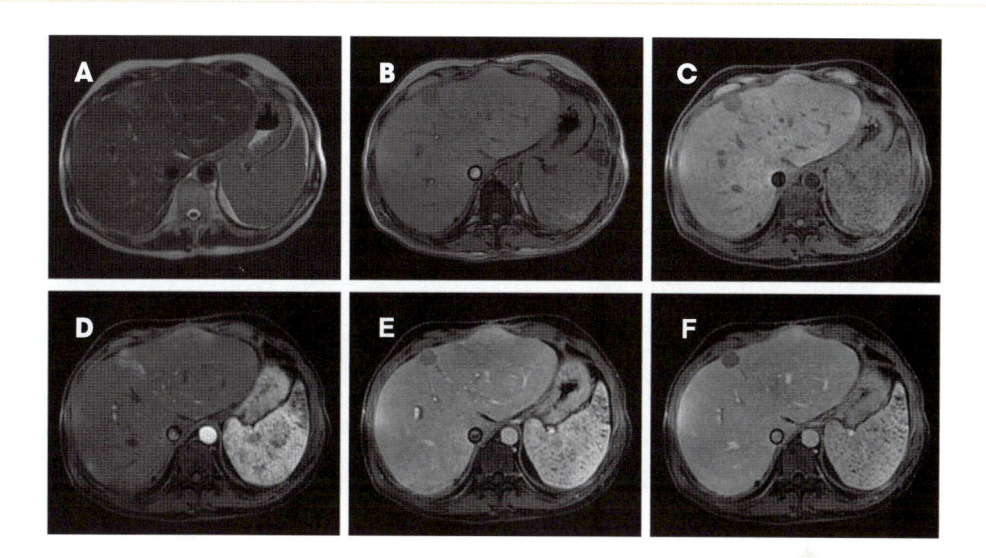

Figure 10-8: Hepatocellular carcinoma (HCC). HCC with a typical slightly hyperintense signal on T2-weighted (A) and hypointense signal on T1-weighted magnetic resonance images, without (B) and with fat suppression (C). On the dynamic contrast-enhanced magnetic resonance imaging (MRI), the HCC shows a classical strong arterial enhancement (D) with a rapid "wash-out" on the portal-venous phase (E), and a thin contrast-enhancing pseudocapsule on the delayed equilibrium phase (F). Moreover, the MRI allows a clearly visualization of the vessel invasion, whereas the tumor thrombus demonstrates in line an arterial enhancement with detectable "wash-out" phenomena.

usually show no arterial contrast enhancement, and dysplastic nodules may exhibit arterial enhancement but without detectable "wash-out" in delayed phases (Figure 10-9D–F). However, overlap of this perfusion pattern with the pattern for HCCs has been reported. First preliminary data suggest that hepatobiliary-specific MR contrast agents allow a more accurate diagnosis of regenerative nodules and dysplastic nodules with, based on their remaining hepatocytic function, detectable contrast uptake, whereas poorly differentiated HCCs usually demonstrate no contrast uptake in the hepatobiliary phase.[59] However, an accurate differentiation between benign dysplastic nodules and early well-differentiated HCCs seems to be also impossible by using hepatobiliary-specific MR contrast agents, and additional clinical studies are warranted. SPIO uptake by HCCs depends on the histological grade of the HCC and the presence of Kupffer cells.[27] Thus, HCCs may show moderate signal loss on T2-weighted images, but classically they appear still hyperintense compared with the surrounding liver parenchyma, which could improve the detection of even small HCC lesions.[27]

MRI provides additional HCC findings that may aid diagnosis and that could be helpful in assessing the prognosis. Thus, a thin pseudocapsule may be visible with a hyperintense signal on T2-weighted images, a hypointense signal on T1-weighted images and delayed hyperintense contrast enhan-cement (Figure 10-8F). An irregular tumor margin seems to be related more to microvascular invasion and poor prognosis.[60] Moreover, macrovascular tumor invasion assessment is critical for tumor classification (e.g., using the TNM system) and optimal treatment evaluation (Figure 10-8). Tumor infiltration into the portal vein is more common than invasion into hepatic veins. Tumor thrombus appears mostly hypointense on T2-weighted images and early postcontrast T1-weighted images, with detectable contrast enhancement in portal-venous phases and possible "wash-out" at delayed imaging. Vessel invasion is a typical finding for HCCs (less frequently

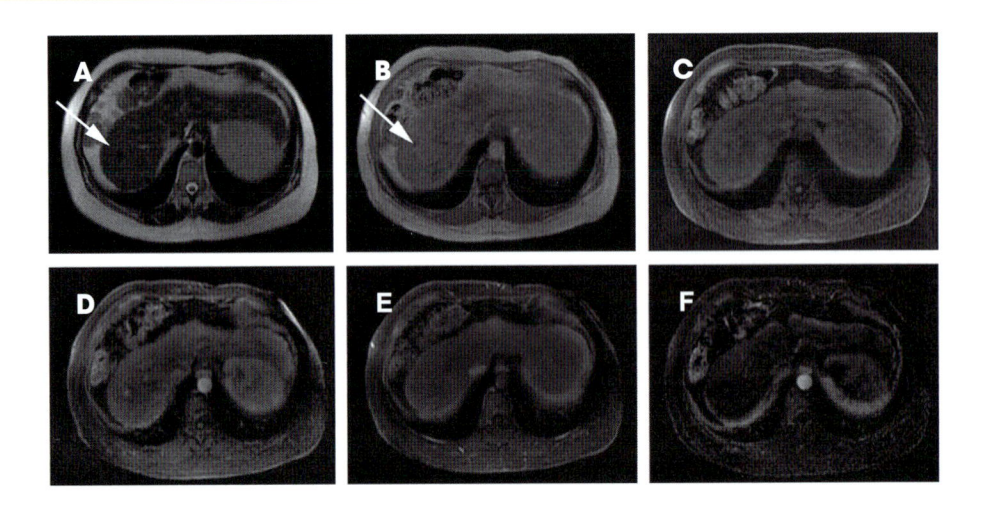

Figure 10-9: Regenerative nodule. Siderotic regenerative nodule in a cirrhotic liver with a slightly hypointense signal on the T2-weighted image (A) and hyperintense signal on precontrast T1-weighted images without (B) and with fat suppression (C). After contrast injection, the regenerative nodule shows no real arterial contrast enhancement (D), as compared with the subtracted image (F). On the delayed phase also, no suspicious "wash-out" was detectable (E).

in combined hepatocholangiocarcinoma) and can be helpful in a few cases for the differential diagnosis of peripheral cholangiocarcinoma.

Fibrolamellar Carcinoma

Fibrolamellar carcinomas (FLCs), which sometimes are called fibrolamellar HCCs, show a distinct imaging pattern compared to conventional HCCs. FLCs usually appear as well-defined, lobulated, larger masses (>5 cm) and may exhibit intrahepatic satellite lesions. In about half of patients, a central scar with radial septa and central calcification can be noticed. At the time of diagnosis, one can frequently observe regional nodal metastasis or, less commonly, pulmonary metastasis.

On conventional US, FLCs usually appear as lobulated, moderately hyperechogenic masses.[61] FLCs show a mostly heterogeneous texture with areas of necrosis and/or hemorrhage, and a central hyperechogenic scar with possible shadowing caused by calcifications. In a case report, CE US showed a strong arterial hyperperfusion with early centripedal filling in the portal-venous phase, and a rapidly centrifugal "wash-out" during late phase imaging, whereas the central irregular region showed only minor to no enhancement.[62]

On noncontrast CT, FLCs typically appear as a large, well-delineated, lobulated, heterogeneous, and hypodense mass with a pronounced hypodense irregular central scar and, possibly, areas of calcification and/or necrosis.[61,63] After contrast injection, FLCs usually show an inhomogeneous arterial enhancement with irregular hypodense central areas. In portal-venous phase, the mass fades to an isodense or hypodense appearance, whereas the central scar exhibits a more delayed enhancement.

On MRI, most FLCs appear heterogeneous and hyperintense on T2-weigthed images and slightly hypointense on T1-weighted images, whereas the central scar appears hypointense on T2- and T1-weighted images (in contrast to the central scar of FNHs which have a hyperintense signal on T2-weighted images).[63] On dynamic CE MRI, FLCs show a strong heterogeneous arterial enhancement, which fades to a more homogeneous enhancement in late phases and a moderate "wash-out" in delayed phases. The central scar usually exhibits a partially delayed enhancement. For hepatobiliary-specific contrast agents and SPIOs, there are only limited data available, but it seems that most FLCs show, based on their histological differentiation, no substantial uptake of these substances.[63]

Cholangiocarcinoma

Cholangiocarcinomas can be classified based on their location as intra- or extrahepatic tumors. Intrahepatic tumors are usually divided into peripheral cholangiocarcinoma, when arising peripherally to the secondary bifurcation of the left or right bile duct, and in hilar cholangiocarcinoma, when arising from the central intrahepatic bile ducts. Extrahepatic cholangiocarcinoma may occur proximally or distally, and are ordinarily separated from ampullary carcinoma of the ampulla of Vater (distal common bile duct at the head of the pancreas and duodenum). On the other hand, cholangiocarcinoma can also be categorized based on their macroscopic manifestations as mass forming, periductal infiltrating, and intraductally growing tumors. Periductal infiltrating cholangiocarcinoma of the perihilar intrahepatic and extrahepatic bile ducts (Klatskin tumor) are clinically classified by Bismuth-Corlette categories. Periductal infiltrating and intraductally growing cholangiocarcinomas normally induce relative early bile duct obstruction with proximal biliary dilation and may be clinically diagnosed by jaundice. Peripheral intrahepatic cholangiocarcinomas are often diagnosed late as large lobular liver masses with only some dilated peripheral bile ducts. At this late tumor stage, liver parenchyma atrophy and capsular retractions of the peripheral liver segments can frequently be observed due to encasement of the bile ducts and portal vein branches.

On conventional US, large mass-forming peripheral cholangiocarcinomas appear mostly as heterogeneous and hyperechogenic, whereas smaller peripheral and perihilar cholangiocarcinomas appear mostly isoechogenic and can be obscured (Figure 10-10A).[64,65] Intraductally growing cholangiocarcinomas occur as a circumscribed stricture or intraluminal polypoid masses. In case of tumor-related bile duct stenosis or obstruction, grayscale US may clearly show the proximal bile duct dilation and tumorous transition zone. However, additional Doppler US could be helpful to distinguish bile ducts

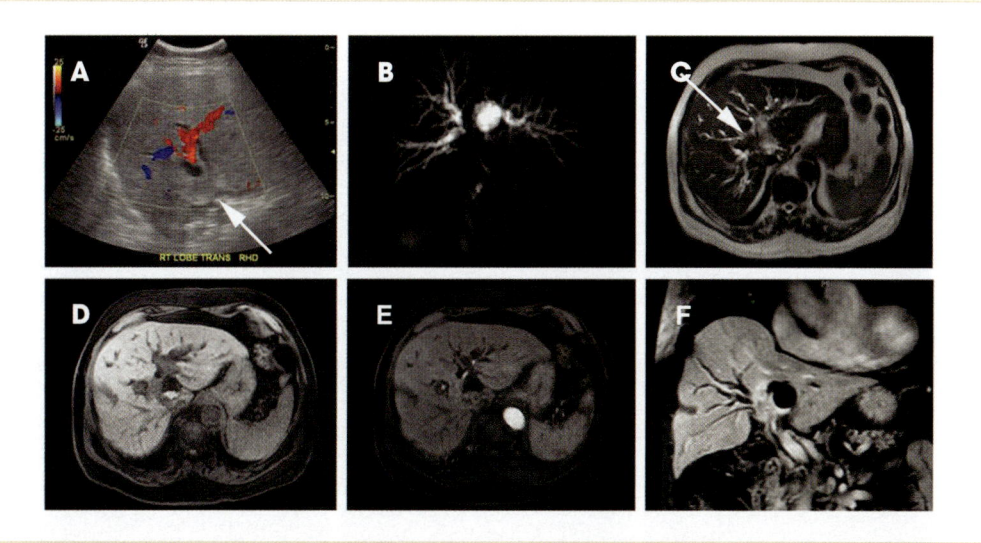

Figure 10-10: Cholangiocarcinoma. Small, periductal infiltrating cholangiocarcinoma at the liver hilus (Klatskin tumors) with a compression of the central bile duct system and an isoechogenic appearance on ultrasonography (A). The MR cholangiopancreatography demonstrates noninvasively the perihilar compression with dilatation of the intrahepatic bile ducts (B). On the anatomic T2-weighted sequence the cholangiocarcinoma appears isointense (C) with a hypointense signal on the T1-weighted image (D). The contrast-enhanced magnetic resonance imaging demonstrates a typical initial moderate, rim-like enhancement (E) with a widely homogenous hyperintense contrast enhancement on the delayed image after 5 min (F).

from adjacent vascular structures and may reveal unspecific intratumoral perfusion. On CE US, large cholangiocarcinomas (>3 cm) show mostly in the arterial phase a peripheral rim enhancement and less commonly a diffuse heterogeneous hyperperfusion or hypoperfusion, whereas small tumors (<3 cm) preferentially show a moderate homogeneous hyperperfusion.[66,67] In portal-venous and late phase imaging, most cholangiocarcinomas can be delineated as hypoenhancing lesions due to the purely intravascular distribution of the microbubbles and, discordantly to CT and MRI, missing late contrast enhancement in the fibrous tumor stroma.

Noncontrast CT usually demonstrates peripheral cholangiocarcinomas as well-delineated, slightly hypodense masses with some dilated peripheral bile ducts and possible granular calcifications (Figure 10-11A).[68] Intraductal and periductal cholangiocarcinomas may only be suspected because of an unclear cholestasis or a diffuse mass at the liver hilus. On CE CT, peripheral cholangiocarcinomas typically show an early peripheral rim enhancement with progressively delayed centripetal accumulation and a hyperdense heterogeneous appearance in extreme late phases (>10 min). Periductal cholangiocarcinomas can show in small tumors a more homogeneous, and in larger tumors a more heterogeneous initially rim-like, delayed enhancement. Intraductal cholangiocarcinomas might be detected by an intraluminal contrast-enhancing polypoid soft tissue. Therefore, three-dimensional MPR may be beneficial, and could improve the depiction of intraluminal masses and/or semicircular or circular bile duct thickening. Moreover, initial data showed that in unclear strictures associated with primary sclerosing cholangitis, FDG-PET-CT might be helpful in the differentiation of benign and malignant obstruction.[69] Otherwise, invasive ERCP diagnosis supported by FISH should be discussed.

On MRI, intrahepatic cholangiocarcinomas usually appear as large lobulated masses with a slightly hyperintense signal on T2-weighted images and a moderately hypointense signal on T1-weighted images (Figure 10-11B and C).[68] Large tumors typically show a heterogeneous texture with areas of fibrosis and/or necrosis. During dynamic CE MRI,

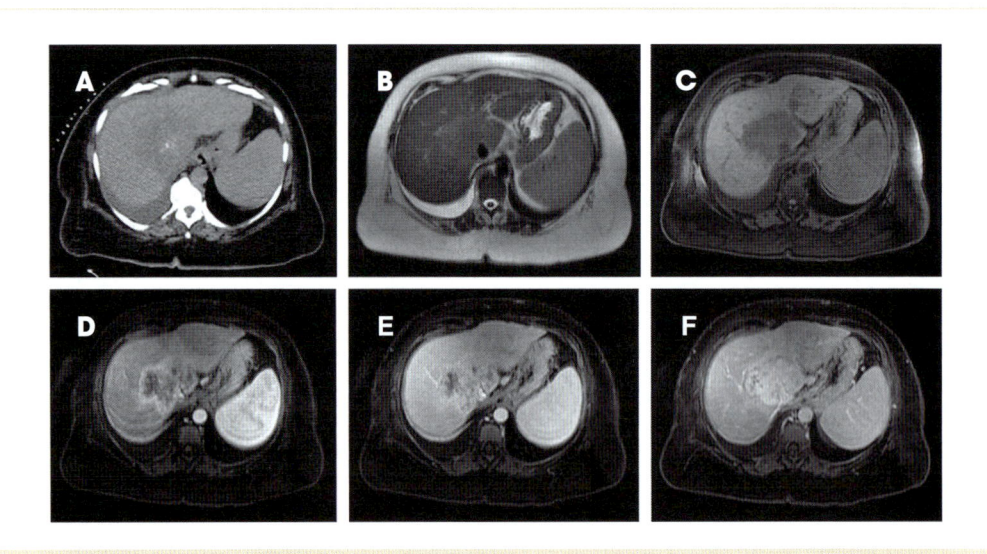

Figure 10-11: Cholangiocarcinoma. Large, mass-forming cholangiocarcinoma with a typical slightly hypodense appearance and some granular calcifications on the noncontrast computed tomography (A). On magnetic resonance imaging, the cholangiocarcinoma appears as a large lobulated masses with a slightly hyperintense signal on T2-weighted images (B) and a moderately hypointense signal on T1-weighted images (C). After contrast injection, the cholangiocarcinoma shows a classical moderate, peripheral rim enhancement on the arterial phase (D) with progressive centripetal enhancement on the equilibrium phase (E), and persistent enhancement in the fibrotic tumor tissue on late phases after 20 min (F).

larger cholangiocarcinomas initially show, for the most part, a moderate peripheral rim enhancement with progressive centripetal increases and delayed persistent enhancements (>10 min) (Figure 10-11D and F). Regions of fibrosis (e.g., the central scar) may even exhibit a late enhancement of extracellular MR contrast agents, whereas areas with cystic or necrotic changes show no enhancement. Periductal infiltrating and intraductally growing tumors can most clearly be depicted by MRCP sequences showing the stricture with associated obstruction, whereas the anatomic T2- and T1-weighted images (with fat suppression after gadolinium injection) reveal the complete tumor size and infiltration of surrounding structures (Figure 10-10).[20] On dynamic CE MRI, these smaller tumors have a more homogeneous, initial rim-like, delayed peak enhancement (Figure 10-10E and F). Cholangiocarcinomas show no substantial uptake of hepatobiliary-specific MR contrast agents and appear relatively hypointense on hepatobiliary phase imaging. On the contrary, dual-contrast MRI with SPIO and nonspecific extracellular MR contrast agents could provide suppression of the normal liver with a improved diagnosis of intrahepatic cholangiocarcinomas on delayed enhanced imaging in the late accumulation phase.

Gallbladder Carcinoma

Gallbladder carcinomas can be depicted as a thickening of the gallbladder wall, focal eccentric mass of the gallbladder wall or polypoid intraluminal mass of the gallbladder. However, at the time of diagnosis in most of the cases large gallbladder carcinomas directly infiltrating the gallbladder fossa and the adjacent liver with focal lymphadenopathy can be noticed.

On conventional US, gallbladder carcinomas can appear as gallbladder wall thickening and masses (Figure 10-12A), or larger polypoid mucosal lesions (>1 cm). Doppler US could demonstrate a detectable hypervascularization. CE US could show an arterial hyperperfusion with "wash-out" phenomena in delayed phases.[66]

Noncontrast CT may show gallbladder stones or calcification of the gallbladder wall (porcelain gallbladder) as possible risk factors. On CE CT, gallbladder carcinomas typically appear as hypovascular infiltrating masses with only moderate contrast enhancement (Figure 10-12B).[70]

On MRI, gallbladder carcinomas appear as slightly hyperintense masses on T2-weighted images with an isointense to hypointense signal on T1-weighted images (Figure 10-12C).[71] On postcontrast T1-weighted images (with fat suppression) a moderate contrast enhancement can usually be noticed, whereas the wall thickening is best seen on T2-weighted images. Infiltration of the gallbladder fossa and adjacent structures (e.g., liver or biliary tract), and regional lymph node metastasis can be clearly seen on postcontrast T1-weighted images with fat suppression and may be helpful for the differential diagnosis (e.g., gallbladder sludge with posture change and absence of contrast enhancement, benign gallbladder polyps [commonly ≤0.6 cm], adenomyomatosis with typically fundal focal wall thickening and multiple intramural microcysts, or (chronic) cholecystitis with a clinical history).[70,72]

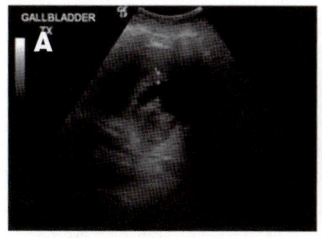

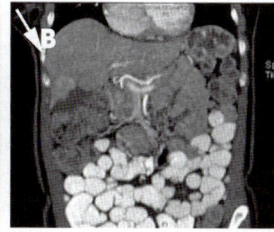

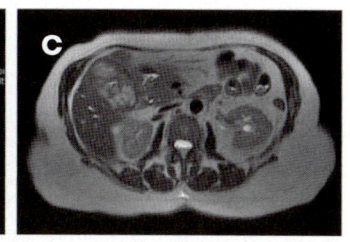

Figure 10-12: Gallbladder carcinoma. Gallbladder carcinomas can be depicted by ultrasonography, computed tomography, or magnetic resonance imaging as a circumscribed thickening of the gallbladder wall (A), focal eccentric mass (B; arrow), or intraluminal mass of the gallbladder with direct infiltration of the liver (C).

Lymphoma

Hepatic lymphoma (predominantly secondary NHL, less frequently infiltration of advanced Hodgkin lymphoma) can appear as a solitary mass, multiple lesions or diffuse infiltration. On the contrary, lymphonodular manifestation of lymphomas at the liver hilus with secondary compression and/or infiltration of the bile duct system and liver capsule can occur.

Conventional US usually shows a hypoechogenic mass or multiple hypoechogenic lesions in focal lymphomas and a diffuse hypoechogenic liver texture in diffuse lymphomas, which can sometimes be difficult to detect and only a measurable hepatomegaly might be indicative. On CE US, hepatic lymphomas may show an inhomogeneous moderate enhancement in the arterial phase with heterogeneous hypoperfusion in late phases.[73]

On noncontrast CT, hepatic lymphomas could appear as a focal hypodense mass or show a diffuse isodense to hypodense appearance of the liver parenchyma with, in some cases, measurable hepatomegaly.[47] On dynamic CE CT scans, hepatic lymphomas may exhibit a moderate heterogeneous enhancement in the arterial phase and appear as isodense to hypodense masses in delayed phases. However, diagnosis of a secondary hepatic lymphoma is often challenging on CT alone and FDG-PET-CT might be helpful.[74] FDG-PET-CT allows a clear visualization and quantification the metabolic activity for detection and follow-up monitoring.

On MRI, focal hepatic lymphoma usually appears moderately hyperintense on T2-weighted images and moderately hypointense on T1-weighted images, whereas diffuse hepatic manifestations tend to be more isointense and are only poorly detectable.[38] On postcontrast T1-weighted images, hepatic lymphomas usually show a moderately inhomogeneous enhancement.

Less Common Malignant Tumors

Rare malignant hepatobiliary tumors include, among others, biliary cystadenocarcinoma, hepatic epithelioid hemangioendothelioma, and hepatic angiosarcoma.

Biliary Cystadenocarcinoma

Biliary cystadenocarcinomas have an appearance that is similar to benign biliary cystadenomas on US, CT, and MRI (see biliary cystadenoma). Thus, no reliable radiological differentiation between these two entities seems possible, and only progressive disease with large soft tissue components may be indicative for a biliary cystadenocarcinoma.

Hepatic Epithelioid Hemangioendothelioma and Hepatic Angiosarcoma

Hepatic epithelioid hemangioendothelioma and hepatic angiosarcoma (i.e., hemangiosarcoma) are rare mesenchymal tumors of vascular origin, whereas epithelioid hemangioendothelioma represents a low-grade to intermediate-grade malignancy between benign hemangioma and angiosarcoma.[75,76] Both tumors mostly show a multifocal appearance but can also occur as a solitary lesion or as a diffuse micronodular infiltrating mass in the liver. For a typical multifocal hepatic epithelioid hemangioendothelioma, most of the lesions are peripherally located with bulging of the liver capsule and, possibly, associated capsular retraction adjacent to the lesion. At the time of diagnosis of hepatic angiosarcoma, lung, bone, and/or regional lymph node metastasis can commonly be noticed.

Conventional US predominantly shows multiple hypoechogenic lesions for both entities, but imaging appearance can also vary from isoechogenic to hyperechogenic; and in diffuse infiltrating tumors, only a heterogeneous liver texture may be detectable.

Noncontrast CT may show well-defined hypodense lesions to complex inhomogeneous masses with calcifications.

On MRI, hepatic epithelioid hem-angioendotheliomas and angiosarcomas appear mostly hyperintense on T2-weigthed and DWI images, and hypointense on T1-weighted images.

On dynamic CE US, CT, and MRI, both tumors demonstrate varying perfusion patterns, which can mimic hemangioma. In the presence of a hemangioma untypical nodular enhancement, chaotic central perfusion discordant to the "blood pool" and missing centripetal complete filling on delayed phases, diagnosis of a hepatic epithelioid hemangioendothelioma or angiosarcoma should be considered. Hepatic epithelioid hemangioendothelioma classically has a "target sign" appearance due to a central nonenhancing sclerotic area, a peripheral hypervascularized rim of cellular proliferation and a thin nonenhancing ring of compressed normal liver parenchyma. However, imaging and perfusion patterns for both tumors are unspecific and the differential diagnosis to exclude other malignant lesions (e.g., hepatic metastasis and lymphoma) may be difficult or impossible.

References

1. Foley WD. BRL, Gay SB, et al. Liver lesion characterization. *Am Coll Radiol (ACR)*. 2006;1–7. www.acr.org [online publication].
2. Izumi N. Diagnostic and treatment algorithm of the Japanese society of hepatology: a consensus-based practice guideline. *Oncology*. 2010;78(suppl 1):78–86.
3. Bruix J, Sherman M. Management of hepatocellular carcinoma. *Hepatology*. 2005;42:1208–1236.
4. Bruix J, Sherman M, Llovet JM, et al. Clinical management of hepatocellular carcinoma. Conclusions of the Barcelona-2000 EASL conference. European Association for the Study of the Liver. *J Hepatol*. 2001;35:421–430.
5. Floriani I, Torri V, Rulli E, et al. Performance of imaging modalities in diagnosis of liver metastases from colorectal cancer: a systematic review and meta-analysis. *J Magn Reson Imaging*. 2010;31:19–31.
6. Wernecke K, Rummeny E, Bongartz G, et al. Detection of hepatic masses in patients with carcinoma: comparative sensitivities of sonography, CT, and MR imaging. *AJR Am J Roentgenol*. 1991;157:731–739.
7. Seitz K, Strobel D, Bernatik T, et al. Contrast-Enhanced Ultrasound (CEUS) for the characterization of focal liver lesions - prospective comparison in clinical practice: CEUS vs. CT (DEGUM multicenter trial). Parts of this manuscript were presented at the Ultrasound Dreilandertreffen 2008, Davos. *Ultraschall Med*. 2009;30:383–389.
8. Seitz K, Bernatik T, Strobel D, et al. Contrast-enhanced ultrasound (CEUS) for the characterization of focal liver lesions in clinical practice (DEGUM Multicenter Trial): CEUS vs. MRI--a prospective comparison in 269 patients. *Ultraschall Med*. 2010;31:492–499.
9. Trillaud H, Bruel JM, Valette PJ, et al. Characterization of focal liver lesions with SonoVue-enhanced sonography: international multicenter-study in comparison to CT and MRI. *World J Gastroenterol*. 2009;15:3748–3756.
10. Wilson SR, Burns PN. Microbubble-enhanced US in body imaging: what role? *Radiology*. 2010;257:24–39.
11. Strobel D, Seitz K, Blank W, et al. Tumor-specific vascularization pattern ofliver metastasis, hepatocellular carcinoma, hemangioma and focal nodular hyperplasia in the differential diagnosis of 1,349 liver lesions in contrast-enhanced ultrasound (CEUS). *Ultraschall Med*. 2009;30:376–382.
12. Wilson SR, Kim TK, Jang HJ, Burns PN. Enhancement patterns of focal liver masses: discordance between contrast-enhanced sonography and contrast-enhanced CT and MRI. AJR *Am J Roentgenol*. 2007;189:W7–W12.
13. Oliva MR, Saini S. Liver cancer imaging: role of CT, MRI, US and PET. *Cancer Imaging* 2004;4 (Spec No A):S42–S46.
14. Hammerstingl RM, Vogl TJ. Abdominal MDCT: protocols and contrast considerations. *Eur Radiol*. 2005;15(suppl 5):E78–E90.
15. Lee SW, Kim HJ, Park JH, et al. Clinical usefulness of 18F-FDG PET-CT for patients with gallbladder cancer and cholangiocarcinoma. *J Gastroenterol*. 2010;45:560–566.
16. Niekel MC, Bipat S, Stoker J. Diagnostic imaging of colorectal liver metastases with CT, MR imaging, FDG PET, and/or FDG PET/CT: a meta-analysis of prospective studies including patients who have not previously undergone treatment. *Radiology*. 2010;257:674–684.
17. Apostolova I, Riethdorf S, Buchert R, et al. SPECT/CT stabilizes the interpretation of somatostatin receptor scintigraphy findings: a retrospective analysis of inter-rater agreement. *Ann Nucl Med*. 2010;24:477–483.
18. Glockner JF. Hepatobiliary MRI: current concepts and controversies. *J Magn Reson Imaging*. 2007;25:681–695.
19. Low RN. Abdominal MRI advances in the detection of liver tumours and characterisation. *Lancet Oncol*. 2007;8:525–535.
20. Vogl TJ, Schwarz WO, Heller M, et al. Staging of Klatskin tumours (hilar cholangiocarcinomas): comparison of MR cholangiography, MR imaging, and endoscopic retrograde cholangiography. *Eur Radiol*. 2006;16:2317–2325.
21. Tanimoto A, Lee JM, Murakami T, et al. Consensus report of the 2nd International Forum for Liver MRI. *Eur Radiol*. 2009;19(suppl 5):S975–S989.
22. Gandhi SN, Brown MA, Wong JG, et al. MR contrast agents for liver imaging: what, when, how. *Radiographics*. 2006;26:1621–1636.

23. Seale MK, Catalano OA, Saini S, et al. Hepatobiliary-specific MR contrast agents: role in imaging the liver and biliary tree. *Radiographics*. 2009;29:1725–1748.
24. Papanikolaou N, Prassopoulos P, Eracleous E, et al. Contrast-enhanced magnetic resonance cholangiography versus heavily T2-weighted magnetic resonance cholangiography. *Invest Radiol*. 2001;36:682–686.
25. Lim JS, Kim MJ, Jung YY, Kim KW. Gadobenate dimeglumine as an intra-biliary contrast agent: comparison with mangafodipir trisodium with respect to non-dilated biliary treedepiction. *Korean J Radiol*. 2005;6:229–234.
26. Tschirch FT, Struwe A, Petrowsky H, et al. Contrast-enhanced MR cholangiography with Gd-EOB-DTPA in patients with liver cirrhosis: visualization of the biliary ducts in comparison with patients with normal liver parenchyma. *Eur Radiol*. 2008;18:1577–1586.
27. Reimer P, Balzer T. Ferucarbotran (resovist): a new clinically appro-ved RES-specific contrast agent for contrast-enhanced MRI of the liver: properties, clinical development, and applications. *Eur Radiol*. 2003;13:1266–1276.
28. Nishie A, Tajima T, Ishigami K, et al. Detection of hepatocellular carcinoma (HCC) using super paramagnetic iron oxide (SPIO)-enhanced MRI: added value of diffusion-weighted imaging (DWI). *J Magn Reson Imaging*. 2010;31:373–382.
29. Macarini L, Marini S, Milillo P, et al. Double-contrast MRI (DC-MRI) in the study of the cirrhotic liver: utility of administering Gd-DTPA as a complement to examinations in which SPIO liver uptake and distribution alterations (SPIO-LUDA) are present and in the identification and characterisation of focal lesions. *Radiol Med*. 2006;111:1087–1102.
30. Shin DS, Jeffrey RB, Desser TS. Pearls and pitfalls in hepatic ultrasonography. *Ultrasound Q*. 2010;26:17–25.
31. Ma X, Holalkere NS, Kambadakone RA, et al. Imaging-based quantification of hepatic fat: methods and clinical applications. *Radiographics*. 2009;29:1253–1277.
32. Bartolotta TV, Taibbi A, Midiri M, Lagalla R. Focal liver lesions: contrast-enhanced ultrasound. *Abdom Imaging*. 2009;34:193–209.
33. Horton KM, Bluemke DA, HrubanRH, et al. CT and MR imaging of benign hepatic and biliary tumors. *Radiographics*. 1999;19:431–451.
34. Schwartz LH. DDR. Magnetic resonance imaging of the liver, pancreas, and biliary tract. In: Blumgart LH, ed. *Surgery of the Liver, Biliary Tract and Pancreas*. Philadelphia, PA: Saunders Elsevier, 2007:306–321.
35. Stark DD, Felder RC, Wittenberg J, et al. Magnetic resonance imaging of cavernous hemangioma of the liver: tissue-specific characterization. *AJR Am J Roentgenol*. 1985;145:213–222.
36. van den Esschert JW, van Gulik TM, Phoa SS. Imaging modalities for focal nodular hyperplasia and hepatocellular adenoma. *Dig Surg*. 2010;27:46–55.
37. Bartolotta TV, Taibbi A, Matranga D, et al. Hepatic focal nodular hyperplasia: contrast-enhanced ultrasound findings with emphasis on lesion size, depth and liver echogenicity. *Eur Radiol*. 2010;20:2248–2256.
38. Semelka RC, Martin DR, Balci NC. Focal lesions in normal liver. *J Gastroenterol Hepatol*. 2005;20:1478–1487.
39. Grazioli L, Morana G, Kirchin MA, Schneider G. Accurate differentiation of focal nodular hyperplasia from hepatic adenoma at gadobenate dimeglumine-enhanced MR imaging: prospective study. *Radiology*. 2005;236:166–177.
40. Paley MR, Mergo PJ, Torres GM, Ros PR. Characterization of focal hepatic lesions with ferumoxides-enhanced T2-weighted MR imaging. *AJR Am J Roentgenol*. 2000;175:159–163.
41. Zheng RQ, Zhang B, Kudo M, et al. Imaging findings of biliary hamartomas. *World J Gastroenterol*. 2005;11:6354–6359.
42. Hohmann J, Loddenkemper C, Albrecht T. Assessment of a biliary hamartoma with contrast-enhanced sonography using two different contrast agents. *Ultraschall Med*. 2009;30:185–188.
43. Luo TY, Itai Y, Eguchi N, et al. Von Meyenburg complexes of the liver: imaging findings. *J Comput Assist Tomogr*. 1998;22:372–378.
44. Lewin M, Mourra N, Honigman I, et al. Assessment of MRI and MRCP in diagnosis of biliary cystadenoma and cystadenocarcinoma. *Eur Radiol*. 2006;16:407–413.
45. Prasad SR, Wang H, Rosas H, et al. Fat-containing lesions of the liver: radio-logic-pathologic correlation. *Radiographics*. 2005;25:321–331.
46. Wang Z, Xu HX, Xie XY, et al. Imaging features of hepatic angiomyolipomas on real-time contrast-enhanced ultrasound. *Br J Radiol*. 2010;83:411–418.
47. Winston C. TJ. Computed tomography of the liver, biliary tract and pancreas. In: Blumgart LH, ed.

48. Kanematsu M, Kondo H, Goshima S, et al. Imaging liver metastases: review and update. *Eur J Radiol.* 2006;58:217–228.
49. Lombardo DM, Baker ME, Spritzer CE, et al. Hepatic hemangiomas vs metastases: MR differentiation at 1.5 T. *AJR Am J Roentgenol.* 1990;155:55–59.
50. Bluemke DA, Sahani D, Amendola M, et al. Efficacy and safety of MR imaging with liver-specific contrast agent: U.S. multicenter phase III study. *Radiology.* 2005;237:89–98.
51. Coakley FV, Schwartz LH. Imaging of hepatocellular carcinoma: a practical approach. *Semin Oncol.* 2001;28:460–473.
52. Baron RL, Peterson MS. From the RSNA refresher courses: screening the cirrhotic liver for hepatocellular carcinoma with CT and MR imaging: opportunities and pitfalls. *Radiographics.* 2001;21(Spec No):S117–S132.
53. Hussain SM, Zondervan PE, IJzermans JN, et al. Benign versus malignant hepatic nodules: MR imaging findings with pathologic correlation. *Radiographics.* 2002;22:1023–1036; discussion 1037–1029.
54. Lee JY, Choi BI, Han JK, et al. State-of-the-art ultrasonography of hepatocellular carcinoma. *Eur J Radiol.* 2006;58:177–185.
55. Sakabe K, Yamamoto T, Kubo S, et al. Correlation between dynamic computed tomographic and histopathological findings in the diagnosis of small hepatocellular carcinoma. *Dig Surg.* 2004;21:413–420.
56. Kelekis NL, Semelka RC, Worawattanakul S, et al. Hepatocel-lular carcinoma in North America: a multiinstitutional study of appearance on T1-weighted, T2-weighted, and serial gadolinium-enhanced gradient-echo images. *AJR Am J Roentgenol.* 1998;170:1005–1013.
57. Kadoya M, Matsui O, Takashima T, Nonomura A. Hepatocellular carcinoma: correlation of MR imaging and histopathologic findings. *Radiology.* 1992;183:819–825.
58. Ito K. Hepatocellular carcinoma: conventional MRI findings including gadolinium-enhanced dynamic imaging. *Eur J Radiol.* 2006;58:186–199.
59. Kudo M. Will Gd-EOB-MRI change the diagnostic algorithm in hepatocellular carcinoma? *Oncology.* 2010;78(suppl 1):87–93.
60. Kuo MD, Gollub J, Sirlin CB, et al. Radiogenomic analysis to identify imaging phenotypes associated with drug response gene expression programs in hepatocellular carcinoma. *J Vasc Interv Radiol.* 2007;18:821–831.
61. McLarney JK, Rucker PT, Bender GN, et al. Fibrolamellar carcinoma of the liver: radiologic-pathologic correlation. *Radiographics.* 1999;19:453–471.
62. Mandry D, Bressenot A, Galloy MA, et al. Contrast-enhanced ultrasound in fibro-lamellar hepatocellular carcinoma: a case report. *Ultraschall Med.* 2007;28:547–552.
63. Ichikawa T, Federle MP, Grazioli L, et al. Fibrolamellar hepatocellular carcinoma: imaging and pathologic findings in 31 recent cases. *Radiology.* 1999;213:352–361.
64. Bloom CM, Langer B, Wilson SR. Role of US in the detection, characterization, and staging of cholangiocarcinoma. *Radiographics.* 1999;19:1199–1218.
65. Hann LE, Greatrex KV, Bach AM, et al. Cholangiocarcinoma at the hepatic hilus: sonographic findings. *AJR Am J Roentgenol.* 1997;168:985–989.
66. Xu HX. Contrast-enhanced ultrasound in the biliary system: potential uses and indications. *World J Radiol.* 2009;1:37–44.
67. Chen LD, Xu HX, Xie XY, et al. Intrahepatic cholangiocarcinoma and hepatocellular carcinoma: differential diagnosis with contrast-enhanced ultrasound. *Eur Radiol.* 2010;20:743–753.
68. Chung YE, Kim MJ, Park YN, et al. Varying appearances of cholangiocarcinoma: radiologic-pathologic correlation. *Radiographics.* 2009;29:683–700.
69. Berr F, Wiedmann M, Mossner J, et al. Detection of cholangiocarcinoma in primary sclerosing cholangitis by positron emission tomography. *Hepatology.* 1999;29:611–613.
70. Levy AD, Murakata LA, Rohrmann CA, Jr. Gallbladder carcinoma: radiologic-pathologic correlation. *Radiographics.* 2001;21:295–314; questionnaire, 549–255.
71. Schwartz LH, Black J, Fong Y, et al. Gallbladder carcinoma: findings at MR imaging with MR cholangiopancreatography. *J Comput Assist Tomogr.* 2002;26:405–410.
72. Corwin MT, Siewert B, Sheiman RG, Kane RA. Incidentally detected gallbladder polyps: is follow-up necessary?—Long-term clinical and US analysis of 346 patients. *Radiology.* 2011;258:277–282.
73. Foschi FG, Dall'Aglio AC, Marano G, et al. Role of contrast-enhanced ultrasonography in primary hepatic lymphoma. *J Ultrasound Med.* 2010;29:1353–1356.

74. Seshadri N, Ananthasivan R, Kavindran R, et al. Primary hepatic (extranodal) lymphoma: utility of [(18)F]fluorodeoxyglucose-PET/CT. *Cancer Imaging*. 2010;10:194–197.

75. Lyburn ID, Torreggiani WC, Harris AC, et al. Hepatic epithelioid hemangioendothelioma: sonographic, CT, and MR imaging appearances. *AJR Am J Roentgenol*. 2003;180:1359–1364.

76. Koyama T, Fletcher JG, Johnson CD, et al. Primary hepatic angiosarcoma: findings at CT and MR imaging. *Radiology*. 2002;222:667–673.

CHAPTER 11

Diagnostic and Therapeutic Approaches for Patients With Liver Tumors

Kimberly Moore Dalal

The workup and treatment of biliary and hepatic neoplasms have undergone major improvements in the last decade. Improvements in ultrasound (US), computed tomography (CT), and magnetic resonance imaging (MRI) scans have allowed for the accurate identification of extremely small lesions and precise delineation of the relationship of benign and malignant tumors to major vasculature. There is now a greater ability to diagnose disease and establish treatment plans, including surgical therapies. Improvements in invasive procedures such as endoscopic retrograde cholangiopancreatography (ERCP), percutaneous transhepatic cholangiography (PTC), and laparoscopic surgery allow for these minimally invasive strategies to evolve from diagnostic and palliative procedures to definitive therapies. Even difficult tumors, such a cholangiocarcinomas, can now be treated with potential for long-term survival.

The choice of tests and the appropriate sequence have become increasingly important in an effort to streamline workups, arrive expeditiously at a therapeutic plan, and minimize cost. As an increasing number of patients are being scanned for various reasons, having a reasoned approach at workup of incidentalomas will be important in diagnosing early cancers for effective treatment and dismissing benign lesions to avoid both morbid invasive procedures and alleviate patient anxiety.

In this chapter, we introduce clinical algorithms for workup and treatment of common symptoms and signs of hepatic and biliary disease as well as the incidentally discovered gallbladder mass and liver mass. In each section, we discuss the most important clinical entities responsible, followed by algorithms for workup of particular presentations that combine efficiency with cost considerations.

Clinical Presentation of Biliary and Liver Disease

Many patients with biliary and liver disease present for medical attention with nonspecific symptoms such as weight loss, malaise, or indigestion. These patients will then be identified to have biliary or liver pathologic findings by blood tests or diagnostic imaging modalities.

Right Upper Quadrant Pain

The symptom of right upper quadrant (RUQ) pain is not specific for biliary and liver disease, although hepatobiliary disease must be entertained in any patient presenting with pain in this quadrant. Patients presenting with RUQ pain and hemodynamic instability must be considered to have a ruptured liver malignancy, ruptured adenoma, or a ruptured liver from trauma. In parts of the world where hepatitis and cirrhosis are endemic, hepatocellular carcinoma (HCC) can present as rupture and abdominal catastrophe in as many as 10% of patients. Rapid history and physical examination should be directed at eliciting symptoms, signs, or history of hepatitis and cirrhosis. Along with urgent resuscitation, imaging by US or CT should be obtained to look for hemoperitoneum and liver mass. An emergent angiogram can be diagnostic and allow for arterial embolization as the definitive life-saving procedure.

RUQ pain and sepsis can be associated with stone disease complicated by infection. However, the differential diagnosis includes peptic ulcer disease, biliary dyskinesia, colonic diverticulitis, pancreatitis, hepatitis, appendicitis, gallbladder malignancy, or hepatic malignancy. We will discuss the workup and treatment of gallstones, segregating the algorithms according to the presence of jaundice, sepsis, and other symptoms.

Jaundice

Jaundice is the only symptom that is pathognomonic for biliary or hepatic disease. The color of the skin is accompanied usually by acholic stool and dark urine with pruritus occurring in one-third of patients. The causes of jaundice can be prehepatic, hepatic, or posthepatic. Most prehepatic and hepatic causes of jaundice, such as hemolysis or acute hepatitis, are not surgical diseases and lack signs of biliary dilatation on imaging. The causes of jaundice that are surgical diseases are generally those with biliary obstruction and ductal dilatation. We will discuss in detail the workup of obstructive jaundice.

The majority of patients who present to a surgeon with a hepatobiliary problem have already undergone a partial workup including imaging for their chief complaint. Following are the common clinical scenarios and their workups.

Jaundice Without Gallstones

In patients presenting with jaundice and no gallstones, the most important consideration is to determine whether the jaundice is obstructive. Nonobstructive jaundice includes most of the prehepatic and hepatic causes of jaundice, which are generally not surgical diseases. The causes of obstructive jaundice should be segregated according to the level of obstruction: only intrahepatic ductal dilatation or both intrahepatic and extrahepatic ductal dilatation. By obtaining fractionated bilirubin levels, hepatitis serologies, and US, the patient with jaundice and without gallstones can be referred to a hepatologist for treatment of medical causes of jaundice or be sent for appropriate workup according to the algorithms in Figures 11-1 and 11-2.

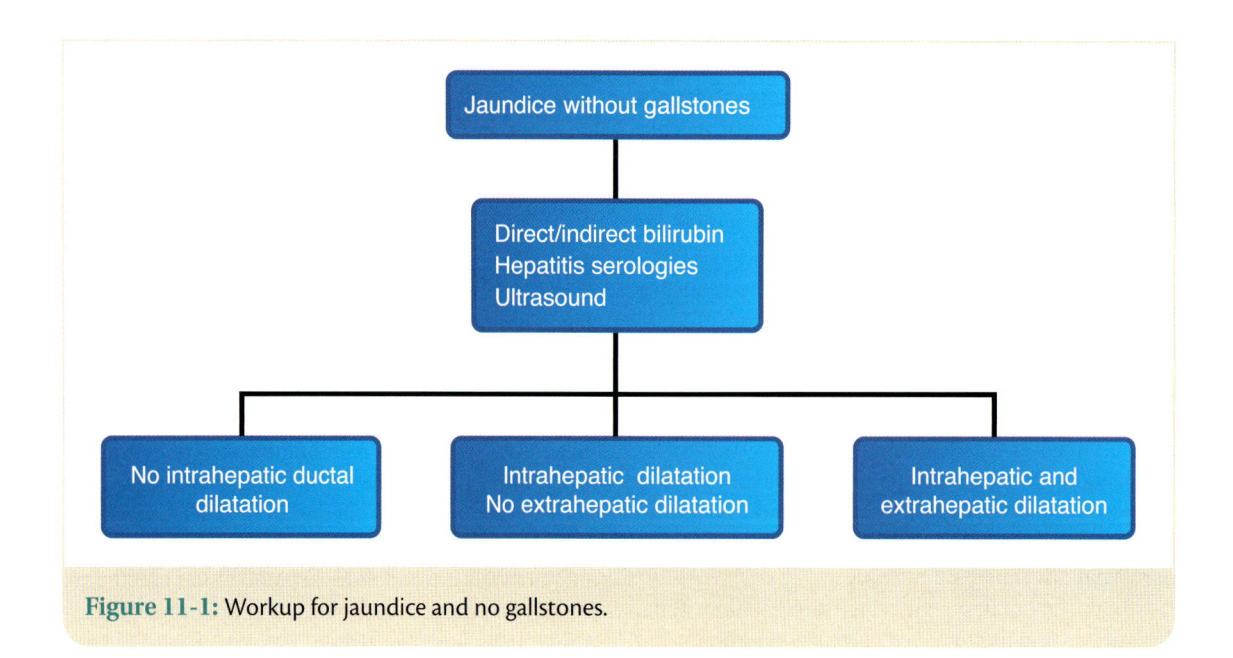

Figure 11-1: Workup for jaundice and no gallstones.

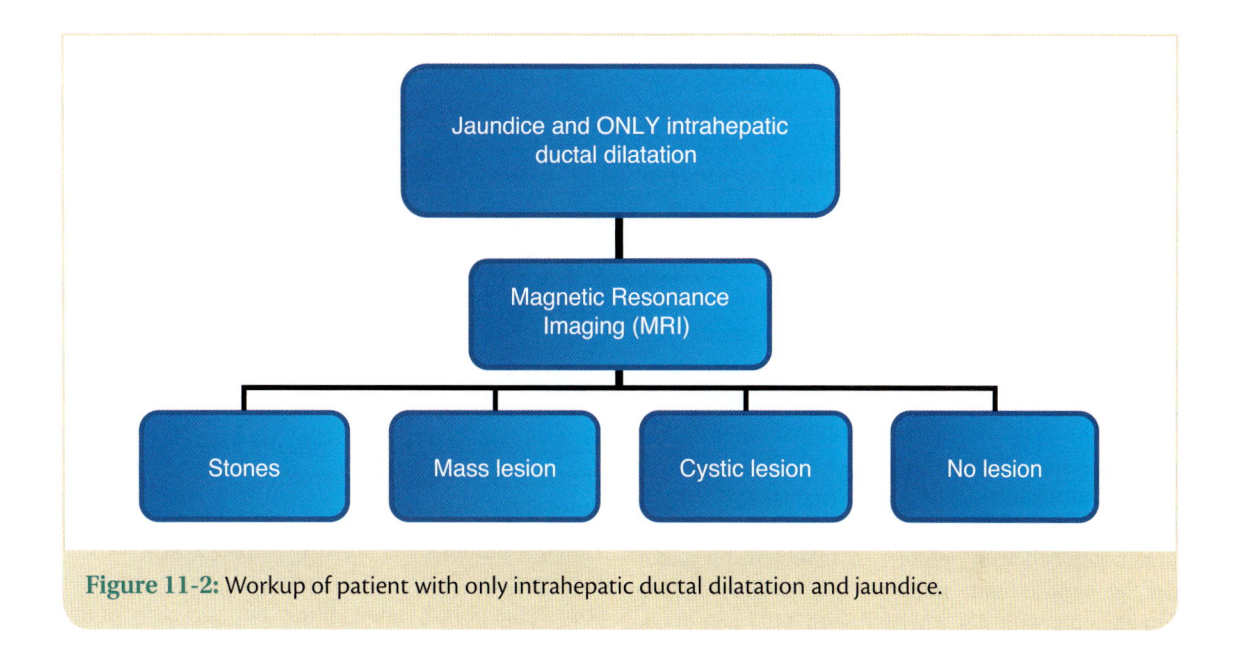

Figure 11-2: Workup of patient with only intrahepatic ductal dilatation and jaundice.

Patients With Only Intrahepatic Ductal Dilatation

Patients with dilated intrahepatic ducts but without extrahepatic ductal dilatation have obstruction in the liver or high in the porta hepatis. The etiology of high biliary obstruction includes stones, mass lesions, cystic lesions, or primary sclerosing cholangitis (PSC). Stones can cause common duct obstruction or intrahepatic ductal obstruction. Mass lesions may be identified either as parenchymal lesions in the liver impinging on the bile duct or as masses growing from the biliary tree; the workup of the hepatic parenchymal lesion is discussed later in this chapter. The most common neoplastic cause of biliary obstruction and jaundice is HCC, which can produce jaundice by both extrinsic compression and intraductal extension. Cholangiocarcinoma may also cause jaundice from high biliary obstruction, either as a small tumor occurring at the hilus of the liver (Klatskin tumor) or as a large one extending to involve the hilus (intrahepatic cholangiocarcinoma). Cystic lesions, both benign and malignant, may also cause jaundice. Benign simple cysts that are large can obstruct the biliary tree, although the more common reason is rapid expansion from a spontaneous bleed into the cyst. Complex cysts resulting from infection (e.g., echinococcal) or malignancy (cystadenocarcinoma) can also cause jaundice. Finally, high biliary stricture can be caused by multifocal or unifocal sclerosing cholangitis. The multifocal form will usually be suspected because of multiple strictures seen on imaging and confirmed by liver biopsy. The unifocal form often is diagnosed only after an extensive liver and biliary resection for presumed cholangiocarcinoma.

Diagnostic Imaging Of Patients With Intrahepatic Ductal Dilatation

The imaging test of choice for a high bile duct obstruction is magnetic resonance cholangiopancreatography (MRCP). This is a specialized MRI in which images are obtained in 1.5-mm overlapping slices. Images are also acquired at various phases after contrast injection to produce a detailed depiction of the arterial, portal venous, and hepatic venous vessels. The most important images are those acquired as delayed T2 images that highlight slow-flowing fluid, which appears very bright relative to the low intensity of the surrounding tissues, allowing for precise depiction of the obstructed biliary tree. An MRCP can identify larger intrahepatic ducts and extrahepatic ducts in 80%–100% of nondilated ducts and 90%–100% in dilated ducts. There is an overall sensitivity and specificity of MRCP of 95% and 97%, respectively, in the diagnosis of biliary obstruction.

Between US and MRCP, most high bile duct obstructions can be diagnosed and even subcentimeter hilar cholangiocarcinomas can be identified with confidence, as shown in Figure 11-3. These masses can be obscured by indwelling biliary stents. Nondecompressed dilated ducts can point to the area of obstruction and highlight the mass involved. Ductal dilatation in both hepatic lobes with a contracted gallbladder or nonunion of the right and left hepatic ducts suggests a Klatskin tumor. In addition to visualization of the tumor, the relationship of the tumor with adjacent vasculature, such as the portal veins and hepatic arteries, can be determined. Importantly, hepatic lobar atrophy indicates either long-standing ductal obstruction of that side or portal venous involvement by tumor. Moreover, atrophy on one side combined with vascular involvement by tumor on the opposite side indicates unresectable cancer. For patients with PSC, MRCP with MRI can document the segmental extent of ductal involvement in surgical planning, assess for intrahepatic metastases, and identify aberrant ductal anatomy. MRCP has the capability to evaluate the bile ducts above and below a structure while identifying intrahepatic mass lesions.

PTC and drainage are preferred over ERCP as palliation for jaundice secondary to high biliary obstruction. Endoscopic decompression is often difficult in high biliary obstruction. In addition, because the liver is often segregated into multiple isolated segments by the obstruction, if ERCP is performed and the liver is incompletely drained, sepsis may ensue from the contaminated, but incompletely drained segments of liver. PTC may be employed late in the disease process because dilated ducts often aid in the diagnosis.

Patients with Both Intrahepatic and Extrahepatic Ductal Dilatation

A finding of extrahepatic ductal dilatation indicates distal bile duct obstruction.

Diagnostic Imaging of Patients with Intrahepatic and Extrahepatic Ductal Dilatation

Patients should be imaged by either ERCP or CT angiography, a thin-cut CT with images acquired not only at the portal venous phase but also early in the arterial phase. The advantage is that it allows visualization and characterization of small periampullary tumors. If stones are noted by MRCP or US, an ERCP should be performed to extract the stone. If a mass is noted, the enhancement pattern may provide clues for diagnosis. A very hypervascular mass may suggest a neuroendocrine tumor. A small mass at the tip of the dilated duct may suggest an ampullary adenoma or carcinoma. From a practical standpoint, however, the exact diagnosis of a resectable neoplasm is not necessary. Most mass lesions that cause painless jaundice will be cancerous or precancerous and deserve resection. The major exceptions are lesions that result from pancreatitis. Thus, the scans should be scrutinized for signs of chronic pancreatitis, such as pancreatic calcifications or pseudocysts. If pancreatitis is suspected, observation may be the most appropriate treatment.

CT angiogram or MRI can assess for local vascular invasion by tumor and for signs of liver and peritoneal metastases. If the periampullary cancer is not resectable, a biopsy should be performed to confirm diagnosis and to aid in planning palliative therapy.

Often jaundice and extrahepatic biliary obstruction will be found with no appreciable mass lesion. ERCP and endoscopic ultrasound (EUS) should be performed to assess the characteristics of the stricture and to determine the presence of a small mass in the head of the pancreas, which can be biopsied by EUS guidance. If it is a long stricture, cancer in

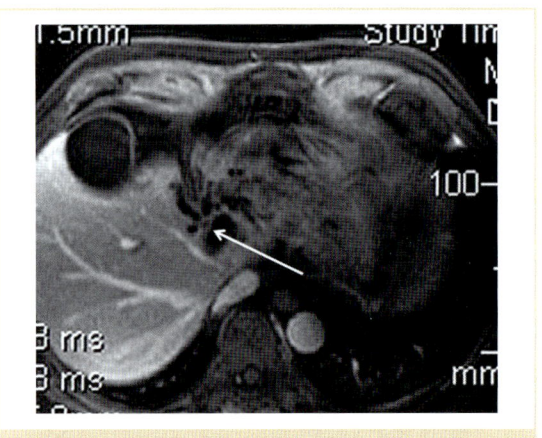

Figure 11-3: Magnetic resonance cholangiopancreatography demonstrating small cholangiocarcinoma (arrow) at hilus of liver.

the form of distal cholangiocarcinoma or pancreatic cancer must be suspected. Short strictures with no appreciable mass may be observed for a short time. ERCP allows placement of biliary stents for palliation (see Figure 11-4).

Gallbladder Polyps

Most gallbladder masses are benign and are found in up to 5% of patients assessed by US. There is no association between the presence of gallbladder polyps and the typical risk factors for gallstones. They are rarely described in children and occur either as a primary disorder or in association with Peutz–Jeghers syndrome, metachromatic leukodystrophy, or pancreato-biliary malunion. Benign polyps can be classified into epithelial tumors (adenoma), mesenchymal tumors (fibroma, lipoma, and hemangioma), or pseudotumors (cholesterol polyps, inflammatory polyps, and adenomyoma).

The majority are cholesterol polyps, which are histologically mucosal deposits of lipid-laden macrophages. These lesions, which comprise 90% of benign lesions, are characteristically multiple (>3), small, and have an intact mucosa. Adenomyomatosis, characterized by mucosal overgrowth, thickening of the muscle wall, and intramural diverticula, does not involve adenomatous changes in the gallbladder epithelium and is not premalignant. The only polyp with malignant potential is the adenoma, which is rare with an incidence of 0.5%. The frequency of the adenoma-to-adenocarcinoma sequence is unknown; however, the risk of malignancy is related to polyp size. In general, gallbladder adenocarcinoma is significantly more likely to be found in polyps of patients older than 50 years, solitary and sessile in nature, and > 1.0 cm in diameter[1] (Figure 11-5).

Gallbladder polyps may cause biliary pain, due to prolapse of the polyp into Hartmann's pouch or from cystic duct obstruction from a detached piece of

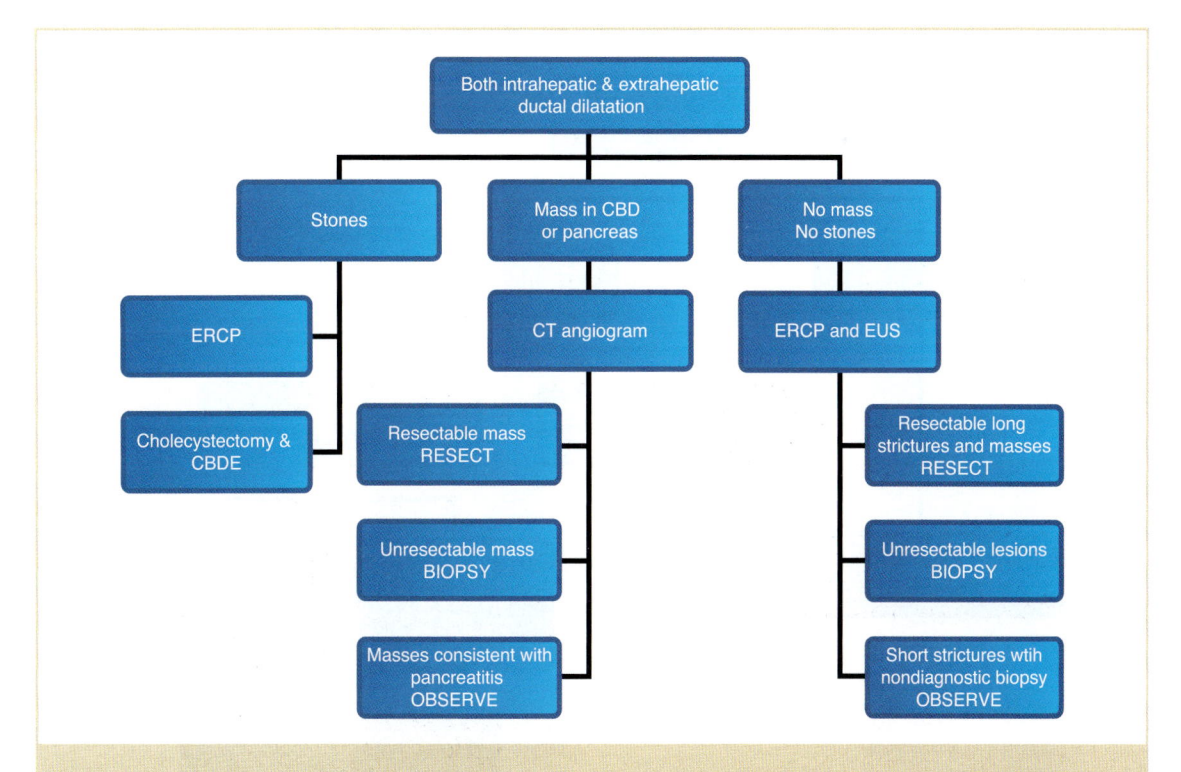

Figure 11-4: Treatment of a patient with both intrahepatic and extrahepatic ductal dilatation. CBDE, common bile duct exploration, ERCP, endoscopic retrograde cholangiopancreatography; CT, computed tomography; EUS, endoscopic ultrasound.

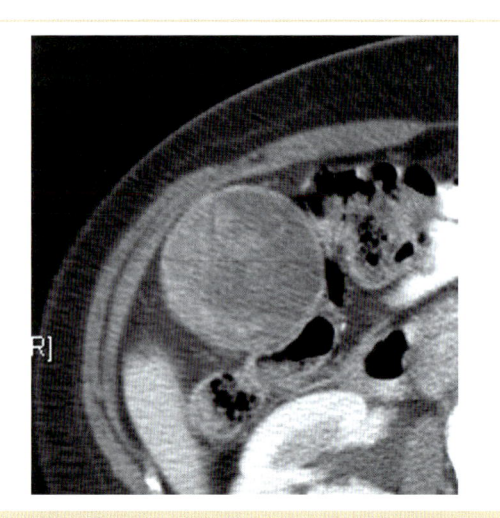

Figure 11-5: Sessile gallbladder polyp seen as incidental finding on computed tomography scan. Also worrisome is the mass that is brightly enhanced on this scan after contrast injection.

Diagnostic Imaging of Patients with Gallbladder Polyps

Figure 11-6 demonstrates the workup and treatment of patients with gallbladder polyps, recognizing that polyps <1 cm followed by imaging have a low rate of subsequent diagnosis of cancer. Abdominal US is the study of choice due to its >90% sensitivity and specificity rates in diagnosing small polyps. CT is most useful in patients with suspected gallbladder cancer as it can provide staging information such as liver involvement or metastasis.

Treatment of Patients with Gallbladder Polyps

Gallbladder cancer has a very poor prognosis, with median survival of <6 months for incompletely resected lesions; therefore, for any solitary

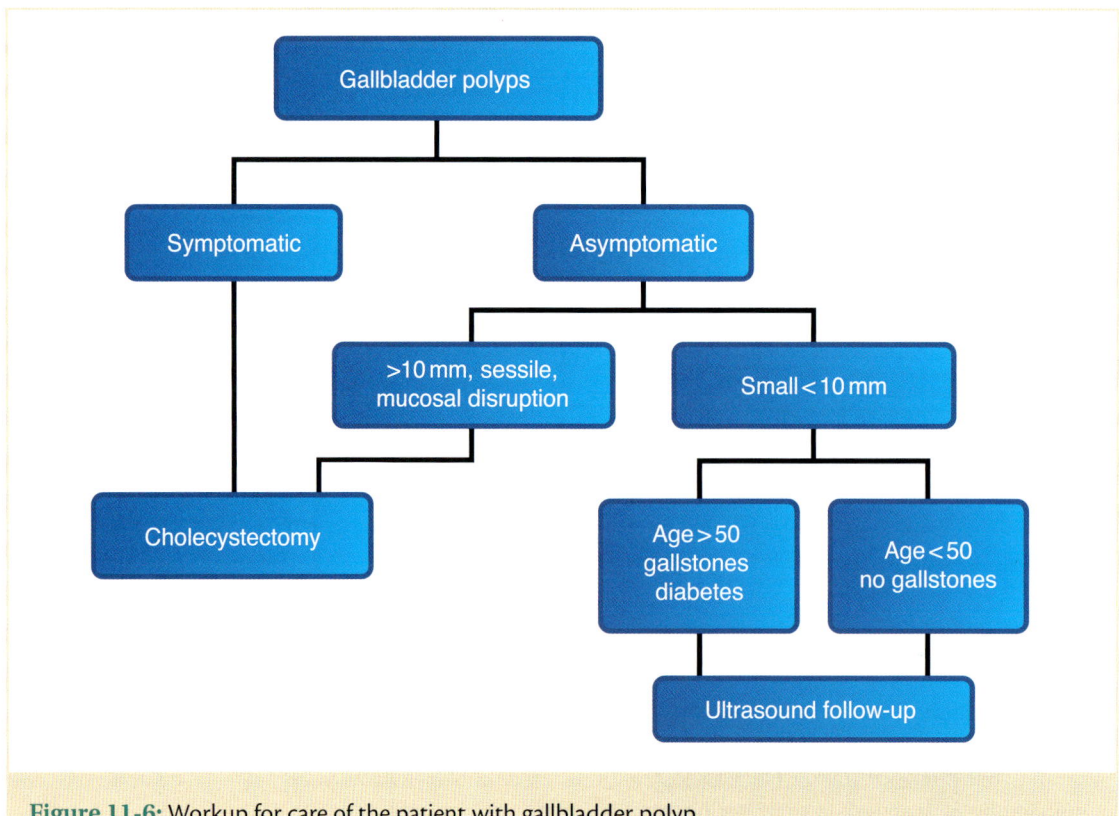

Figure 11-6: Workup for care of the patient with gallbladder polyp.

polyp >1.0 cm in diameter, the recommended treatment is open cholecystectomy to include removal of the entire connective tissue layers of the gallbladder bed to expose the liver surface. This aggressive approach is also considered for patients with fewer than three polyps, regardless of size, or denuded mucosa. Patients should undergo preoperative staging with CT scan or EUS. For lesions >1.8 cm, an extended cholecystectomy with lymph node dissection and partial hepatic resection of the gallbladder bed should be considered.

For patients with symptomatic polyps (i.e., biliary colic, pancreatitis) or patients with polyps and concomitant gallstones, cholecystectomy should be performed because gallstones are a risk factor for gallbladder cancer in patients with gallbladder polyps. In addition, gallbladder polyps arising in the setting of PSC are frequently malignant and should be removed. Asymptomatic patients with polyps <1.0 cm should be followed up by US every six months for two examinations, then yearly; any suspicious findings or growth should result in cholecystectomy.

Liver Mass

Many patients are found to have liver masses on imaging performed as staging for a malignancy or as workup for a symptom, and increasingly more are discovered incidentally on imaging performed for another reason. It is most important to determine (1) whether there is a history of malignancy, (2) whether the lesion is new, and (3) what are the characteristics of the lesion.

Workup of Patients with History of Malignancy

A new hepatic lesion in a patient with a prior malignancy is assumed to be metastatic disease until proven otherwise. Appropriate serum tumor markers should be assayed to aid in diagnosis (e.g., carcinoembryonic antigen [CEA], CA19-9, CA15.3, CA125). On US, metastases from adenocarcinoma are often multiple and hypoechoic when compared with normal liver parenchyma. On triphasic (unenhanced, arterial, and portal venous phase) CT of the liver, metastatic liver lesions from the colon, stomach, and pancreas are usually lower attenuation in contrast to the brighter surrounding parenchyma. Hypervascular metastases, such as metastases from neuroendocrine tumors, renal cell cancer, breast cancer, thyroid cancer, melanoma, and sarcoma, rapidly enhance on the arterial phase. On MRI, metastatic lesions appear as low-signal areas on T1-weight images and moderately high signal on T2-weighted images. These metastases enhance and are best seen on arterial phase images with the characteristic feature of ring of enhancement after contrast administration and heterogeneous washout on delayed imaging. An MRI also assists in delineating vascular involvement and extrahepatic lesions. Figure 11-7 demonstrates the algorithm for workup and treatment of patients with liver mass and a history of malignancy.

Colorectal Cancer Metastases

Patients with a history of colorectal cancer (CRC) or neuroendocrine cancers are treated very differently than others because surgical resection and cytoreduction in these diseases have been proven to have survival benefit.

Diagnostic Imaging of Patients with History of Colorectal Cancer

For the patient with a history of CRC, staging includes helical CT and 18-fluorodeoxyglucose positron emission tomography (PET).[2] Metastatic CRC hepatic metastases are usually hypovascular on CT. PET scans can identify hypermetabolic CRC liver metastases and radiographically occult extrahepatic disease. A triple-phase contrast-enhanced CT and a PET scan significantly reduces the number of futile laparotomies when compared with CT only or the combined PET/CT without intravenous contrast, which decreases the detection of small metastases. Of note, chemotherapy may alter the sensitivity of PET for detecting metastases due to decreased metabolic activity. Preoperative liver MRI and intraoperative ultrasound (IOUS) are used to optimally assess number, size, and proximity of tumors to the portal vein, hepatic arteries, and hepatic veins as well as biliary structures. An MRI is particularly important in patients with steatohepatitis from chemotherapy in which the fatty liver may obscure liver metastases on CT. IOUS can identify subcentimeter metastases and detect unexpected tumors, resulting in modification of the proposed resection in over half of the patients undergoing segmental liver resection. Diagnostic

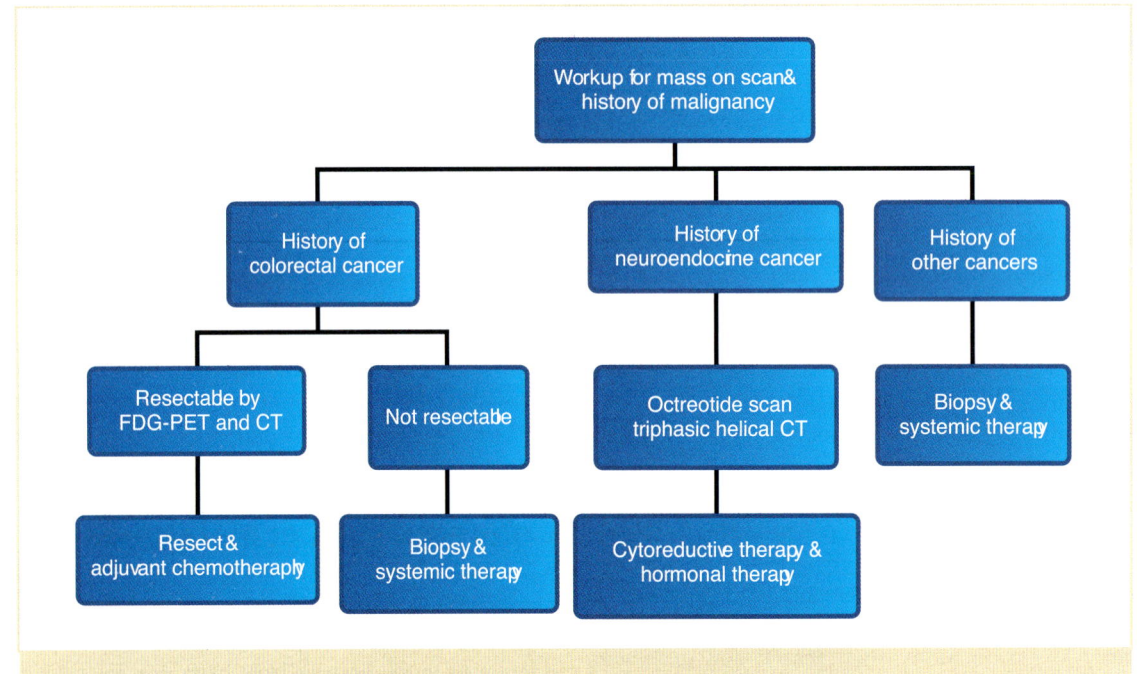

Figure 11-7: Workup for liver mass in patients with history of malignancies. FDG-PET, 18-fluorodeoxyglucose positron emission tomography; CT, computed tomography.

laparoscopy can be used to evaluate patients who may have peritoneal disease on preoperative imaging.

For new lesions with characteristic appearances of metastases in someone with a history of CRC, one may proceed to resection without a biopsy. If the lesions appear unresectable, a biopsy is performed to confirm stage IV disease before the patient is referred for chemotherapy (see Figure 11-7).

Treatment of Patients with History of Colorectal Cancer

Most surgeons aggressively approach hepatic CRC metastases. Surgical resection offers the greatest chance for cure in patients with liver-isolated CRC metastases, with five-year survival rates of 24%–58% and a surgical mortality rate <5%. Ten-year survivors following resection appear to be cured. Criteria for resectability have been expanded to include any patient in whom all disease can be resected with a negative margin and who has adequate hepatic reserve. Concurrent resection of hepatic and extrahepatic disease in well-selected patients has been associated with long-term survival. The primary tumor should be resected for cure. In addition, there is no difference in five-year overall survival or recurrence rates whether the tumor-free margin is 1–4 mm, 5–9 mm, or >10 mm. Absolute unresectability is defined as nontreatable extrahepatic disease, inability to tolerate surgery, involvement of >70% of the liver or six segments.[3] There should be no radiographic evidence of hepatic artery, major bile duct, main portal vein, or celiac/paraaortic lymph node involvement.

Neoadjuvant chemotherapy with FOLFOX (5-FU, leucovorin, oxaliplatin), CAPOX (5-FU, leucovorin, capecitabine), or FOLFIRI (5-FU, leucovorin, irinotecan) with or without bevacizumab or with cetuximab (for wild-type *K-ras* only) can downstage patients with initially unresectable colorectal hepatic metastases in 12%–33% of patients permitting a complete resection, leading to five-year survival rates of 30%–35%. Radiographic assessment should be performed at six-week intervals after starting chemotherapy. Importantly, radiographic completely responding lesions contain viable tumor, and resection is still necessary. A supermagnetic iron oxide–enhanced MRI may preoperatively detect sinusoidal obstruction "blue liver" in patients with oxaliplatin-containing regimens, which predisposes patients to postoperative complications.

Initial surgery, rather than neoadjuvant chemotherapy for medically fit patients with four or few lesions in the same hepatic lobe and no portal lymph node involvement, may be a reasonable approach, followed by six months of systemic chemotherapy containing oxaliplatin. Resection is preferred over local ablation strategies (cryosurgery, radiofrequency ablation [RFA], microwave ablation [MWA]). For incompletely resected metastatic disease, RFA/MWA or cryosurgery can be used. Staged resection is often used in bilobar disease, which may require sizeable hepatic resections, and this may be performed with or without portal vein embolization (PVE). If the future liver remnant is <20% in a patient with a normal liver or <40% in a cirrhotic liver, PVE should be considered. PVE is used to induce compensatory hypertrophy in the future liver remnant, which may decrease postoperative morbidity and mortality.[4] Four weeks after PVE, there can be an increase in liver volume of 10%–12%.[5] Volumetric assessment of the liver with CT imaging should be performed before PVE and before surgery.

Neuroendocrine Metastases

For a patient with a history of neuroendocrine tumor, workup consists of a triphasic helical CT and an octreotide scan. On CT, these tumors are hypervascular and enhance during the arterial phase images, confirming the diagnosis and determining the extent of hepatic disease. The degree of arterial enhancement also predicts the response of these lesions to treatment by arterial embolization. The octreotide scan provides whole-body assessment of disease and potential response to hormonal therapy. After staging, the patient can be treated by cytoreduction (surgery and/or ablation) and hormonal therapy.

History of Other Malignancy

For patients with a history of any other malignancy (e.g., gastric, pancreas, renal cell, breast, thyroid, melanoma), percutaneous needle biopsy should be performed after a triphasic helical CT or MRI is performed to rule out a hemangioma to prevent hemorrhage. Although some patients may undergo surgical treatment because of a favorable clinical course characterized by long disease-free interval, limited metastases, and response to systemic therapy, most patients will be treated only by systemic therapy.[6]

Workup of Patients with No History of Malignancy

In patients with no history of cancer, workup is directed at determining premalignant or malignant entities. Lesions may be congenital (simple cysts, choledochal cysts, polycystic disease, hemangioma, focal nodular hyperplasia [FNH]), infectious (echinococcal cysts, pyogenic abscesses, amebic abscesses), primary neoplasms (adenoma, HCC, intrahepatic cholangiocarcinoma), or metastatic disease.

A thorough history should be obtained, including questions directed at exposure to viral hepatitis or chemical injury to the liver, such as past blood transfusions, tattoos, illicit intravenous drug use, sexual promiscuity, alcohol use, past medications, and metabolic liver disease such as hereditary hemochromatosis, as etiologic factors for HCC. Patients should be asked about any symptoms of infection or travel history that may indicate other infectious causes for liver masses. Intrahepatic cholangiocarcinoma should be considered in patients with a liver mass in the setting of chronic cholestatic liver disease, such as PSC, longstanding choledochocele, intrahepatic lithiasis from parasitic diseases of the bile ducts, or exposure to thorotrast for radiologic procedures. Clinical features of liver disease such as pruritus, jaundice, spider telangiectasias, splenomegaly, gynecomastia, and testicular atrophy should be investigated. Hepatitis serologies and tumor markers such as α-fetoprotein (AFP), CA19-9, and CEA should be considered. The workup algorithm is outlined in Figure 11-8.

Diagnostic Imaging of Patients with No History of Malignancy

US is useful for determining whether the lesion is cystic or solid and can delineate septations within cysts. Widely available and noninvasive, US is helpful in screening patient with cirrhosis at three- to six-month intervals for the presence of HCC and detecting portal vein patency and vascular invasion in staging patients with HCC. Biopsy of hepatic lesions as well as RFA/MWA and cryoablation can be performed under US guidance.

The best test for characterization of a liver tumor is MRI.[7] Compared with CT, an MRI has superior

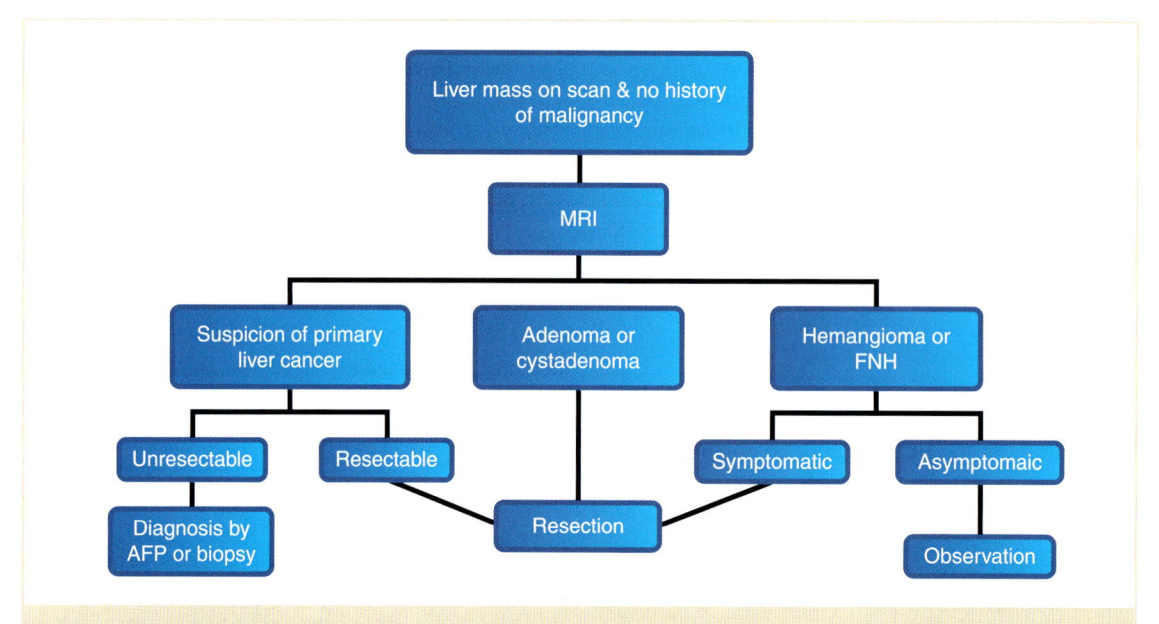

Figure 11-8: Workup for liver mass in patients with no history of prior malignancy. MRI, magnetic resonance imaging; FNH, fibronodular hyperplasia; AFP, α-fetoprotein.

lesion-to-liver contrast, without the use of ionizing radiation, and is more specific than CT for characterizing hemangiomas and focal fatty infiltration. An MRI is also useful for identifying hypervascular liver lesions, including hemangioma, FNH, adenoma, HCC, and hypervascular metastases, such as islet cell carcinoma, carcinoid tumors, thyroid tumors, renal cell carcinoma, and melanoma[8] (Table 11-1). On noncontrast T1-weighted images, water has a low-signal intensity (i.e., dark), whereas lesions with fat, protein, hemorrhage, and melanin are high in signal and appear bright. In-phase and out-of-phase T1-weighted images are used to detect fatty lesions, such as hepatic adenomas. On T2-weighted images, water has a high intensity and appears bright. Fat suppression, commonly performed on T2-weighted images, improves visualization of regions bordered by fat. Gadopentetate dimeglumine (Gd-BOPTA) is a dynamic contrast agent that improves the characterization on T1-weighted images and can help determine lesion vascularity and identify hemangiomas.[9] After administration of contrast, images are taken at 20 (arterial phase), 60 (portal venous), and 120 (equilibrium phase) seconds and sometimes at one hour after injection. Although allergic reaction are uncommon, there is a rare disorder called nephrogenic systemic fibrosis, which is seen in patients with moderate-to-severe kidney failure, and this can have chronic and unremitting course that may lead to death.

Hepatic Cystic Lesions

Most hepatic cysts are found incidentally and have a benign course. Simple cysts contain clear fluid that does not communicate with the intrahepatic biliary tree. More commonly found in the right lobe and in women, cysts may present with abdominal discomfort or nausea. Larger cysts are more likely to be symptomatic and cause complications such as hemorrhage, rupture, infection, or biliary obstruction.

Simple cysts must be differentiated from echinococcal cysts, cystadenomas, and cystadenocarcinomas. Large, complex cysts can be simple cysts that have undergone spontaneous hemorrhage or echinococcal cysts. Echinococcal cysts are caused by the larval form of *Echinococcus granulosus*, acquired from infected dogs. Often asymptomatic, they can cause symptoms due to enlargement or complications such as rupture into the biliary tree. For patients native to or have traveled to the Mediterranean or South America, an ELISA echinococcal serology test should be performed. The most

TABLE 11-1: MR Characteristics of Hypervascular Liver Masses

	T1 Weighted	T2 Weighted	Arterial Phase	Portal Venous Phase	Delayed Phase	1 h Delayed	Other
Hemangioma	↓	↑↑	↑	↑	↑	Variable	
Focal nodular hyperplasia	↓	↑	↑	Isointense	↑	↑	
Adenoma	↑	↑	↑	↓	↓	↓	Heterogeneous In- and out-of-phase
Hepatocellular carcinoma	Variable	↑	↑	↓	↓	↓	Heterogeneous
Cholangio-carcinoma	↓	↑	↑	↑	↑	↓	
Metastases	↓	↑↑	↑	↓	↓	↓	

↑ = increased signal, ↑↑ = greatly increased signal, ↓ = decreased signal

common complex cystic masses seen in the United States are either cystadenomas, which are premalignant, or cystadenocarcinomas. Cystadenocarcinomas are rare, usually found in the elderly, and arise from malignant transformation of a cystadenoma.

Diagnostic Imaging of Patients with Hepatic Cystic Lesions

Simple cysts appear as a unilocular, fluid-filled space with a well-defined thin wall without septations but with increased through-transmission on US. A cystadenoma is a hypoechoic lesion with thickened, irregular walls, septations, and internal echoes representing debris or wall nodularity. On CT, a cystadenocarcinoma may have septations and thickened, irregular walls with masses protruding from the internal cyst lining. Echinococcal cysts may have calcifications. MRI demonstrates cysts as well-defined low-attenuation lesions on T1-weighted images and very bright lesions on T2-weighted images, with no enhancement after contrast administration. Aspiration is not required for diagnosing cysts.

Treatment of Patients with Hepatic Cystic Lesions

Asymptomatic simple cysts do not require therapy. Cysts >4 cm in diameter should be monitored 3 months after diagnosis then again at 6–12 months up to two years to assure stability. If symptomatic, laparoscopic wide unroofing (fenestration) or cyst resection has been associated with low recurrence and complication rates. Polycystic disease should undergo fenestration only when severely symptomatic. Prior to fenestration of symptomatic simple cysts, US should be performed to ensure no suggestions of mass in the wall or within the cyst, indicating a cystadenoma. A frozen section of the wall should be sent at the time of fenestration; if positive for cystadenoma, complete excision of the cyst should be undertaken, as malignant transformation of the cyst lining has been described in 15% of patients with cystadenomas. Complex cysts should be completely excised and can be enucleated. Cystadenocarcinomas should be removed through formal liver resection to reduce the risk of recurrence.

Hepatic Solid Masses

Solid masses in patients with no history of cancer may be benign (hemangioma, fibronodular hyperplasia [FNH], adenoma, pyogenic or amebic abscess) or malignant (HCC, intrahepatic cholangiocarcinoma, metastases with unknown primary). Patients with solid tumors should have hepatitis serologies as well as AFP, CA19-9, and CEA levels assessed.

Hemangioma

Hemangioma is the most common solid, benign liver tumor, predominantly seen in women aged 30–50 years and typically discovered incidentally. Giant hemangiomas (>5 cm) can present with abdominal symptoms such as RUQ discomfort or fullness. Hemangiomas of moderate or large size are nearly always diagnosed (Figure 11-9). Giant hemangiomas in children have been associated with high output cardiac failure, hypothyroidism, and Kasabach–Merritt syndrome, a consumptive coagulopathy.

Adenoma

Hepatic adenoma is a benign epithelial liver tumor arising in a noncirrhotic liver, most commonly seen in premenopausal women older than 30 years who have used oral contraceptives (OCPs) for more than two years and also in patients with type 1 glycogen storage diseases. More than half of patients present with upper abdominal discomfort, and one-third of patients have a hepatic adenoma discovered incidentally (Figure 11-10). There is potential for malignant transformation in up to 13% of patients and significant risk of rupture (due to a lack of fibrous capsule), which is increased during pregnancy. An elevated AFP should raise concern that malignant transformation has occurred.

Fibronodular Hyperplasia

One of the most important benign lesions to diagnose is FNH (Figure 11-11) because these lesions do not require resection if asymptomatic. FNH is thought to be a hyperplastic response to an anomalous artery. Like hepatic adenoma, FNH affects 5%–7% of the population, most commonly in women aged between 20 and 50 years, and is diagnosed incidentally. FNH does not rupture and is not premalignant; pregnancy is safe.

Abscesses

Hepatic pyogenic abscesses develop due to local spread from peritoneal infections or hematogenous seeding. Patients may present with RUQ abdominal discomfort, fever, chills, malaise, anorexia, and

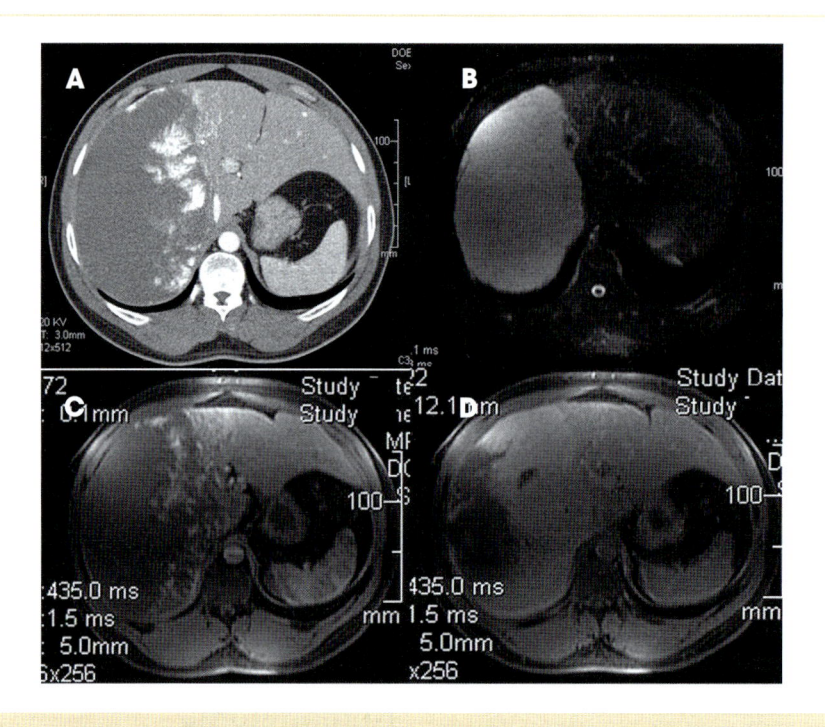

Figure 11-9: Classic appearance of hemangioma on CT (A) and magnetic resonance imaging (B–D). Lesion is very bright on T2 (B) and shows nodular enhancement that fills in from the periphery with increasing time after gadolinium injection (C–D).

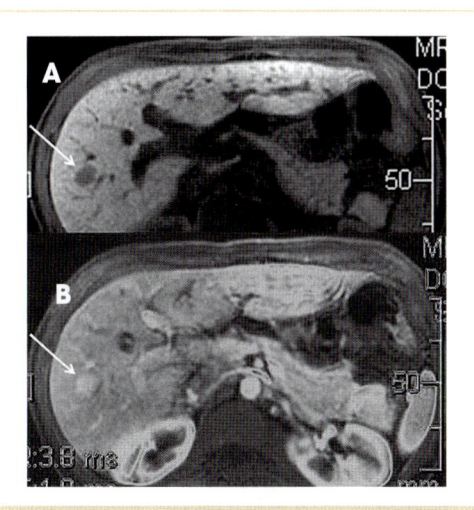

Diagnostic and Therapeutic Approaches for Patients with Liver Tumors

Figure 11-10: Magnetic resonance imaging finding for an adenoma. This is an exophytic lesion (A) with a heterogeneous enhancing pattern after contrast injection (B).

weight loss. Half of patients will have hepatomegaly or splenomegaly. Laboratory work demonstrates leukocytosis with elevation of liver function tests.

Amebic abscesses occur mainly in the right hepatic lobe and result from ingestion of cysts of *Entamoeba histolytica*, which invade colonic mucosa and mesenteric venules, then migrate to the liver via the portal vein. Patients usually present with RUQ pain and up to two weeks of fever, associated with diarrhea. Diagnosis is made by ELISA testing.

Hepatocellular Carcinoma

HCC should be suspected in patients with previously compensated cirrhosis who develop ascites, encephalopathy, jaundice, or variceal bleeding. Symptoms are vague and include upper abdominal discomfort, weight loss, early satiety, or palpable mass. Life-threatening intraperitoneal bleeding due to tumor rupture occurs in 10% of patients and may require emergent angiography and embolization, which should be followed by formal staging,

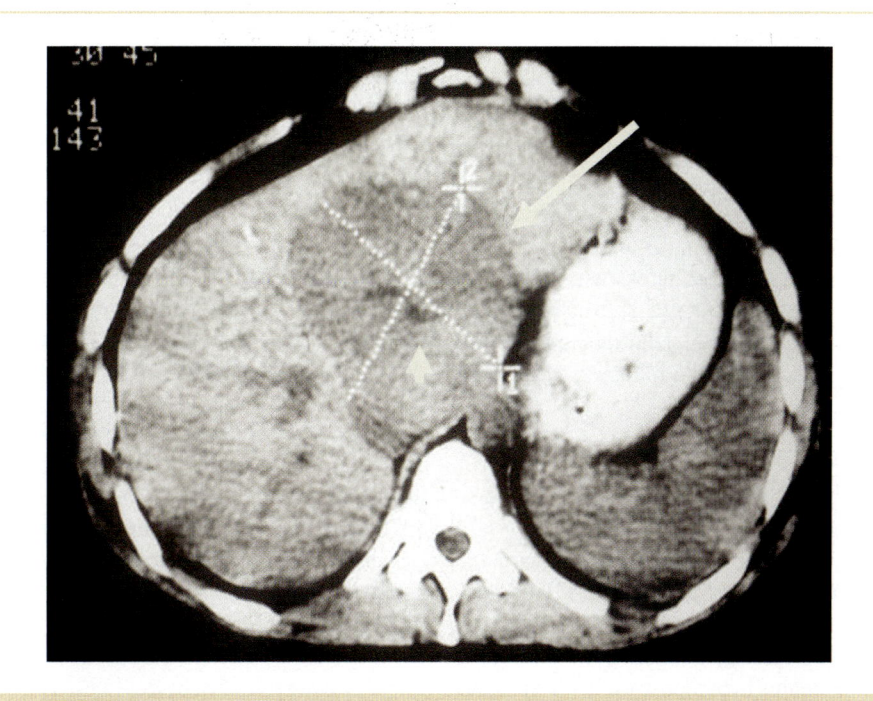

Figure 11-11: Computed tomographic appearance of a fibronodular hyperplasia lesion. The lesion has a central scar and may be confused with a fibrolamellar hepatocellular carcinoma. The long arrow points to a lesion, and the short arrow points to a central scar.

laparoscopic exploration, and attempt at resection. An increase in of serum AFP in cirrhotic should raise suspicion of HCC; serum levels >400 µg/L in a patient with a hypervascular liver mass is diagnostic of HCC. Of note, a normal AFP level can be seen in up to 40% of patients with HCC and in the majority of patients with fibrolamellar HCC, a variant of HCC.

Cholangiocarcinoma

A solitary mass accompanied with no other primary site of cancer is likely to be an intrahepatic cholangiocarcinoma. Intrahepatic cholangiocarcinomas may cause dull RUQ discomfort, weight loss, elevated alkaline phosphatase, and bilirubin. Patients with PSC and cholangiocarcinoma tend to present with declining performance status and increasing cholestasis. These tumors are usually associated with high CA19-9 and/or CEA levels. However, up to one-third of patients with symptoms and cholangiogram suggestive of a bile duct malignancy will have a benign fibrosing disease or another malignancy with metastases with biliary obstruction.

Metastases with Unknown Primary

Hypovascular masses on T1- and T2-weighted images on MRI or multiple masses are likely to be metastases; they are most conspicuous on portal venous phase images. A search for a primary site of cancer should be undertaken. Colonoscopy, upper endoscopy, mammography, pancreas assessment by cross-sectional imaging, and full skin examination are performed. If a metastasis is suspected with no site of primary tumor, a needle biopsy may be indicated.

Diagnostic Imaging of Patients with Benign Hepatic Solid Lesions

Hemangioma typically appears as a well-demarcated homogeneous hyperechoic mass on US. CT demonstrates peripheral nodular enhancement in the early phase, followed by centripetal "filling in" during the late phase, and remains hyperdense on delayed scans. An MRI is the most sensitive and specific study for hemangiomas. If a mass is well circumscribed, homogenous, very bright on T2-weighted images (Figure 11-9), shows early peripheral, nodular, and interrupted enhancement immediately after injection of contrast and progresses to complete filling, it is a hemangioma. Hemangiomas have a very low risk of rupture and are not premalignant. Liver biopsy can result in iatrogenic rupture and is not recommended.

Hepatic adenomas are often large, in the right hepatic lobe, hyperechoic on US, and have a central hypoechoic area, which corresponds to hemorrhage. These are pushing, hypervascular masses with heterogeneous enhancement patterns after contrast injection, as seen on CT. On MRI, adenomas have hyperintense T1-weighted signal intensity due to high glycogen and lipid content, and the central hemorrhage is often visualized. Depiction of intralesional fat with in- and out-of-phase sequences distinguishes adenomas from FNH. After contrast administration, there is heterogeneous hypervascularity in arterial phase, washout on delayed images, and hypointensity on one-hour delayed images using Gd-BOPTA, which distinguishes hepatic adenoma from FNH. Distinguishing an adenoma from a well-differentiated HCC can be difficult and unnecessary, as most adenomas should be resected. A needle biopsy is not recommended due to bleeding risks, and most needle biopsies are nondiagnostic.

US can identify the central scar of FNH in only 20% of cases. On CT, these lesions are well circumscribed and exhibit a central scar and can be confused with fibrolamellar HCC. On MRI, FNH appears as a very homogeneous lesion that exhibits early contrast enhancement and becomes isointense with surrounding parenchyma on delayed contrast images (Figure 11-12). A central scar is classically present and appears hypointense on T1 and hyperintense on T2 due to blood vessels or edema within the myxomatous tissue. The central scar enhances on delayed imaging as contrast gradually diffuses into the tissues. On one-hour delayed images with Gd-BOPTA, FNH may appear hyperintense and may also have a peripheral, ring-type delayed enhancement pattern. Occasionally, diagnostic doubt still exists after an MRI, and an angiogram can distinguish FNH from an adenoma or HCC.

For pyogenic abscesses, US may show single or multiple round hypoechoic areas, and the portal vein may be thrombosed. CT may reveal an area of rim-like enhancement.

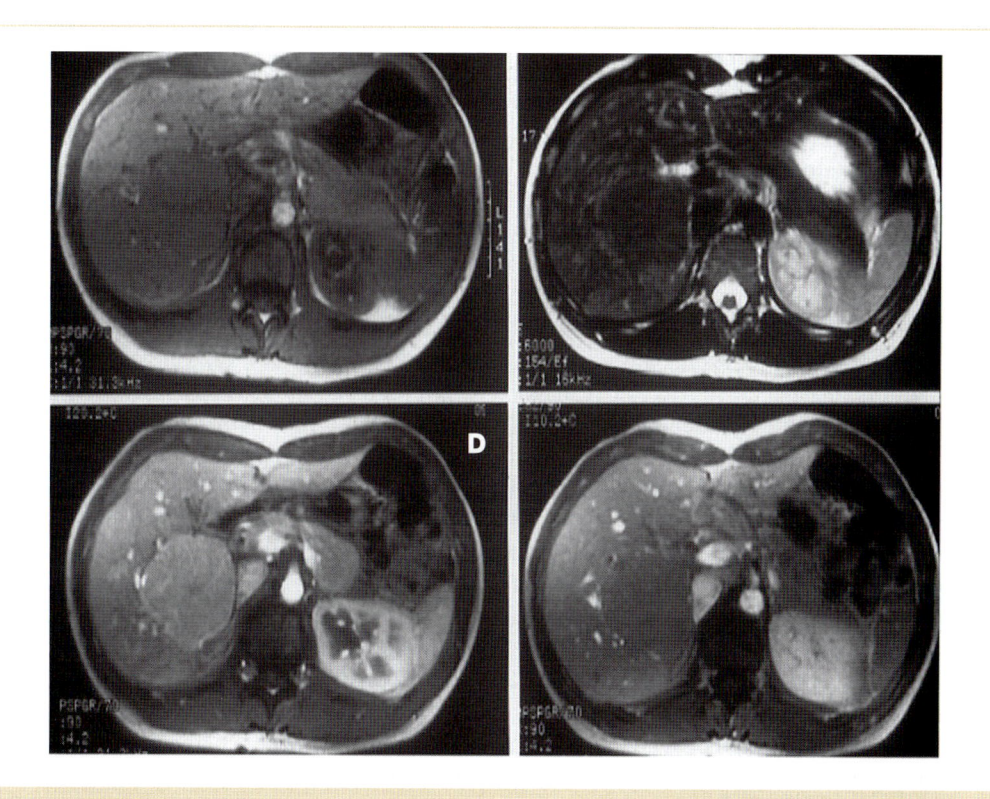

Figure 11-12: Magnetic resonance imaging appearance of a fibronodular hyperplasia lesion in the right liver, seen on T1-weighted (A) and T2-weighted (B) images. The lesion is very homogenous. After contrast injection (C and D), the tumor is initially bright (C) but then becomes almost isodense with surrounding parenchyma (D).

Diagnostic Imaging of Patients with Malignant Solid Lesions

With 60% sensitivity and 97% specificity for HCC, US typically reveals a mass with poorly defined margins and coarse, irregular internal echoes. Small tumors are often hypoechoic, and as they grow, become isoechoic or hyperechoic.[10] Helical CT can detect 30%–40% more tumor nodules on arterial phase imaging than does conventional CT, which may miss small HCCs that are often isodense to the liver in the portal venous phase.[11] In a cirrhotic, any dominant nodule that is not a hemangioma should be considered HCC until proven otherwise. For noncirrhotic patients, the diagnosis of HCC should be considered for any hypervascular hepatic mass that is not clearly a hemangioma or FNH. In patients with cirrhosis, perihepatic lymphadenopathy, especially involving the porta hepatis and portacaval space, may represent benign nodal enlargement. The rare lymph node metastasis portends a worse outcome.

An MRI has 81% sensitivity and 85% specificity in detecting HCC.[12] HCC is generally isointense or hyperintense (if >1.5 cm, due to lipid, copper, or glycogen) on T1-weighted images and hyperintense on T2-weighted images. Of note, the fibrolamellar variant of HCC is heterogeneous on T2 sequences, and the central fibrotic scar is hypointense on both T1 and T2 images. In the cirrhotic liver, an MRI can characterize HCC, regenerative nodules, and fatty infiltration (with in- and out-of-phase techniques); HCC tends to be hyperintense on T2 images while regenerative nodules remain low in signal intensity. Venous washout increases the specificity for HCC as regenerative nodules do not wash out. Fatty metamorphosis in a cirrhotic nodule is also suspicious for HCC. On diffusion-weighted images, well-differentiated tumors are isointense while moderate- to poorly-differentiated tumors are hyperintense.

If the lesion is hypervascular, has increased T2 signal intensity on MRI, demonstrates venous invasion, or is associated with an AFP >400 ng/mL, it is HCC until proven otherwise, and biopsy is not required.[13] Percutaneous biopsy should be performed only when diagnostic imaging results are uncertain, and the result would have an impact on management. Risks of biopsy include bleeding and spread of tumor along the needle track.[14] If biopsy is negative for HCC, patients should undergo US or CT scans every 3–6 months.

Chest CT and bone scan are recommended to complete the staging evaluation as 10%–20% of patients present with extrahepatic spread to lung, abdominal lymph nodes, and bone. PET is not generally recommended for the diagnosis or staging of patients with HCC.

Diagnosis of cholangiocarcinoma is challenging, particularly in patients with PSC. Initial transabdominal US confirms biliary ductal dilatation, localizes the site of obstruction 94% of the time, and excludes gallstones. Intrahepatic cholangiocarcinoma appears as a mass on US. Proximal lesions cause dilatation of the intrahepatic ducts, and more distal lesions also result in dilation of the extrahepatic ducts. Duplex US allows evaluation of portal vein or hepatic artery involvement as well as invasion, which preclude resectability. On contrast-enhanced triple-phase helical CT, cholangiocarcinomas are hypodense on the portal venous phase and hyperattenuated on delayed images. Dilation of the ducts within an atrophied hepatic lobe and a hypertrophic contralateral lobe suggest invasion of the portal vein. Abdominal lymphadenopathy is common in PSC and does not necessarily indicate malignant involvement.

MRCP is the imaging technique of choice for cholangiocarcinoma as it can image intrahepatic lesions as well as create a three-dimensional image of the biliary tree; however, it may understage disease in 20% of patients. Cholangiocarcinomas appear as hypointense on T1-weighted images and hyperintense on T2-weighted images. Dynamic images show peripheral enhancement followed by progressive and concentric filling after contrast administration and pooling of contrast on delayed images. MRCP should be performed before biliary drainage as to evaluate biliary pathology before it is collapsed.

Cholangiography may be indicated if preoperative drainage of the biliary tree is needed. ERCP is preferred in patients with PSC because the stricturing of the intrahepatic biliary tree is challenging for a percutaneous approach. Although ERCP and PTC techniques can be used to obtain brush cytology of the bile ducts, only 30% of cases will demonstrate positive cytology for cholangiocarcinoma. Endoscopic biopsy has 43%–88% sensitivity; however, a negative test does not rule out malignant disease. Combining cytology with an abnormal CA 19-9 leads to a sensitivity of 88% and specificity of 97%. Because cholangiocarcinoma appears histologically similar to metastatic breast, lung, and pancreas, immunohistochemistry with cytokeratin stains is very important in establishing the diagnosis. Tissue diagnosis is often difficult to obtain, but it is most valuable in strictures of clinically indeterminate origin, when patient or surgeon is reluctant to proceed with surgery without a tissue diagnosis, or prior to chemotherapy or radiation.

EUS may allow for visualization of the local extent of the primary tumor and status of regional lymph nodes as well as fine-needle aspiration that avoids contamination of the biliary tree. PET may be useful in screening patients with PSC for cholangiocarcinoma as it can identify tumors >1 cm and occult metastases. Finally, staging laparoscopy can identify the majority of patients with unresectable disease reducing the number of unnecessary laparotomies. However, true unresectability can be determined only after abdominal exploration.

Treatment for Solid Benign Liver Tumors

Treatment recommendations for patients with benign liver tumors are based on their malignant potential and risk of rupture and hemorrhage (Table 11-2). Twenty-five percent of adenomas will present as bleeding from rupture. Bleeding appears to be related to tumor size, is increased with pregnancy, and is associated with mortality of up to 20%. Moreover, between 15% and 25% of adenomas will degenerate into HCC on follow-up. Thus, resection is recommended for adenomas because they may be difficult to distinguish from well-differentiated HCC, may be complicated by rupture and bleeding, and

TABLE 11-2: Behavior of Various Benign Tumors

Tumor	Malignant Potential	Spontaneous Hemorrhage
Focal nodular hyperplasia	No	No
Hemangioma	No	Rare
Cystadenoma	Yes	No
Adenoma	Yes	Yes

may undergo malignant transformation. In women with adenomas <5 cm in diameter with OCP use, regression may ensue with discontinuation of the medication. However, despite regression, malignant transformation has been documented; therefore, we recommend resection of all adenomas regardless of size. Pregnancy should be avoided if surgical resection is not pursued. If discovered during pregnancy, resection should ideally be performed during the second trimester to reduce risks to both mother and fetus. Surgical options include enucleation, resection, and rarely liver transplantation (in whom resection is not possible due to tumor size/location). For patients who present with intraperitoneal bleeding, preoperative embolization may control bleeding and allow for a more controlled definitive resection.

Conversely, hemangiomas and FNH need no therapy unless symptoms arise as these two tumors have no malignant potential. Resection of hemangioma is generally indicated only if they are symptomatic, if it is not possible to rule out cancer, or if the patient develops Kasabach–Merritt syndrome. A giant hemangioma in a subcapsular lesion may be closely followed up. Extrahepatic ligation of the main arterial supply may be prudent before attempting enucleation of a hemangioma. Hepatic artery embolization alone may be complicated by abscess formation, and there is no evidence of long-term efficacy. Liver resection is another option for surgically treating hemangiomas. Orthotopic liver transplantation has been used to successfully treat patient with unresectable giant hemangiomas associated with Kasabach–Merritt syndrome.

Resection of FNH is considered in symptomatic patients or when hepatic adenoma or HCC cannot be definitively excluded. It is reasonable to obtain follow-up imaging in 6–12 months in women who continue OCPs because patients taking these medications tend to have larger, more vascular lesions.

Treatment for Solid Malignant Liver Tumors

Unfortunately, most patients with HCC present with unresectable disease, with a median survival following diagnosis of 6–20 months.[15] The mainstay of therapy for HCC is surgical resection; however, only 10%–30% of patients are candidates for resection due to tumor extent or underlying liver dysfunction, reflected by the Child-Pugh classification (Table 11-3). Large tumor size does not impact survival when vascular invasion is absent. In fact, patients with T2 tumors (solitary tumor with vascular invasion or multiple tumors, none >5 cm), single HCCs >5 cm or even >10 cm in diameter, may benefit from resection as long as liver function permits.[16] Patients should have liver-only disease, no radiographic evidence of hepatic vasculature invasion or portal hypertension, and should have well-preserved hepatic function. For patients with cirrhosis, surgical resection is most safely performed in patients with Child-Pugh class A disease; however, some patients may develop rapid hepatic decompensation following surgery due to limited functional hepatic reserve.[17] Assessment of volume and function of residual liver should be addressed by hepatic volumetry.[18] PVE, used to induce compensatory hypertrophy, should be considered if the future liver remnant is <20% in a patient with a normal liver or <40% in a patient with a cirrhotic liver.

Intraoperatively, laparoscopy and IOUS may improve selection of patients for curative resection.[19] IOUS guides segmental or nonanatomic resection as it can determine the size of the primary tumor and portal or hepatic vein involvement, which precludes curative resection. In this way, 16% of planned laparotomies can be aborted due to unresectable disease detected on laparoscopy.[19]

In the noncirrhotic liver, an anatomical resection should be performed as up to two-thirds of functional parenchyma can be resected safely. For cirrhotic patients, <25% of liver should be removed because liver regeneration is impaired in cirrhotics. The Pringle maneuver for vascular inflow occlusion is tolerated in cirrhotics up to 60 minutes. Ultrasonic dissector and vascular staplers as well as harmonic scalpel can limit blood loss.[20] Laparoscopic surgery is feasible and safe in this population and can provide

TABLE 11-3: Child-Pugh Classification of Liver Functional Status
Scoring: 5–6 points = A, excellent hepatic reserve; 7–9 points = B, moderate hepatic reserve; 10–15 points = C, low hepatic reserve.

	Points 1	Points 2	Points 3
Albumin (g/dL)	>3.5	2.8–3.5	<2.8
Bilirubin (mg/dL)	<2	2–3	>3
Prothrombin time (sec prolonged)	1–3	4–6	>6
Encephalopathy	None	Controlled	Dense
Ascites	None	Controlled	Refractory

decreased complications, blood transfusion, and length of hospital stay. The 30-day operative mortality is three times as high in cirrhotic (15%) as in noncirrhotics (5%), mostly due to postoperative liver failure.[21] Five-year recurrence-free survival is 32%–62%, and five-year survival rates are as high as 90%.[22]

Other treatment options for HCC include liver transplantation for unresectable patients with a solitary HCC <5 cm, up to three separate lesions none >3 cm, no evidence of gross vascular invasion, and no regional nodal or distant metastases. RFA/MWA is reasonable for patients who do not meet resectability criteria and have liver-only disease. The best outcomes are in patients with a single tumor <4 cm in diameter with only Child-Pugh class A or B severity.[23] Transcatheter arterial chemoembolization (TACE), often used for the treatment of large, unresectable HCC, involves the injection of a chemotherapeutic agent with or without lipiodol or procoagulant material into the hepatic artery, the blood supply to HCC. Absolute contraindications for TACE include portal vein thrombosis, encephalopathy, and biliary obstruction. Cryoablation has been used most frequently in patients deemed unresectable intraoperatively and where RFA may be limited by collateral thermal damage. Although chemotherapy has not been used routinely for patients with advanced HCC except within a clinical trial, Sorafenib, a multitargeted tyrosine kinase inhibitor, has been shown to significantly improve survival rates in patients with advanced HCC. There is an ongoing clinical trial investigating Sorafenib in the adjuvant setting.[24]

If a cholangiocarcinoma is diagnosed, resection is the treatment of choice. Cholangiocarcinomas have an average five-year survival rate of 5%–10%. Intrahepatic cholangiocarcinomas have a resectability rate of 91%, and this rate has increased over time due to more aggressive operative strategies.[25] Criteria for resectability include absence of retropancreatic and paraceliac nodal metastases or distant liver metastases; absence of invasion of the portal vein or main hepatic artery; absence of extrahepatic adjacent organ invasion; and absence of disseminated disease. Ultimately, however, resectability is determined at surgery.

Nonoperative biliary drainage is performed in patients with serum bilirubin >10 mg/dL, deferring definitive operative management until bilirubin levels are <3 mg/dL. Stent placement should follow high-quality imaging to assess unresectability. Preoperative PVE for patients with a predicted postoperative liver remnant volume of <25% is employed to induce lobar hypertrophy to increase the limits of safe resection. Main prognostic factors are histologic margin status and lymph node involvement. Three-year overall survival is 22%–60%, and 3-year disease-specific survival is 6%–41%.

If unresectable for anatomic reasons or lack of hepatic reserve, a biopsy is performed to document diagnosis, and RFA/MWA or systemic therapy with 5-FU-based chemoradiotherapy may be administered.

References

1. Lee KF, Wong J, Li JC, et al. Polypoid lesions of the gallbladder. *Am J Surg.* 2004;188(2):186.
2. Akhurst T, Kates TJ, Mazumdar M, et al. Recent chemotherapy reduces the sensitivity of [18F]

fluorodeoxyglucose positron emission tomography in the detection of colorectal metastases. *J Clin Oncol.* 2005;23:8713.
3. Poston GJ, Adam R, Alberts S, et al. OncoSurge: a strategy for improving resectability with curative intent in metastastic colorectal cancer. *J Clin Oncol.* 2005;23:7175.
4. Palavecino M, Chun YS, Madoff DC, et al. Major hepatic resection for hepatocellular carcinoma with or without portal vein embolization: perioperative outcome and survival. *Surgery.* 2009;145:399.
5. Abulkir A, Limongelli P, Healey AJ, et al. Preoperative portal vein embolization for major liver resection: a meta-analysis. *Ann Surg.* 2008;247:49.
6. Weitz J, Blumgart LH, Fong Y, et al. Partial hepatectomy for metastases from noncolorectal, nonneuroendocrine carcinoma. *Ann Surg.* 2005;241(2):269.
7. Semelka RC, Martin DR, Balci NC. Focal lesions in normal liver. *J Gastroenterol Hepatol.* 2005;20(10):1478.
8. Silva AC, Evans JM, McCullough AE, et al. MR imaging of hypervascular liver masses: a review of current techniques. *Radiographics.* 2009; 29(2):385.
9. Ros PR, Freeny PC, Harms Se, et al. Hepatic MR imaging with ferumoxides: a multicenter clinical trial of the safety and efficacy in the detection of focal hepatic lesions. *Radiology.* 1995;196:481.
10. Ishiguchi T, Shimamoto K, Fukatsu H, et al. Radiologic diagnosis of hepatocellular carcinoma. *Semin Surg Oncol.* 1996;12:164.
11. Baron R, Oliver J III, Dodd GD, et al. Hepatocellular carcinoma: evaluation with biphasic, contrast-enhanced, helical CT. *Radiology.* 1996;199:505.
12. Colli A, Fraquelli M, Casazza G, et al. Accuracy of ultrasonography, spiral CT, magnetic resonance, and alpha-fetoprotein in diagnosing hepatocellular carcinoma: a systematic review. *Am J Gastroenterol.* 2006;101:513.
13. Wu JT. Serum alpha-fetoprotein monitoring in Chinese patients with chronic hepatitis B virus infection: role in the early detection of hepatocellular carcinoma. *Hepatology.* 1989;9:110.
14. Bruix J, Sherman M, Llovet JM, et al. Clinical management of hepatocellular carcinoma. Conclusions of the Barcelona-2000 EASL conference. European Association for the Study of the Liver. *J Hepatol.* 2001;35:421.
15. A new prognostic system for hepatocellular carcinoma: a retrospective study of 425 patients: the Cancer of the Liver Italian Program (CLIP) investigators. *Hepatology.* 1998;28:751.
16. Bruix J, Sherman M. Practice Guidelines Committee, American Association for the Study of Liver Diseases. Management of hepatocellular carcinoma. *Hepatology.* 2005;42:1208.
17. Bruix J, Castells A, Bosch J, et al. Surgical resection of hepatocellular carcinoma in cirrhotic patients: prognostic value of preoperative portal pressure. *Gastroenterology.* 1996;111:1018.
18. Abdalla EK, Hicks ME, Vauthey JN. Portal vein embolization: rationale, technique and future prospects. *Br J Surg.* 2011;88:165.
19. Lo Cm, Lai EC, Lieu CL, et al. Laparoscopy and laparoscopic ultrasonography avoid exploratory laparotomy in patients with hepatocellular carcinoma. *Ann Surg.* 1998;227:527.
20. Hodgson WJ, Morgan J, Byme D, DelGuercio LR. Hepatic resections for primary and metastatic tumors using the ultrasonic surgical dissector. *Am J Surg.* 1992;163:246.
21. Bozzetti F, Gennari L, Regalia E, et al. Morbidity and mortality after surgical resection of liver tumors. Analysis of 229 cases. *Hepatogastroenterology.* 1992;39:237.
22. Fong Y, Sun RL, Jarnagin W, Blumgart LH. An analysis of 412 cases of hepatocellular carcinoma at a Western center. *Ann Surg.* 1999;229:790.
23. Tanabe KK, Curley SA, Dodd GD, et al. Radiofrequency ablation: the experts weigh in. *Cancer.* 2004;100:641.
24. Clinical trial information. http://clinicaltrials.gov/ct2/show/NCT00692770. Accessed July 15, 2008.
25. Endo I, Gonen M, Yopp AC, et al. Intrahepatic cholangiocarcinoma: rising frequency, improved survival, and determinants of outcome after resection. *Ann Surg.* 2008;248:84.

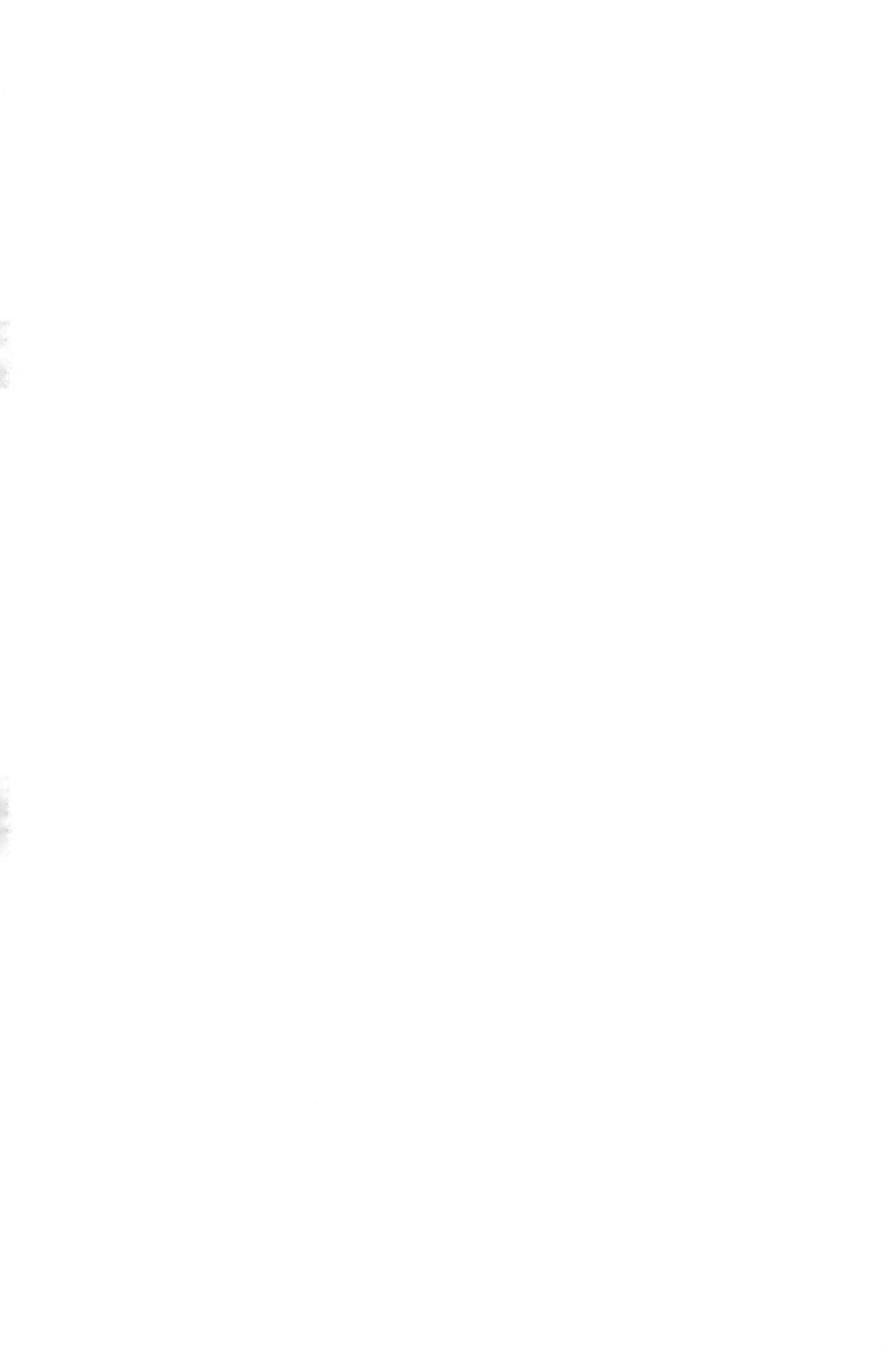

IV SECTION

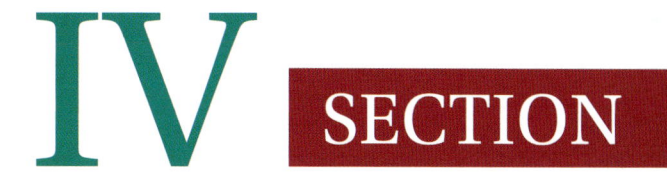

Surgical Therapies

Yuman Fong

CHAPTER 12

Techniques for Hepatic Resection

Clifford S. Cho

Introduction

The past three decades have witnessed enormous progress in the field of hepatic surgery. Rare procedures once associated with significant risk of operative mortality have become commonplace, with resections of up to 85% of functional hepatic parenchyma presently being performed with operative mortality rates of less than 2%.[1–3] However, safe conduct of hepatic resection demands a thorough appreciation of relevant hepatic anatomy and operative strategies; these will be the subject of this chapter.

Hepatic anatomy

Figure 12-1[4] demonstrates segmental anatomy of the liver. The right and left hemilivers are separated by the principal scissura (Cantlie's line), through which the middle hepatic vein courses. The location of the principal scissura may be identified along an imaginary line between the gallbladder fossa and inferior vena cava. The right hemiliver consists of Couinaud's segments V through VIII and is nourished by the right portal vein and right hepatic artery. The right scissura (along which the right hepatic veins courses) separates the right anterior section (segments V and VIII) from the right posterior section (segments VI and VII). The venous drainage of the right hemiliver enters both the right and middle hepatic veins. An accessory right hepatic vein is often seen coursing more inferiorly into the vena cava, and large accessory right hepatic veins can often sustain the entire venous drainage of the right hemiliver after ligation of the main right and middle hepatic veins. The left hemiliver consists of segments II through IV and is nourished by the left portal vein and left hepatic artery. The left scissura (along which the left hepatic vein courses) separates segments II from segments III and IV, whereas the externally visible falciform ligament separates segments II and III from IV. The venous drainage of the left hemiliver enters the left and middle hepatic veins, which typically form a short common trunk before entering the vena cava. Segment I (the caudate lobe) resides between the portal vein and inferior vena cava and typically receives its vascular inflow from both the right and left hepatic arteries and portal veins; its venous drainage enters directly into the inferior vena cava.

The portal vein and hepatic artery bifurcate below the hilus of liver. On the right side, the right portal vein and hepatic artery and hepatic duct enter the hepatic parenchyma as a triad after a very short extrahepatic course. In contrast, the left portal vein and hepatic duct follow a longer extrahepatic course along the undersurface of segment IV before joining with the left hepatic artery as they enter the umbilical fissure. The fibrous Glissonian capsule envelops the portal triad structures as they pass into the hepatic parenchyma; *en masse* control of these strictures through pedicle ligation (vide infra) takes advantage of this anatomic relationship.[5]

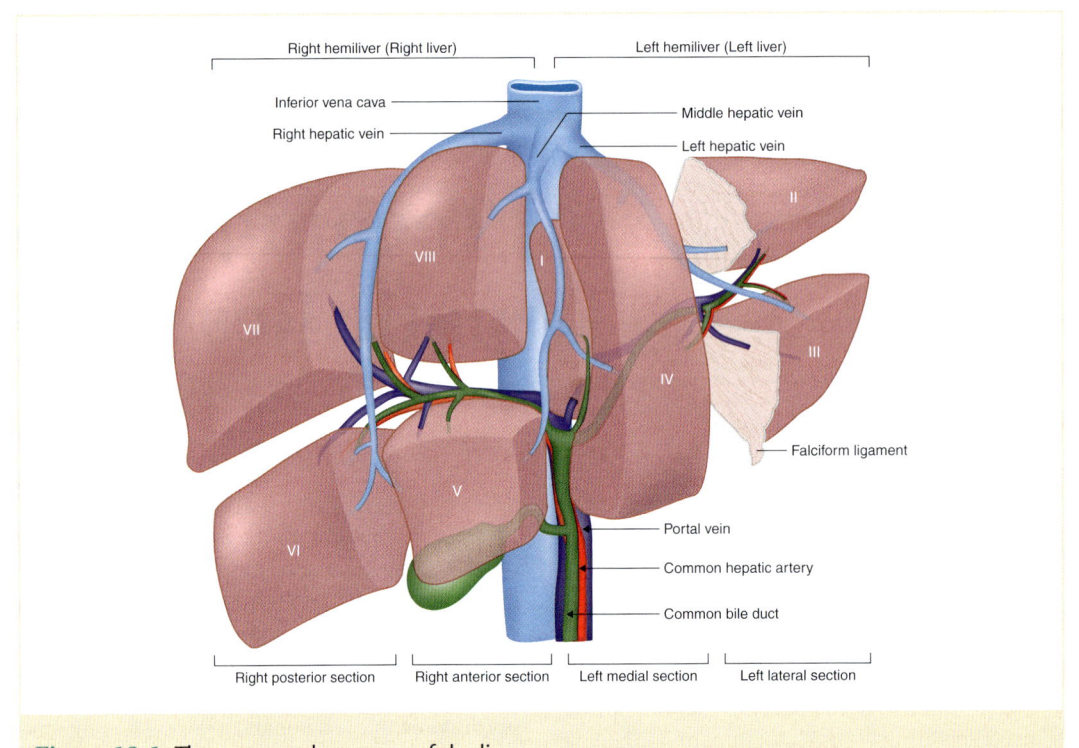

Figure 12-1: The segmental anatomy of the liver.

Preoperative Considerations

Cirrhosis

Because of the significantly increased risk of postoperative hepatic failure, the presence of cirrhosis generally mandates some adjustment in operative strategy. Resections that may be well tolerated in patients with normal hepatic function may prove fatal for patients with hepatic functional decompensation. Therefore, careful assessment of hepatic function is necessary during the preoperative assessment of patients with cirrhosis.

A number of assays have been advocated for the purpose of quantifying hepatic functional deficits for patients with cirrhosis. Many of these measure the ability of the liver to metabolize or clear dyes and substrates (e.g., indocyanine green dye, aminopyrine, and lidocaine).[6–8] Direct and indirect measurements of various parameters of portal hypertension have also been used to estimate the likelihood of postoperative hepatic failure.[9,10] In the United States, the Child–Pugh classification system is the most widely used system for quantifying the extent of cirrhosis-induced hepatic dysfunction, as major hepatic resections for patients with Child–Pugh scores of 8 or higher are associated with extreme morbidity and mortality.[11,12]

Chemotherapy-Associated Hepatotoxicity

Advancements in systemic chemotherapy have broadened the indications for partial hepatectomy as a potentially curative intervention for patients with hepatic metastases from colorectal adenocarcinoma. The efficacy of contemporary oxaliplatin- and irinotecan-based chemotherapeutic regimens have enabled patients with technically unresectable metastases to become downstaged to resectability; as a result, more and more patients undergoing hepatic metastasectomy have been heavily pretreated with systemic chemotherapy. Unfortunately, the improved response rates associated with these newer agents have come at the cost of new hepatotoxicities that can affect the safety and feasibility of hepatic resection.[13,14] Oxaliplatin has been associated with sinusoidal obstruction and dilatation[15] and irinotecan has been linked with hepatic steatosis[16]; both agents have been associated with steatohepatitis, which is a clear risk factor for heightened postoperative morbidity.[17,18]

For this reason patients with a history of heavy systemic chemotherapeutic treatment who are being evaluated for possible hepatic resection must be screened for signs of chemotherapy-associated hepatotoxicity. Steatosis, splenomegaly, and thrombocytopenia have also been associated with chemotherapy-associated hepatotoxicity. The presence of low attenuation in the liver compared with the spleen for computed tomography (CT) imaging or signal dropout on out-of-phase sequences for magnetic resonance imaging (MRI) is suggestive of hepatic steatosis; however, a normal CT or MRI scan does not exclude the possibility of clinically significant steatosis, and percutaneous biopsy may be indicated for patients who have been heavily treated with chemotherapy.[19] Like cirrhosis, chemotherapy-associated hepatotoxicity may handicap the ability of a patient to tolerate a major hepatic resection, and its diagnosis may mandate alterations in operative strategy or the use of preoperative adjuncts like portal vein embolization (PVE) (vide infra).

Portal Vein Embolization

The ability to offer hepatic resection as a therapeutic maneuver is often restricted by issues related to hepatic parenchymal volume and function. It is evident that partial hepatectomy must be undertaken in a manner that will leave patients with a minimal future liver remnant (FLR) capable of sustaining postresection hepatic hypertrophy and preserved hepatic function. In patients with functionally normal livers, aggressive hepatic resections that leave FLR volumes of 20% are routinely well tolerated. However, in patients with underlying hepatic parenchymal dysfunction from steatosis, cirrhosis, or chemotherapy-induced hepatotoxicity, FLR volumes as high as 50% may be needed.[20] Preoperative PVE is now being incorporated as a useful preoperative intervention to increase FLR size, intended to minimize the risk of acute postoperative hepatic failure.[21–23]

We routinely calculate hepatic volumetrics for patients with underlying liver diseases and patients who have received intensive chemotherapy on whom major hepatectomy (extended right hemihepatectomy or more) is contemplated. If the calculated anticipated FLR is deemed to be too small, PVE is typically undertaken at least one month before planned hepatic resection. The portal vein ipsilateral to the side of the liver to be resected is accessed percutaneously, and particle- and coil-based embolization is undertaken with care taken to ensure complete cessation of flow throughout the involved portal circulation. In patients with preserved hepatic function, PVE should result in ipsilateral parenchymal atrophy and compensatory contralateral hypertrophy that generally peaks at four weeks (Figure 12-2). Thus, if repeat imaging performed one month after PVE confirms satisfactory hypertrophy with no new lesions within the planned liver remnant, operative resection is undertaken. In contrast, the absence of satisfactory hypertrophy at the time of repeat imaging may be indicative of significant underlying parenchymal dysfunction that would predict a high likelihood of posthepatectomy liver failure;

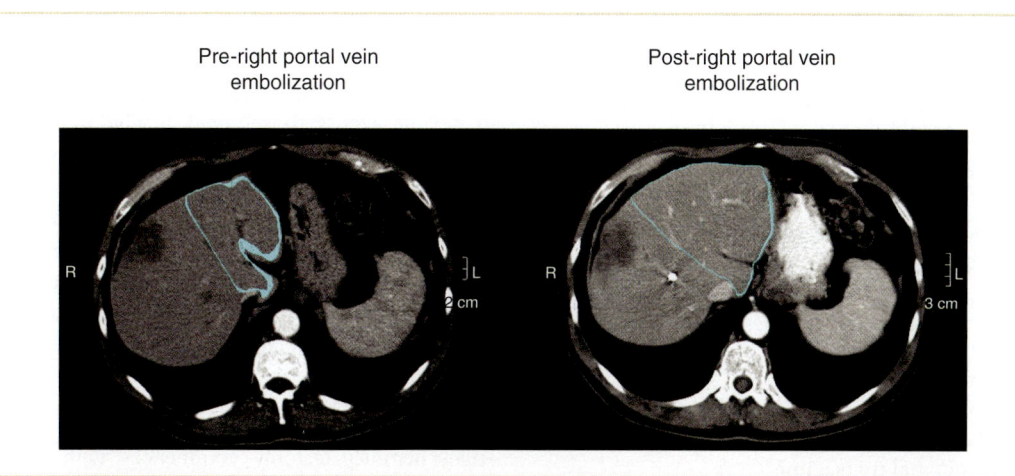

Figure 12-2: Portal vein embolization. A 63-year-old man with bilateral hepatic rectal adenocarcinoma metastases initially presented with an anticipated FLR of 16.8%. Following right PVE, his anticipated FLR increased to 31.9%, permitting an uncomplicated extended right hemihepatectomy.

major hepatic resection is typically not offered under these circumstances. Early concerns regarding the potential oncological ramifications of delaying operative intervention for one month to accommodate PVE have been allayed by recent observations that systemic chemotherapy can be continued following PVE without significantly impairing hepatic hypertrophy.[24]

Operative Preparation

Before undertaking major resections, we routinely place a central venous catheter for intraoperative monitoring of central venous pressures. Most of the blood loss encountered during partial hepatectomy is a result of venous bleeding from the major hepatic veins or vena cava. Thus, by maintaining central venous pressures of less than 5 mm Hg during hepatic parenchymal transaction, operative bleeding may be minimized.[25] Patient positioning in a 15° Trendelenberg position increases venous return and enhances cardiac output, allowing for better hemodynamic tolerance of low central venous pressures.

When positioning the patient, consideration should be given to the possible need for right thoracotomy in the event that maximal access to the suprahepatic vena cava is required. We therefore favor positioning the patient with the arms extended laterally to provide easier access to the right upper quadrant and chest. A crossbar permitting placement of self-retaining retractors to elevate the costal margin in an anterocephalad manner should be utilized. Ring-based self-retaining retractors may also be used; however, care should be taken to prevent the positioning of the rings from hindering lateral access that might impede posterior dissection of the retrohepatic vena cava.

Operative Conduct

The conduct of partial hepatectomy may be organized into the following steps:

1. Incision
2. Exploration
3. Mobilization
4. Inflow control
5. Outflow control
6. Parenchymal transaction

The details of each step will be described for various common resective procedures performed: right hemihepatectomy, left hemihepatectomy, right trisectionectomy, left trisectionectomy, and left lateral sectionectomy.

Right Hemihepatectomy

Right hemihepatectomy is the most common hepatic resective procedure and involves extirpation of segments V through VIII.

Step 1: Incision

Our preference is to begin with an upper midline incision extending from the xiphoid to several centimeters above the umbilicus (Figure 12-3). Preliminary exploration of the liver and peritoneal cavity may be undertaken through this incision to evaluate extent of disease. In selected cases, operative exploration can also begin with laparoscopy. If resection is to be undertaken, a right subcostal extension typically affords sufficient access for all right- or left-sided resections. The ligamentum teres is ligated and divided; the proximal tie may then be left long and used as a handle to facilitate elevation of the left hemiliver and full exposure of the umbilical fissure. The falciform ligament is divided with electrocautery from the edge of the ligamentum teres to the confluence of the hepatic veins. In very limited cases, a right thoracoabdominal incision may also be used if maximal access to the suprahepatic vena cava is needed.

Step 2: Exploration and Intraoperative Hepatic Ultrasonography

Careful bimanual palpation of all accessible liver surfaces and intraoperative hepatic ultrasonography are performed to confirm the anatomic location of preoperatively identified tumors. To facilitate hepatic exploration, the hepatogastric ligament is divided to permit access to segment I. The porta hepatis is then inspected by passing a finger through the opened lesser sac and out the foramen of Winslow. Suspiciously enlarged or firm portal lymph nodes may be excised and submitted for frozen section pathological analysis. The entire abdominal cavity is also inspected for evidence of extrahepatic disease that may contraindicate partial hepatectomy.

Step 3: Liver Mobilization

Right hemihepatectomy commences with mobilization of the right hemiliver. This requires division of the retroperitoneal and diaphragmatic attachments of the right hemiliver, beginning with division of the right triangular ligament (Figure 12-4). Care must be taken

Techniques for Hepatic Resection 273

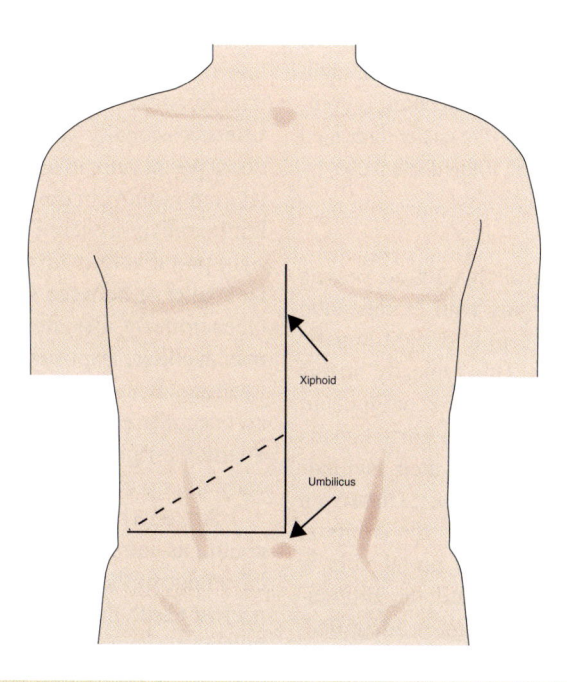

Figure 12-3: Suggested incisions for open partial hepatectomy. A subcostal incision (dotted line) or a vertical upper midline incision with a right lateral extension (solid line) permit excellent visualization of and access to the entire liver. (Reprinted with kind permission of Springer Science + Business Media.[36])

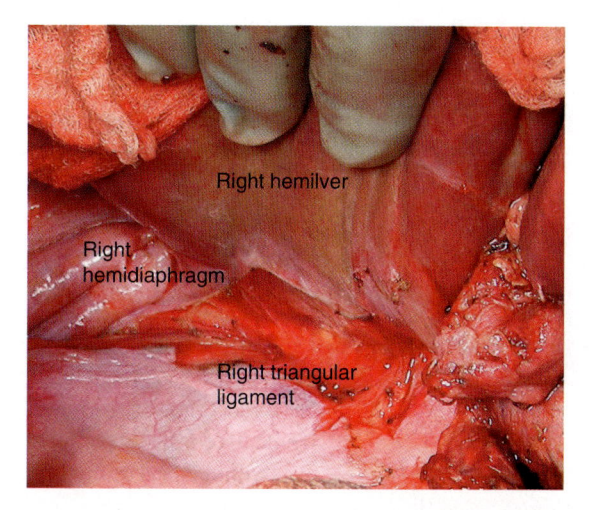

Figure 12-4: Mobilization of the right hemiliver. The retroperitoneal and diaphragmatic attachments of the right hemiliver are divided, as the right hemiliver is elevated and rotated medially. (Reprinted with kind permission of Springer Science + Business Media.[36])

to avoid injury to the right adrenal gland and right hemidiaphragm. This dissection proceeds up to the retrohepatic vena cava behind the liver and to the right hepatic vein above the liver. Once mobilization is completed, the entire right hemiliver may be easily displaced out of the right upper quadrant and rotated medially.

Step 4: Inflow Control

The classic approach to control the inflow vessels for right hemihepatectomy begins with extrahepatic dissection of the right portal vein and right hepatic artery within the porta hepatis. This typically begins with cholecystectomy, after which the peritoneum overlying the right lateral aspect of the porta hepatis is incised. The cystic duct stump is elevated, facilitating identification of the common bile duct. Dissection then proceeds along the plane between the common bile duct and portal vein. The main portal vein is followed in a cephalad direction until the bifurcation of the right and left portal veins is identified. The right portal vein is then encircled with a vessel loop (Figure 12-5). The right hepatic artery can also be identified as it courses posterior to the common hepatic duct and is also encircled with a vessel loop. Transient occlusion of the encircled right portal vein and right hepatic artery should result in clear ischemic demarcation of the right hemiliver (Figure 12-6); absence of clear demarcation should prompt further exploration of the porta hepatis to verify one's interpretation of the portal structures. The left portal vein occasionally arises from the right anterior sectional portal vein; inadvertent division of the right portal vein in this circumstance will render the remnant left hemiliver ischemic. Once properly identified, the right portal vein is ligated and divided with a vascular stapler or between vascular clamps (Figure 12-7). Occasionally, division of the right hepatic artery may facilitate exposure of the right portal vein for ligation. Owing to the enormous variability that may be encountered in the biliary anatomy, we generally divide the right hepatic duct higher and intrahepatically, after parenchymal transection has begun.

An alternative approach to right-sided inflow control is intrahepatic pedicle ligation, which takes advantage of the presence of the thick capsule of connective tissue that enshrouds the vascular inflow and biliary outflow structures inside the hepatic parenchyma. By avoiding portal dissection, this approach minimizes the risk of inadvertent compromise of the contralateral inflow and biliary structures. In this approach, the most inferior venous structures between the liver and inferior vena cava are divided, and hepatotomies are made in sites A and B (Figure 12-8). Hepatotomy A is made along the caudate process, and hepatotomy B is made along the base of the gallbladder fossa. Both hepatotomies involve full-thickness incisions through which small intrahepatic biliary and vascular structures are crushed and ligated. Both hepatotomies must be deep enough to permit finger dissection or clamp placement around the right hepatic pedicle, and temporary occlusion of the portal inflow (the Pringle maneuver) may limit bleeding during this dissection. Umbilical tape is passed around the pedicle with the assistance of a long curved clamp to permit downward retraction. Once visualized, the tape is pulled medially to retract the left-sided pedicle away, and the right pedicle may be transected with a stapler. Because intrahepatic pedicle ligation avoids dissection near the porta hepatis, this approach cannot be used for extirpation of tumors that are in proximity (within 2 cm) of the hepatic hilus.

Step 5: Outflow Control

Vascular control of the venous drainage of the right hemiliver begins by mobilizing the liver off the retrohepatic vena cava. The liver is elevated off the

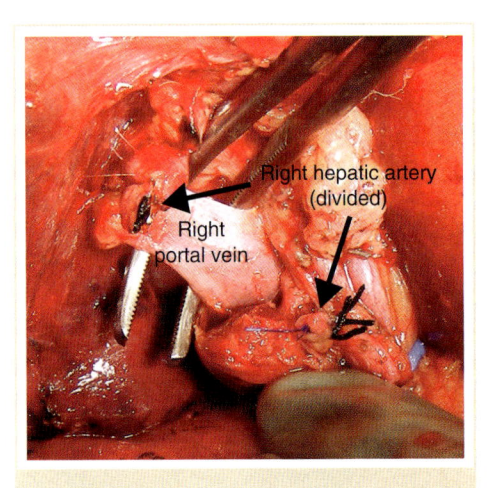

Figure 12-5: Right hepatic inflow control. The exposed right portal vein is demonstrated following division of the right hepatic artery. (Reprinted with kind permission of Springer Science + Business Media.[36])

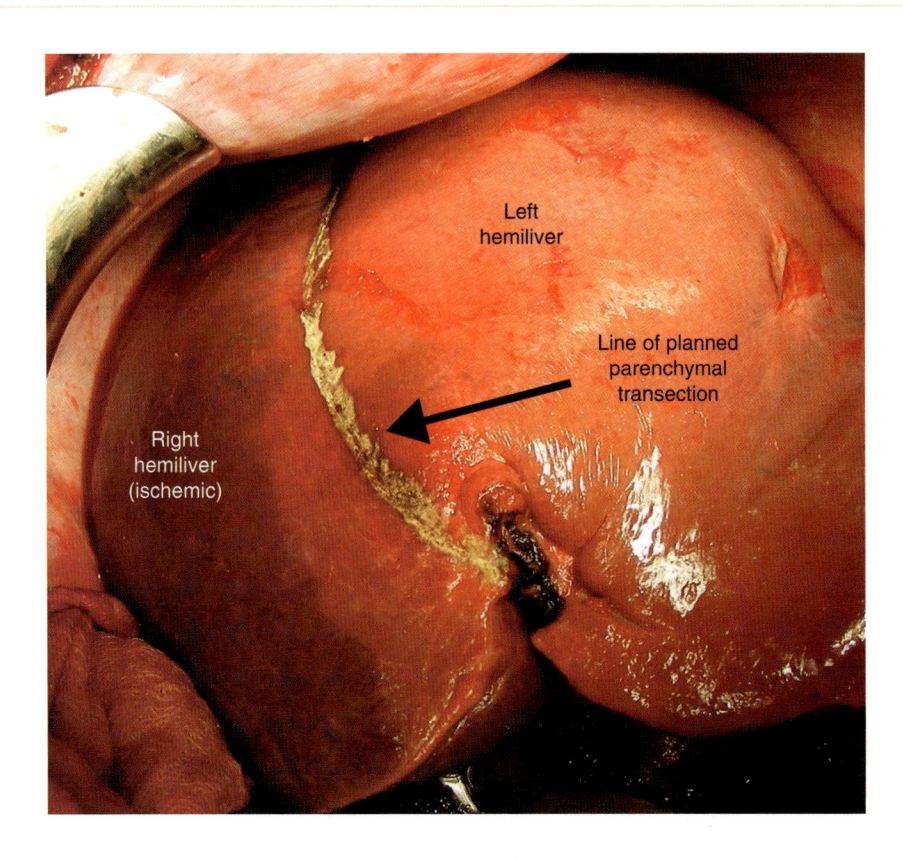

Figure 12-6: Ischemic demarcation of the right hemiliver. Following division of the right portal vein and right hepatic artery, the right hemiliver becomes visibly ischemic and the line of planned parenchymal transection along the principal scissura (Cantlie's line) is marked with electrocautery. (Reprinted with kind permission of Springer Science + Business Media.[36])

vena cava, and numerous venous structures between the liver and vena cava are serially ligated and divided between vascular clips or ligatures (Figure 12-9). This dissection proceeds from the inferior aspect of the liver up to the confluence of the hepatic veins. The inferior vena caval ligament is a segment of hepatic parenchyma that often bridges the liver and retroperitoneum just to the right of the right hepatic vein; division of this ligament with electrocautery or a stapler is usually necessary to fully visualize the right hepatic vein, which is then encircled and divided with a stapler or between vascular clamps (Figures 12-9 and 12-10). We prefer to introduce the stapler along the vena cava and encircle the right hepatic vein from below.

The middle hepatic vein typically converges with the left hepatic vein as they enter the vena cava; thus, attempts to control the middle hepatic vein can risk injury to the venous outflow of the planned liver remnant. We typically do not undertake control of the middle hepatic vein extrahepatically, as it can be safely divided intrahepatically after parenchymal transection.

Occasionally, the presence of a large tumor at the dome of the liver may impede access to the hepatic veins and vena cava; consideration should be given to extend the incision into the chest with a right thoracoabdominal extension so as to permit full access to the suprahepatic vena cava.

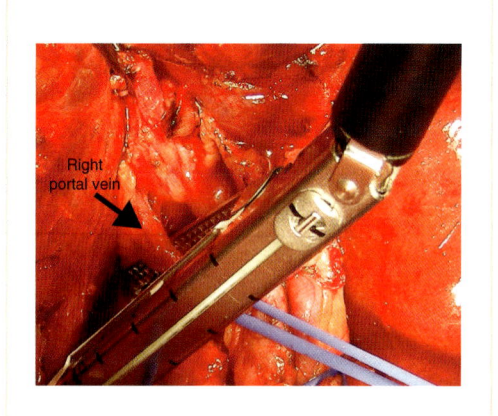

Figure 12-7: Division of the right portal vein. Stapled transection of the right portal vein is demonstrated. Care is taken to retract the left portal vein to avoid inadvertent injury. (Reprinted with kind permission of Springer Science + Business Media.[36])

Step 6: Parenchymal Transection

Parenchymal transection begins with placement of stay sutures of 0 chromic along either side of the planned plane of dissection (along the principal scissura). These stay sutures provide hemostasis along the anterior liver margin and permit elevation of the liver above the level of central venous pressure, limiting venous back-bleeding. Transection can be performed with or without intermittent hepatic inflow occlusion (Pringle maneuver). A number of methods have been advocated for division of hepatic parenchyma. We generally utilize the rapid and cost-effective technique of blunt clamp dissection. In this approach, Glisson's capsule is divided sharply or with a harmonic scalpel (Figure 12-11). A Kelly clamp is then used to crush the liver parenchyma; the soft parenchyma dissects away, exposing only vascular and biliary structures (Figure 12-12). These structures are divided between vascular clips and ligatures (Figure 12-13). The middle hepatic vein may be encountered during transection and may be divided intrahepatically with a vascular stapler (Figure 12-14A and B). In most

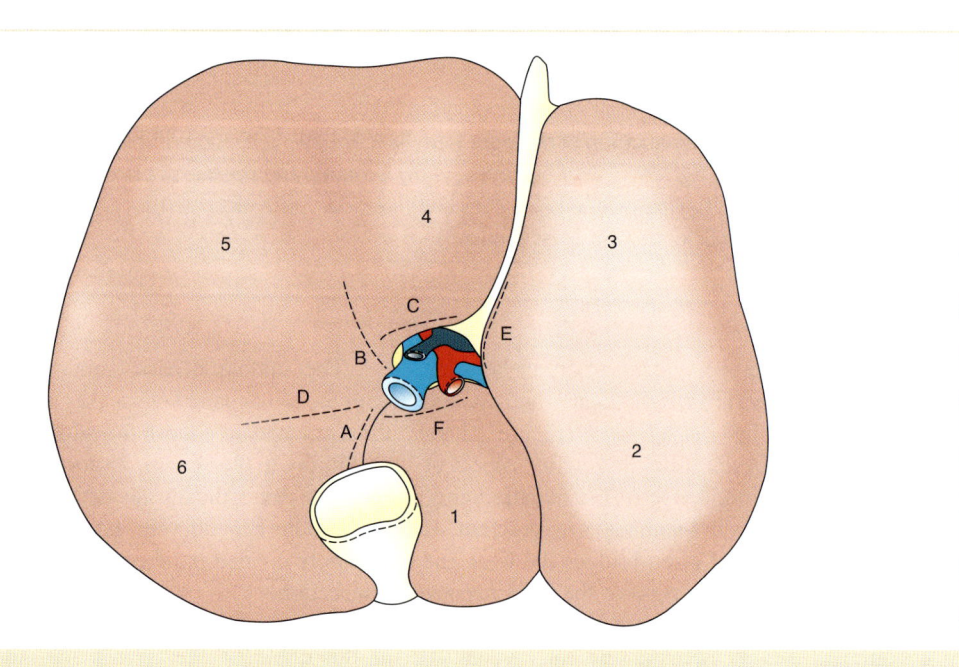

Figure 12-8: Hepatotomy sites for intrahepatic pedicle ligation. Hepatotomies at A and B permit access to the right portal pedicle. A and D permit access to the right posterior portal pedicle, whereas B and D permit access to the right anterior portal pedicle. Hepatotomies at C and F permit access to the left portal pedicle if segment I is to be resected; C and E permit access to the left portal pedicle if segment I is to be spared.

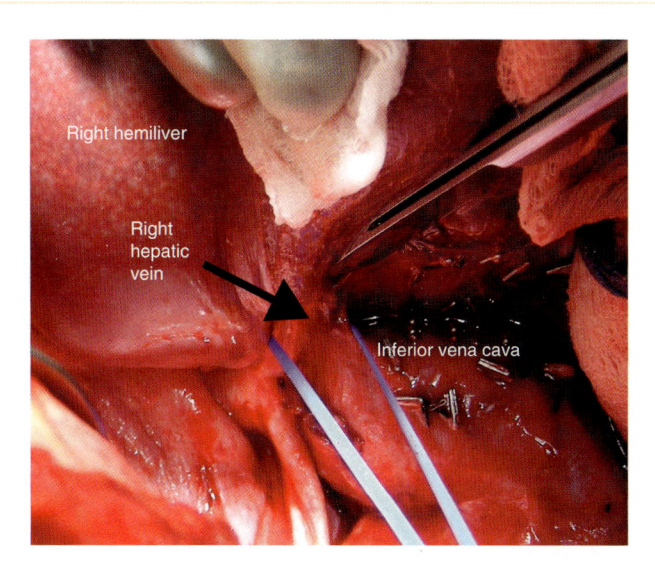

Figure 12-9: Right hepatic outflow control. Multiple direct draining veins from the inferior vena cava are divided, and the right hepatic vein is encircled. (Reprinted with kind permission of Springer Science + Business Media.[36])

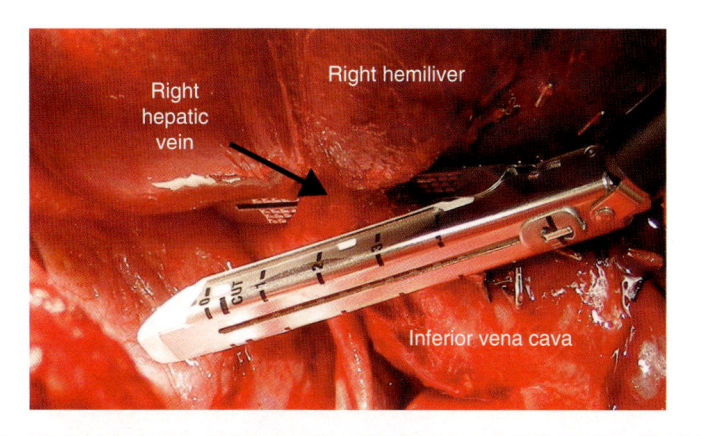

Figure 12-10: Division of the right hepatic vein. Stapled transection of the right hepatic vein is demonstrated. (Reprinted with kind permission of Springer Science + Business Media.[36])

circumstances, the transection can be completed in its entirety in less than 30 minutes.

In patients with cirrhosis or severe steatosis, blunt clamp dissection may be suboptimal due to easy tearing of vascular and biliary structures. In these circumstances, alternative dissection techniques using the LigaSure, water-jet dissection, or staplers may be employed.

Once the specimen is removed, the cut liver surface is carefully inspected for evidence of bleeding or bile leakage. Large vessels or bile leaks are controlled with suture or clip ligation; light bleeding can be controlled with an argon beam coagulator. We do not place operative drains unless a biliary-enteric anastomosis has been made or a bile leak persists.[26]

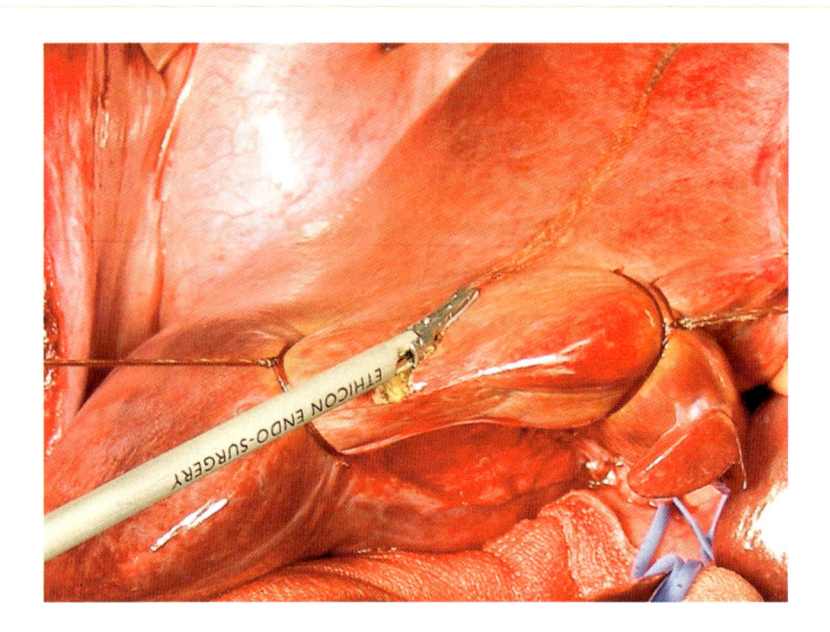

Figure 12-11: Parenchymal transection. The harmonic scalpel may also be used to initiate parenchymal transection. (Reprinted with kind permission of Springer Science + Business Media.[36])

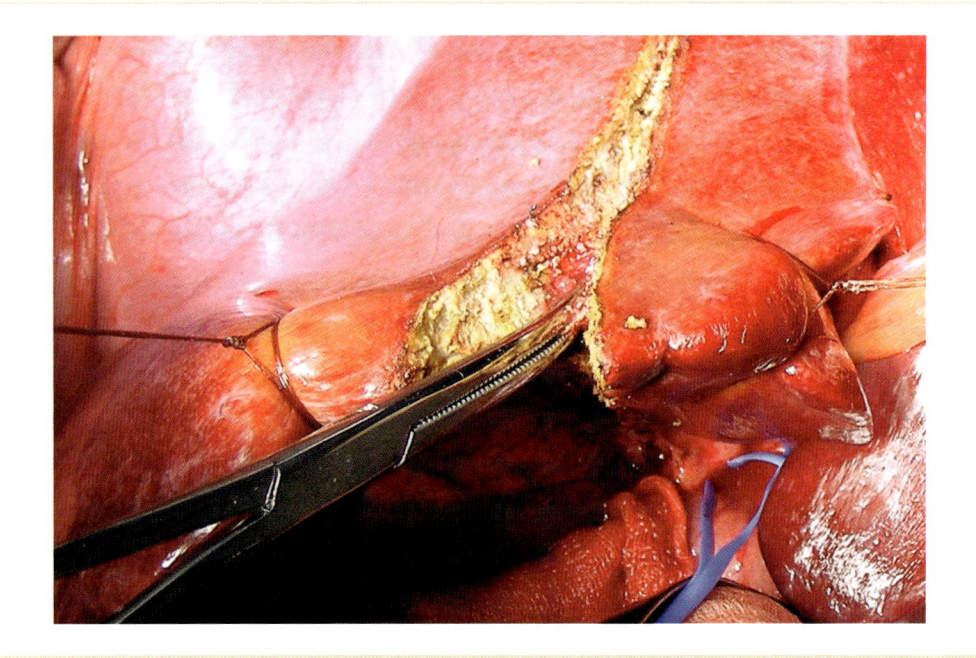

Figure 12-12: Parenchymal transection using blunt clamp dissection. A Kelly clamp may be used to crush the hepatic parenchyma. (Reprinted with kind permission of Springer Science + Business Media.[36])

Techniques for Hepatic Resection

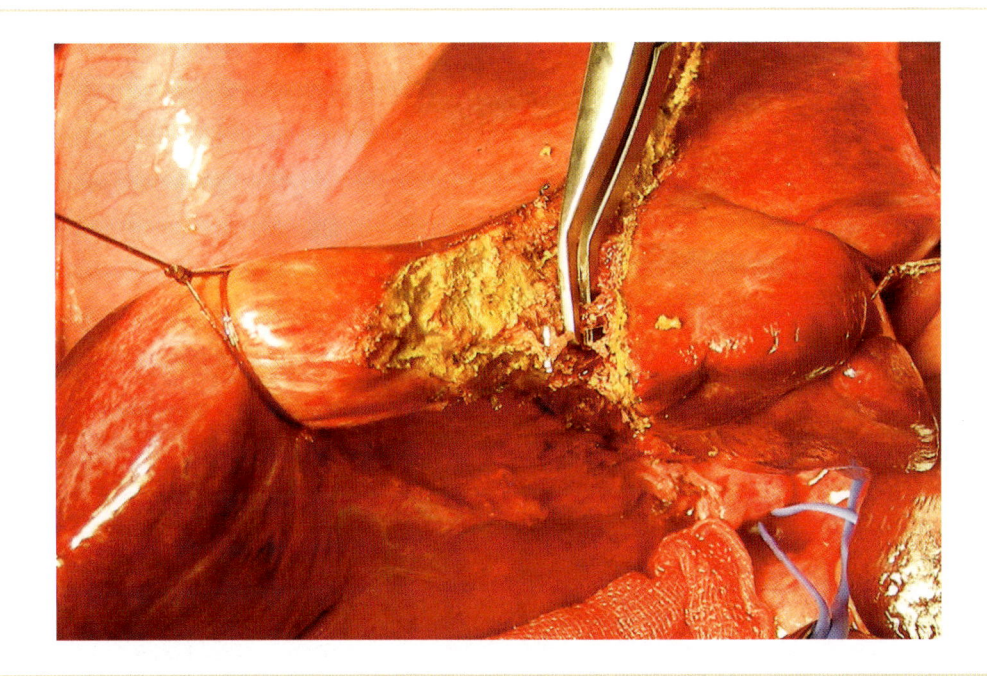

Figure 12-13: Parenchymal transection using blunt clamp dissection. Blunt crushing of the hepatic parenchyma exposes biliary and vascular structures, which may then be divided between ligature clips. (Reprinted with kind permission of Springer Science + Business Media.[36])

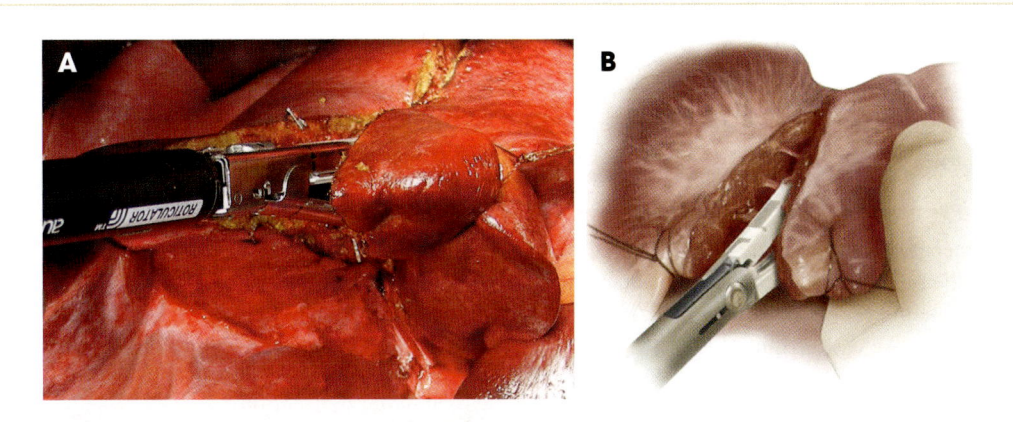

Figure 12-14: (A) Stapled parenchymal transection. Larger venous structures may be divided intrahepatically using a stapling device. (Reprinted with kind permission of Springer Science + Business Media.[36]) (B) Alternatively, the blood vessels seen after clamp crushing can be transected with a bipolar coagulating instrument after visual inspection to be sure the vessels are less than 5 mm in width. (With permission from Patrlj L, Tuorto S, Fong Y. *J Am Coll Surg* 2010;210:39–44 and Elsevier Inc.[37])

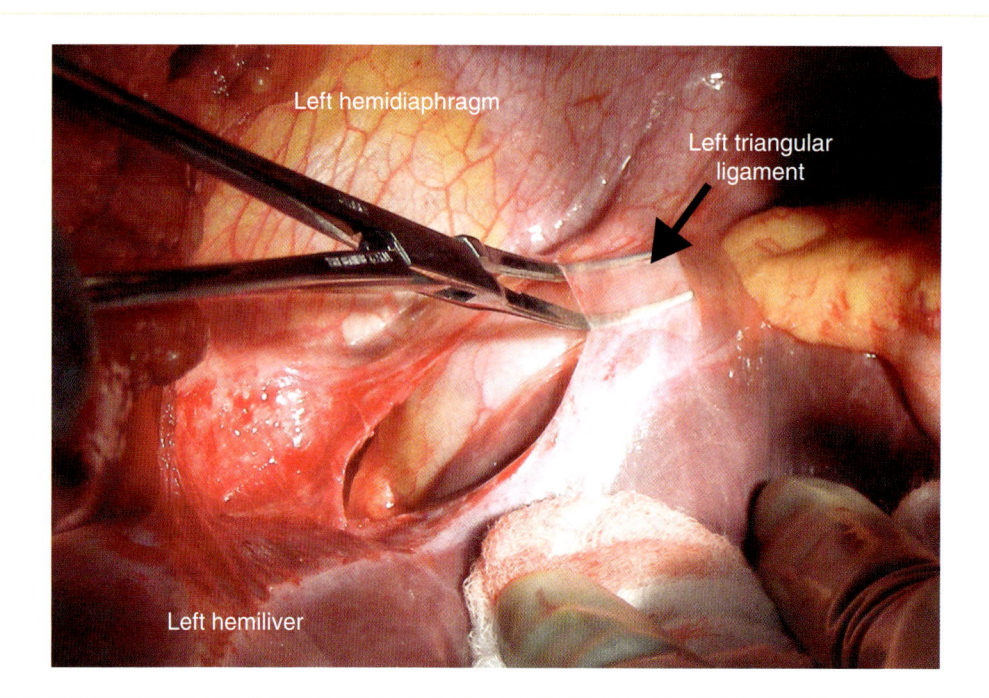

Figure 12-15: Mobilization of the left hemiliver. The diaphragmatic attachments of the left hemiliver are divided as the left lateral section is rotated to the right. (Reprinted with kind permission of Springer Science + Business Media.[36])

Left Hemihepatectomy

Left hemihepatectomy involves extirpation of segments II through IV.

Steps 1 and 2

Incision and exploration are similar to that described above for right hemihepatectomy.

Step 3: Liver Mobilization

Left hemihepatectomy commences with mobilization of the left hemiliver. The diaphragmatic attachments of the left lateral section are divided so as to permit easy rotation toward the right (Figure 12-15). The lesser sac is entered by dividing the hepatogastric ligament. This permits access to the ligamentum venosum, which runs between segments I and II; this is divided close to the liver toward its superior attachment to the left hepatic vein.

Step 4: Inflow Control

In contrast to right hemihepatectomy, we generally begin dissection along the base of the umbilical fissure to identify and divide the left hepatic artery as it joins the left portal vein and hepatic duct (Figure 12-16). The hilar plate is lowered by dividing the peritoneal reflection of the hepatic hilus along the undersurface of segment IV. In this fashion, the left portal vein may be identified and circumferentially dissected. There is generally a short branch to segment I that emanates from the proximal left portal vein (Figure 12-17); if segment I is to be spared, the left portal vein is divided distal to this branch with a stapler or between vascular clamps. Satisfactory ischemic demarcation of the left hemiliver can be confirmed at this point (Figure 12-18). As with right hemihepatectomy, we generally prefer to divide the left hepatic duct intrahepatically after initiation of parenchymal transection.

Intrahepatic pedicle ligation is also a viable option for left hemihepatectomy. The left pedicle may be isolated between hepatotomy sites C and E (Figure 12-8); alternatively, if segment I is to be resected, the proximal left pedicle may be isolated between hepatotomy sites C and F (Figure 12-8). The left pedicle is retracted with umbilical tape in preparation for stapled ligation.

Step 5: Outflow Control

In most patients, the left and middle hepatic veins form a common trunk as they enter the vena cava. However, left hemihepatectomy can often be performed without sacrificing the middle hepatic vein. It is therefore useful to isolate and divide the left hepatic vein in isolation. This maneuver is facilitated by retracting the left lateral section downward or toward the right to visualize the junction between the left and middle hepatic veins (Figure 12-19). The umbilical vein may occasionally be found in this junction as well and is typically taken with the left hepatic vein. The left hepatic vein may then be divided using a stapler passed from above or between vascular clamps. If the middle hepatic vein is to be taken as well, the common trunk of the middle and hepatic veins may be isolated in a similar fashion.

Step 6: Parenchymal Transection

Parenchymal transection proceeds in a similar manner to that described for right hemihepatectomy.

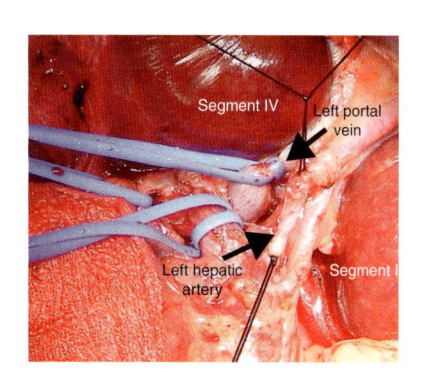

Figure 12-16: Left hepatic inflow control. The exposed left portal vein and hepatic artery are demonstrated along the base of segment IV. (Reprinted with kind permission of Springer Science + Business Media.[36])

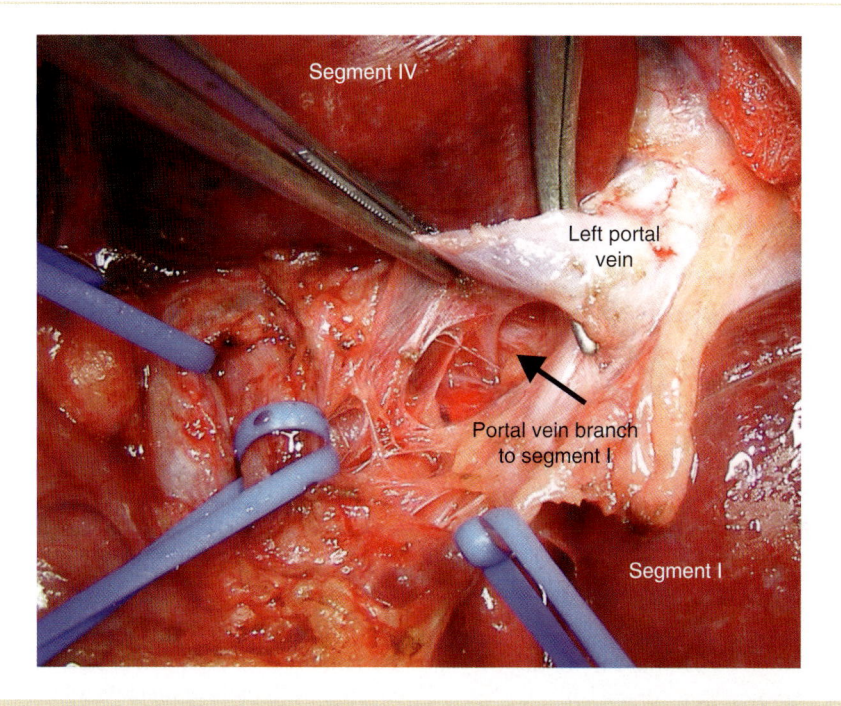

Figure 12-17: Left hepatic inflow control. The portal vein branch to segment I is demonstrated. Care should be taken to divide the left portal vein distal to this branch if segment I is to be spared. (Reprinted with kind permission of Springer Science + Business Media.[36])

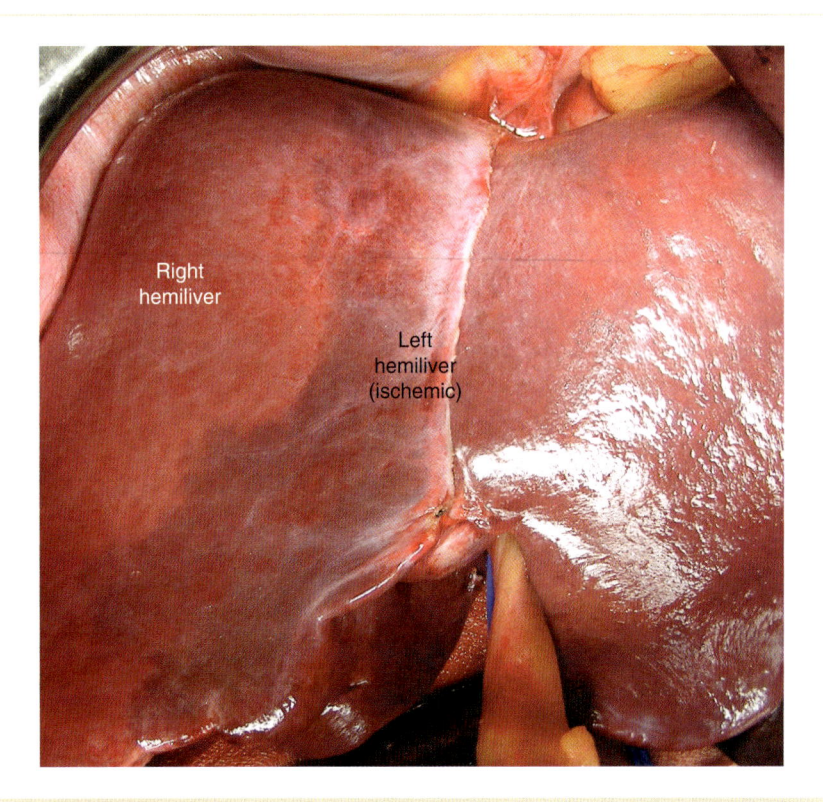

Figure 12-18: Ischemic demarcation of the left hemiliver. Following division of the left portal vein and left hepatic artery, the left hemiliver becomes visibly ischemic. (Reprinted with kind permission of Springer Science + Business Media.[36])

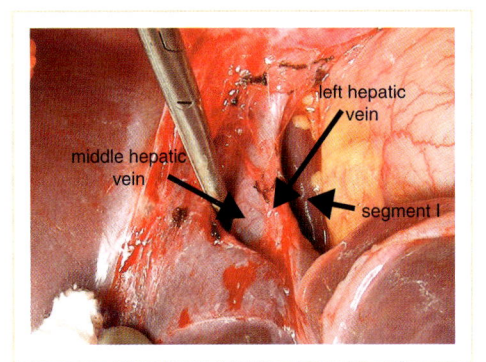

Figure 12-19: Left hepatic outflow control. Division of the ligamentum teres facilitates access to the left hepatic vein. The common trunk of the left hepatic vein and middle hepatic vein is demonstrated here. (Reprinted with kind permission of Springer Science + Business Media.[36])

Left Lateral Sectionectomy

Left lateral sectionectomy involves extirpation of segments II and III.

Steps 1 Through 3

The initial conduct of left lateral sectionectomy is performed in an identical manner to that undertaken for left hemihepatectomy. In many patients, this can be performed through a vertical midline incision with or without a short lateral extension.

Step 4: Inflow Control

The inflow to the left lateral section is secured within the umbilical fissure. The umbilical fissure is often covered by hepatic parenchyma; this is divided with electrocautery to permit access to the inflow vessels to the left hemiliver. The ligamentum teres is retracted anterocaudally to permit full exposure of the umbilical fissure, where the inflow vessels to segments II and III are seen along the left of the fissure

Techniques for Hepatic Resection

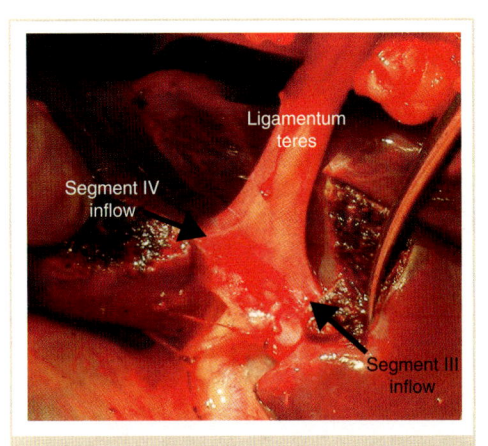

Figure 12-20: Left hepatic segmental inflow control. Elevation of the ligamentum teres facilitates visualization of the portal inflow to segments II–IV. (Reprinted with kind permission of Springer Science + Business Media.[36])

and the inflow vessels to segments IVA and IVB are found along the right of the fissure (Figure 12-20). The inflow vessels to segments II and III along the left of the umbilical fissure are suture ligated and divided (Figure 12-21), rendering the left lateral section visibly ischemic (Figure 12-22).

Step 5: Outflow Control

Outflow control can be performed extrahepatically as with left hemihepatectomy; alternatively, we often divide the left hepatic vein intrahepatically after parenchymal transection.

Step 6: Parenchymal Transection

Parenchymal transection proceeds by dividing the liver along a plane just to the left of the falciform ligament (Figure 12-23). The left hepatic vein may be taken intrahepatically.

Right Trisectionectomy

Right trisectionectomy involves extirpation of segments IV through VIII. This is undertaken in much the same manner as conventional right hemihepatectomy, with the additional need to control the vascular inflow to segment IV.

Steps 1 Through 5

The initial conduct of right trisectionectomy is identical to that undertaken for right hemihepatectomy.

In addition to securing the inflow to the right hemiliver, the inflow to segment IV is controlled within the umbilical fissure. The umbilical fissure is often covered by a segment of hepatic parenchyma; this is divided with electrocautery to permit access to the inflow vessels to the left hemiliver. The ligamentum teres is retracted anterocaudally to permit full exposure of the umbilical fissure, where the inflow vessels to segments II and III are seen along the left of the fissure and the inflow vessels to segments IVA and IVB are found along the right of the fissure. The latter structures are suture ligated and then divided. Satisfactory inflow control is verified when ischemic demarcation of segments IV through VIII is observed. Outflow control is also performed in a fashion similar to that employed for right hemihepatectomy. The middle hepatic vein is routinely taken during right trisectionectomy, and we generally divide this structure intrahepatically after parenchymal transection.

Step 6: Parenchymal Transection

Parenchymal transection proceeds by dividing the liver to the right of the falciform ligament; the plane of transection continues toward the right hepatic vein, and the middle hepatic vein is divided as parenchymal transection proceeds along the dome of the liver near its insertion into the vena cava. Throughout transection, care should be taken to avoid inadvertent injury to the left hepatic vein.

Left Trisectionectomy

Left trisectionectomy, or resection of segments II–V and VIII, is a difficult procedure used for extirpation of large left-sided tumors that cross the principal scissura. There are three major technical challenges in this operation. One rests in the need to preserve the right hepatic vein as the sole venous outflow of the remnant right posterior section; the plane of parenchymal transection is the right scissura, risking inadvertent injury to the right hepatic vein (which runs along the right scissura). Another challenge is because the origin of inflow to segment VII often arises from the right anterior pedicle (or from the junction between the right anterior and posterior pedicles), introducing the potential for inadvertently devascularizing the inflow to half of the intended liver remnant. Finally, the enormous variability in biliary anatomy raises the risk of iatrogenic biliary injury. Because of these variables, it is especially important that assiduous attention be paid to preoperative imaging in anticipation of this operative endeavor.

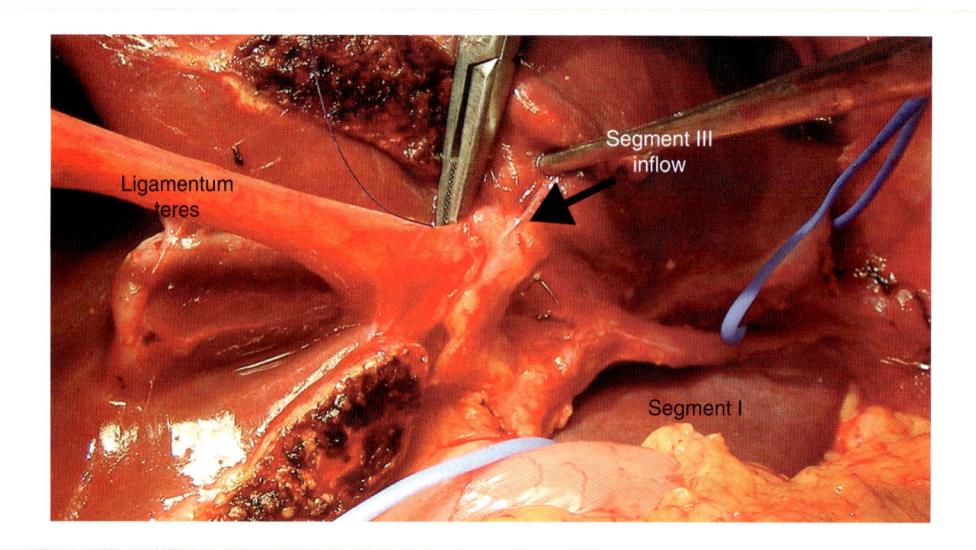

Figure 12-21: Left hepatic segmental inflow control. Suture ligation of the portal inflow to segment III is demonstrated. (Reprinted with kind permission of Springer Science + Business Media.[36])

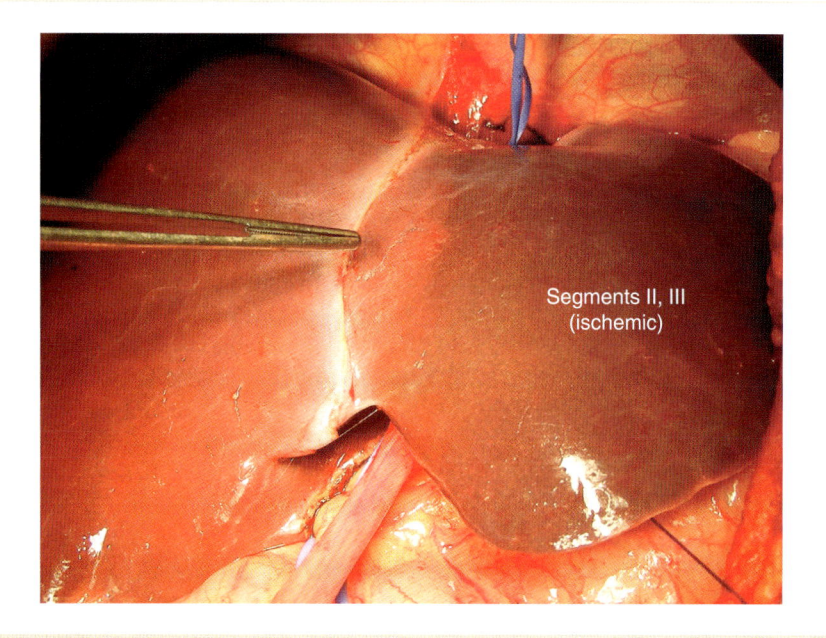

Figure 12-22: Ischemic demarcation of the left lateral section. Following division of the inflow to segments II and III, the left lateral section becomes visibly ischemic. (Reprinted with kind permission of Springer Science + Business Media.[36])

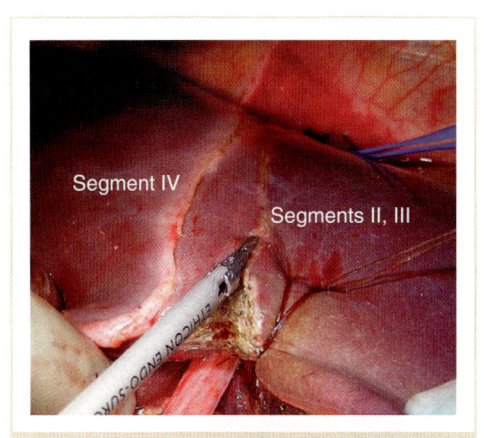

Figure 12-23: Left lateral sectionectomy parenchymal transection. (Reprinted with kind permission of Springer Science + Business Media.[36])

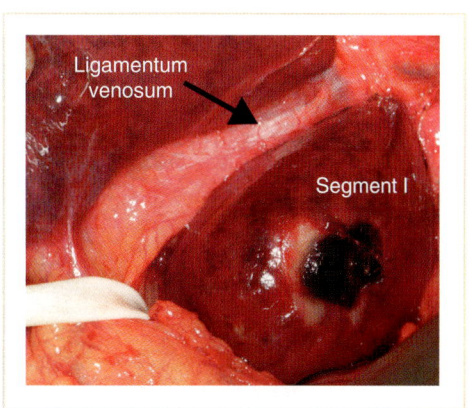

Figure 12-24: Segment I. Division of the hepatogastric ligament along the ligamentum venosum permits exposure of segment I.

Steps 1 Through 3

The initial conduct of this operation proceeds in a manner identical to that of right and left hemihepatectomy. Both the right and left hemilivers are mobilized.

Steps 4 and 5

Initial vascular control of inflow and outflow proceeds in a manner similar to that undertaken for left hemihepatectomy.

Step 6: Parenchymal Transection

It is critical to understand that the plane of dissection along the right scissura (along the plane of the right hepatic vein) runs horizontally or parallel to the operating room floor. The transection plane may be highlighted by occluding the right anterior pedicle to induce ischemic demarcation of segments V and VIII. In circumstances where the tumor is not in proximity to the hepatic hilus, this can be achieved by intrahepatic right anterior pedicle ligation (as described above for right hemihepatectomy). Importantly, if segment VII becomes ischemic during transient occlusion of the right anterior pedicle, additional dissection will be needed to identify and protect the vascular inflow to segment VII (which often emanates from the right anterior pedicle or from the junction between the right anterior and posterior pedicles). Parenchymal transection then proceeds along the line of ischemic demarcation, and great care is taken to avoid injury to the right hepatic vein.

Segmentectomy I

Resection of the caudate lobe requires a close familiarity with the anatomic relationships between segment I and the remainder of the liver and local vascular structures. Segment resides between the middle and left hepatic veins superiorly and the inferior vena cava posteriorly and the porta hepatis anteriorly. In addition, the anterior surface of the left half of segment I is covered by the gastrohepatic ligament.

Steps 1 Through 3

The initial exposure and mobilization are performed in a manner similar to that undertaken for left hemihepatectomy. The left lateral section is fully mobilized, and the gastrohepatic ligament is divided along the ligamentum venosum to expose the caudate lobe (Figure 12-24).

Step 4: Inflow Control

The inflow to segment I is found along the base of the umbilical fissure and is taken as it emanates from the left portal vein (Figure 12-17).

Step 5: Outflow Control

A unique anatomic aspect of segment I is that its venous drainage directly enters the inferior vena cava through several short veins found along its posterior aspect. To access these vessels, a fibrous attachment that is often found between segment

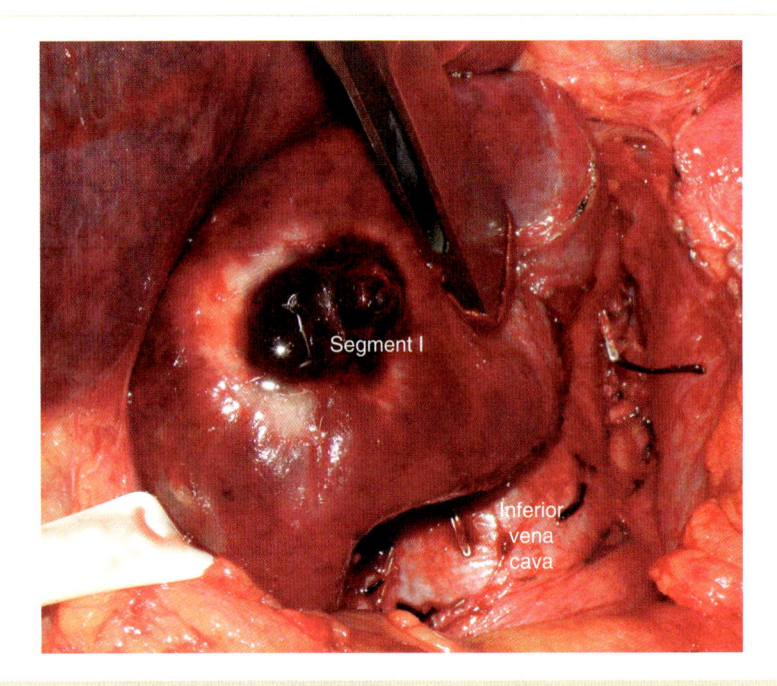

Figure 12-25: Mobilization of segment I. The fibrous attachments between the left lateral margin of segment I and the retroperitoneum is divided, and the numerous veins directly draining segment I into the inferior vena cava are divided.

I and the retroperitoneum along the left lateral aspect of the inferior vena cava is divided (Figure 12-25). The veins are then serially divided between clips and ligatures. Of note, these vessels can also be accessed from the right side as is performed for right hemihepatecomy during mobilization of the right hemiliver (Figure 12-9).

Step 6: Parenchymal Transection
Once the caudate lobe has been fully mobilized off the inferior vena cava, parenchymal transection proceeds along a plane running from the right aspect of the left portal vein superiorly to the right aspect of the inferior vena cava inferiorly (Figure 12-26). During dissection, care must be taken to avoid injury to the right and middle hepatic veins, as they course in close anterior proximity to the cephalad portion of segment I.

Operative Strategies

Two-Stage Hepatectomy
In patients with extensive bilateral hepatic tumors for whom a single-stage resective procedure would result in an insufficient FLR volume, operative therapy may best be undertaken in a staged fashion.[27,28] In this approach, therapy is initially directed at the side of the liver that is less involved with disease. This is generally performed using laparoscopic wedge resection with or without ablation, or with percutaneous ablation, in an attempt to eradicate all disease from that hemiliver. Because the anticipated recovery following these procedures is generally brief, PVE of the contralateral hemiliver (the side that is more involved with disease) can be undertaken before discharge. Four weeks after PVE, repeat imaging is undertaken to assess for postembolization hypertrophy and to confirm that the hypertrophied hemiliver remains clear of disease. If both of these criteria are met, operative intervention is completed by resecting the embolized hemiliver and clearing all remaining foci of disease. The strategy of two-stage hepatectomy has proven to be very effective in permitting complete resection for patients who would otherwise be considered unresectable and has broadened the ability to offer surgical therapy for patients with hepatic metastases.[27,28]

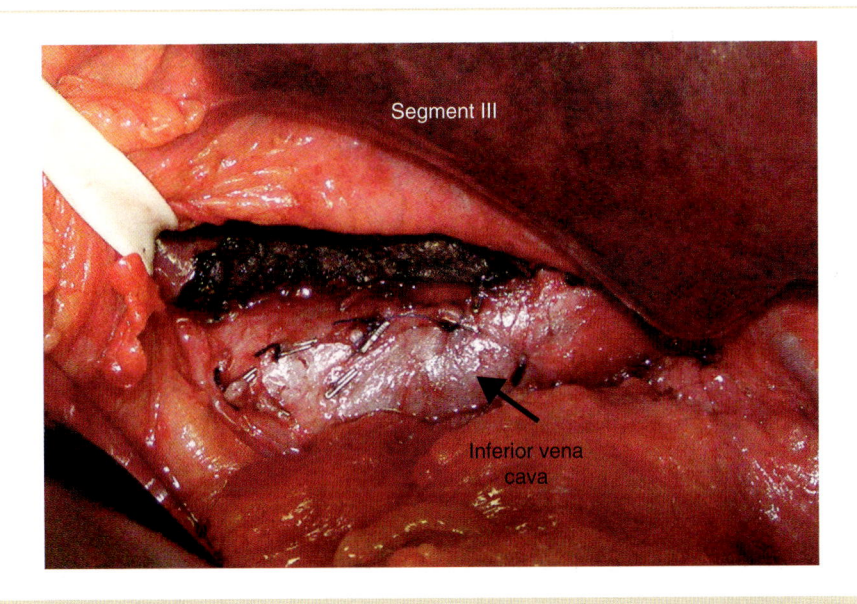

Figure 12-26: Segmentectomy I. The exposed vena cava following resection of segment I is demonstrated.

Nonanatomic Resections

An important operative distinction exists between anatomic and nonanatomic resections. Anatomic resections involve the formal control of the inflow to the segment(s) to be resected, with the planes of parenchymal transection taking place between hepatic Counaud's segments. In contrast, nonanatomic resections are performed by transecting the hepatic parenchyma around the lesion to be removed, without specific regard for intersegmental planes. Retrospective analyses have identified lower rates of positive margins with anatomic resection, although this is likely to be influenced by the generally larger resection specimens that result from anatomic resections.[29] A clear advantage of anatomic resections is the lower blood loss that is generally encountered when specific inflow control and intersegmental dissection are performed. For this reason, lesions that are located deep within the liver parenchyma are often not amenable to nonanatomic resection.

There are several circumstances in which nonanatomic resections are favored. One is in the setting of cirrhosis, where effort must be expended to preserve as much hepatic parenchyma as possible.[12,30] In the management of hepatic neuroendocrine metastases, where operative resections are not uncommonly undertaken for relief of hormonal symptoms and the likelihood of recurrence is very high, lesions are typically resected in a nonanatomic fashion without the need for wide resection margins.[31] In addition, benign tumors for which there is no concern for recurrent disease (such as hepatic adenomas or symptomatic hemangiomata or cysts) are typically resected in a nonanatomic fashion.

Laparoscopic Partial Hepatectomy

The use of laparoscopy has proven very useful for hepatic wedge resection and biopsy procedures, and its implementation for major hepatectomies is now increasing. The success of major laparoscopic liver resections continues to be driven by advances in technology, particularly with respect to instruments used for parenchymal transection. Laparoscopic partial hepatectomy requires a close familiarity with hepatic anatomy and open resections, as well as ready access to high-quality instrumentation for laparoscopic ultrasonography. Each of the various major hepatectomy operations has now been performed laparoscopically, but routine use of major laparoscopic liver resections presently remains limited to a relatively small number of centers worldwide.[32,33]

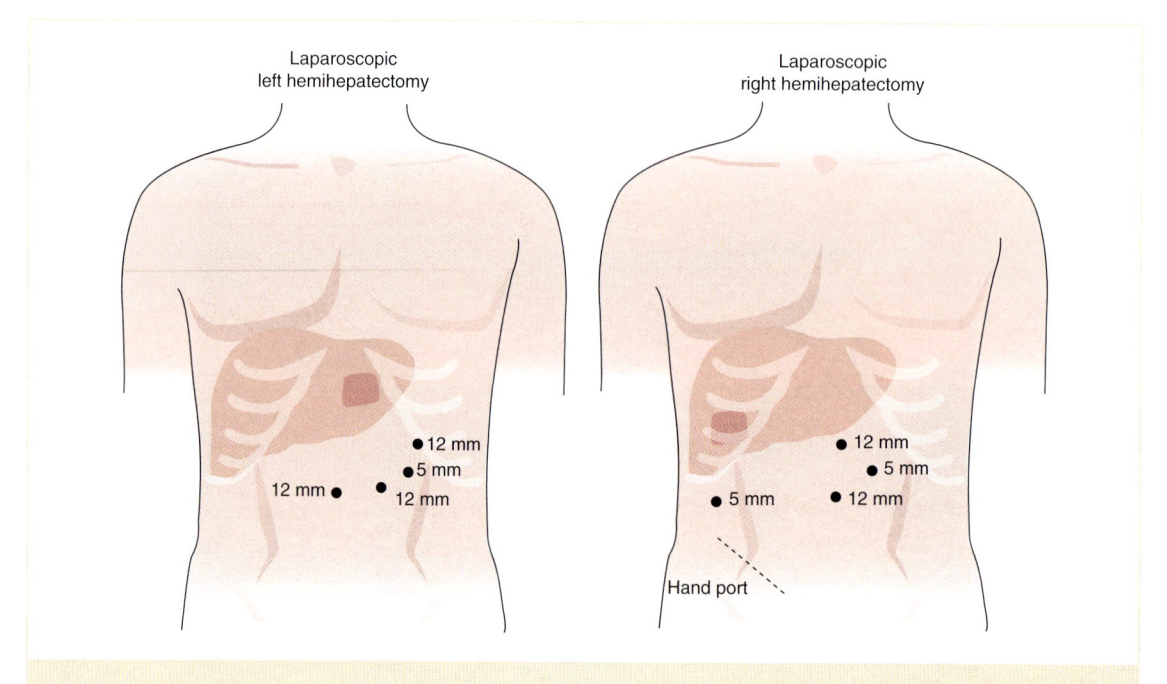

Figure 12-27: Laparoscopic partial hepatectomy port site incisions. Suggested port site incisions for laparoscopic left and right hemihepatectomy are illustrated.

Suggested port placements for laparoscopic resection of left- and right-sided hepatic tumors are shown in Figure 12-27. Alternative placement of ports shown for laparoscopic right hemihepatectomy is shown in Figure 12-28. Laparoscopic partial hepatectomy is undertaken in much the same manner as used for traditional open resections. The operation begins with a careful laparoscopic ultraonographic examination to verify the location of tumors and their anatomic relationships to important biliary and vascular structures. Liver mobilization is then undertaken in a standard fashion using electrocautery or an energy device. We have found that mobilization of the right hemiliver is facilitated by the laparoscopic approach, which affords much clearer visualization of the retrohepatic space (Figure 12-29). Use of the handport provides a number of advantages. The ability to insert a hand facilitates retraction of the liver, which is particularly useful during right hemihepatectomy. This also allows for easy compression of the liver parenchyma in the event that untoward bleeding should be encountered. Furthermore, the incision at the handport site provides easy access for stapler insertion and for specimen removal. We also place a sponge into the peritoneal cavity through the handport; this allows for absorption of blood and cleansing of the laparoscopic camera. We generally divide the inflow and outflow intrahepatically using the stapler after initiation of parenchymal transection. Parenchymal transection is undertaken using a laparoscopic harmonic scalpel or bipolar energy device. Larger venous structures are divided using a laparoscopic stapler. When difficulty is encountered during isolation and division of the right hepatic vein, it is often useful to place the stapler through the handport incision as would be performed during open resection.

The Anterior Approach and Hanging Maneuver

Conduct of the right hemihepatectomy typically involves full mobilization of the right hemiliver off the right hemidiaphragm and retroperitoneum. In circumstances where the right-sided tumor is very

Techniques for Hepatic Resection 289

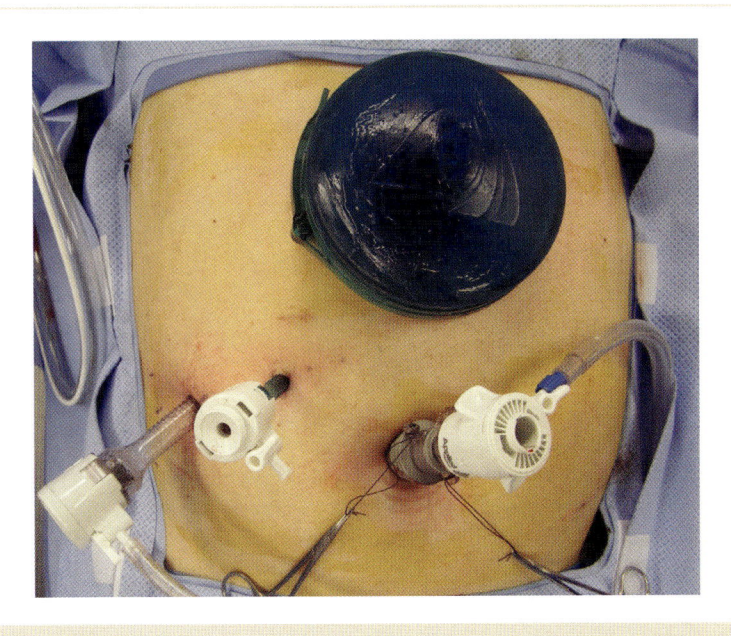

Figure 12-28: Laparoscopic right hemihepatectomy. Alternative port placements for laparoscopic right hemihepatectomy are demonstrated.

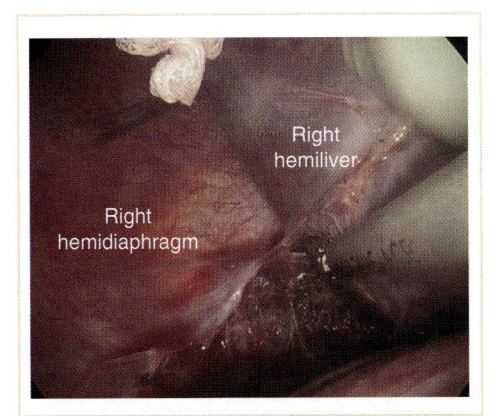

Figure 12-29: Laparoscopic mobilization of the right hemiliver. Visualization of the retrohepatic space is facilitated by laparoscopy.

large or vascular or invasive into the surrounding extrahepatic tissues, early mobilization of the right hemiliver may result in excessive bleeding or risk of tumoral rupture. In this circumstance, an anterior approach has been advocated, in which parenchymal transection is initiated along the anterior surface of the liver and extended posteriorly toward the inferior vena cava.[34] The hepatic inflow and outflow vessels are divided as they are encountered within the hepatic parenchyma, and resection is completed as the remaining attachments of the right hemiliver to the inferior vena cava, retroperitoneum, and diaphragm are divided.

The hanging maneuver is a variation of the anterior approach in which blunt dissection is carried out along the anterior surface of the inferior vena cava[35] (Figure 12-30). Dissection begins along the retrohepatic space from its cephalad aspect by passing a clamp downward between the right and middle

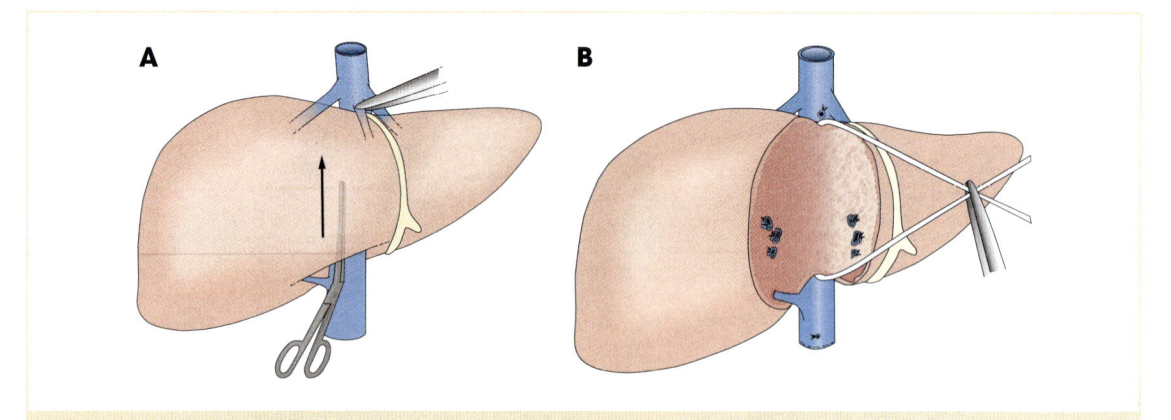

Figure 12-30: The hanging maneuver. Passage of a long blunt vascular clamp along the anterior surface of the inferior vena cava to a point between the right and middle hepatic veins permits passage of an umbilical tape (A). Elevation of the umbilical tape can greatly facilitate anterior resection (B).

hepatic veins. Dissection along this plane is also performed from its caudal aspect between the caudate lobe and inferior vena cava, with care taken to avoid injury to small venous vessels between these two structures. By completing this tunneled dissection, an umbilical tape can be passed and used to suspend the liver anteriorly, facilitating the anterior approach parenchymal transection.

References

1. Fan ST, Lo CM, Liu CL, et al. Hepatectomy for hepatocellular carcinoma: toward zero hospital deaths. *Ann Surg*. 1999;229:322–330.
2. Belghiti J, Hiramatsu K, Benoist S, et al. Seven hundred forty-seven hepatectomies in the 1990s: an update to evaluate the actual risk of liver resection. *J Am Coll Surg*. 2000;191:38–46.
3. Jarnagin WR, Gonen M, Fong Y, et al. Improvement in perioprative outcome after hepatic resection analysis of 1,803 consecutive cases over the past decade. *Ann Surg*. 2002;236:397–406.
4. Strasberg SM, Belghiti J, Clavien PA, et al. The Brisbane 2000 terminology of liver anatomy and resection. *HPB*. 2000;2:333–339.
5. Launois B, Jamieson GG. The importance of Glisson's capsule and its sheaths in the intrahepatic approach to resection of the liver. *Surg Gynecol Obstet*. 1992 174:7–10.
6. Lau H, Man K, Fan ST, et al. Evaluation of preoperative hepatic function in patients with hepatocellular carcinoma undergoing hepatectomy. *Br J Surg*. 1997;84:1255–1259.
7. Fan ST, Lai EC, Lo CM, et al. Hospital mortality of major hepatectomy for hepatocellular carcinoma associated with cirrhosis. *Arch Surg*. 1995;130:198–203.
8. Ercolani G, Grazi GL, Calliva R, et al. The lidocaine (MEGX) test as an index of hepatic function: its clinical usefulness in liver surgery. *Surgery*. 2000;127:464–471.
9. Bruix J, Castells A, Bosch J, et al. Surgical resection of hepatocellular carcinoma in cirrhotic patients: prognostic value of preoperative portal pressure. *Gastroenterology*. 1996;111:1018–1022.
10. Yin XY, Lu MD, Huang JF, et al. Significance of portal hemodynamic investigation in prediction of hepatic functional reserve in patients with hepatocellular carcinoma undergoing operative treatment. *Hepatogastroenterology*. 2001;48:1701–1704.
11. Franco D, Capussotti L, Smadja C, et al. Resection of hepatocellular carcinomas: results in 72 European patients with cirrhosis. *Gastroentology*. 1990;98:733–738.
12. Wu CC, Ho WL, Yeh DC, et al. Hepatic resection of hepatocellular carcinoma in cirrhotic livers: is it unjustified in impaired liver function? *Surgery*. 1996;120:34–39.
13. Karoui M, Penna C, Amin-Hashem M, et al. Influence of preoperative chemotherapy on the risk of

major hepatectomy for colorectal liver metastases. *Ann Surg.* 2006;243:1–7.
14. Fong Y, Bentrem DJ. CASH (chemotherapy-associated steatohepatitis) costs. *Ann Surg.* 2006;243:8–9.
15. Rubbia-Brandt L, Audard V, Sartoretti P, et al. Severe hepatic sinusoidal obstruction associated with oxaliplatin-based chemotherapy in patients with metastatic colorectal cancer. *Ann Oncol.* 2004;15:460–466.
16. Vauthey JN, Pawlik TM, Ribero D, et al. Chemotherapy regimen predicts steatohepatitis and an increase in 90-day mortality after surgery for hepatic colorectal metastases. *J Clin Oncol.* 2006;24:2065–2072.
17. Cleary JM, Tanabe KT, Lauwers GY, et al. Hepatic toxicities associated with the use of preoperative systemic therapy in patients with metastatic colorectal adenocarcinoma to the liver. *Oncologist.* 2009;14:1095–1105.
18. Kooby DA, Fong Y, Suriawinata A, et al. Impact of steatosis on perioperative outcome following hepatic resection. *J Gastrointest Surg.* 2003; 7:1034–1044.
19. Cho CS, Curran S, Schwartz LH, et al. Preoperative radiographic assessment of hepatic steatosis with histologic correlation. *J Am Coll Surg.* 2008;206:480–488.
20. Shirabe K, Shimada M, Gion T, et al. Postoperative liver failure after major hepatic resection for hepatocellular carcinoma in the modern era with special reference to remnant liver volume. *J Am Coll Surg.* 1999;188:304–309.
21. Makuuchi M, Thai BL, Takayasu K, et al. Preoperative portal embolization to increase safety of major hepatectomy for hilar bile duct carcinoma: a preliminary report. *Surgery.* 1990;107:521–527.
22. Lee KC, Kinoshita H, Hirohashi K, et al. Extension of surgical indications for hepatocellular carcinoma by portal vein embolization. *World J Surg.* 1993;17:109–115.
23. Azoulay D, Castaing D, Krissat J, et al. Percutaneous portal vein embolization increases the feasibility and safety of major liver resection for hepatocellular carcinoma in injured liver. *Ann Surg.* 2000;232:665–672.
24. Covey AM, Brown KT, Jarnagin WR, et al. Combined portal vein embolization and neoadjuvant chemotherapy as a treatment strategy for resectable hepatic colorectal metastases. *Ann Surg.* 2008;247:451–455.
25. Melendez JA, Arslan V, Fischer ME, et al. Perioperative outcomes of major hepatic resections under low central venous pressure anesthesia: blood loss, blood transfusions, and the risk of postoperative renal dysfunction. *J Am Coll Surg.* 1998;187: 620–625.
26. Fong Y, Brennan MF, Brown K, et al. Drainage is unnecessary after elective liver resection. *Am J Surg.* 1996;171:158–162.
27. Jaeck D, Oussoultzoglou E, Rosso E, et al. A two-stage hepatectomy procedure combined with portal vein embolization to achieve curative resection for initially unresectable multiple and bilobar colorectal liver metastases. *Ann Surg.* 2004;240: 1037–1049.
28. Wicherts DA, Miller R, de Haas RJ, et al. Long-term results of two-stage hepatectomy for irresectable colorectal cancer liver metastases. *Ann Surg.* 2008;248:994–1005.
29. DeMatteo RP, Palese C, Jarnagin WR, et al. Anatomic segmental hepatic resection is superior to wedge resection as an oncologic operation for colorectal liver metastases. *J Gastrointest Surg.* 2000;4:178–184.
30. Cho CS. Surgical resection of hepatocellular carcinoma: less is more? *J Surg Res.* 2009; 157:155–157.
31. Cho CS, Labow DM, Tang L, et al. Histologic grade is correlated with outcome after resection of hepatic neuroendocrine neoplasms. *Cancer.* 2008;113:126–134.
32. Nguyen KT, Gamblin TC, Geller DA. World review of laparoscopic liver resection – 2,804 patients. *Ann Surg.* 2009;250:831–841.
33. Buell JF, Cherqui D, Geller DA, et al. The international position on laparoscopic liver surgery: the Louisville Statement 2008. *Ann Surg.* 2009;250:825–830.
34. Lai EC, Fan ST, Lo CM, et al. Anterior approach for difficult major right hepatectomy. *World J Surg.* 1996;20:314–317.
35. Belghiti J, Guevera OA, Noun R, et al. Liver hanging maneuver: a safe approach to right hepatectomy without liver mobilization. *J Am Coll Surg.* 2001;193:109–111.
36. Russ AJ, Cho CS. Hepatic procedures. In: Chen H, ed. *Illustrative Handbook of General Surgery*. London, UK: Springer-Verlag; 2010:249–278.
37. Patrlj L, Tuorto S, Fong Y. Combined blunt-clamp dissection and LigaSure ligation for hepatic parenchyma dissection: postcoagulation technique. *J Am Coll Surg* 2010;210:39–44.

CHAPTER 13

Liver Transplantation for Malignant Tumors

Vatche G. Agopian & Henrik Petrowsky

Introduction

Liver transplantation appears as an attractive surgical approach to treat hepatobiliary cancers. The rational behind this concept is that many hepatobiliary cancers, especially hepatocellular cancer (HCC), are multifocal. The complete removal of the liver during transplantation achieves tumor-free margins, treats parenchymal and vascular invasion, and corrects the underlying liver disease. Conversely, liver transplantation requires life-long immunosuppression, which is associated with a significantly higher risk of tumor recurrence. Today, the main indications for liver transplantation are primary hepatobiliary malignancies with HCC, the most common tumor type (Figure 13-1). Because chronic inflammatory liver disease is the background of HCC in the majority of cases, liver transplantation simultaneously treats the tumor and underlying liver disease. During the last decade, liver transplantation challenged liver resection for the treatment of unresectable cholangiocarcinoma (CCA). Although liver transplantation for CCA accounted for only 4% of all hepatobiliary cancers (Figure 13-1), there is growing evidence that orthotopic liver transplantation (OLT) offers long-term survival or cure in well-selected patients. Other

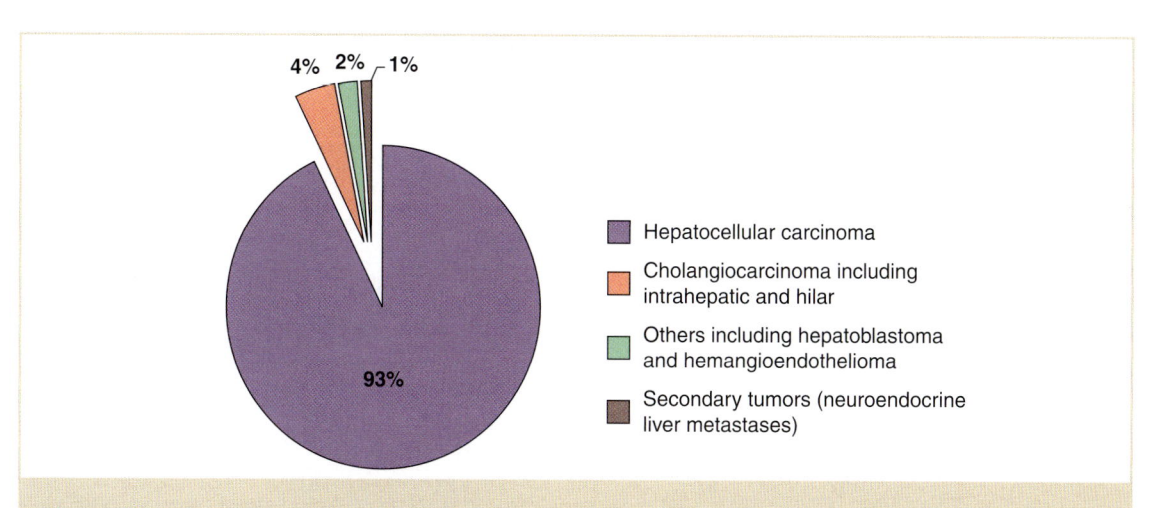

Figure 13-1: Distribution frequencies of liver transplantation for hepatobiliary cancer in the United States from 2003 to 2010. (Adapted from SRTR database.)

rare primary hepatobiliary neoplasias are epithelioid hemangioendothelioma and hepatoblastoma, which may represent excellent indications for OLT. Liver transplantation for liver metastases is contraindicated and is only exceptionally justified for liver metastases from neuroendocrine tumors (NETs). Today, approximately 1% of all OLTs for hepatobiliary malignancies were performed for metastatic NETs (Figure 13-1). Although the initial experience of OLT for NETs was disappointing, an improved and better selection offers posttransplant long-term survival or cure for patients with unresectable liver metastases from NETs.

Liver Transplantation for Hepatocellular Carcinoma

Scope of the Problem

Hepatocellular carcinoma is the third leading cause of cancer-related deaths worldwide, and its incidence is increasing secondary to chronic hepatitis B virus and hepatitis C virus infections.[1] In 2008, approximately 750,000 new cases of HCC were reported worldwide, with 13,300 cases in North America. In the United States, the incidence of hepatitis C virus–related HCC is expected to double in the next 20 years.[2] The prognosis for untreated HCC is dismal, with a five-year survival rate below 10% (Figure 13-2).[3] HCC develops almost exclusively in patients with cirrhosis, adding significant complexity to the optimal treatment algorithms. In recent years, there has been significant progress in both the understanding and treatment of patients with HCC. The current armamentarium for treatment of patients with HCC includes radiologic-directed local regional therapies, surgical resection, liver transplantation, and chemotherapy. Surgical resection has been the treatment of choice in patients with preserved hepatic function and small tumors. However, patients with advanced cirrhosis (Child-Turcotte-Pugh class B and C) with portal hypertension and multifocal tumors are not candidates for surgical resection. In these patients, OLT has become the gold-standard therapy, yielding the best oncologic outcomes and restoring normal hepatic function. However, liver transplantation for HCC should be offered to patients with early-stage tumors with a low risk of recurrence, maximizing oncologic and patient outcomes in an era of significant donor scarcity.

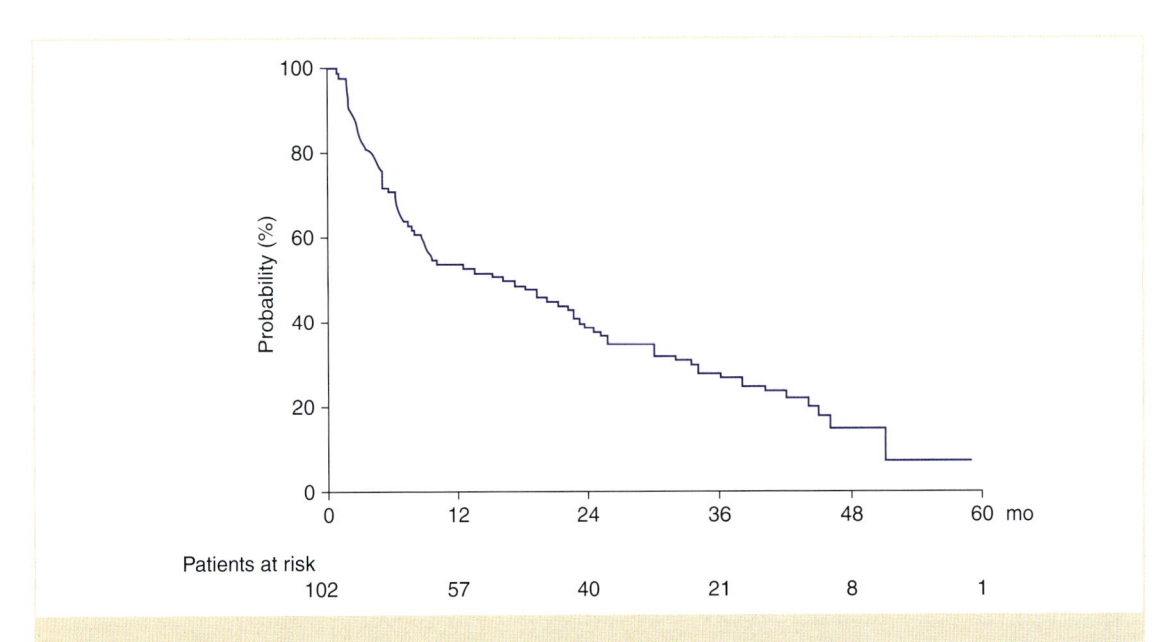

Figure 13-2: Overall survival probability of 102 patients with untreated hepatocellular cancer. (Reprinted from Llovet JM, Bustamante J, Castells A, et al. *Hepatology*. 1999;29:62–67[3] with permission from John Wiley and Sons.)

Patient Selection Based on Tumor Burden

Liver transplantation appears to be the ideal therapy for HCC because it involves removing the entire liver, resulting in negative resection margins. However, the early experience with transplant yielded dismal results. Although the short-term posttransplant survival was reasonable, the recurrence rates, and therefore long-term outcomes, were quite poor. Limitations of donor availability and its impact on all potential liver recipients require that liver transplant be considered only for those patients who have a predicted survival comparable with non-HCC transplant recipients. *Bismuth* was one of the first to consider that tumor burden may serve as a surrogate for tumor biology when they demonstrated that patients with small uninodular or binodular tumors <3 cm had much better outcomes with transplant than resection (83% vs. 18%). This group also found that patients with diffuse form HCC, more than two nodules >3 cm, or those patients with portal venous thrombus had a much higher rate of recurrence leading to poor long-term outcomes.[4]

In 1996, Mazzaferro et al. reported in a landmark study their experience with 48 patients with cirrhosis and unresectable HCC who underwent OLT.[5] This study found a four-year actuarial survival rate of 85% and recurrence-free survival rate of 92% in those patients who met a predetermined criterion (Figure 13-3). In patients who exceeded criteria on explant pathology, actuarial and recurrence-free survival was significantly worse at 50% and 59%, respectively. These standards became the basis for the Milan criteria; defined by a single tumor <5 cm, or three or fewer tumors all individually <3 cm (Figure 13-4). The Milan criteria have subsequently been adopted by the United Network for Organ Sharing (UNOS) as selection criteria for HCC patients evaluated for transplant. The survival benefits of these criteria have been demonstrated in numerous studies.[6,7] The excellent outcomes of HCC patients within the criteria led many to believe that perhaps the Milan criteria was too restrictive, and reasonable outcomes could be established with even more inclusive standards.[8]

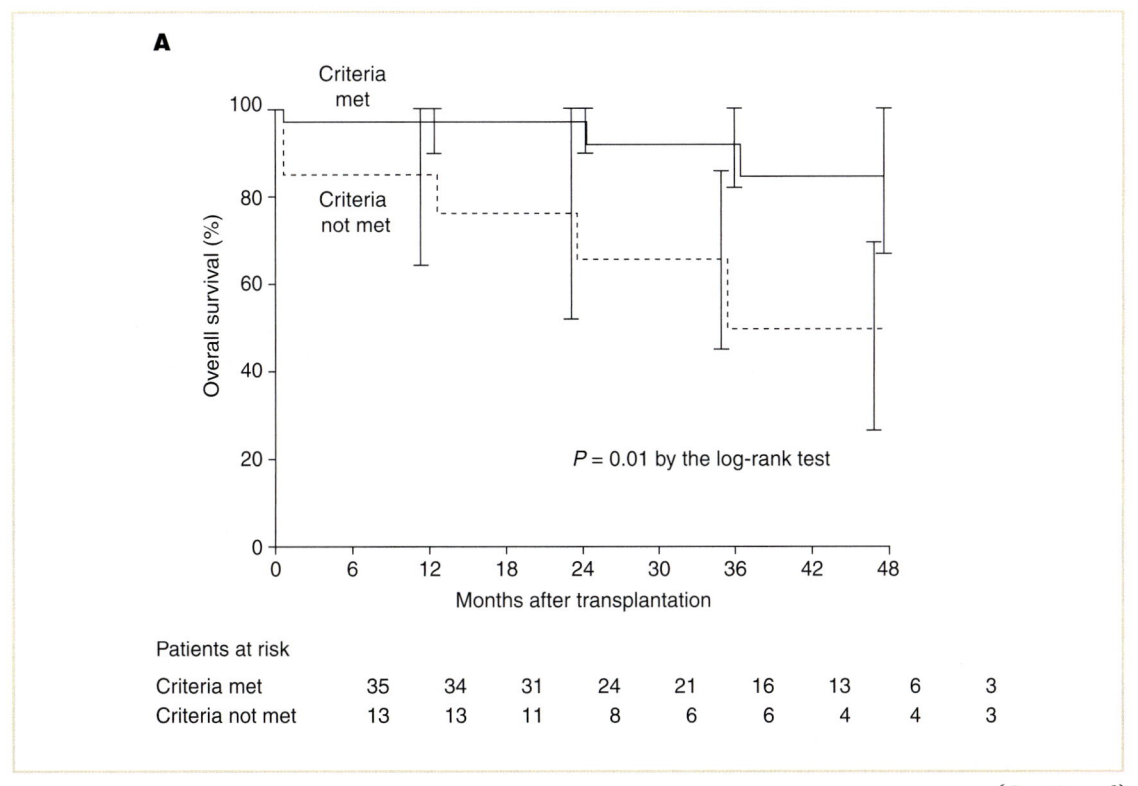

(Continued)

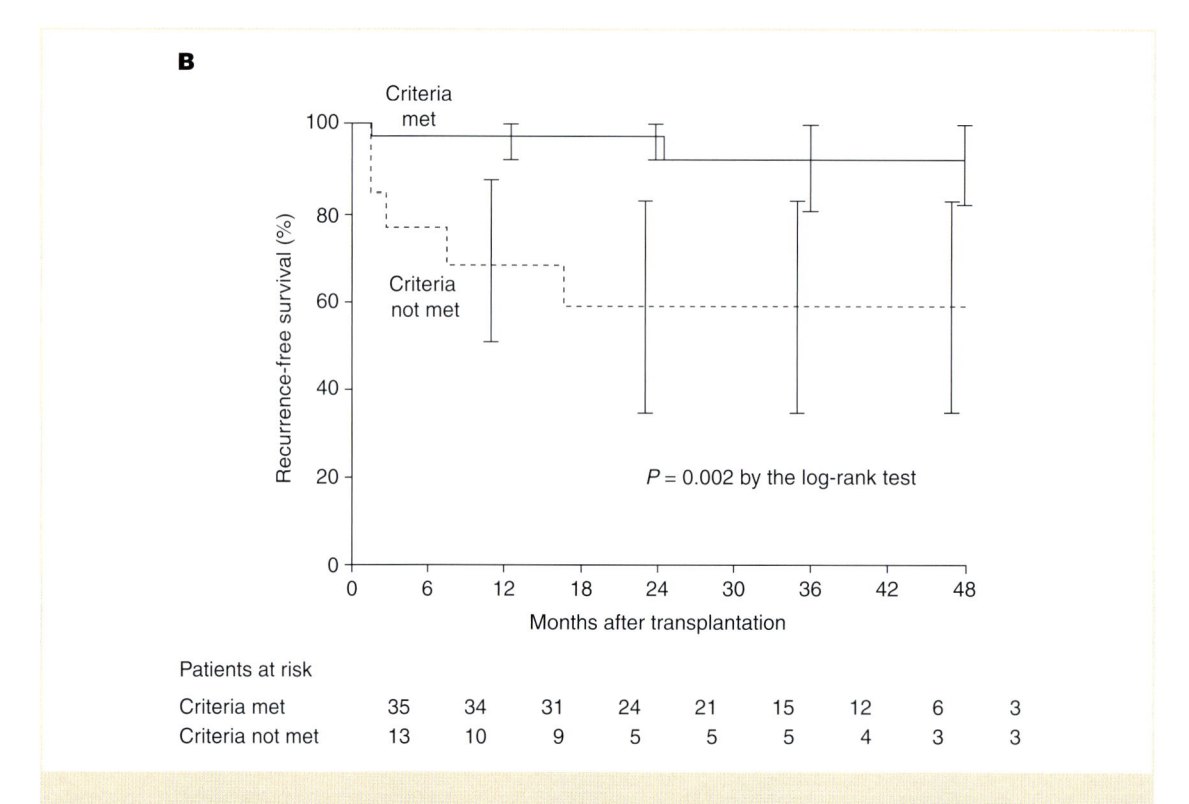

Figure 13-3: Overall survival (A) and recurrence-free survival (B) of patients after liver transplantation for hepatocellular cancer within and outside the Milan criteria. (Reprinted from Mazzaferro V, Regalia E, Doci R, et al. *N Engl J Med.* 1996;334:693–699 © 1996,[5] Massachusetts Medical Society. All rights reserved.)

The University of California, San Francisco (UCSF) group used expanded tumor burden criteria and demonstrated excellent results. They proposed the following criteria: solitary tumor ≤6.5 cm, three or fewer nodules ≤4.5 cm, and total tumor diameter ≤8 cm (Figure 13-4). This established the UCSF criteria and demonstrated a survival rate of 90% and 75% at one and five years, respectively, compared with 50% one-year survival for those with tumors exceeding those limits.[8] However, this study was based on explant biology, something that could not reasonably be established prior to transplant. In 2007, the same group subsequently validated these good outcomes using the same size criteria but based on the measurements taken on preoperative imaging.[9]

The largest experience to date to assess the efficacy of OLT for HCC and evaluate previously established criteria was reported from the University of California, Los Angeles liver transplant center.[10] This study looked at 467 transplants for HCC with an overall one-, three-, and five-year survival of 82%, 65%, and 52%, respectively. Their analysis found that patients meeting the Milan criteria had similar survival to those patients meeting UCSF criteria by both preoperative imaging and explant biology (Figure 13-5). However, they confirmed that tumors beyond UCSF criteria portended survival below 50%. A multivariate analysis demonstrated that tumor number, lymphovascular invasion, and poor differentiation independently predicted poor survival.

These landmark studies have all played a role in the wide acceptance of liver transplantation as an appropriate treatment for hepatocellular carcinoma. Despite this, there are no generally accepted guidelines, and much controversy remains. In December 2010, an international consensus conference with experts from around the world convened in Zurich, Switzerland with the aim of reviewing the current practice regarding liver

Liver Transplantation for Malignant Tumors

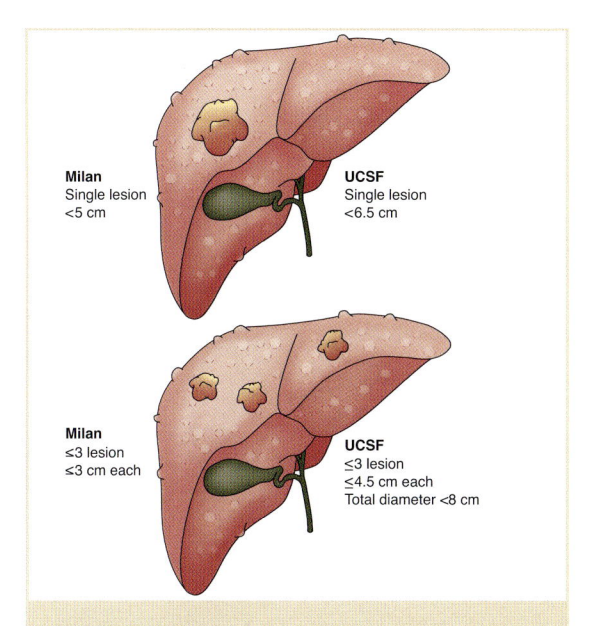

Figure 13-4: Milan (single lesion ≤5 cm or no more than three lesions ≤3 cm) and University of California, San Francisco (UCSF) criteria (single lesion ≤6.5 cm or no more than three lesions ≤4.5 cm and a total diameter of 8 cm) for patients with hepatocellular cancer and undergoing liver transplantation.

transplantation for HCC and developing internationally accepted statements. A total of 37 final statements and recommendations were made covering assessment of candidates for liver transplantation, criteria for listing in cirrhotic and noncirrhotic patients, role of tumor downstaging, management of patients on the waiting list, role of living donation, and posttransplant management. Seventeen of these position statements were made as "strong" recommendations and are summarized in Table 13-1.

Radiologic Criteria for HCC

The purpose of any cancer staging system is to accurately predict prognosis of patients and help determine what treatment is most appropriate. Many of the important prognostic factors for HCC (vascular invasion, satellite nodules, lymph node metastasis, degree of differentiation) are not available prior to pathologic examination of the explanted liver. As many patients with HCC and cirrhosis do not undergo biopsies, staging systems used to guide therapy prior to liver transplantation rely mainly on imaging criteria. The international consensus conference made the strong recommendation that contrast-enhanced computer tomography (CT) or magnetic resonance imaging (MRI) with washout on portal venous or delayed imaging is the best noninvasive test to diagnose and stage cirrhotic patients suspected of having HCC (Table 13-1). Extrahepatic staging should include a chest CT scan. Furthermore, preoperative assessment of the size of the largest tumor or total diameter of the tumors should be the main consideration in selecting patients with HCC for transplantation, with the Milan criteria serving as the benchmark.[11]

Model for End-Stage Liver Disease

In the United States, the model for end-stage liver disease (MELD) is a scoring system that was originally designed to predict the survival of patients with liver failure undergoing transjugularintrahepatic portosystemic shunt (TIPS) procedure.[12] However, MELD was subsequently shown to be an excellent predictor of survival in patients with end-stage liver disease awaiting liver transplantation and, as such, was adopted by UNOS in 2002 for prioritizing deceased donor organ allocation for liver transplantation. Because so many of the patients with HCC have well-compensated cirrhosis, this scoring system does not reasonably assess their true risk of death on the waiting list. With this in mind, the first MELD exception criteria for HCC were established.[13] This initial scoring system assumed a 15% risk of disease progression within three months for stage I disease; therefore, these patients were given a MELD score of 24. For patients with stage II disease, a 30% risk of progression was assumed; this cohort received a MELD of 29. In addition, for each three months that patients remained on the wait list, they were assessed another 10% risk, and therefore, the score was increased. This allocation system led to a dramatic swing in the number of transplants performed for HCC from 7% to 22%.[14] The system was felt by many to give too

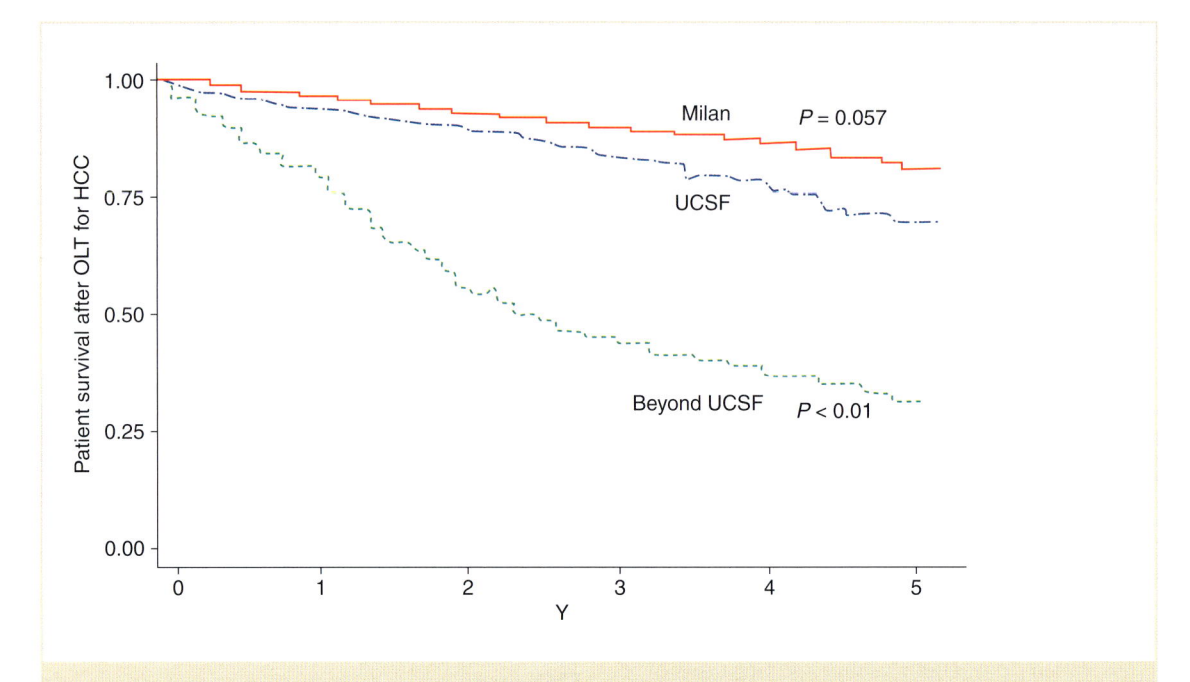

Figure 13-5: Survival estimate by pathological explant examination of hepatocellular cancer (HCC) in a series of 467 patients undergoing orthotopic liver transplantation (OLT) at the University of California, Los Angeles (UCLA) within Milan (red) and UCSF (blue) criteria and beyound UCSF (green) criteria.. UCSF, University of California, San Francisco. (Reprinted from Duffy JP, Vardanian A, Benjamin E, et al. *Ann Surg.* 2007;246:502–509[10] with permission from Lippincott Williams & Wilkins.)

great advantage to HCC patients relative to those with decompensated cirrhosis whose MELD score was physiologic.[15] The allocation for MELD was revised in 2003, resulting in stage I disease receiving a MELD score of 20 and stage II a score of 24. This alteration led to decrease from 22% to 14% of all transplants performed for HCC. A pathologic review of explanted livers found that those with presumed stage I HCC had no demonstrable tumor 31% of the time.[14] Therefore, the exception points were further modified to exclude those with stage I HCC. The current guidelines for MELD score for patients with HCC are as follows: Points are awarded for a tumor burden within Milan criteria, tumors within UCSF, but greater than Milan must be downstaged to Milan; 22 points are awarded for single tumors ≥2 and ≤5 cm or 2–3 tumors ≥1 and ≤3 cm with an automatic increase for every three months spent on the wait list (Figure 13-6).[16]

Listing Criteria for Liver Transplantation in HCC

To guarantee an accurate preoperative evaluation, specific guidelines must be met for listing patients with HCC for OLT. Patients must be assessed radiologically to evaluate the number and size of tumors and to rule out extrahepatic disease and vascular involvement. Definitive tissue diagnosis is not required, but if no biopsy is available, one of the following must be fulfilled: AFP > 200 mg/mL, arteriogram confirming the tumor or arterial enhancement followed by portal venous washout on CT or MRI, or a history of locoregional treatment. Those patients with no demonstrable tumor on imaging may be given MELD exception points if their AFP is >500 mg/mL. Patients with tumors <2 cm or patients beyond Milan criteria can be listed for transplant, but they will receive no additional MELD points for the tumor. All patients must be deemed unresectable,

TABLE 13-1: Strong Recommendations From the International Consensus Conference on Liver Transplantation for HCC

	Level of Evidence
Assessment of candidates with HCC for liver transplantation	
1. When considering treatment options for patients with HCC, the Barcelona Clinic Liver Cancer (BCLC) staging system is the preferred staging system to assess the prognosis of patients with HCC	2b(P)
2. The TNM system (7th ed) including pathological examination of the explanted liver should be used for determining prognosis after transplantation with the addition of assessment of microvascular invasion	2b(P)
3. Either dynamic CT or dynamic MRI with the presence of arterial enhancement followed by washout on portal venous or delayed imaging is the best noninvasive test to make a diagnosis in cirrhotic patients suspected of having HCC and for preoperative staging	1b(D)
4. Extrahepatic staging should include CT of the chest and CT or MRI of the abdomen and pelvis	3b(D)
5. For patients with lesions ≤10 mm, noninvasive imaging does not allow an accurate diagnosis and should not be used to make a decision for or against transplantation	1b(D)
Criteria for listing candidates with HCC in cirrhotic livers for DDLT	
6. Preoperative assessment of the size of the largest tumor or total diameter of tumors should be the main consideration in selecting patients with HCC for liver transplantation	2a(P)
7. The Milan criteria are currently the benchmark for the selection of HCC patients for liver transplantation and the basis for comparison with other suggested criteria	2a(P)
8. Biomarkers other than α-fetoprotein cannot yet be used for clinical decision making regarding liver transplantation for HCC	2b(P)
9. Indication for liver transplantation in HCC should not rely on microvascular invasion because it cannot be reliably detected prior to transplantation	2b(P)
Role of downstaging	
10. Liver transplantation after successful downstaging should achieve a 5-year survival comparable with that of HCC patients who meet the criteria of liver transplantation without requiring downstaging	5(P)
11. Criteria for successful downstaging should include tumor size and number of viable tumors	4(P)
Managing patients on the waiting list	
12. Periodic waiting-list monitoring should be performed by imaging (dynamic CT, dynamic MRI, or contrast-enhanced ultrasonography) and α-fetoprotein measurements	5(P)
13. Patients found to have progressed beyond criteria acceptable for listing for liver transplantation should be placed on hold and considered for downstaging	5(P)
14. Patients with progressive disease in whom locoregional intervention is not considered appropriate, or is ineffective, should be removed from the waiting list	5(P)
Role of LDLT	
15. LDLT must be restricted to centers of excellence in liver surgery and liver transplantation to minimize donor risk and maximize recipient outcome	NA
16. In patients following LDLT for HCC outside the accepted regional criteria for DDLT, retransplantation for graft failure using a deceased donor organ is not recommended	5(P)
Posttransplant management	
17. Liver transplantation is not an appropriate treatment for recurrent HCC	NA

Abbreviations: CT, computed tomography; DDLT, deceased donor liver transplantation; HCC, hepatocellular carcinoma; LDLT, living donor liver transplantation; MRI, magnetic resonance imaging; TNM, tumor node metastasis. (D) diagnosis; (P) prognosis;
Source: Adapted from Clavien et al.[11]

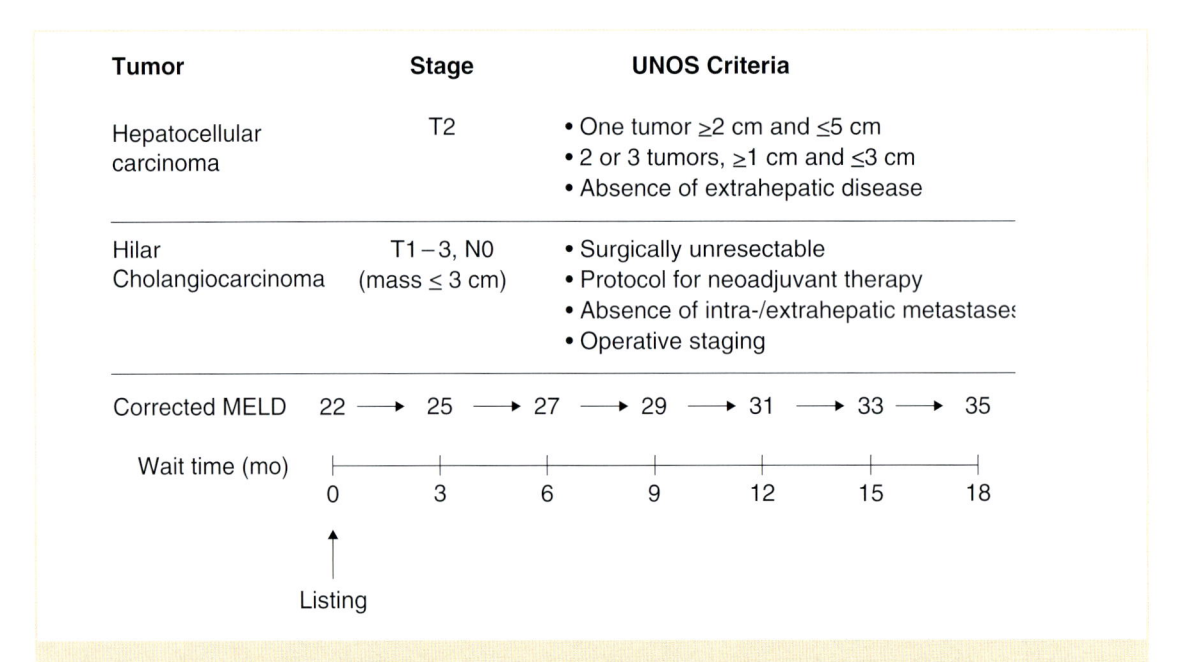

Tumor	Stage	UNOS Criteria
Hepatocellular carcinoma	T2	• One tumor ≥2 cm and ≤5 cm • 2 or 3 tumors, ≥1 cm and ≤3 cm • Absence of extrahepatic disease
Hilar Cholangiocarcinoma	T1–3, N0 (mass ≤ 3 cm)	• Surgically unresectable • Protocol for neoadjuvant therapy • Absence of intra-/extrahepatic metastases • Operative staging

Corrected MELD: 22 → 25 → 27 → 29 → 31 → 33 → 35

Wait time (mo): 0, 3, 6, 9, 12, 15, 18

Listing (at 0)

Figure 13-6: United Network for Organ Sharing (UNOS) criteria for assignment for additional model for end-stage liver disease (MELD) priority points for hepatocellular cancer and cholangiocarcinoma according to the Organ Procurment and Transplantation Network (OPTN) Policy 3.6. Patients with a laboratory MELD below 22 who meet these criteria will receive a MELD score of 22 at time of listing. There is a 10% increase of accrual MELD score every three months.

and there must be documentation of the tumor every three months by CT or MRI to assure that there has been no progression of disease beyond the established criteria.

Wait List Management for HCC

Patients with unresectable HCC who are on the wait list for transplantation must be carefully followed up for disease progression with periodic imaging (dynamic CT/MRI) and α-fetoprotein levels. Patients found to have progressed beyond listing criteria should be placed on hold and considered for downstaging, whereas patients with progressive disease despite locoregional therapy should be removed from the list.[11] Because of the obligate time spent on the wait list with an initial relatively low MELD score, patients with HCC are at risk for tumor progression while awaiting accrual of exception points (Figure 13-6). This progression leads to poor outcome following transplantation or drop out secondary to disease progression beyond acceptable transplantation criteria. Therefore, local treatment of the tumor to control progression is commonly pursued in transplant centers that anticipate a significant wait time. Local treatment options include transcatheter arterial chemoembolization (TACE), percutaneous radiofrequency ablation (RFA), or percutaneous ethanol injection.

TACE is a selective embolization of the arterial inflow feeding the hepatoma with chemotherapeutic agents, usually cisplatin of doxorubicin. This embolization results in ischemic insult to the tumor in combination with localized chemotherapy that has little systemic effect. TACE has been shown to lead to complete necrosis, in some cases, and size reduction in 50% of patients with HCC.[17] TACE can be used with three treatment effects in mind: limiting wait list drop out, improving posttransplant results by decreasing recurrence, and downstaging HCC that is beyond established criteria; so patients in this population can be transplanted (Figure 13-7).

There is reasonable evidence that TACE can be effectively used as a bridge to transplant. A series of 54 patients at the Mayo clinic treated with TACE

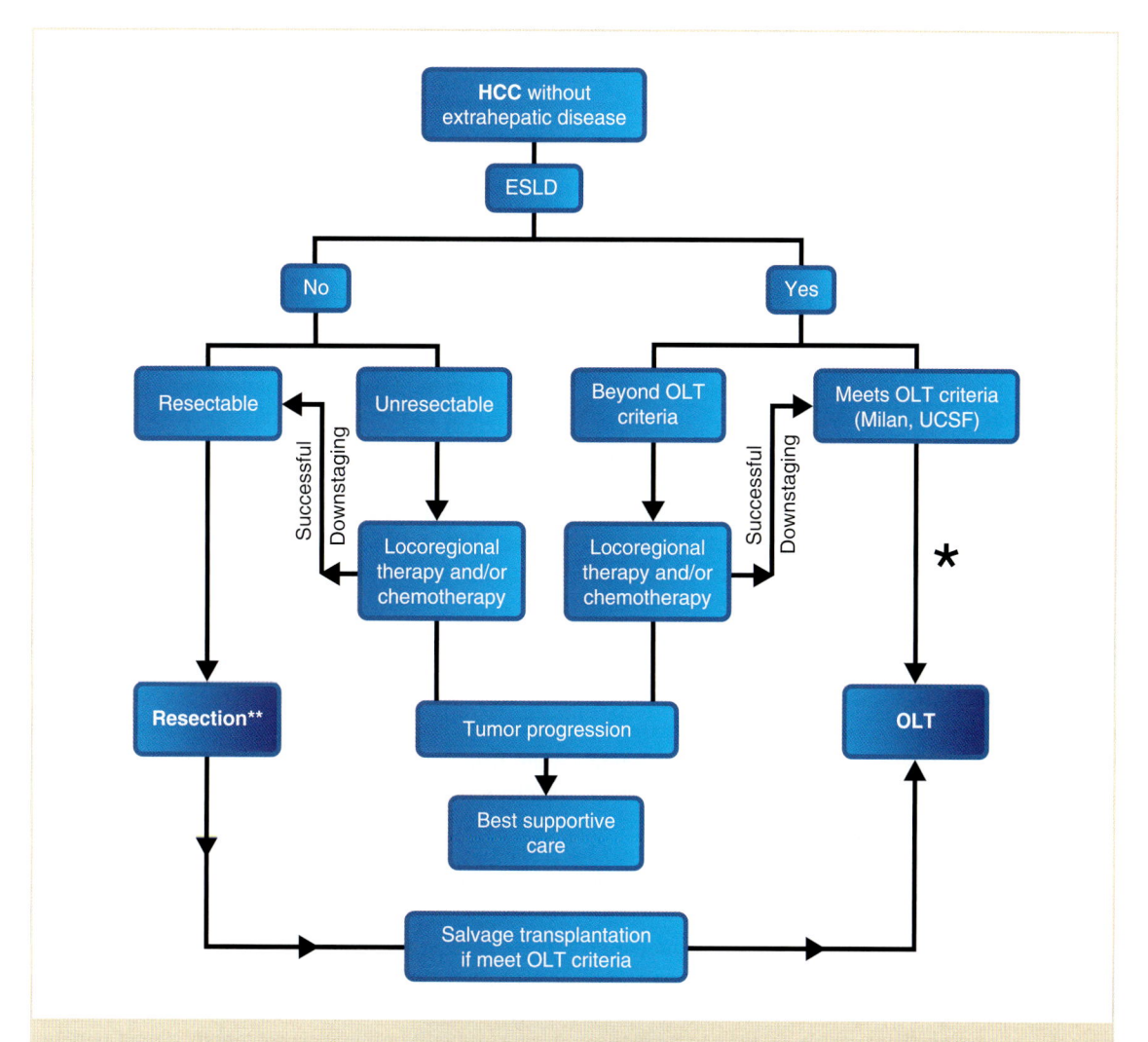

Figure 13-7: Treatment algorithm of hepatocellular cancer (HCC) without extrahepatic tumor involvement. (*) Patients with HCC on the waiting list will be reimaged every three months. Locoregional therapies (transcatheter arterial chemoembolization, radiofrequency ablation, percutaneous ethanol injection) are used as bridging procedures to control the tumor burden within Milan or University of California, San Francisco (UCSF) criteria. (**) Patients who recur after primary resection are candidates for salvage liver transplantation as far the tumor burden meets orthotopic liver transplantation (OLT) criteria. ESLD, end-stage liver disease.

had a dropout rate of 14% which compares favorably with the Barcelona Liver Cancer study group who reported a 38% 12-month dropout probability with observation alone.[18,19] Another study of 116 patients with HCC listed for OLT and treated with TACE found a dropout rate of 2.9% in patients within Milan criteria and 12% in patients outside of Milan criteria, but within UCSF criteria. However, this study also found that patients who were downstaged to Milan criteria fared worse posttransplant, with a five-year survival of only 25%.[20] The evidence is not overwhelming because there has not been a randomized controlled trial to assess dropout rates with and without TACE, but the evidence does favor intervention particularly because TACE is well tolerated with a low rate of complications and side effects.

Percutaneous ethanol injection is the therapy with the least amount of experiential data in the bridge to transplant setting. It is a modality with an attractive side effect and complication profile, in theory, but it is seldom mentioned in the published data. It is an effective treatment option for liver tumors with up to 80% necrosis in small tumors.[21] It is less invasive than most, utilizing a fine needle that may limit the theoretical concern of track seeding. However, it requires multiple treatment sessions and has been largely replaced in most centers with RFA, and therefore, it is unlikely to accumulate any notable data to bolster its use as a bridging therapy.

Radiofrequency ablation is another effective treatment option for liver tumors that is being used as a bridge to transplant for patients with HCC. University of California, Los Angeles reported its experience with 52 consecutive patients with 87 tumors. They had a dropout rate of 5.8% at 12 months due to tumor progression with a three-year survival of 76% for 41 patients from this group that made it to transplant with no recurrences within the established follow-up time period.[22] Mazzaferro et al. reviewed their experience with RFA pretransplant and found no dropout due to tumor progression with a three-year survival of 83%.[23] RFA will be discussed in greater detail in other chapters, but it can be used safely and effectively for bridging patients with small tumors awaiting transplant.

The greatest benefit of any treatment modality used as a bridge to transplant is seen with longer wait times. In those centers that are able to rush patients with HCC to transplant, there is little convincing evidence that pretreatment with any of the aforementioned options provides a survival or recurrence benefit. With this in mind, fast-tracking patients with aggressive tumor biology and at the edge or beyond Milan criteria may be associated with increased recurrence. Most centers are treating HCC patients with a bridging therapy prior to transplant, but at this time, there is no evidence to suggest which is superior.

Living Donor Liver Transplantation for HCC

The number of patients on the liver transplant wait list continues to increase annually, while the number of viable donors remains static. There are currently over 16,000 patients on the waiting list for liver transplantation in the United States, while only 4734 patients received a liver transplant in 2011 (UNOS database). Because of the shortage of deceased donors, living donor liver transplant (LDLT) has become an increasingly utilized modality for treatment of patients with decompensated cirrhosis and those with unresectable HCC, particularly in Asian countries where there is a very limited availability of deceased donor organs, the use of a right or left hemi-liver from a healthy donor may be the only viable option. Overall, outcomes for all patients undergoing LDLT are comparable with the results with deceased donors.[24] A number of studies have demonstrated a survival benefit for LDLT in the setting of HCC.[25] The concern is the risk to the living donor, with morbidity rates as high as 40%. Many have also expressed a concern for LDLT for patients who are outside of the established Milan or UCSF criteria both in terms of recipient outcomes and donor risk. One must consider if there is a selection bias for those patients with established wait time on the transplant list. This may result in selection of favorable tumor biology as those with more aggressive tumors drop out prior to transplant.[26] This important selection factor may be lost if LDLT is rushed, and those with unfavorable tumor biology are transplanted before they can declare themselves with aggressive tumor progression.

According to the 2010 international consensus conference guidelines, LDLT for HCC is acceptable for patients with HCC who have an expected five-year survival similar to comparably staged patients receiving a deceased donor liver. However, two strong recommendations were made: (1) LDLT must be restricted to centers of excellence in liver surgery and liver transplantation to minimize donor risk and maximize recipient outcome and (2) in patients following LDLT for HCC outside the accepted regional criteria for deceased donor liver transplantation, retransplantation for graft failure using a deceased donor organ is not recommended (Table 13-1).

Resection Versus Transplantation for HCC

Currently, liver transplantation is the best therapy option for cirrhotic patients with small HCC. A recently published systematic review on the treatment of HCC analyzed eight studies that compared survival for resection and OLT.[27] The five-year disease-free survival rate was significantly higher for OLT compared with resection in seven of eight studies (Figure 13-8). Unfortunately, OLT can be offered only to a small proportion of patients due to organ shortage and tumor stage beyond accepted criteria. Therefore, liver resection remains the primary surgical therapy for HCC in cirrhotic patients with well-preserved liver function (Child-Turcotte-Pugh class A) and absence of portal hypertension (Figure 13-7).[28] Belghiti proposed that liver resection can be used in conjunction with OLT in three clinical scenarios of small HCC[29]: (1) as primary treatment with salvage transplantation for recurrence (Figure 13-9B), (2) as a diagnostic tool to gain histopathological tumor characteristics for appropriate selection for OLT, and (3) as bridge treatment before OLT to control the tumor burden in patients meeting the Milan[5] or UCSF[8] criteria (Figure 13-4).

Liver resection versus liver transplantation as primary therapy for patients with small HCC and adequate hepatic reserve is hotly debated. The approach of primary resection with salvage transplantation for recurrence has been mainly practiced in geographic regions with a low donation rate and a high incidence of HCC (Figure 13-9B).[30] The rational behind this approach is that longer waiting times after listing increase the risk for tumor progression beyond the accepted criteria for transplantation. Although resection does not correct the underlying liver disease, several authors report comparable overall survival for primary resection and primary OLT for transplantable HCC.[31-33] The *Hong-Kong* group reported that the majority of patients (79%) with small HCC who recurred after resection were still candidates for salvage OLT.[34] Conversely, the strategy of first-line resection and salvage OLT has no clinical significance in geographic regions, such the United States, due to the low proportion of patients with HCC on the waiting list (10%) and a relatively short median time of listing-to-transplantation (three months).[30] Therefore, the choice whether primary OLT or primary resection with salvage OLT should be used for the treatment of small HCC is determined by geographic factors rather than the preferred attitude of the transplant center toward either approach (Figure 13-9).

Another advantage of the primary resection approach is related to pathological information of the resection specimen.[29] Microvascular and macrovascular invasion as well as satellite nodules are important prognostic factors that are associated with inferior outcome. This information can be considered for acceptance or denial of patients for salvage liver transplantation in the case of recurrent tumor disease.

It has been also proposed that liver resection can be used as bridge therapy before OLT.[29] However, this strategy only makes sense if the patient on the waiting list would keep their priority even after complete tumor resection. In the United States where additional MELD priority points are assigned to patients with HCC within Milan criteria (Figure 13-6), a complete tumor resection would result in losing additional priority points for HCC and the priority on the waiting list. Therefore, listed patients with HCC are mainly managed with locoregional therapies such as TACE and RFA to control the tumor burden during the waiting time.

Patients with large HCC exceeding the Milan or UCSF criteria have a more unfavorable outcome than those with small tumors.[5,8] In the United States, patients outside the accepted HCC criteria can be principally transplanted based on the physiological MELD score but do not receive any additional priority points. A comparative study of patients with HCC exceeding the Milan criteria was performed for a cohort undergoing resection ($n = 94$) versus OLT ($n = 92$).[35] The mean maximal tumor size was 10 cm for the resection group and 6.4 cm for the OLT group. Both groups had an overall survival rate of 66%.

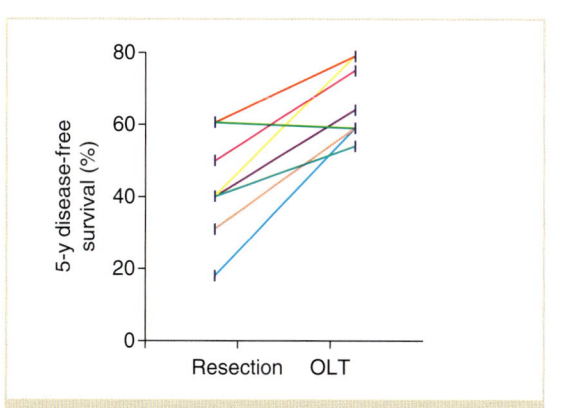

Figure 13-8: Five-year disease-free survival in eight studies comparing resection versus orthotopic liver transplantation (OLT) for the treatment of hepatocellular cancer. Each study is represented by a different color. (Data were extracted from Rahbari et al.,[27] Table 3.)

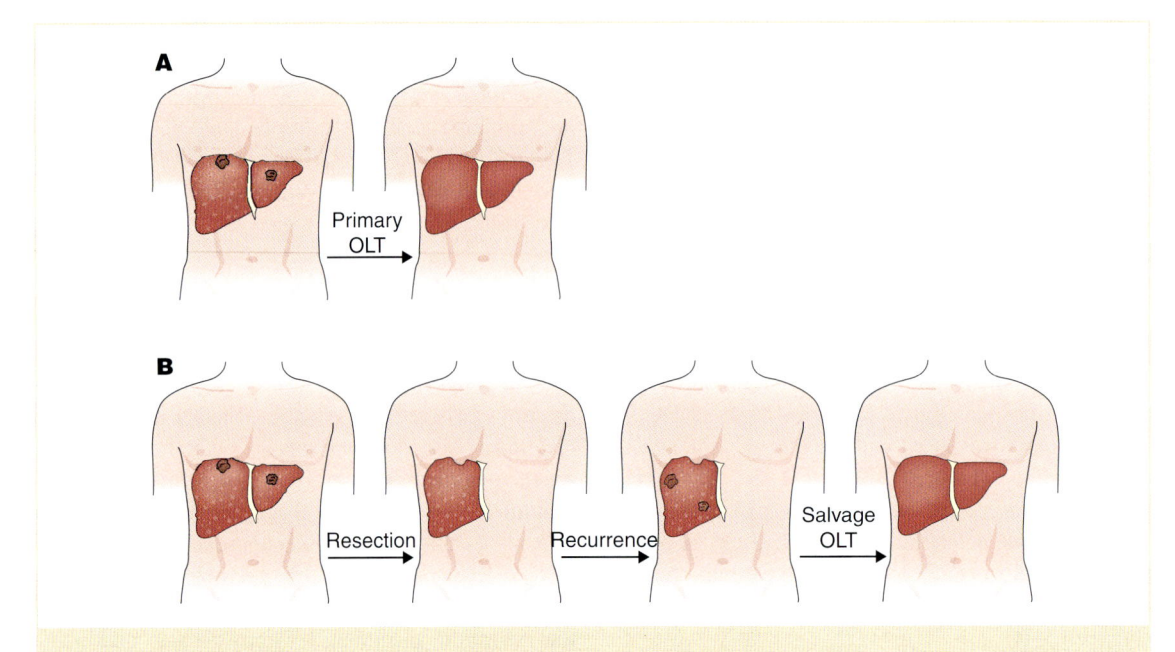

Figure 13-9: Liver transplant strategies for hepatocellular cancer (HCC). This figure illustrates primary orthotopic liver transplantation (OLT) (A) and primary resection with salvage OLT (B) as two different treatment approaches of transplantable HCC.

Although this study has certain limitations in regards to comparability, the results imply that resection and OLT in patients with HCC beyond the Milan criteria have probably similar outcomes.

Liver Transplantation For Cholangiocarcinoma

Scope of the Problem

CCA is an epithelial bile duct malignancy that can arise from the intrahepatic and extrahepatic biliary tree (Figure 13-10). CCA involving the bifurcation of the hepatic ducts, whether they arise from the intrahepatic or extrahepatic biliary tree, is called hilar tumors (also known as perihilar or Klatskin tumors) and are classified according to the Bismuth–Corlette classification system.[36,37] CCA arising from the bile duct posterior to the duodenum are termed distal CCA. CCAs account for approximately 3% of all gastrointestinal malignancies, with a reported incidence of one or two cases per 100,000 population in the United States.[38]

The treatment of CCA is extremely challenging because of the critical location of the tumor in proximity to vital structures, the inherent aggressive nature of the disease, and the lack of effective adjuvant therapy. Operative treatment with complete extirpation of the tumor (R0 resection) has been the only therapy offering any chance of cure; however, this is only achieved in 20%–40% of hilar and intrahepatic CCA and 50% of distal CCA.[39] Resection is further limited in patients with underlying liver disease and inadequate hepatic functional reserve. In the group of patients who are not surgical candidates for resection because of locally advanced disease prohibiting R0 resection or underlying liver disease, the use of total hepatectomy with regional lymphadenectomy followed by OLT has evolved as a promising therapy with excellent long-term recurrence-free survival in appropriately selected patients with hilar and peripheral CCA.

Patient Selection

Patients with hilar and intrahepatic CCA must meet several strict criteria to be candidates for liver transplantation. The predominant consideration is that the tumor must be deemed surgically unresectable, either secondary to extensive local involvement or underlying liver disease.[40] Preoperative imaging with contrast-enhanced CT or MRI is essential in providing an assessment of tumor extent, bile duct

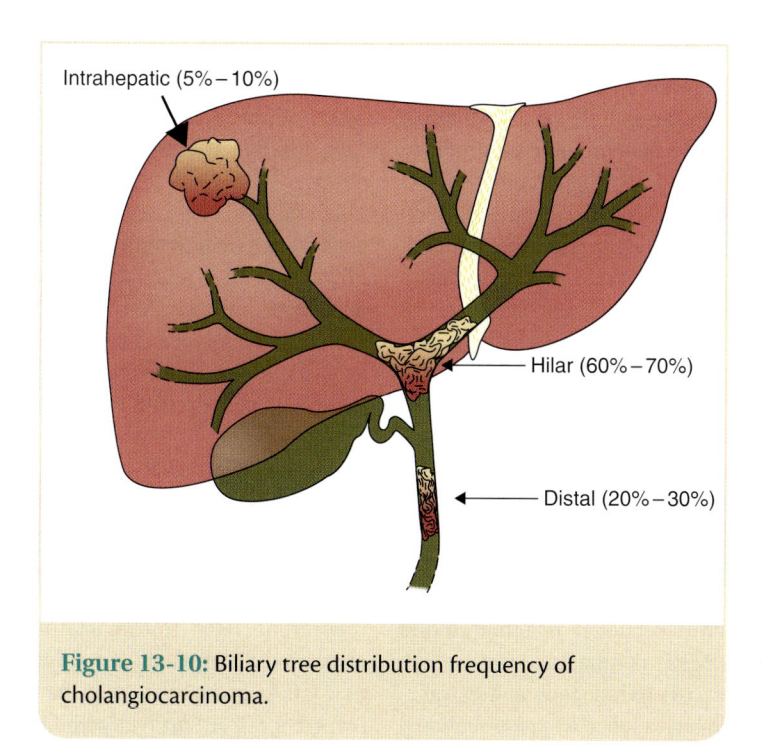

Figure 13-10: Biliary tree distribution frequency of cholangiocarcinoma.

obstruction, vascular involvement, and hepatic lobar atrophy. For both hilar and intrahepatic CCA, extensive local involvement characterized by either bilateral or contralateral involvement of the portal vein, hepatic artery, and/or secondary biliary radicles is a contraindication to surgical resection.[41] Furthermore, nonsatellite hepatic metastases and lymph node metastases beyond the portal vein and celiac axis may preclude surgical resection.[39,42–44]

An underlying liver disease such as cirrhosis or primary sclerosing cholangitis (PSC) might be another selection criterion for OLT. Even if the CCA tumor is technically resectable, patients with end-stage or significant underlying liver disease might not tolerate an extended radical resection. In addition, patients with CCA on the background of PSC remain at risk after surgical resection for de novo and recurrent tumor disease. Similar to OLT for HCC, liver transplantation for CAA in patients with PSC would treat tumor and underlying liver disease.

It is of paramount importance to rule out extrahepatic tumor involvement because locoregional lymph node or distant metastases demonstrate a contraindication for OLT. Recently, the role of combined positron emission tomography (PET) and CT has been evaluated in the preoperative staging of CCA. PET/CT has a higher sensitivity (58%–100%) for detecting distant metastases than conventional CT (0%–25%).[45–47] In one study, PET/CT led to a change in surgical management in 8 of 48 patients (17%) due to new findings.[47] PET/CT has also emerged as a prognostic tool in patients with CCA undergoing OLT. In a small series of 14 patients undergoing OLT for hilar CCA, recurrence-free survival was 100% for PET-negative patients ($n = 5$), whereas 7 of 9 patients (78 %) with PET-positive lesions developed tumor recurrence after OLT.[48] Based on the published experience, PET/CT should be integrated as mandatory imaging modality in the workup for patients with CCA who are evaluated for OLT.

MELD-Based Allocation

Since 2002, liver organ allocation in the United States has been performed using the MELD scoring system that predicts the risk of mortality on the waiting list.[13] However, most patients with unresectable CCA who are liver transplant candidates do not have underlying liver disease, and hence, their MELD score would not accurately reflect their risk of mortality on the wait list. In November 2009, the Organ Procurement and Transplantation Network/UNOS Liver and Intestinal Organ Transplantation Committee met to agree on criteria for assigning MELD exception points in hilar CCA. The criteria were published as

Organ Procurement and Transplantation Network/UNOS policy 3.6.[16] (Figure 13-6)

The criteria drafted were as follows: (1) All transplant centers must have a written protocol submitted to the Organ Procurement and Transplantation Network/UNOS Liver and Intestinal Organ Transplantation Committee including the center's selection criteria, administration of neoadjuvant therapy, and operative staging in patients with CCA to exclude those patients with regional hepatic lymph node metastases, intrahepatic metastases, and/or extrahepatic disease. (2) Candidates must satisfy diagnostic criteria for hilar CCA including a malignant-appearing stricture on cholangiography and one or more of the following: carbohydrate antigen 19-9 of ≥100 U/mL, a biopsy or cytology result demonstrating malignancy, or aneuploidy. The tumor should be considered unresectable on the basis of technical considerations or underlying liver disease. (3) If cross-sectional imaging studies (CT scan, ultrasound, MRI) demonstrate a mass, the mass should be ≤3 cm. (4) Intrahepatic and extrahepatic metastases should be excluded by cross-sectional imaging of the chest and abdomen at the time of initial exception and every three months before the score increases. (5) Regional hepatic lymph node involvement and peritoneal metastases should be assessed by operative staging after completion of neoadjuvant therapy and before liver transplantation.

Patient with hilar CCA meeting these criteria are listed with a MELD score of 22 points. Candidates undergo surveillance imaging of the chest and abdomen every three months to exclude progression of disease beyond listing criteria. If there is no evidence of progression, a 10% increase in the MELD score is awarded during each three-month interval until transplantation (Figure 13-6). For patients with intrahepatic CCA, UNOS has not currently adopted any criteria that allow for the allocation of MELD exception points. In these circumstances, the transplant center can apply to the regional review board that may then grant MELD exception points on a patient-by-patient basis.

Neoadjuvant Therapy

Historical experience with OLT for CCA was disappointing because of the universal recurrence and subsequent mortality, leading many centers to consider CCA a contraindication for OLT.[49–52] In 1989, the University of Pittsburgh was the first to report a disappointing two-year survival of 30% and recurrence rates of 60% in patients with PSC and CCA who underwent OLT.[52] In the mid-1990s, a significant survival benefit was reported for unresectable patients with CCA who underwent palliative radiation, with two-year survivals of 48% versus 0% in patients not treated with radiation. Furthermore, 14% of patients who underwent radiation and no further treatment survived five years. The realization that radiation therapy may have tumor-suppressing effects in CCA led the University of Nebraska to pioneer the use of neoadjuvant radiation therapy before OLT (Table 13-2).[53] The neoadjuvant protocol included 6000 cGy of transhepatic intrabiliary brachytherapy with iridium-192 wires and subsequent daily intravenous infusion of 5-fluorouracil until transplantation. At a median follow-up of 7.5 years, 45% (5/11) of patients had tumor-free survival. These positive reports of liver transplantation with neoadjuvant chemoradiation paved the way for the development of "CCA protocols" that have yielded excellent recurrence-free survival with OLT for CCA.

With the apparent benefits of chemotherapy and radiation therapy prior to OLT, the Mayo Clinic group developed a neoadjuvant protocol in 1993 for the treatment of unresectable hilar CCA combining external beam radiation therapy with brachytherapy, 5-fluorouracil chemosensitization, and a staging operation followed by OLT.[54,55] Eligible patients included only those with early-stage hilar CCAs above the level of the cystic duct that were deemed locally unresectable, with intrahepatic CCAs and gallbladder carcinomas specifically being excluded. Furthermore, the upper limit of tumor size for inclusion was 3 cm. Eligible patients received external beam radiation therapy to a dose of 4500 cGy followed by intrabiliary brachytherapy to a dose of 2000–3000 cGy with iridium-192 wires placed either endoscopically or via a transhepatic route. Systemic intravenous 5-fluorouracil was administered as a chemosensitizing agent followed by oral capecitabine (Xeloda) after radiation therapy until transplantation (Table 13-2).

Recurrence and Survival after Orthotopic Liver Transplantation

The Mayo group reported their outcome of 65 patients undergoing OLT with neoadjuvant treatment in 2006.[55] OLT for hilar CCA resulted in a favorable one- and five-year overall survival rate of 91% and 76%, respectively (Table 13-2).[56] The five-year recurrence-free survival rate was 60% in this study. After a mean follow-up of 32 months post-OLT, there was a 17% overall recurrence rate with a median time to recurrence of 22 months (range: 7–65 months). Important risk factors for recurrence of CCA post-OLT included age, CA 19-9 levels > 100 U/mL, mass on cross-sectional imaging, and explant pathology revealing perineural invasion, advance tumor grade, and a residual tumor >2 cm.

The excellent outcomes with the Mayo protocol has been attributed to the highly rigorous selection bias of patients with favorable biology, in particular the selection of patients with small tumors without pathologic nodal disease. More recent studies have provided justification for the expansion of inclusion criteria for liver transplantation in CCA. Hong et al. reported a 24-year experience in treating CCAs at the University of California, Los Angeles.[57] Of 132 patients diagnosed with CCA, 75 had metastatic disease at presentation and 57 were eligible for surgical therapy. Among the surgical candidates, 38 patients underwent OLT and 19 patients underwent radical bile duct resection with partial hepatectomy. The five-year tumor recurrence-free survival was significantly higher in the OLT versus resection group (38% vs. 0%). Importantly, tumor size >3 cm for hilar tumors and >5 cm for intrahepatic CCA was not a predictor of worse outcome on multivariate analysis. This study challenged the generally accepted notion that liver transplantation for CCA be restricted only to early-stage and small hilar tumors. In 2011, Hong et al. proposed a prognostic scoring system for risk stratification of patients with intrahepatic and hilar CCA who may benefit from OLT.[58] They reported on 40 patients who underwent OLT for locally advanced intrahepatic and hilar CCA and identified 7 multivariate factors predictive for tumor recurrence: multifocal tumor, perineural invasion, infiltrative growth pattern, lack of neoadjuvant and adjuvant therapy, history of PSC, hilar tumors, and lymphovascular invasion. Each of these independent predictors

TABLE 13-2: Results of Liver Transplantation for Cholangiocarcinoma

Author	Period	n	Adjunctive Therapy	Recurrence Rate (%)	Patient Survival (%) 2 yr	3 yr	5 yr
Steiber[45]	1980–1988	10	Adjuvant	60	30	–	–
Goldstein[42]	1984–1992	17	Adjuvant	78	21	–	–
Mayer[8]	1968–1997	207	Adjuvant	51	48	–	23
Shimoda[46]	1984–2000	25	Adjuvant	41	–	35	–
Sudan[47]	1987–2000	11	Neoadjuvant	18	–	–	30
Rables[48]	1988–2001	59	Adjuvant	46	–	–	42 (Intrahepatic) 30 (Hair)
Ghali[9]	1996–2003	10	None	80	–	30	–
Heimbach[49]	1993–2006	65	Neoadjuvant	17	–	–	76
Becker[44]	1987–2005	280	–	–	–	–	38
Morris-Stiff[50]	1981–2004	13	–	–	–	–	46
Hong[1]	1985–2009	38		41	52	38	32
			None	40	27	20	20
			Neoadjuvant and adjuvant	28	88	75	47
			Adjuvant	50	58	33	33

Source: Reprinted from Rana et al.,[56] Table 2, with permission from Lippincott Williams & Wilkins.

was then assigned risk score points ranging from 1 to 4, proportional to their hazard ratio. Patients were then assigned to low-risk (0–3 points, $n = 11$), intermediate-risk (4–7 points, $n = 15$), and high-risk (8–15 points, $n = 14$) categories based on the summation of risk points. The five-year tumor recurrence-free patient survival was significantly higher in the low-risk group (78%) compared with the intermediate-risk (19%) and high-risk (0%) groups, with a survival benefit seen in the intermediate-risk group compared with the high-risk group (Figure 13-11). Based on these findings, a University of California, Los Angeles treatment protocol for unresectable intrahepatic and hilar CCA was developed (Figure 13-12).[58] Inclusion criteria include tumor size ≤8 cm for intrahepatic and ≤3.5cm for hilar CCA, with disease confined to the operative field for total hepatectomy and regional lymphadenectomy as well as absence of metastatic disease. A tumor biopsy is obtained prior to neoadjuvant therapy to ascertain the important predictive indices. Patients then receive locoregional therapy with stereotactic body radiation for a total dose of 40 Gy fractionated into five treatment sessions followed by infusional chemotherapy with 5-fluorouracil followed by oral capecitabine until transplantation. Tumor surveillance is performed with serum tumor marker CA 19-9 levels every three months as well as imaging with CT or MRI. Once an appropriate organ is identified, patients undergo a surgical staging laparotomy followed by OLT if there is no progression of disease beyond the operative field.

Resection Versus Transplantation for Cholangiocarcinoma

Complete tumor extirpation to negative margins (R0 resection) offers the only chance for long-term survival in CCA. Advances in the preoperative management of patients and aggressive operative approaches have allowed for curative resection in patients who would otherwise not be candidates for resection. However, a significant number of patients with CCA present with locally advanced disease precluding resection. In these patients, neoadjuvant chemoradiation followed by total hepatectomy with OLT has allowed for the prospect of cure. However, concerns

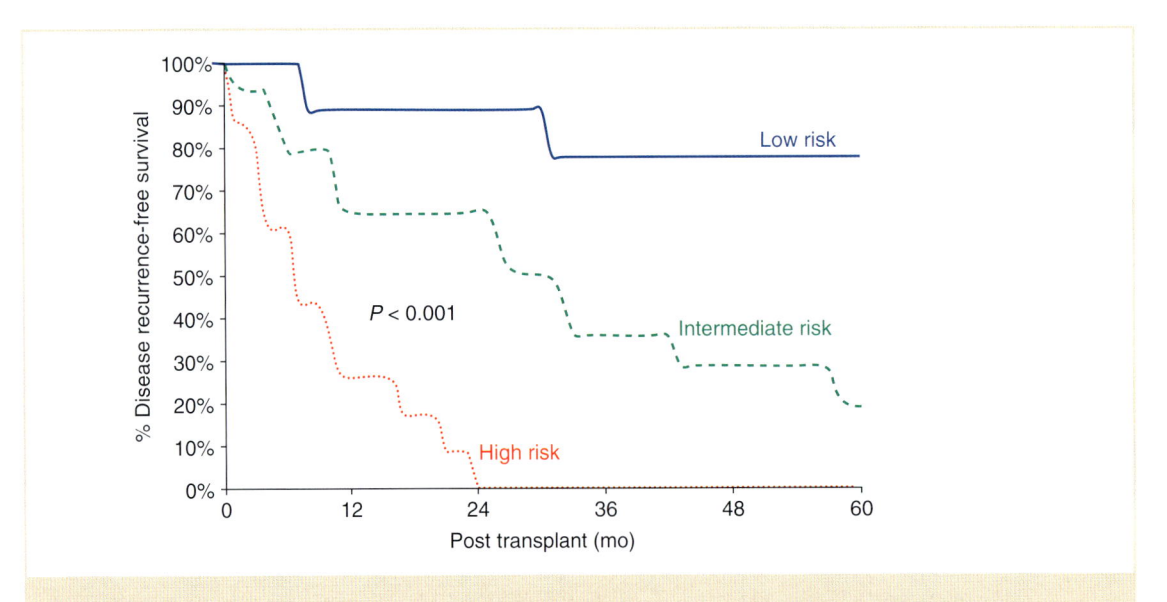

Figure 13-11: Recurrence-free survival in locally advanced intrahepatic and hilar cholangiocarcinmoa. Risk score points were assigned to following independent predictors: 4 points for multifocality, 4 points for perineural invasion, 3 points for infiltrative tumor growth pattern, 3 points for no neoadjuvant therapy, 2 points for history of primary sclerosing cholangitis, 1 point for hilar cholangiocarcinoma, and l point for lymphovascular invasion. Patients were stratified into low (0–3 points), intermediate (4–7 points), and high (8–18 points) risk groups. (Reprinted from Hong JC, Petrowsky H, Kaldas FM, et al. *J Am Coll Surg.* 2011;212:514–520 with permission from Elsevier Inc and the American College of Surgeons © 2011.)

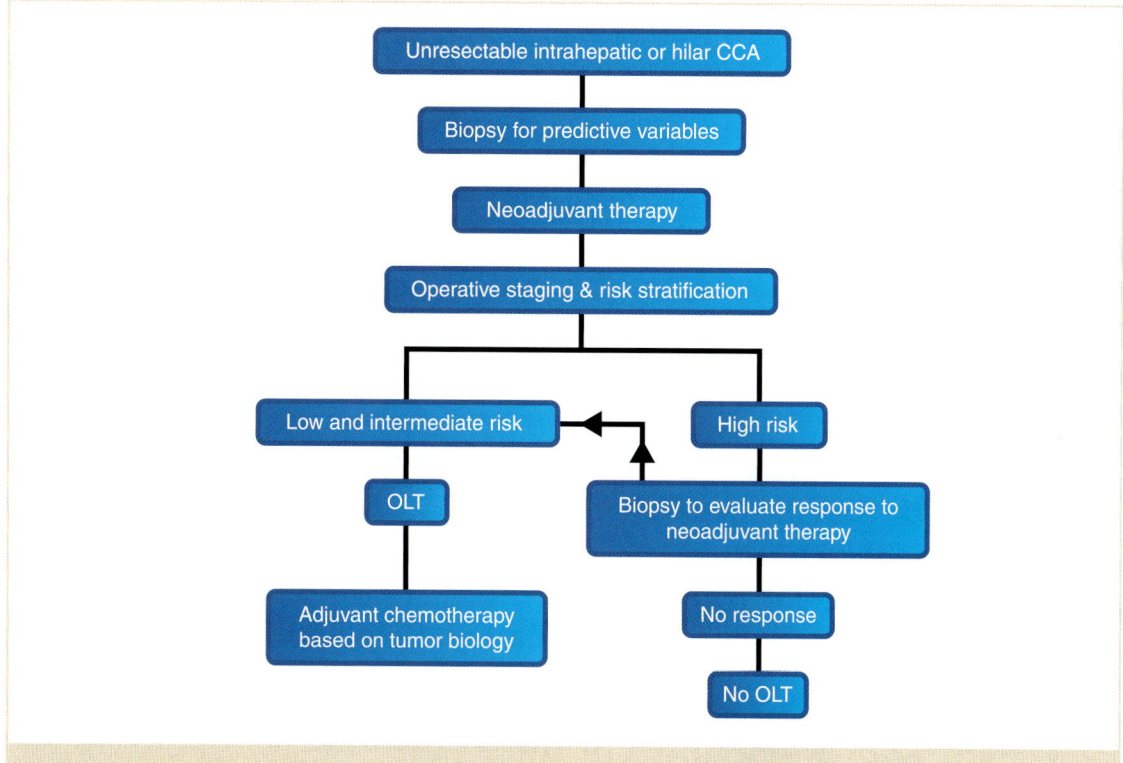

Figure 13-12: Treatment algorithm of the University of California Los Angeles for orthotopic liver transplantation (OLT) candidates with unresectable intrahepatic and hilar cholangiocarcinoma. CCA, cholangiocarcinoma. (Reprinted from Hong JC, Petrowsky H, Kaldas FM, et al. *J Am Coll Surg.* 2011;212:514–520 with permission from Elsevier Inc and American College of Surgeions © 2011.)

over limited donor resources and tumor recurrence after transplantation have raised questions about the appropriateness of transplantation in these patients.

In 2005, Rea et al. reported a large comparative experience of resection versus transplantation for hilar CCA.[59] Seventy-one patients entered the Mayo Clinic transplant treatment protocol and received neoadjuvant chemoradiation as well as operative staging, with 36 undergoing transplantation. Fifty-four patients underwent exploration for resection, with 26 (48%) undergoing resection and 28 (52%) being found to have unresectable disease. The five-year patient survival was 82% after transplantation and 21% after resection, with significantly fewer recurrences after transplantation versus resection (13% vs. 27%). Although patients undergoing liver transplantation were a highly selected group with small hilar tumors without pathologic nodal involvement, they fared better than the subgroup of resection patients who were node negative and had negative margins. This study was one of the first to suggest that liver transplantation with neoadjuvant therapy may have greater efficacy than resection in selected patients with localized, node-negative hilar CCA.

Recently, Hong et al. reported a large comparative experience of resection versus transplantation for CCA.[57] In this study, 57 patients with hilar and intrahepatic CCA underwent surgical therapy, with 38 patients undergoing liver transplantation and 19 undergoing radical resection. The five-year tumor recurrence-free survival rate was significantly better after OLT compared with resection (33% vs. 0%). Furthermore, significant independent predictors of survival were identified, which included having a hilar tumor, multifocal tumor, perineural invasion, and resection as surgical therapy. Importantly, they found that tumor size ≥3 cm for hilar and ≥5 cm for intrahepatic CCA was not a predictor of worse outcome. This study was one of the first to show that the survival benefit of OLT for CCA was not limited only to patients with small, node-negative hilar tumors. Rather, in selected patients with locally advanced hilar or intrahepatic CCA, reasonable outcomes with a prospect of cure may be achieved.

In summary, surgical resection remains the preferred treatment option for patients with preserved liver function who present without locally advanced disease that precludes R0 resection. In patients with locally advanced hilar or intrahepatic CCA who are not resection candidates, protocols utilizing neoadjuvant chemoradiation followed by OLT have emerged as a viable treatment option that can provide excellent long-term recurrence-free survival in appropriately selected patients.

Liver Transplantation for Liver Metastases from Neuroendocrine Tumors

Scope of the Problem

NET is a very rare disease with a geographic- and race-varying incidence of 2–6.5 per 100,000 persons per year.[60] NETs originate in the majority (70%–80%) in the gastrointestinal tract, and the second most affected primary site is the lung in 20%–30% of all cases. Among NETs arising from the gastrointestinal tract, tumors originating from small intestine, appendix, and rectum have the best survival compared with pancreatic NETs regardless of therapy (five-year survival: 64%–88% vs. 27%–35%).[60] Functionally, NETs are divided into hormone-active (functioning) and hormone-inactive (nonfunctioning) tumors. A simpler categorization is the classification into carcinoid versus noncarcinoid tumors. In many cases, the diagnosis of NET is delayed, and the disease is often diagnosed in the metastatic phase when the patient has become symptomatic. The liver is the most involved organ for distant metastases from the primary NET site followed by bone and lung. Because 80% of liver metastases are bilobar and multinodular,[61] liver resection often fails in achieving complete and curative resection. In contrast to HCC, the nontumorous liver parenchyma in patients with NET metastases is not cirrhotic. Although the initial experience with OLT was disappointing, the concept of liver transplantation appears reasonable and attractive as best oncological operation for unresectable NET metastases in well-selected patients.

Patient Selection

Liver transplantation for metastases from NETs is less defined compared with HCC (Figure 13-4). However, patients with liver metastases from carcinoid and noncarcinoid NETs who are unresectable should be evaluated for OLT. Some authors suggest that it is important to select only those patients for OLT whose primary NET drains into the portal vein (Figure 13-13). The rational behind this principle is that the liver is as filter organ for metastases

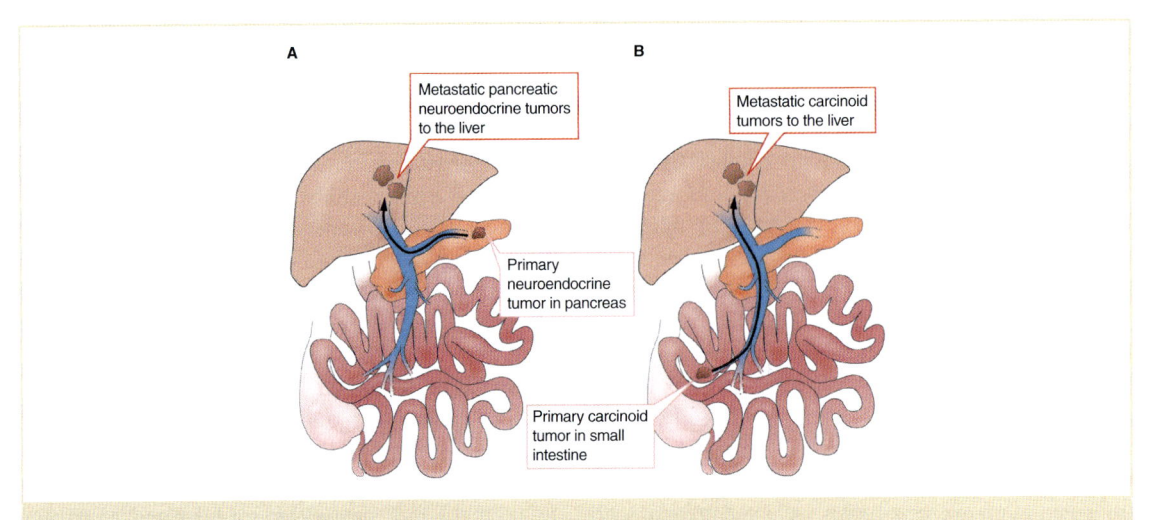

Figure 13-13: Portal venous drainage of primary neuroendocrine tumor originating from the pancreas (A) or small intestine (B).

from primary NETs and that the establishment of extrahepatic metastatic disease is less likely compared with primary NETs from nongastrointestinal origin. Conversely, patients with primary NET in organs (esophagus, lower rectum, lungs, adrenals, and others) that do not drain through the portal venous system should probably not be considered for OLT (Table 13-3).[62] Similar to HCC and CCA, extrahepatic metastatic tumor disease of NETs is considered as contraindication for OLT. Therefore, one of the most important aspects of the workup for OLT is to rule out any extrahepatic tumor disease. During the past decade, PET/CT using new radiolabeled tracers (^{18}F-DOPA, ^{68}Ga-DOTATOC) has shown diagnostic superiority to standard imaging including CT, MRI, and somatostatin receptor scintigraphy.[63,64] Therefore, PET/CT with neuroendocrine specific tracers should be a mandatory diagnostic tool especially for the detection of extrahepatic metastases.

There is general consensus that the primary extrahepatic NET should be resected before OLT.[62,65] This should be done as separate surgery instead of performing a complex simultaneous resection and OLT procedure because the combined approach is associated with a higher postoperative complication rate. The advantage of a two-stage approach is the possibility to observe the natural course of the metastatic tumor disease. In contrast to patients who progress after primary resection, patients with stable disease or partial response to medical therapies are potential candidates for OLT. This concept is supported by the findings of two recently studies in which longer wait time was associated with significantly better posttransplant outcome (Figure 13-14).[66,67]

TABLE 13-3: Proposed Selection Criteria for OLT for Metastatic Neuroendocrine Tumors

Indications	Contraindications
• Unresectable • Absence of extrahepatic metastatic disease • Portal venous drainage of primary NET • Stable tumor disease for at least 2 mo (preferable 6 mo)	• Extrahepatic metastatic disease • Poor differentiation • High Ki-67 index (≥20%) • Severe comorbidities precluding OLT

Abbreviation: NET, neuroendocrine tumor; OLT, orthotopic liver transplantation.

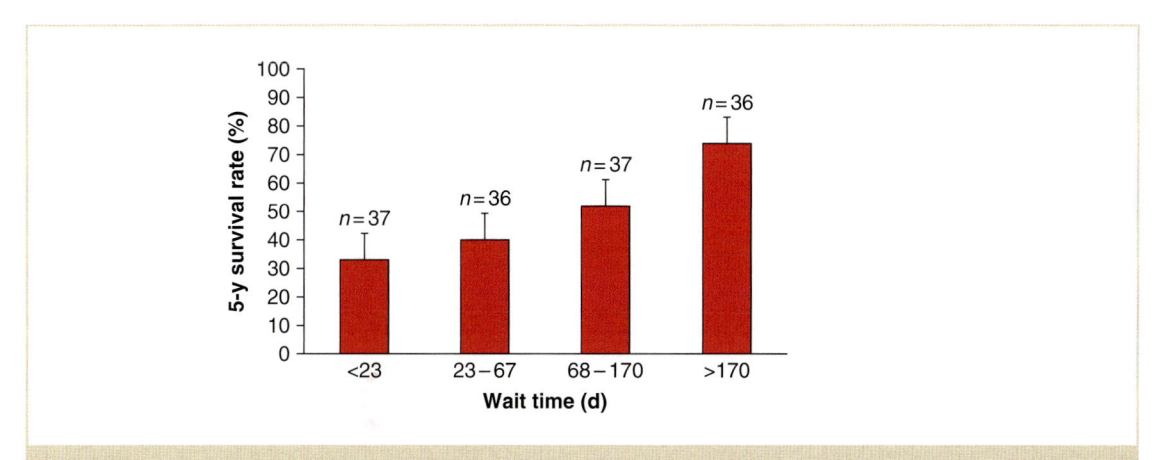

Figure 13-14: Five-year survival rate of patients who underwent orthotopic liver transplantation for neuroendocrine tumors according to wait time after listing. (Data are presented as mean ± standard error of the mean and were extracted from Gedaly et al.,[66] Table 2.)

Although age has been proposed as selection criteria by several authors,[62] there is no study that demonstrated that advanced age is an independent predictor of reduced survival after liver transplantation for NETs. The mean or median age in the most transplant series is ranging between 45 and 47 years. A recently published analysis showed that younger patients (<55 years) had a superior five-year post-transplant survival rate than patients older than 55 years; however, this survival benefit was not statistically significant in the univariate analysis.[66] Therefore, advanced age (>55 years) should not be considered as an absolute contraindication for liver transplantation. The tumor expression of the nuclear protein Ki-67 has been proposed as a prognostic marker for both liver resection and liver transplantation.[68,69] Although other authors could not confirm the findings on Ki-67,[70] most authors consider patients with highly proliferating liver tumors (Ki-67 index ≥20%) as high risk group for tumor recurrence after transplantation, who will not benefit from OLT.[61,69,71] Furthermore, patients with poorly differentiated high-grade NETs should not be considered for OLT due to the poor outcome. Table 13-3 summarizes proposed criteria for OLT in patients with NET metastases.

The development of carcinoid heart disease is associated with an inferior prognosis compared with patients without carcinoid heart disease. Approximately 20% of patients with carcinoid NETs have carcinoid heart disease at time of diagnosis.[72] The main manifestation of carcinoid heart disease affects the right-sided valves. Therefore, a careful cardiac workup with echocardiography is mandatory for patients who are evaluated for OLT regardless of age.

MELD-Based Allocation

In the United States, patients with NET metastases are listed according to their laboratory MELD score. These MELD score are usually low because the nontumorous tissue is noncirrhotic and the liver function is well preserved. In contrast to HCC and hilar CCA, there is no official UNOS policy for the assignment of additional MELD priority points to patients with NETs.[65] However, the assignment of additional MELD priority points is managed by the Regional Review Boards on a case-by-case basis.

Recurrence and Survival After OLT

Recurrence of NET after liver transplantation is common, and the reported five-year recurrence-free survival ranges from 9% to 77%. In a French series, the five-year recurrence-free survival was 17% for a mixed patient population that included carcinoid and noncarcinoid tumors as well as primary tumors with portal or systemic drainage,[73] while an Italian series, which included only carcinoids with primary tumors exclusively drained through the portal system, reported a five-year recurrence-free survival of 70%.[62] This demonstrates that appropriate patient selection is the most important key factor for favorable outcome after OLT. Furthermore, the significant risk for tumor recurrence after OLT implies to manage immunosuppression with low levels of calcineurin inhibitors and early withdrawal of steroids and mycophenolate.

The majority of the multicenter series on OLT for NETs reported a one-, three-, and five-year survival rate of 52%–81%, 52%–65%, and 47%–49%, respectively (Table 13-4).[62,66,67,74,75] These survival figures are comparable with those achieved for patients with HCC (Figure 13-15). A recently published analysis of the UNOS database revealed a comparable three-year survival for patients with NETs (36%) versus for patients with HCC (70%) who were transplanted after 2003.[66] The impact of the primary tumor type (carcinoid vs. noncarcinoid) on survival has been controversially discussed. Although two studies demonstrated significantly inferior survival for noncarcinoids compared with carcinoids,[70,73] this finding was not confirmed by the recently published analysis of the UNOS database.[66] Therefore, the opinion that OLT should not be offered to patients with noncarcinoid tumors has to be revised.[62,65] It is more important to take Ki-67 score and differentiation into account when patients with noncarcinoid NETs are considered for OLT. A patient with unresectable noncarcinoid NET having a Ki-67 score <10% and being well differentiated should not be denied for OLT based on the primary tumor type.

The authors of the 85-case French multicenter study have developed a risk score model for patients who undergo OLT for NET.[67] The multivariate analysis revealed that the primary tumor site in duodenum or pancreas and hepatomegaly

TABLE 13-4: Multicenter Studies on Liver Transplantation for Metastatic NETs

Author, Year	Study Centers	Study Period	Patients (n)	1-y survival (%)	3-y survival (%)	5-y survival (%)
Bechstein and Neuhaus, 1994[74]	International	1988–1993	30	52	52	—
Lehnert, 1998[75]	International	1981–1997	103	68	53	47
Jamil, 2002[76]	United Kingdom	—	29	79	—	24
Mazzaferro 2007[62]	Italy	1987–2006	24	—	—	90
Le Treut 2008[67]	French	1989–2005	85	72	59	47
Gedaly 2011[66]	United States	1988–2008	150	81	65	49

Abbreviation: NET, neuroendocrine tumor.

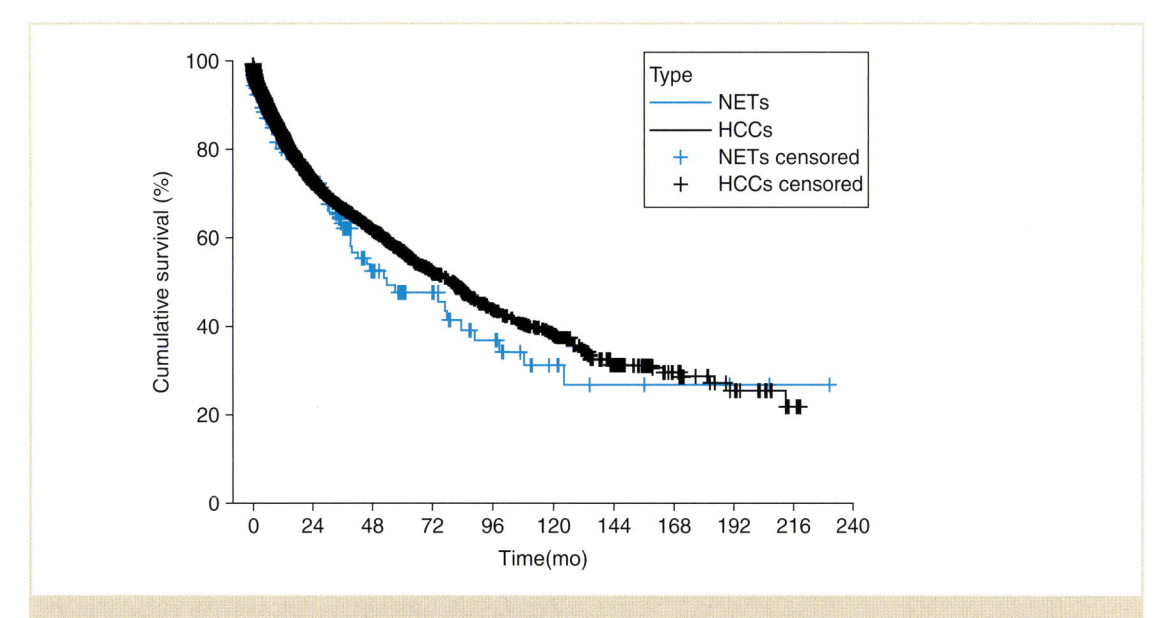

Figure 13-15: Overall survival of patients after orthotopic liver transplantation with neuroendocrine tumors (NETs) (n = 150) versus hepatocellular carcinoma (n = 4693); Mantel-Cox log-rank test, $P = 0.23$. HCC, hepatocellular cancer. (Reprinted from Gedaly R, Daily MF, Davenport D, et al. *Arch Surg*. 2011;146: 953–958 with permission from American Medical Association © 2011. All rights reserved.)

were independent predictors for reduced survival. A score of 1 was assigned to each variable. Patients with a score of 0 and 1 had a favorable survival after OLT (68% at five years), whereas patients with a score of 2 (hepatomegaly and primary tumor site in duodenum or pancreas) had a poor survival after OLT (12% at five years). Based on the presented studies, there is evidence that better patient selection results in better outcome after OLT for NETs. In well-selected patients who are not amenable to resection, OLT offers cure or long-term survival.

References

1. Parkin DM, Bray F, Ferlay J, Pisani P. Global cancer statistics, 2002. *CA Cancer J Clin.* 2005;55:74–108.
2. Altekruse SF, McGlynn KA, Reichman ME. Hepatocellular carcinoma incidence, mortality, and survival trends in the United States from 1975 to 2005. *J Clin Oncol.* 2009;27:1485–1491.
3. Llovet JM, Bustamante J, Castells A, et al. Natural history of untreated nonsurgical hepatocellular carcinoma: rationale for the design and evaluation of therapeutic trials. *Hepatology.* 1999;29:62–67.
4. Bismuth H, Chiche L, Adam R, et al. Liver resection versus transplantation for hepatocellular carcinoma in cirrhotic patients. *Ann Surg.* 1993;218:145–151.
5. Mazzaferro V, Regalia E, Doci R, et al. Liver transplantation for the treatment of small hepatocellular carcinomas in patients with cirrhosis. *N Engl J Med.* 1996;334:693–699.
6. Cillo U, Vitale A, Bassanello M, et al. Liver transplantation for the treatment of moderately or well-differentiated hepatocellular carcinoma. *Ann Surg.* 2004;239:150–159.
7. Hemming AW, Cattral MS, Reed AI, et al. Liver transplantation for hepatocellular carcinoma. *Ann Surg.* 2001;233:652–659.
8. Yao FY, Ferrell L, Bass NM, et al. Liver transplantation for hepatocellular carcinoma: expansion of the tumor size limits does not adversely impact survival. *Hepatology.* 2001;33:1394–1403.
9. Yao FY, Xiao L, Bass NM, et al. Liver transplantation for hepatocellular carcinoma: validation of the UCSF-expanded criteria based on preoperative imaging. *Am J Transplant.* 2007;7:2587–2596.
10. Duffy JP, Vardanian A, Benjamin E, et al. Liver transplantation criteria for hepatocellular carcinoma should be expanded: a 22-year experience with 467 patients at UCLA. *Ann Surg.* 2007;246:502–509.
11. Clavien PA, Lesurtel M, Bossuyt PM, et al. Recommendations for liver transplantation for hepatocellular carcinoma: an international consensus conference report. *Lancet Oncol.* 2012;13:e11–e22.
12. Malinchoc M, Kamath PS, Gordon FD, et al. A model to predict poor survival in patients undergoing trans-jugular intrahepatic portosystemic shunts. *Hepatology.* 2000;31:864–871.
13. Wiesner R, Edwards E, Freeman R, et al. Model for end-stage liver disease (MELD) and allocation of donor livers. *Gastroenterology.* 2003;124:91–96.
14. Wiesner RH, Freeman RB, Mulligan DC. Liver transplantation for hepatocellular cancer: the impact of the MELD allocation policy. *Gastroenterology.* 2004;127(5 suppl 1):S261–S267.
15. Sharma P, Balan V, Hernandez JL, et al. Liver transplantation for hepatocellular carcinoma: the MELD impact. *Liver Transpl.* 2004;10:36–41.
16. http://optn.transplant.hrsa.gov/PoliciesandBylaws2/policies/pdfs/policy_8.pdf. Accessed March 2012.
17. Lo CM, Ngan H, Tso WK, et al. Randomized controlled trial of transarterial lipiodol chemoembolization for unresectable hepatocellular carcinoma. *Hepatology.* 2002;35:1164–1171.
18. Llovet JM, Fuster J, Bruix J. Intention-to-treat analysis of surgical treatment for early hepatocellular carcinoma: resection versus transplantation. *Hepatology.* 1999;30:1434–1440.
19. Maddala YK, Stadheim L, Andrews JC, et al. Drop-out rates of patients with hepatocellular cancer listed for liver transplantation: outcome with chemoembolization. *Liver Transpl.* 2004;10:449–455.
20. Millonig G, Graziadei IW, Freund MC, et al. Response to preoperative chemoembolization correlates with outcome after liver transplantation in patients with hepatocellular carcinoma. *Liver Transpl.* 2007;13:272–279.
21. Vilana R, Bruix J, Bru C, et al. Tumor size determines the efficacy of percutaneous ethanol injection for the treatment of small hepatocellular carcinoma. *Hepatology.* 1992;16:353–357.
22. Lu DS, Yu NC, Raman SS, et al. Radiofrequency ablation of hepatocellular carcinoma: treatment success as defined by histologic examination of the explanted liver. *Radiology.* 2005;234:954–960.
23. Mazzaferro V, Battiston C, Perrone S, et al. Radiofrequency ablation of small hepatocellular carcinoma in cirrhotic patients awaiting liver transplantation: a prospective study. *Ann Surg.* 2004;240:900–909.
24. Olthoff KM, Merion RM, Ghobrial RM, et al. Outcomes of 385 adult-to-adult living donor liver transplant recipients: a report from the A2ALL Consortium. *Ann Surg.* 2005;242:314–323.
25. Sarasin FP, Majno PE, Llovet JM, et al. Living donor liver transplantation for early hepatocellular carcinoma: a life-expectancy and cost-effectiveness perspective. *Hepatology.* 2001;33:1073–1079.
26. Kulik L, Abecassis M. Living donor liver transplantation for hepatocellular carcinoma. *Gastroenterology.* 2004;127(5 suppl 1):S277–S282.
27. Rahbari NN, Mehrabi A, Mollberg NM, et al. Hepatocellular carcinoma: current management and perspectives for the future. *Ann Surg.* 2011;253:453–469.

28. Clavien PA, Petrowsky H, DeOliveira ML, Graf R. Strategies for safer liver surgery and partial liver transplantation. *N Engl J Med.* 2007;356:1545–1559.
29. Belghiti J. Resection and liver transplantation for HCC. *J Gastroenterol.* 2009;44(suppl 19):132–135.
30. Cucchetti A, Vitale A, Gaudio MD, et al. Harm and benefits of primary liver resection and salvage transplantation for hepatocellular carcinoma. *Am J Transplant.* 2010;10:619–627.
31. Cherqui D, Laurent A, Mocellin N, et al. Liver resection for transplantable hepatocellular carcinoma: long-term survival and role of secondary liver transplantation. *Ann Surg.* 2009;250:738–746.
32. Chua TC, Saxena A, Chu F, Morris DL. Hepatic Resection for transplantable hepatocellular carcinoma for patients within milan and UCSF criteria. *Am J Clin Oncol.* 2012;35:141–145.
33. Margarit C, Escartin A, Castells L, et al. Resection for hepatocellular carcinoma is a good option in Child-Turcotte-Pugh class A patients with cirrhosis who are eligible for liver transplantation. *Liver Transpl.* 2005;11:1242–1251.
34. Poon RT, Fan ST, Lo CM, et al. Long-term survival and pattern of recurrence after resection of small hepatocellular carcinoma in patients with preserved liver function: implications for a strategy of salvage transplantation. *Ann Surg.* 2002;235:373–382.
35. Canter RJ, Patel SA, Kennedy T, et al. Comparative analysis of outcome in patients with hepatocellular carcinoma exceeding the milan criteria treated with liver transplantation versus partial hepatectomy. *Am J Clin Oncol.* 2010;34:466–471.
36. Bismuth H, Corlette MB. Intrahepatic cholangioenteric anastomosis in carcinoma of the hilus of the liver. *Surg Gynecol Obstet.* 1975;140:170–178.
37. de Groen PC, Gores GJ, LaRusso NF, et al. Biliary tract cancers. *N Engl J Med.* 1999;341:1368–1378.
38. Vauthey JN, Blumgart LH. Recent advances in the management of cholangiocarcinomas. *Semin Liver Dis.* 1994;14:109–114.
39. Hemming AW, Reed AI, Fujita S, et al. Surgical management of hilar cholangiocarcinoma. *Ann Surg.* 2005;241:693–699.
40. Schulick RD. Criteria of unresectability and the decision-making process. *HPB.* 2008;10:122–125.
41. Petrowsky H, Hong JC. Current surgical management of hilar and intrahepatic cholangiocarcinoma: the role of resection and orthotopic liver transplantation. *Transplant Proc.* 2009;41:4023–4335.
42. Ebata T, Nagino M, Kamiya J, et al. Hepatectomy with portal vein resection for hilar cholangiocarcinoma: audit of 52 consecutive cases. *Ann Surg.* 2003;238:720–727.
43. Rajagopalan V, Daines WP, Grossbard ML, Kozuch P. Gallbladder and biliary tract carcinoma: a comprehensive update, Part 1. *Oncology.* 2004;18:889–896.
44. Tsao JI, Nimura Y, Kamiya J, et al. Management of hilar cholangiocarcinoma: comparison of an American and a Japanese experience. *Ann Surg.* 2000;232:166–174.
45. Jadvar H, Henderson RW, Conti PS. [F-18]fluorodeoxyglucose positron emission tomography and positron emission tomography: computed tomography in recurrent and metastatic cholangiocarcinoma. *J Comput Assist Tomogr.* 2007;31:223–228.
46. Kim JY, Kim MH, Lee TY, et al. Clinical role of 18F-FDG PET-CT in suspected and potentially operable cholangiocarcinoma: a prospective study compared with conventional imaging. *Am J Gastroenterol.* 2008;103:1145–1151.
47. Petrowsky H, Wildbrett P, Husarik DB, et al. Impact of integrated positron emission tomography and computed tomography on staging and management of gallbladder cancer and cholangiocarcinoma. *J Hepatol.* 2006;45:43–50.
48. Kornberg A, Kupper B, Thrum K, et al. Recurrence-free long-term survival after liver transplantation in patients with 18F-FDG non-avid hilar cholan-giocarcinoma on PET. *Am J Transplant.* 2009;9:2631–2636.
49. Goldstein RM, Stone M, Tillery GW, et al. Is liver transplantation indicated for cholangiocarcinoma? *Am J Surg.* 1993;166:768–771.
50. Meyer CG, Penn I, James L. Liver transplantation for cholangiocarcinoma: results in 207 patients. *Transplantation.* 2000;69:1633–1637.
51. Robles R, Figueras J, Turrion VS, et al. Spanish experience in liver transplantation for hilar and peripheral cholangiocarcinoma. *Ann Surg.* 2004;239:265–271.
52. Stieber AC, Marino IR, Iwatsuki S, Starzl TE. Cholangiocarcinoma in sclerosing cholangitis. The role of liver transplantation. *Int Surg.* 1989;74:1–3.
53. Sudan D, DeRoover A, Chinnakotla S, et al. Radiochemotherapy and transplantation allow long-term survival for nonresectable hilar cholangiocarcinoma. *Am J Transplant.* 2002;2:774–779.
54. Hassoun Z, Gores GJ, Rosen CB. Preliminary experience with liver transplantation in selected patients with unresectable hilar cholangiocarcinoma. *Surg Oncol Clin N Am.* 2002;11:909–921.
55. Heimbach JK, Gores GJ, Haddock MG, et al. Liver transplantation for unresectable perihilar

cholangiocarcinoma. *Semin Liver Dis.* 2004;24: 201–207.
56. Rana A, Hong JC. Orthotopic liver transplantation in combination with neoadjuvant therapy: a new paradigm in the treatment of unresectable intrahepatic cholangiocarcinoma. *Curr Opin Gastroenterol.* 2012;28:258–265
57. Hong JC, Jones CM, Duffy JP, et al. Comparative analysis of resection and liver transplantation for intrahepatic and hilar cholangiocarcinoma: a 24-year experience in a single center. *Arch Surg.* 2011;146:683–699.
58. Hong JC, Petrowsky H, Kaldas FM, et al. Predictive index for tumor recurrence after liver transplantation for locally advanced intrahepatic and hilar cholangiocarcinoma. *J Am Coll Surg.* 2011;212:514–520.
59. Rea DJ, Heimbach JK, Rosen CB, et al. Liver transplantation with neoadjuvant chemoradiation is more effective than resection for hilar cholangiocarcinoma. *Ann Surg.* 2005;242:451–458.
60. Ramage JK, Ahmed A, Ardill J, et al. Guidelines for the management of gastroenteropancreatic neuroendocrine (including carcinoid) tumours (NETs). *Gut.* 2012;61:6–32.
61. Gregoire E, Le Treut YP. Liver transplantation for primary or secondary endocrine tumors. *Transpl Int.* 2010;23:704–711.
62. Mazzaferro V, Pulvirenti A, Coppa J. Neuroendocrine tumors metastatic to the liver: how to select patients for liver transplantation? *J Hepatol.* 2007;47:460–466.
63. Frilling A, Sotiropoulos GC, Radtke A, et al. The impact of 68Ga-DOTATOC positron emission tomography/computed tomography on the multimodal management of patients with neuroendocrine tumors. *Ann Surg.* 2010;252:850–856.
64. Schiesser M, Veit-Haibach P, Muller MK, et al. Value of combined 6-[18F]fluorodihydroxyphenylalanine PET/CT for imaging of neuroendocrine tumours. *Br J Surg.* 2010;97:691–697.
65. Punch J, Gish RG. Model for end-stage liver disease (MELD) exception for uncommon hepatic tumors. *Liver Transpl.* 2006;12(12 suppl 3): S122–S123.
66. Gedaly R, Daily MF, Davenport D, et al. Liver transplantation for the treatment of liver metastases from neuroendocrine tumors: an analysis of the UNOS database. *Arch Surg.* 2011;146: 953–958.
67. Le Treut YP, Gregoire E, Belghiti J, et al. Predictors of long-term survival after liver transplantation for metastatic endocrine tumors: an 85-case French multicentric report. *Am J Transplant.* 2008;8: 1205–1213.
68. Ahmed A, Turner G, King B, et al. Midgut neuroendocrine tumours with liver metastases: results of the UKINETS study. *Endocr Relat Cancer.* 2009;16:885–894.
69. Rosenau J, Bahr MJ, von Wasielewski R, et al. Ki67, E-cadherin, and p53 as prognostic indicators of long-term outcome after liver transplantation for metastatic neuroendocrine tumors. *Transplantation.* 2002;73:386–894.
70. van Vilsteren FG, Baskin-Bey ES, Nagorney DM, et al. Liver transplantation for gastroenteropancreatic neuroendocrine cancers: Defining selection criteria to improve survival. *Liver Transpl.* 2006;12:448–456.
71. Amarapurkar AD, Davies A, Ramage JK, et al. Proliferation of antigen MIB-1 in metastatic carcinoid tumours removed at liver transplantation: relevance to prognosis. *Eur J Gastroenterol Hepatol.* 2003;15:139–143.
72. Bhattacharyya S, Toumpanakis C, Caplin ME, Davar J. Analysis of 150 patients with carcinoid syndrome seen in a single year at one institution in the first decade of the twenty-first century. *Am J Cardiol.* 2008;101:378–381.
73. Le Treut YP, Delpero JR, Dousset B, et al. Results of liver transplantation in the treatment of metastatic neuroendocrine tumors. A 31-case French multicentric report. *Ann Surg.* 1997;225:355–364.
74. Bechstein WO, Neuhaus P. Liver transplantation for hepatic metastases of neuroendocrine tumors. *Ann N Y Acad Sci.* 1994;733:507–514.
75. Lehnert T. Liver transplantation for metastatic neuroendocrine carcinoma: an analysis of 103 patients. *Transplantation.* 1998;66:1307–1312.
76. Jamil A, Taylor-Robinson S, Millson C, et al. Orthotopic liver transplantation for the treatment of metastatic neuroendocrine tumours—analysis of all UK patients. *Gut.* 2002;50:1e–25e.

SECTION V

Ablative Therapies

Damian E. Dupuy

CHAPTER 14

Ablation Therapy for Hepatocellular Carcinoma

Jason D. Iannuccilli & Damian E. Dupuy

Introduction

Hepatocellular carcinoma (HCC) is the sixth leading cause of cancer-related death worldwide, accounting for over 500,000 deaths per year.[1] Its incidence varies widely by geographic location, with the highest incidence noted in Eastern Asia and Japan, particularly, in the People's Republic of China, where the number of new cases approaches 137,000 per year.[2,3] The incidence of HCC is on the rise in many developed western countries. In the United States, there has been an approximate 80% increase in the annual incidence of HCC during the last few decades alone, now accounting for about 8500 new cases of liver cancer each year with an estimated annual healthcare expenditure of approximately $455 million.[4,5]

HCC is a locally aggressive tumor that predominantly occurs in the setting of chronic liver disease and cirrhosis. Diagnosis typically occurs late within the course of the disease, and median survival is approximately 6–20 months.[6] The mainstay of treatment is surgical resection; however, many patients are ineligible for invasive therapy as a result of advanced stage of disease at the time of diagnosis or underlying liver dysfunction. Fortunately, less-invasive treatment options exist in addition to systemic medical therapies that have been shown to be effective in disease palliation and cure. These treatments include catheter-based therapies such as selective bland arterial embolization, intra-arterial chemoinfusion, combination chemoembolization, and selective arterial radioembolization, as well as various chemical and thermal ablation techniques. In recent decades, these locoregional therapies have led to major breakthroughs in management of unresectable disease and are often used in combination with greater success than when used alone.[7] This chapter will discuss the role of current thermal and chemical ablation techniques in the management of HCC. Catheter-based therapies and targeted radiotherapy will be discussed separately in additional chapters of this book.

Tumor Staging

Current treatment algorithms for HCC are complex and depend on tumor stage, underlying liver function, and the presence and severity of comorbid disease. Partial hepatectomy remains the gold standard for potentially curative treatment of HCC; however, only 10%–20% of patients are eligible for surgical resection. This is usually due to unfavorable anatomic location of the tumor within the liver, size or number of liver lesions, compromised liver function, and inadequate reserve or comorbid medical conditions that put the patient at high risk for life-threatening surgical complications.[8–10] Some patients with poor liver function due to underlying cirrhosis may benefit from orthotopic liver transplantation for cure. However, this treatment is limited in its applicability by scarcity of liver donors. Locoregional therapies, therefore, play an important role in minimally invasive management of HCC in patients who are ineligible for surgery, as a palliative or curative measure or as a bridge to liver transplantation.[11] HCC is particularly well suited to treatment with locoregional therapy because the tumor often remains localized to the liver, and distant metastasis is typically not seen until very late in the course of the disease. Patients most often die of liver failure secondary to local tumor growth and mass effect, rather than extrahepatic disease.[8]

Consideration of therapeutic options for HCC begins with appropriate tumor staging. Accurate staging provides prognostic data and allows for stratification of patients into two groups, those with tumor anatomy conducive to surgical resection versus those with surgically unresectable disease. A number of staging systems currently exist for HCC, some of which rely mostly on imaging and clinical parameters to assess disease extent, and others that utilize pathologic data for determining tumor burden.[12] Staging systems that rely on imaging and clinical parameters are more applicable in determining appropriate therapeutic options in most patients, since the majority of patients with HCC have anatomic or physiologic contraindications to surgery at the time of diagnosis.

There are currently no universal criteria regarding the tumor size and eligibility for surgical resection; however, many surgeons restrict eligibility for partial hepatectomy to patients with tumors ≤ 5 cm in diameter. Anatomic location and overall extent of the tumor, however, are more important when determining surgical treatment options. Based on the most recent modifications to the AJCC/UICC staging system, most consider stage IIIB, IIIC, and IV disease to be inoperable. These stages are defined by the presence of tumor in both hepatic lobes, invasion of a major portal or hepatic vein, direct invasion of extrahepatic organs other than the gallbladder, tumor rupture, and nodal or distant metastatic disease.[13,14]

Anatomical tumor staging alone has a limited role in determining appropriate treatment of HCC, as most patients with HCC also have cirrhosis, and complex interactions between these disease processes have major implications on prognosis following treatment. Assessment of underlying liver function as a measure of hepatic reserve is therefore critical prior to consideration of surgical resection or locoregional therapy.

The Barcelona Clinic Liver Cancer (BCLC) staging system incorporates variables related to anatomic tumor stage, liver function, and physical status of the patient to provide prognostic data based on published response rates to various treatments and has become the most widely accepted staging system for HCC. This system groups patients with hepatic malignancy into one of five prognostic categories, which is then used to establish an appropriate treatment strategy[6,15]:

- *Very early stage disease:* Patients with well-compensated liver function (Child-Pugh class A), World Health Organization (WHO) performance status class 0, and a single tumor <2 cm in size, without evidence of macroscopic vascular invasion or extrahepatic metastasis. A five-year survival rate of up to 90% has been reported in this patient population.

- *Early stage disease:* Patients with compensated liver function (Child-Pugh class A or B), WHO performance status class 0, and a solitary tumor of ≤ 5 cm, or up to 3 tumor nodules < 3 cm in size, without evidence of macroscopic vascular invasion or extra-hepatic metastasis. A five-year survival rate of between 50% and 75% has been reported in this patient population.

- *Intermediate stage disease:* Patients with compensated liver function (Child-Pugh class A or B), WHO performance status class 0, and a solitary tumor of >5 cm or multinodular HCC, without evidence of macroscopic vascular invasion or extra-hepatic metastasis. Survival may exceed 50% at three years.

- *Advanced stage disease:* Patients with compensated liver function (Child-Pugh class A or B), WHO performance status class <2, and tumor demonstrating macroscopic portal vein invasion or extrahepatic spread. Overall survival has been reported at <10% at three years.

- *Terminal stage disease:* Patients with severe hepatic decompensation (Child-Pugh class C) or WHO performance status > 2. Prognosis within this group of patients is grim, with one-year survival rates at <10%.

Patients with early stage HCC have been shown to benefit from treatment with surgical resection or ablation therapy with the possibility of long-term cure. Published data for five-year survival in these patients ranges from 50% to 75%.[16] Surgical resection is generally performed whenever possible. However, there currently exists no concrete data from randomized controlled trials to support either surgical resection or ablation as the optimal first-line treatment for early stage disease. Patients with BCLC intermediate or advanced stage disease are generally not considered candidates for surgery or ablation treatment, but may be candidates for catheter-based locoregional therapies as a primary method of treatment, or as a bridging therapy to liver transplantation. Locoregional therapy is generally performed in patients with terminal stage disease as a palliative measure for relief of tumor-related pain or symptoms from tumor mass effect.[7,9]

Local Ablation Therapies for HCC

The overall goal of image-guided tumor ablation therapy is twofold: (1) to achieve complete eradication of all malignant cells within a designated area and (2) to minimize destruction of surrounding normal tissue within the treated region. Similar to surgical resection of malignant lesions for cure, image-guided ablation therapy of malignant neoplasms aims to achieve a 1.0 cm margin of cell death around the target lesion so as to minimize risk of recurrence due to sparing of malignant cells at the periphery of the lesion.[17,18]

Locoregional ablation therapies for HCC rely either on thermal or chemical induction of cell disruption, which leads to tissue coagulation necrosis. Currently available thermal ablation techniques include radiofrequency ablation (RFA), microwave coagulation therapy, laser ablation, and cryoablation. Chemical ablation is most often achieved by targeted injection of absolute ethanol or acetic acid. Each ablation technique is associated with its own advantages and disadvantages, and the most appropriate choice of therapy is determined predominantly by the size and morphology of the target lesion, as well as its proximity to adjacent nontarget tissues that may inadvertently become damaged in the treatment process. In this section, the basic physics of available thermal and chemical ablation techniques will be discussed, along with their associated technical considerations and current applications in treatment of HCC.

Chemical Ablation

Percutaneous Ethanol Injection

Basic principles

Percutaneous ethanol injection (PEI) therapy was first introduced into clinical practice in 1983 for treatment of small HCCs in patients who are not candidates for surgical resection due to poor functional hepatic reserve. This technique, due to its inexpensive application and technical simplicity, was rapidly accepted and has since become the most studied minimally invasive locoregional therapy for unresectable HCC worldwide.

When absolute ethanol is injected into tissues in sufficiently high concentration, it induces tissue necrosis as a result of cellular dehydration, cell membrane lysis, protein denaturation, and microvascular occlusion leading to ischemic tissue necrosis.[19] Small nodular-type HCCs in the setting of underlying cirrhosis are particularly suitable for treatment with PEI because the tumor itself tends to be relatively homogeneous and soft in comparison to the firm fibrotic tissue of the surrounding cirrhotic liver. This enables relatively selective and uniform distribution of ethanol throughout the targeted tumor, with limited spread to the surrounding liver parenchyma[20] (Figure 14-1). The overall effectiveness of this technique depends heavily on the size and morphology of the treated tumor. Lesions > 3 cm in size and those with irregular shape, internal septations, necrosis, or peripheral daughter nodules tend to result in less homogeneous distribution of ethanol throughout the tumor mass and greater rates of undertreatment and local recurrence.[21–24]

Treatment of HCC with PEI may be performed using multiple treatment sessions or a single session in which a large volume of ethanol is injected, usually achieving adequate tumor coverage through multiple separate needle punctures. Multiple treatment sessions are usually necessary to ensure complete coagulation necrosis of the targeted tumor.[7,9] Typical treatment schedules include once or twice weekly injections of small amounts (1–8 ml) of ethanol for a total of 4–12 treatments. The number of treatment sessions and amount of ethanol injected per session vary according to the size and morphology of the treated tumor. Use of multipronged needles has also been reported to aid in distribution of ethanol and minimize the number of needle punctures required for adequate

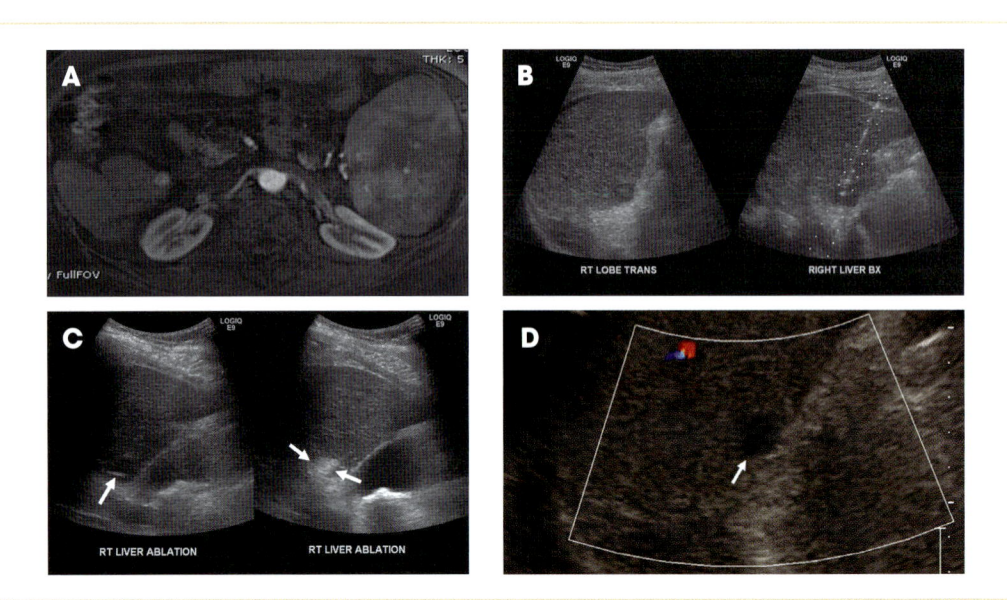

Figure 14-1: (A) Axial T1 VIBE image at 20 seconds after dynamic gadolinium injection of the liver in a patient with NASH cirrhosis shows a 1.7 cm hypervascular mass in segment 6 (arrow). (B) Transverse grey scale ultrasound image of the right lobe shows the heterogeneous liver parenchyma and focal hypoechoic lesion in the posterior aspect of segment 6 (left image) that was biopsied under ultrasound guidance (right image) confirming the diagnosis of hepatocellular carcinoma. (C) Under ultrasound guidance a 20 G Chiba needle was inserted in the posterior aspect of the mass (arrow) (left image). Two 7-mL injections of absolute ethanol were instilled into the mass. The microbubbles within the ethanol are visualized as a region of increased echogenicity (arrows) that completely fill the HCC (right image). (D) Month after the ablation the patient developed worsening renal failure form his underlying liver disease that prevented contrast MRI follow-up. A one-year follow-up color Doppler ultrasound image shows a small residual cystic appearing hypovascular mass on color Doppler ultrasound consistent with successful treatment (arrow).

treatment.[25] Single treatment strategies involve infusion of a large volume of ethanol (60–150 cc) into the targeted lesion through multiple injections over the course of approximately 30 minutes. This approach must be performed under general anesthesia and is associated with higher rates of complication, requiring inpatient postprocedural monitoring. As a result, it has largely been abandoned in favor of new safer and more effective thermal ablation strategies.[7]

Technique

Percutaneous ethanol ablation can be performed under the guidance of CT, ultrasound, or magnetic resonance imaging (MRI), but it is most frequently performed via real-time ultrasound guidance whenever possible (Figure 14-1). Limited visualization of the targeted lesion by patient body habitus, excessive bowel gas, or location of the targeted lesion within the dome of the liver are the factors that may preclude the safe and effective use of ultrasound. The procedure is usually performed under local anesthesia, but treatment of deep liver lesions often requires the additional use of conscious sedation to effectively manage procedure-related pain. Sterile or clean operating conditions are established, with the overlying skin appropriately prepped and draped. Real-time ultrasound guidance is provided with a 3.5- or 5-MHz curved-array transducer to direct a 20- or 22-gauge end-hole or conical-tipped needle with multiple side holes into the target lesion. Use of real-time imaging serves to ascertain the correct position of the needle within the target lesion and enables real-time monitoring for secondary signs of tissue necrosis as an early indicator of the effectiveness of the procedure. Ethanol is typically infused at the most distal tumor margin first, and subsequent injections proceed proximally to avoid incomplete visualization of the tumor margin by artifact from microbubbles of gas suspended in the injection.

The appropriate volume of ethanol which should be administered to achieve adequate tissue necrosis depends on the volume of the target tissue lesion. The appropriate dose can be approximated by the following formula: $V = (4/3)\pi(r + 0.5)^3$, where V is the total volume of ethanol to be infused and r is the radius of the target lesion in centimeters, with the addition of 0.5 cm to provide a safety margin that ensures appropriate destruction of a small amount of surrounding normal liver tissue. Most tumors, however, are not shaped as a perfect sphere, and this formula only represents an approximation of an appropriate ethanol dose. Most treatment sessions do not exceed an injected volume of 8 cc, and the total calculated therapeutic dose of ethanol is usually administered over multiple treatment sessions which specifically target residual tumor.[7,9,26]

When real-time ultrasound imaging is performed to monitor percutaneous ethanol ablation, several sonographic changes can be seen within the target tissue lesion that serves as secondary markers for assessing the margins of the ablation zone. Prior to injection, the ethanol preparation is usually agitated within the syringe to form a small microbubble suspension, which can be seen by ultrasound as the solution is locally infiltrated into the target tissue. These microbubbles cause echogenic artifact within the target lesion, the extent of which approximates the margins of the ablation zone. As these microbubbles are reabsorbed in tissue (usually within one minute), the echogenic artifact resolves, and the needle tip is again visualized within the lesion. Secondary measures of therapeutic efficacy also include visualization of cessation of blood flow within the lesion by color-Doppler analysis during and after the injection.

Patients undergoing multisession percutaneous ethanol ablation with small doses of ethanol (1–8 cc) per treatment may be treated as outpatients and discharged after appropriate postprocedure monitoring of vital signs for two to four hours. Patients who experience no complications are typically discharged to home with oral narcotics for pain control. Appropriate clinical follow-up for additional treatment or assessment of treatment response is scheduled with the radiologist or referring clinician. Following complete treatment, appropriate imaging may be performed to assess treatment response or lab testing may be performed to monitor serum AFP as a marker of disease activity.

Results

Several retrospective and observational studies have provided indirect evidence that PEI improves the natural history of HCC. In patients with Child-Pugh class A cirrhosis, 5-year survival rates in these studies ranged from 39% to 78%, and 10-year survival rates are reported to reach 15.8%.[20,27–33] The overall survival rate of patients with small HCC ≤ 2 cm treated with PEI was shown to be significantly higher than that of patients with tumors larger than 2 cm in size. Other factors influencing long-term survival in these patient populations included severity of underlying liver dysfunction and serum AFP levels.[31,32]

Early studies comparing the efficacy of PEI to surgical resection for treatment of early-stage HCC in Japan showed no significant difference in one- and three-year survival rates for patients treated with either modality, but five-year survival for PEI (37%) was relatively poor in comparison to surgical resection (51%).[34] Survival outcomes vary according to size of the treated tumor, however, and investigators have shown that five-year survival rates for primary HCC ≤ 3 cm in size are comparable to those achievable with surgical resection.[28,35–37] A recent prospective randomized controlled trial conducted in Taiwan comparing the effects of PEI and surgical resection in patients with small HCC ≤ 3 cm in size confirmed no significant difference in survival or recurrence rates between these two treatments at up to 59 months of follow-up; however, tumor size larger than 2 cm and α-fetoprotein levels >200 ng/mL correlated with higher recurrence rate, and Child-Pugh class B liver cirrhosis correlated with shorter overall survival within both treatment groups.[38]

PEI treatment of HCC is reported to achieve complete coagulative necrosis in 70% to 80% of solitary tumors ≤ 3 cm, and in nearly 100% of tumors < 2 cm in size; however, overall efficacy decreases to approximately 50% for tumors ranging between 3 and 5 cm.[7,9,39] It is speculated that larger tumors are more likely to be incompletely treated because there is a greater likelihood of irregular morphology, internal septations, necrosis, or peripheral daughter nodules in association with larger tumors, which tend to result in less homogeneous distribution of ethanol throughout the tumor mass.[21–24]

Complications and contraindications

Right upper quadrant pain and fever are common in the immediate posttreatment period due to tumor necrosis and are usually effectively managed with analgesics. The rate of severe complications related to PEI treatment for HCC is reportedly low, ranging from 1.7% to 4.6%, with overall mortality rates reported at 0.1%–0.7%.[22,28] Observed complications with this treatment include peritoneal hemorrhage, transient renal insufficiency, and hepatic decompensation. Risk of procedure-related complication in most studies appears to increase relative to the size of the treated tumor. Infarction of liver segments adjacent to the targeted tumor has also been reported in rare cases, usually in the setting of previous arterial chemoembolization treatment.[40,41] Metastatic tumor seeding of extrahepatic tissues along the needle tract has been reported by some investigators,[42,43] but large scale clinical studies have demonstrated that rates of occurrence of this complication are negligible, ranging from 0.65% to 1.5%.[22,28,43]

Although PEI has been the most utilized and studied technique for treatment of non-surgical HCC, its clinical use is now being abandoned in favor of thermal ablation techniques. Its current use appears to be limited to the treatment of small (<3 cm) early stage surgically unresectable tumors that are unable to be treated by other minimally invasive thermal ablation techniques, such as lesions located in close proximity to organs that may be easily damaged by the thermal effects of the therapy, such as the colon or gallbladder. PEI treatment of tumor thrombus within the portal vein has also been reported as a palliative measure.[7] Contraindications to use of PEI therapy for HCC include tumors whose overall volume is greater than 30% of the total liver volume, extrahepatic disease, and in patients with severe underlying liver dysfunction (Child-Pugh class C cirrhosis with prothrombin time >40% of normal or platelet count > 40,000/μL).[20,44]

Percutaneous Acetic Acid Injection

Basic principles

Ethanol is a popular agent for chemical ablation due to its widespread availability, low cost, and the ease at which it is able to be stored and used. Several other chemical agents have also been effectively used for percutaneous ablation therapy, such as acetic acid, sodium tetradecyl sulfate (STS), polidocanol, sodium morrhuate, and doxycyline. Although not extensively studied in clinical practice, percutaneous acetic acid injection has been successfully performed for treatment of small (<3 cm), surgically unresectable HCC.[45–49]

Technique

Clinical indications for treatment and the technique by which acetic acid is administered are identical to those of PEI; however, the dose of acetic acid necessary to induce coagulation necrosis within the target tumor is notably lower than that of ethanol. Early histopathologic dose-response studies performed in rats indicate that the cytotoxic effects of acetic acid plateau at a concentration of 50% (8 mmol/L).[45] Initial clinical applications report excellent radiologic–histopathologic correlation for tumor kill with administered 50% acetic acid doses of approximately 1/3 the calculated ethanol dose required for treatment.[46]

Results

An initial early randomized controlled trial comparing PAI and PEI treatment in patients with HCC < 3 cm and similar degree of underlying liver dysfunction showed greater local tumor recurrence with ethanol compared with acetic acid (37% vs. 8%, $P < 0.001$) at 23 and 29 months after treatment. A significant and substantial difference in cancer-free and overall survival was also observed, with one- and two-year overall survival rates of 100% and 92% in the acetic acid group and 83% and 63% in the ethanol group, respectively.[49] A subsequent meta-analysis study comparing PEI and PAI therapy for early HCC showed no significant difference in complication rates and recurrence-free or overall survival between these groups, but acknowledges that this analysis is highly prone to selection bias due to the limited number of patients studied.[50]

Complications and contraindications

Potential complications and contraindications for PAI are similar to those of PEI; however, some authors report transient hemoglobinuria immediately after treatment with PAI, even with small volumes (5–10 mL) of 50% acetic acid. This usually spontaneously clears with normal voiding and does not affect the serum creatinine level; however, alkalinizing the urine prior to the procedure by administering intravenous fluids containing bicarbonate may be of some preventative benefit.[47,48] Unlike PEI, percutaneous acetic acid injection for treatment of HCC has not been extensively studied in clinical practice; however, applications for its use appear to be similar and limited to the treatment of small (<3 cm) early-stage surgically unresectable tumors that are unable to be treated by other minimally invasive thermal ablation techniques.

Thermal Ablation

Overview

Thermal ablation therapy relies on controlled alteration of tissue temperature to induce irreversible cell injury, resulting in cell death, and coagulative tissue necrosis. Thermal ablation may be accomplished by application of cytotoxic levels of heat or by freezing tissue to achieve cell death. Currently available thermal ablation techniques that have been successfully used to treat HCC include RFA, microwave ablation, cryoablation, and laser ablation therapy, each of which is discussed in further detail later.

The effectiveness of thermal ablation hinges on adequate delivery of heat to the target tissue. Although it has been shown that critical temperatures required for cell death vary depending on heating time and the type of tissue being heated, it is commonly accepted that optimal temperatures for ablation lie within the range of 50–100°C.[51–53] At these temperatures, irreversible cell injury occurs on the basis of denaturation of enzymatic proteins within the cytoplasm and histones required to maintain the tertiary structure of DNA. This process is referred to as "coagulation necrosis" and results in cell death over the course of several days.

Patient selection

Potential candidates for liver thermal ablation therapy include: (1) patients who are poor surgical candidates due to inadequate liver function from underlying cirrhosis or prior partial hepatectomy, (2) patients who are poor surgical candidates due to comorbid underlying medical conditions, (3) patients who are ineligible for surgical resection due to anatomic distribution of the tumor, (4) patients in need of control of local tumor burden as a bridge to liver transplantation, and (5) patients with tumors that are eligible for surgical resection but locoregional therapy is favored according to the "test of time approach" to limit unnecessary hepatectomy.[11] Most patients with HCC fall within categories 1–4, while category 5 applies more to the use of thermal ablation for treatment in patients with hepatic metastasis from some other primary malignant source, in which close imaging surveillance may reveal rapid progression of previously occult multifocal disease that would otherwise preclude segmental hepatectomy for cure.

In general, locoregional thermal ablation therapy is considered a reasonable treatment option in patients with HCC confined to the liver that do not meet criteria for surgical resection. In patients with underlying cirrhosis, thermal ablation treatment is usually restricted to those with Child-Pugh class A or B disease severity. Although there is currently no concrete data to suggest an absolute tumor size beyond which thermal ablation should not be performed, the best outcomes to date appear to be associated with treatments of a single tumor ≤ 5 cm.[39,54,55]

Patients with limited HCC may be candidates for orthotopic liver transplantation (OLT); however, waiting times for donor organs may range from several months to a year. Current eligibility for OLT as treatment of limited HCC is based on the Milan criteria, which include patients with a single HCC up to 5 cm in size, or those with up to three HCCs with no single HCC larger than 3 cm.[56] Should an existing tumor grow while a patient awaits a donor liver, the patient may become ineligible for a potentially curative surgery on the basis of these criteria. Percutaneous thermal ablation and transcatheter therapies have been utilized to control tumor burden in this setting as a bridge to liver transplantation.

Radiofrequency Ablation

Basic principles

RFA utilizes an alternating current created between a conducting electrode inserted within the target lesion and a grounding source to produce thermal energy at the electrode tip. The RF electrode consists of a thin 21–14-gauge needle that is electrically insulated along all but the distal 1–3 cm tip that is in direct electrical contact with the target tissue. The grounding source may be in the form of an adherent electrical grounding pad placed on the patient's skin (monopolar array) or a separate grounding lead incorporated into the conducting electrode itself (bipolar array).

When radiofrequency pulses (<1 MHz) are applied by the generator, an oscillating current is created between the conducting electrode and the grounding source. Tissue heating occurs as energy is transferred from the oscillating current of electrons to the ionic molecules of the tissue itself on account of natural resistance to conductance of the electric current due to tissue interactions. This process of frictional heating of tissue is referred to as "ionic agitation."[17] Electrons are most concentrated at the electrode tip, which is positioned within the target lesion, resulting in the greatest amount of heat transfer at the electrode tip itself. When sufficient heat energy has been transferred and local tissue achieves cytotoxic temperatures in the range of 50–100°C, cell death and coagulation necrosis ensues. Temperature decreases in a radial fashion with increasing distance from the electrode tip, thereby achieving an effective "sphere of coagulation" that is proportionate in size to the amount of current applied to the tissue. By manipulating the amount of current applied to the tissue, the operator can control the extent of tissue damage in a predictable manner.[17,18,51]

The extent of coagulation necrosis induced during thermal ablation is directly proportional to the amount of heat energy deposited in the tissue. Overall heat deposition is in turn dependent on the strength of the RF source, and the amount of local heat loss that occurs within the target tissue before thermal damage is sustained. The amount of heat loss depends on local tissue interactions.[17] This basic relationship, derived from Pennes' bioheat equation, serves as the fundamental principle that drives thermal ablation therapy.

Temperature is the sole parameter governing tissue destruction in all thermal ablation therapies, and an understanding of how heat interacts with tissue to cause cell death is therefore necessary to effectively and safely employ thermal ablation techniques. In general, increasing the amount of RF current being passed through the electrode increases the amount of heat energy deposited within the target tissue, but this relationship is not without limitation.

Living cells can generally tolerate mild elevation of temperature to around 42°C based on their innate mechanisms of homeostasis, but become more susceptible to cellular damage when temperatures reach hyperthermic levels within the range of 42–45°C. Irreversible cell damage occurs at temperatures ranging from 46–50°C, and the time required for induction of coagulation necrosis begins to decrease as temperature increases to a ceiling level of 105°C. At this point, higher temperatures result in tissue boiling and vaporization. This results in an increase in local electrical impedance within the vaporized tissue, thus effectively shielding more peripheral tissues from obtaining the maximal cytotoxic level of heat deposition that is required for cell death. The induced "sphere of coagulation" within the target tissue therefore becomes much smaller than that which would have been achieved at slightly lower temperatures.[17,51,52] The primary goal of effective thermal ablation therapy is therefore to achieve and maintain cytotoxic temperatures (50°–100°C) throughout the entire volume of the target tissue lesion.

Overcoming limitations of heat deposition in tissue

The relationship between tissue heating and cell death is complicated by multiple, often tissue-specific factors that prevent adequate heating of the entire volume of a tumor. Heterogeneous tissue heating occurs from a number of different factors. As previously mentioned, there is a rapid decrease in the amount of heat deposited in tissues at greater distances from the conducting electrode, largely owing to innately high resistance of tissue to conductance of both the electron current and generated heat. The total amount of energy deposited within the tissue is also limited by tissue vaporization effects at high temperatures. Tissue vaporization leads to local gas formation that subsequently acts as a local insulator, preventing the further spread of heat.[17,18,51,52] Advancements in device design and technique, however, have overcome many of these limitations, creating larger zones of heat distribution and reducing treatment time.

The amount of energy deposition that can be achieved with a single conducting RF electrode (i.e., a monopolar electrode) effectively produces a region of coagulation necrosis which measures only 1.6 cm in maximum diameter.[57] Allowing for at least a 0.5-cm treatment margin beyond the edge of the tumor, the effective kill zone of a monopolar electrode is too small to adequately treat most tumors. Placement of multiple conducting electrodes within the target lesion with overlapping treatment zones will increase the zone of thermal coverage; however, this technique is time consuming and difficult to employ in a clinical setting as it is often technically challenging to accurately place each probe in three-dimensional space to assure that the entire lesion will be successfully treated. The development of umbrella-shaped, multiprobe arrays was designed to overcome this problem. These electrodes are composed of as many as 12 hooked arrays, or tines, in a complex geometric configuration, which simultaneously conduct current through the target tissue to create larger zones of coagulation necrosis that can measure up to 3–5 cm in diameter.[51,52]

Energy deposition in tissue and volume of coagulation necrosis can also be increased by using bipolar arrays, as opposed to the traditional monopolar electrode design. With bipolar electrodes, a grounding electrode is located either adjacent to (within 5 cm) or on the same probe as the conducting electrode, thereby eliminating the need for grounding pads on the surface of the patient. With this design, heat is generated not only at the tip of the conducting electrode but also around the grounding electrode, thereby generating larger (up to 3 cm in diameter), more elliptical zones of coagulation necrosis than those that can be achieved with a monopolar device.[51,52,58] Use of bipolar electrodes also eliminates the need for surface grounding pads on the patient's skin, which thereby eliminates the risk of grounding pad burns.

Tissue vaporization effects at high temperatures within the immediate vicinity of the conducting electrode can be minimized by the use of internally cooled electrodes. These devices consist of two internal lumens through which chilled perfusate is circulated, creating a "heat-sink" effect that removes heat from the tissue closest to the electrode tip. By minimizing the amount of charring and vaporization of tissue adjacent to the conducting electrode tip, resistance of local tissue to conductance of RF current and heat is minimized, creating larger zones of coagulation necrosis. Early studies comparing the size of coagulation zones induced by internally cooled versus standard electrodes in muscle and liver show increases in coagulation diameter from a baseline of 1.8 cm to up to 5.4 cm, but treatment times were significantly longer for the internally cooled electrode technique.[59,60]

In addition to use of internally cooled electrodes, delivering pulsed RF energy currents to target tissue instead of continuous application allows partial cooling of tissue adjacent to the electrode tip during short periods of low energy deposition. This allows for greater energy deposition by enabling greater heat dispersion and results in larger zones of tissue coagulation necrosis. Pulsed RF deposition has also shown synergistic effects when utilized with internally cooled electrodes, resulting in even larger regions of coagulation necrosis than those that can be achieved by either technique alone.[51,61]

It is now a well-known phenomenon that heat deposition within a target tissue lesion does not conform to the uniform predictable distribution that would be expected for the particular shape and type of conducting electrode used during thermal ablation. This phenomenon can be attributed to local heat loss within the tissue, the extent of which varies in location according to tissue specific factors. Overall degree of heat loss within the target tissue depends on both the type of tissue being ablated, and the degree of vascular flow within the tissue itself.[17] It has been shown that heat conduction within tissues can be improved by injection of saline solution or iron-based compounds into the target lesion, thereby increasing the ionicity of the tissue, resulting in greater electrical conductivity and current flow. The overall result is a larger region of coagulation necrosis for a given amount of applied RF energy, and the actual coagulation diameter is influenced by the volume and concentration of saline infused.[62]

Increased vascular flow within a lesion also reduces the extent of coagulation necrosis by acting as a "heat-sink" shunting heat away from the target lesion. Reduction of blood flow to the lesion via angiographic balloon occlusion or particle embolotherapy of a feeding artery may therefore potentiate the effects of thermal ablation therapy.[63,64] The notoriously heterogeneous distribution of heat within a target lesion and the high likelihood of incomplete treatment by thermal ablation modalities alone has led to various combination therapies for minimally invasive tumor treatment that combine external beam radiation, chemotherapy, embolotherapy, or direct ethanol injection with thermal ablation techniques to enhance tissue eradication and cell death. Use of these additional therapies prior to thermal ablation increases the sensitivity of tumor cells to heat and leads to a greater number of cell deaths.[52]

RFA technique

RFA of HCC may be performed via a percutaneous, laparoscopic, or open surgical approach depending on clinical circumstances. The percutaneous approach is the least invasive and is performed most commonly in patients with underlying cirrhosis and surgically unresectable disease. Combination segmental hepatectomy and intraoperative ultrasound-guided local ablation therapy has been shown to be an effective treatment strategy for multinodular HCC.[65]

Prior to scheduling a percutaneous ablation procedure, each patient is seen in formal outpatient consultation in an office setting where the case history, a focused physical examination, and pertinent imaging studies are reviewed. At this time, complete assessment of underlying liver function, tumor stage, and physical status of the patient is assessed, and the feasibility and appropriateness of RFA is determined and discussed with the patient. This consultation routinely includes a discussion on the risks and benefits of the procedure, as well as potential alternative treatment options. Potential side effects of RFA are also discussed. If necessary, additional preprocedural imaging or laboratory studies are ordered. A complete review of all available imaging studies is performed, and an appropriate approach to the target lesion is planned. In general, most patients who are healthy enough to undergo computed tomography (CT)-guided needle biopsy are good candidates for RFA.

All patients undergo an overnight fast prior to a planned ablation procedure, to minimize risk of aspiration on account of sedation used during the procedure itself. Patients may take any necessary cardiac or antihypertensive medications on the morning of the scheduled procedure with a small quantity of water. Insulin-dependent diabetic patients should administer half of their usual morning insulin dose to avoid hyperglycemia. Each patient undergoes an abridged physical examination and a repeat discussion on issues relating to informed consent immediately prior to a scheduled procedure. An intravenous line is then placed for administration of sedative medications and fluids in the perioperative period. At our institution, we do not routinely administer prophylactic antibiotics prior to ablation therapy in the liver, but will do so in the setting of underlying biliary obstruction, an indwelling biliary stent, or prior surgery resulting in an enteroenteric anastomosis.

Patients are then brought to the CT or ultrasound suite and appropriately positioned on the gantry or examination table. Technical staff place grounding pads in an appropriate location on the patient to direct the RF current and thus prevent damage to adjacent vital structures within the target area. After initial CT or ultrasound imaging is performed, and the target lesion is confirmed and appropriately visualized, the skin overlying the planned entry site for the RF probe is then marked. When utilizing CT-guidance, this site is mapped on the patient's skin by a computer-guided laser grid based on information obtained by preliminary CT images. Horizontal and vertical laser lights in the CT gantry correspond to the x- and y-axes from the software generated grid on the workstation monitor, and a ruler can be placed to match the desired skin entry site as determined by information on the source images. The area is then prepped and draped in sterile fashion and local buffered lidocaine anesthesia is administered both intradermally and to the deeper soft tissues adjacent to the target lesion with a 25-gauge skin needle and 22-gauge spinal needle, respectively. A small skin incision is made at the skin entry site using a #11 scalpel blade. For ultrasound-guided procedures, direct visualization is then performed as the RF electrode is placed through the skin incision and advanced along the planned trajectory to a predetermined location within the target lesion. Multiple additional conducting electrodes may be placed in this fashion to assure adequate volume of coagulation and complete treatment of the target lesion. When using CT-guidance, CT-fluoroscopy is initiated and an image is taken with the spinal needle in place to identify proper table position and needle angle. Repositioning can be performed with the spinal needle if necessary. The spinal needle is then exchanged for the RF electrode, which is advanced along the same trajectory by approximately 1/2–1/3 the distance to the target lesion. A CT-fluoroscopic image is then obtained, and the RF electrode angle in the x, y, and z plane is corrected as necessary before advancing any further. This technique is followed until the tip of the RF electrode is successfully placed at a predetermined location within the target lesion. For lesions larger than 2 cm in diameter, larger electrodes or several overlapping ablation zones may be needed to insure adequate thermocoagulation of the target lesion.

Depending upon the RF equipment used, each ablation should be carried out according to the manufacturer's specifications regarding target temperatures [e.g., Cool-tip electrode (Covidien,

Boulder, CO) and Starburst/Talon electrode (Angiodynamics/Rita Medical Systems Inc., Mountain View, CA)] and/or electrical impedance [Leveen electrode (Boston Scientific, Watertown, MA)]. Just before and during RF heating, patients are administered intravenous midazolam (0.5–1 mg doses) and fentanyl (25–50 mcg doses) for conscious sedation and analgesia. Patient vital signs and an EKG tracing are continuously monitored throughout the procedure to ensure an adequate and safe level of conscious sedation. Appropriate levels of sedation and analgesia vary on a case-by-case basis according to lesion size and location. Occasionally, general anesthesia may need to be used in pediatric patients or patients who may not tolerate the RF heating with conscious sedation alone.

Following the ablation procedure, the patient is monitored by nursing staff in a postprocedure recovery room for one to two hours prior to being discharged from the department. Vital signs are routinely monitored for signs of early complication. Patients who receive general anesthesia or conscious sedation require longer monitoring until the effects of sedative medications have completely resolved. Patients undergoing sedation are not permitted to drive a motor vehicle in the postprocedure period and are discharged only under the care of a friend or relative that may provide transportation home. Discharge instructions are given to the patient both verbally and in writing. Patients are advised to take acetaminophen for minor pain and to avoid aspirin or NSAIDS to minimize risk of bleeding. Contact phone numbers for the department and for a radiologist on call are provided, and the patient is instructed to call in the event of excessive pain, progressive swelling, bruising, or fever to >100.5 F in the postprocedure period. Patients are usually allowed a trial of solid and liquid intake under supervision, prior to leaving the department. If appropriate, patients are allowed to resume their normal diet approximately two hours following the procedure.

RFA devices

There are currently four major commercial manufacturers of RF tumor ablation systems within the United States. Each of these manufacturers has focused electrode design on one of three alternative strategies for energy application. The Valley Lab/Covidien (Boulder, CO) device consists of internally cooled electrodes, which use a pulsed RF energy algorithm to minimize excessive heat deposition that could lead to tissue vaporization and decreased volume of coagulation necrosis.[61] Two other manufacturers (Radiotherapeutics, Boston Scientific, Watertown, MA, and Angiodynamics/RITA Medical Systems Inc., Mountain View, CA) utilize a deployable array RF electrode that consists of 10–16 small wires (tines) deployed through a 14–17 gauge needle once it is appropriately positioned within the target lesion under imaging guidance. Use of multitined devices result in heat deposition over larger tissue volumes, but require longer treatment times. The Radiotherapeutics device uses incremental increases in RF energy to avoid tissue vaporization and charring and achieve larger ablation zone diameters. The RITA Star-Burst-XL configuration utilizes a multitined approach, but the device is designed to minimize excessive heat deposition by gradually extending the tines in incremental fashion to achieve larger ablation zones in the realm of 3–5 cm in diameter.[52]

Multitined devices often must be eccentrically placed within a target lesion to appropriately include the entirety of the lesion within the treatment zone. When deployed, the tines of the Radiotherapeutics, Boston Scientific Device (LeVeen electrode) curve back toward the needle, and this device is therefore initially deployed at the more inferior margin of the target lesion. In contrast, the RITA electrode tines course in a forward and lateral direction, so this device is deployed at the superomedial margin of the target lesion. The Cool-tip system (ValleyLab/Covidien, Boulder, Colorado) utilizes a single or triple-cluster internally cooled electrode (no tines), the tip of which is usually positioned at the distal tumor margin. By using internally cooled RF electrodes, this device can achieve a volume of induced thermocoagulation measuring up to 4–7 cm in diameter.[59] The device's single or cluster RF electrode contains a thermocouple embedded within its tip, which is used to measure intratumoral temperature and automated feedback modulates applied RF energy to reduce tissue boiling.[52]

With increased understanding of RF principles and continued advancement in technology of RF tumor ablation systems, the paradigms upon which current commercially available systems are based are continually changing. Each method of delivering RF energy to tissue has its share of merits and drawbacks, and manufacturers are committed to ongoing development and improvement in design of RF electrodes and generators. Currently used methodologies are still somewhat experimental, and as of this writing, there is no clearly discernable difference in effectiveness or complication rates of any one device over the others.

Results

In the United States, RFA is currently the most widely used technique for in situ liver tumor destruction.[11] Results of RFA for early, surgically unresectable HCC vary depending on tumor size, location, and to a lesser extent, the presence or absence of tumor encapsulation.[26,55,66–69] Although there is no currently established threshold tumor diameter at which RFA treatment of HCC becomes unsuccessful, results within the current literature suggest that the probability of complete ablation diminishes with tumor diameter > 5 cm, with optimal treatment results noted in tumors < 3 cm in size (Figure 14-2).[66] The complete ablation rate of tumors < 3 cm in size is reported to be approximately 90% by imaging follow-up criteria (Figures 14-3 and 14-4).[70–74] One study conducted a more definitive analysis of 47 HCC nodules treated by RFA in 24 explanted human liver specimens and showed complete necrosis in 83% of tumors < 3 cm in size. Results of this study also showed 36% sensitivity and 100% specificity of posttreatment CT or MRI for detection of residual or recurrent tumor.[75] The presence of underlying liver cirrhosis or a well-defined tumor capsule has also been shown to improve the effectiveness of thermal ablation. This observation is presumably due to the so-called "oven effect," in which underlying liver fibrosis or a fibrous capsule serves as a local thermal insulator around the tumor, allowing for higher achievable peak tissue temperatures and longer cytotoxic temperature duration during treatment (Figure 14-5).[26] Proximity of tumors to large (> 3 mm diameter) vessels within

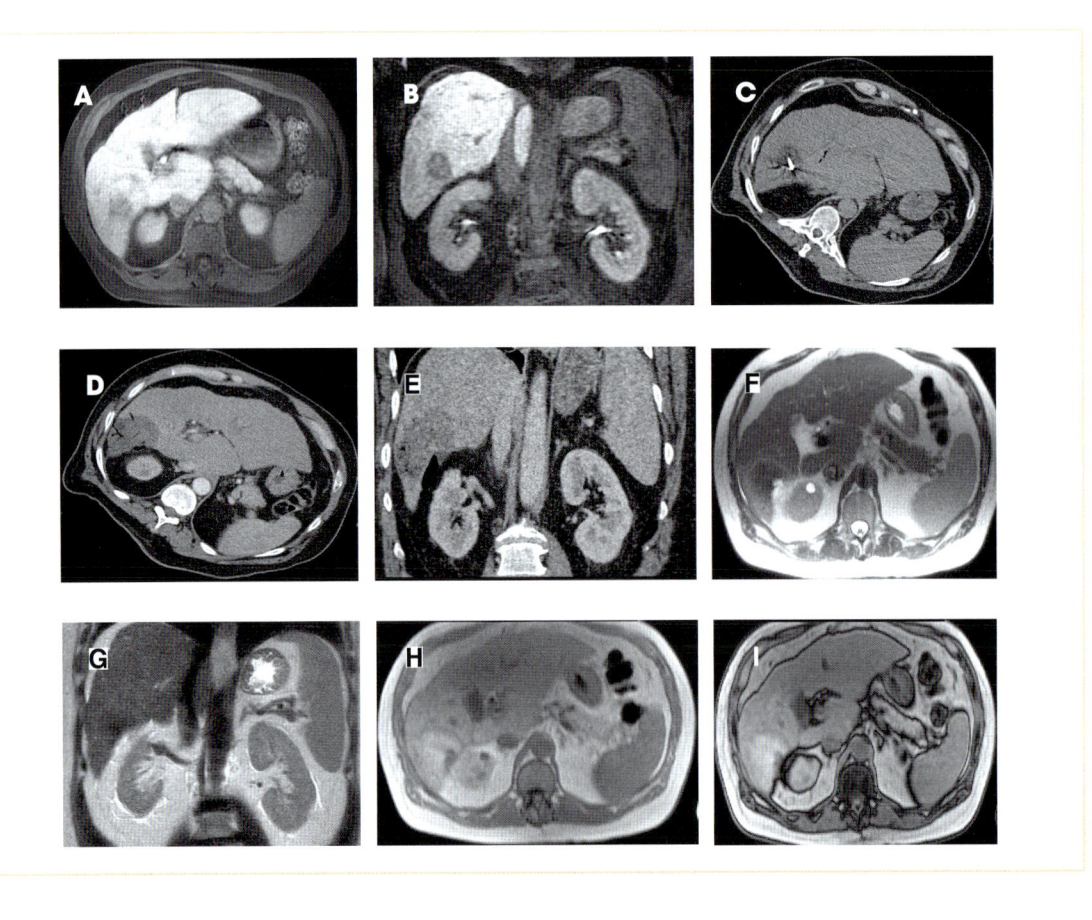

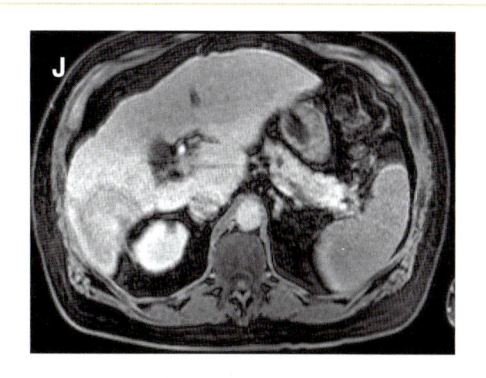

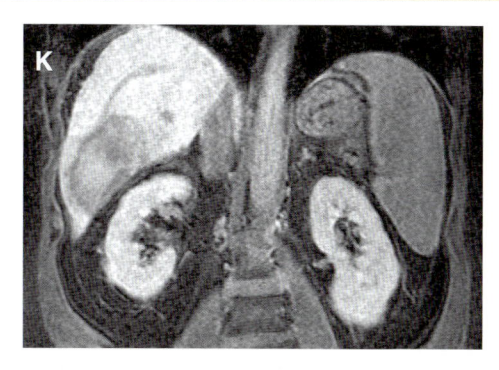

Ablation Therapy for Hepatocellular Carcinoma 331

Figure 14-2: (A–B) Axial and coronal post-Eovist T1 VIBE images (15-min delay) showing 3.8 cm HCC within segment 6. (C) Noncontrast axial CT image acquired at 8 min of 16-min duration treatment using 2.5 cm active tip cluster RF electrode and power range of 80–150 W. (D–E) Axial and coronal portal venous phase enhanced CT images following RFA using two overlapping treatment zones. (F–G) Axial and coronal T2 HASTE posttreatment images showing clearly demarcated T2 dark ablation zone (desiccated tissue). (H-I) Axial T1 in- and out-of-phase images showing T1 hyperintense regions of coagulative necrosis within the treatment zone. (J–K) Axial and coronal post-Eovist T1 VIBE images (18–20 min delay) showing well-demarcated ablation zone adequately encompassing the treated lesion.

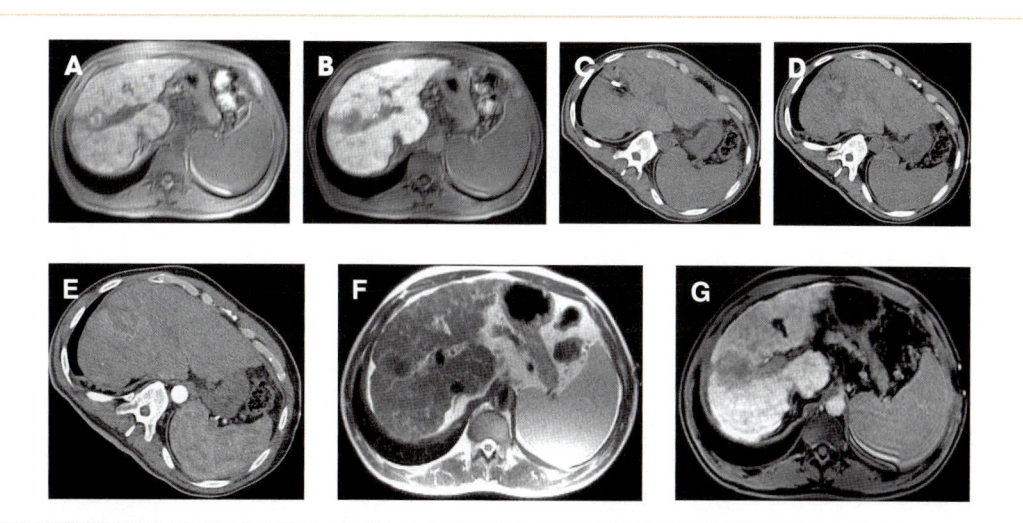

Figure 14-3: (A) Axial T1 VIBE fat-saturated and (B) post-Eovist T1 VIBE images (20-min delay) showing 2.2 cm HCC within segment 8. (C) Noncontrast axial CT image acquired at 6 minutes of 16 minute duration treatment using 2.5 cm active tip cluster RF electrode and power range of 80–137 W. (D) Axial noncontrast posttreatment CT image showing hypodense treatment zone with central hyperdensity corresponding to coagulative necrosis. (E) Axial arterial phase enhanced CT images following RFA using two overlapping treatment zones, showing thin enhancing rim of hyperemic normal liver parenchyma. (F) Axial T2 HASTE posttreatment image showing clearly demarcated T2 dark ablation zone (desiccated tissue). (G) Axial post-Eovist T1 VIBE image (18-min delay) showing well-demarcated ablation zone adequately encompassing the treated lesion.

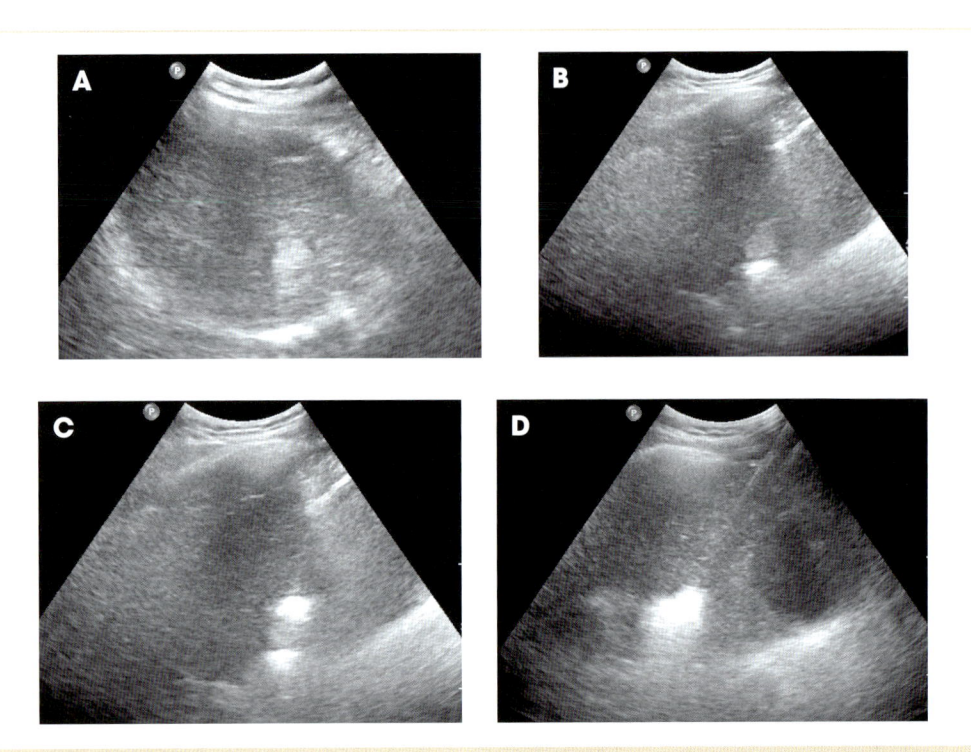

Figure 14-4: Appearance of thermal ablation zone by ultrasound: (A) Grayscale ultrasound image showing hyperechoic 2.2 cm HCC within segment 8. (B) 3 cm active tip single RF electrode placed; at 2 minutes of treatment with 100 W, echogenic microbubbles are visualized at the electrode tip. (C) At 6 minutes of treatment with 120 W, echogenic microbubbles are also visualized at the proximal margin of the 3 cm active tip. (D) At 12 minutes of treatment at maximum power of 160 W, distal and proximal echogenic ablation fronts coalesce, completely masking the underlying lesion. Cytotoxic temperature of 84°C was achieved.

the liver has been shown to diminish treatment effectiveness due to the "heat sink" effect of blood flow, which effectively shunts heat away from the adjacent tumor tissue.[76]

Published systematic reviews of overall treatment effectiveness of RFA for surgically unresectable HCC are somewhat limited in their ability to establish accurate long-term survival statistics due to difficulties in interpretation of the overall data as a result of variation in the outcome measurements, techniques, approaches, and RF electrode designs utilized in cohort studies to date. Several large cohort studies report overall five-year survival rates ranging from 33% to 58% for patients with surgically unresectable early-stage HCC treated with RFA.[67–69,77–80] For patients meeting the Milan criteria awaiting liver transplantation, use of RFA as a bridging therapy to slow progression of disease has been reported to yield four-year overall and disease free survival rates of 85% and 92% respectively.[56] This data was derived from observational studies only, however, and the impact of RFA as a bridging therapy to liver transplantation on the overall survival of patients with HCC is still not well defined. Currently most would agree that it is useful, but there is no level I, II-1, and II-2 evidence to show that it decreases the dropout rate from transplant lists, prolongs patient survival, or decreases tumor recurrence rate after liver transplantation.[8]

Reported survival rates of patients with HCC treated by RFA have improved to such a degree that RFA is beginning to challenge partial hepatectomy as a first line treatment for patients with surgically resectable disease. A small number of randomized controlled trials comparing RFA versus surgical resection as primary treatment of a solitary HCC ≤

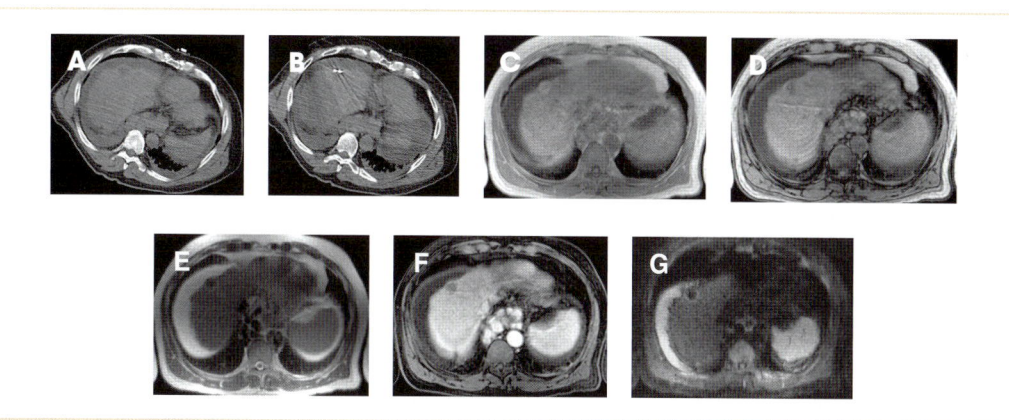

Figure 14-5: The "Oven Effect": (A) Noncontrast axial CT image showing cirrhotic liver with 2.2 cm hypodense HCC within segment 8 at the liver dome. Perihepatic fluid represents artificial ascites induced by infusion of sterile D5W into the peritoneal cavity for thermal protection of the adjacent diaphragm. (B) Noncontrast axial CT image showing placement of two single 3 cm active tip RF electrodes along the medial and lateral aspects of the targeted mass, approximately 1 cm apart. (C–D) Following 16 min treatment at 80–164 W, cytotoxic temperature of 84°C was achieved. Axial T1 in- and out-of-phase images showing T1 hyperintense regions of coagulative necrosis within the treatment zone. The treatment zone is approximately the same size as the treated lesion, with very little thermal damage to surrounding normal liver parenchyma due to fibrous encapsulation. (E) Axial T2 HASTE image showing clearly demarcated T2 dark ablation zone (desiccated tissue) corresponding to the exact size of the treated lesion. (F) Axial post-Eovist (10 cc) T1 VIBE arterial phase image showing thin rim of reactive hyperemia without nodularity, and (G) no restricted diffusion within the lesion to suggest residual tumor.

5 cm showed no significant difference in overall and disease-free survival outcomes between the two treatments with follow-up intervals as long as four years after therapy.[55,81] Several nonrandomized controlled trials showed similar results.[82–84] One nonrandomized comparative study of 200 patients showed significantly better overall and disease-free survival rates in surgically treated patients versus those treated with RFA when tumor size was > 3 cm.[85]

Several randomized controlled trials have been conducted to investigate the therapeutic benefits of RFA versus PEI for treatment of small surgically unresectable HCC.[70–74,86,87] Meta-analyses of these studies show significant survival benefit for RFA versus PEI treatment of small unresectable HCC (mean size, 2.5 cm) in patients with Child-Pugh class A cirrhosis up to four years after therapy.[86,87] In these study populations, RFA was shown to have significantly lower rates of local recurrence at the treatment site. The overall rate of adverse events was higher with RFA; however, there was no significant difference in rates of major complications between therapies.[86,87] RFA has also been shown to achieve complete tumor ablation with fewer treatment sessions when compared to chemical ablation techniques.[71]

Transcatheter arterial chemoembolization (TACE) is commonly used for treatment of surgically unresectable HCC, predominantly in patients with multinodular disease or as palliative therapy in local control of tumor burden to prolong life or bridge patients awaiting liver transplantation. Although RFA has been utilized in the treatment of multinodular disease, the best results have been observed in patients with solitary tumors <3 cm in size. It is still unknown as to whether RFA or TACE is more effective in improving survival of patients with unresectable HCC that is amenable to either treatment, as there has been no randomized controlled trial to date that directly compares these two treatments. An early prospective nonrandomized trial comparing efficacy of TACE, laparoscopic RFA, and conservative treatment for HCC in patients with Child-Pugh class B or C cirrhosis demonstrated improved overall survival and fewer complications with laparoscopic RFA treatment as compared with TACE or conservative management.[88] A subsequent retrospective analysis of 91 patients with unresectable HCC (median tumor size of 3 cm) treated with TACE or RFA that was amenable to either treatment showed similar overall survival and time to disease progression in both groups.[89] These authors concluded that RFA and TACE were equally efficacious in treating patients with small early-stage surgically unresectable HCC.

Complications and contraindications

RFA is considered a relatively safe, minimally invasive locoregional therapy for treatment of tumors within the liver. The overall rate of major complications associated with this procedure is reported to range between 2.2% and 3.1%, with an estimated mortality rate of 0.1%–0.5%.[90–97] Reported major complications include hepatic failure, intraperitoneal hemorrhage, hepatic abscess, bile duct injury, local skin burns, tumor seeding, and gastrointestinal perforation. Minor complications include subcapsular hematoma, reactive pleural effusion, and partial liver infarction. Reported rate of occurrence for minor complications ranges from 0.82% to 4.7%.[93] Sepsis and liver failures are the most common causes of procedure-related mortality in large surveys. Progression to complete liver failure was more common in patients with Child-Pugh class B or C cirrhosis, and the presence of underlying biliary obstruction appears to increase the risk for posttreatment sepsis.[97,98] In most studies, the risk of major complication appears to increase with size of the treated tumor, and tumors < 3 cm in size are associated with the lowest risk for major treatment-related complications.[97,98]

Postablation syndrome is a transient self-limited symptom complex of low-grade fever, right upper quadrant pain, anorexia, and general malaise that is commonly experienced in up to 37% of patients treated with RFA.[93,99] It is felt to occur as a response to the transient systemic release of circulating immunomodulators released during tumor cell death. Symptoms may persist for up to two weeks following treatment, and total duration depends on the volume of tumor necrosis within the liver. Significant predictors of occurrence in the posttreatment period include tumor volume >4.5 cm in diameter, ablated tissue volume of 6.5 cm in diameter, or postablation aspartate aminotransferase levels > 350 IU/L.[99]

The incidence of tumor seeding along the needle tract following percutaneous RFA treatment of HCC has been reported to range from 0% to 12.5%.[100–102] This complication has been reported to be related to subcapsular tumor location, poor differentiation of underlying tumor histology, and high AFP levels (> 100 ng/mL).[100] One particular study showed that use of a cooled-tip RF electrode was associated with a low risk of neoplastic seeding, and this complication was more likely to be related to prior percutaneous biopsy than to thermal ablation treatment.[102]

There are currently no commonly agreed-upon criteria by which to establish definite contraindications to RFA treatment of surgically unresectable HCC. Current recommendations for use of RFA as a primary treatment modality are based on the most favorable published outcomes from cumulative experience in multiple centers, which advocate for treatment of small (<3 cm), solitary tumors in patients with good underlying liver function (Child-Pugh class A). Although size and number of tumor lesions within the liver have been shown to be related to efficacy of therapy and overall rate of complication, neither criterion has been shown to represent an absolute contraindication to RFA treatment at this time. Relative contraindications to RFA treatment are more related to tumor location and risk of thermal injury to adjacent nontarget tissues, as well as underlying liver function and the presence of biliary obstruction that may predispose to posttreatment sepsis.[103]

Suggested criteria for relative contraindications to RFA treatment of HCC include: (1) tumor located <1 cm from the main biliary duct (due to risk of delayed stenosis), (2) intrahepatic bile duct dilatation, (3) anterior exophytic location of the tumor (due to the risk of tumor seeding), (4) bilioenteric anastomosis, (5) irreversible coagulopathy, and (6) Child-Pugh class B or C cirrhosis.[98,103] Although risk for injury to the biliary tree is present with centrally located tumors, it appears as though reported rates of this complication are low, ranging from 0.1% to 1.0%.[97] Changes in the imaging appearance of the biliary tree are frequent following RFA of HCC; however, this has been shown to be of no clinical significance in the majority of cases.[104] The presence of ascites has also been considered by some to be a contraindication to percutaneous RFA treatment of HCC; however, a more recent retrospective study showed no increased risk for procedure-related complications in this patient population.[105]

Caution must be used when using RFA or microwave ablation (MWA) in patients with implantable cardiac pacemakers or automated internal cardiac defibrillators. Pacemakers are susceptible to interference by energy in the radiofrequency and microwave spectrum (10^9–10^{11} Hz).[106,107] According to manufacturers, pacemakers are at risk for malfunction from external electrical activity within 15 cm of the leads. Careful positioning of grounding pads may help to direct the flow of current away from the cardiac device and minimize the chance of interaction. The following preliminary guidelines are therefore suggested for patients with pacemakers and defibrillators undergoing tumor ablation procedures: (i) coordinate treatment with cardiac electrophysiologists to interrogate and program pacemakers to automatic pacing modes and turn off defibrillators during the ablation procedure; (ii) provide an external pacing/defibrillation system for emergency use; (iii) appropriately place grounding pads to direct current away from the pacemaker/defibrillator device and its leads; and (iv) where possible position electrodes and antennae >5 cm from pacemaker/defibrillator leads.[108]

Microwave Coagulation Therapy

Basic principles

Microwave energy is a form of electromagnetic radiation that ranges in frequency from 0.3 to 300 GHz and can be used as an energy source for percutaneous thermal tissue ablation. Microwave coagulation therapy (MCT) antennae and generators are similar to RFA; however, they use a different part of the electromagnetic spectrum. Unlike RFA, where the inserted electrode functions as the active energy source, MCT utilizes inserted applicators that function as antennas for transmission of applied energy ranging in frequency from 915 to 2450 MHz. At these oscillation frequencies, the electrical charge of a microwave changes polarity nearly two billion times per second, which in turn causes rotation of polar molecules (i.e., water molecules) within tissue. The higher the applied microwave energy, the greater the rotational forces on water molecules within tissue. It is this vigorous movement of water molecules against frictional forces that generates heat within tissue during MCT. When the amount of heat generated reaches cytotoxic levels in the range of 50°C–100°C, cell death and coagulation necrosis ensue.[109,110]

MCT is one of the most recent advances in the field of thermal ablation technology and, similar to RFA, can be performed open, laparoscopically, or percutaneously. The potential advantages of microwave technology compared with RFA include more uniform production of higher intratumoral temperatures, improved heat convection profiles, and the ability to achieve synergistic effects by use of multiple antennae, all of which result in larger tumor ablation volumes. MCT is also associated with shorter ablation times and less procedural pain. This technique does not require the use of grounding pads, which decreases the time required for patient preparation and eliminates the risk of inadvertent patient injury from grounding pad-related skin burns.[111–113]

MCT achieves a larger zone of tissue heating than RFA through use of transmitting antennae that create a broad field of power density deposition which can measure up to 2 cm in radius from the antenna itself. With RFA, the zone of tissue heating is limited to a few millimeters surrounding the active electrode tip, and the remainder of the ablation zone is heated via thermal conduction.[114] The greater radius of heat deposition associated with MCT has the potential to allow for more uniform tumor kill within the ablation zone than that which can be achieved with RFA. MCT is also less susceptible to the "heat sink" effect of flowing blood within nearby vessels.[111]

MCT technique

The preprocedural workup, patient preparation, and planning of an appropriate image-guided approach to MWA in the liver is the same as that which has been previously described for RFA. MCT can be performed percutaneously, laparoscopically, or as an alternative to segmental hepatectomy during open laparotomy. Depending on whether the percutaneous or surgical approach is performed, a single or multiple thin (14.5-gauge) microwave antennae are passed under CT or ultrasound guidance into the tumor, and the antennae are then electrically coupled to the microwave generator with a coaxial cable. Application of electrical energy from the generator results in emission of electromagnetic microwaves from the exposed, noninsulated portion of the antenna. Each generator is capable of producing 30–140 W of power at a frequency of 915 or 2450 MHz. Since application of microwave energy within tissue does not require the use of a grounding pad, the procedure is not associated with risk of grounding pad burns.

During the procedure, temperatures within the ablation zone may be monitored by a separately placed thermocouple sensor to confirm appropriate cytotoxic levels of heat deposition within the target tissue. For tumors >3.0 cm in size, multiple MCT antennae can be placed within the target lesion to create a larger zone of thermocoagulation. Antennae should ideally be spaced 1.5–2 cm apart, and depending upon the length of the active tip spherical zones of ablation measuring approximately 4.5–6 cm can be achieved in a single 7–15 minute treatment. The central microwave emission point ("feed point") is at the middle of the active tip in most systems and this should ideally be centered within the tumor mass being treated (Figure 14-6).

MCT devices

Currently, in the United States, there are six commercially available microwave systems that utilize either a 915-MHz (Evident, Covidien, Boulder, CO; MicrothermX, BSD Medical, Salt Lake City, UT; Avecure, Medwaves, San Diego, CA) or 2450-MHz (Certus 140, Neuwave, Madison, WI; Amica, Hospital Service, Rome, Italy; Acculis MTA, Microsulis Medical Limited, Hampshire, UK) generator and straight antennae with varying active tips of 0.6–4.0 cm. Perfusion of the antennae shaft is required in five of the six systems either with room temperature fluid or carbon dioxide to reduce conductive heating of the nonactive portion of the antenna, thus preventing damage to the skin and tissues proximal to the active tip. A single applicator is used with a single generator in four of the systems. Two of the systems have the ability to power up to three antennas with a single generator. Since most of the microwave systems are newly FDA approved, there is no published data at this time on their differences in safety or effectiveness. Perceived advantages of MW over RF include a greater convection profile and less heat sink effects that may reduce local recurrences and larger resultant ablative volume when using multiple applicators simultaneously that will allow faster treatment of larger tumors.

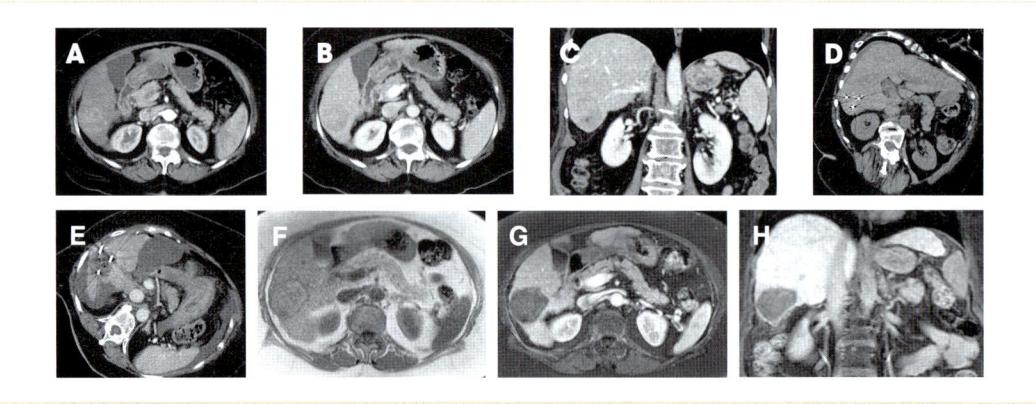

Figure 14-6: Large treatment zone achieved with microwave ablation: (A) Axial arterial phase postcontrast CT image showing large 4.6 cm hyper-enhancing mass in segment 6, which demonstrates contrast washout on axial (B) and coronal (C) portal-venous phase imaging, compatible with HCC. (D) Axial reformatted noncontrast CT image showing placement of three microwave antennae in cluster formation, approximately 1.5 cm apart within the lesion. (E) Axial portal-venous phase contrast-enhanced CT image showing large hypodense, nonenhancing thermal ablation zone encompassing the targeted lesion. Perihepatic fluid represents iatrogenic ascites induced via infusion of sterile D5W into Morrison's pouch for thermal protection of the right kidney. (F) Axial T1-weighted image performed at one month posttreatment showing hyperintense regions of coagulative necrosis within the treatment zone. (G-H) Axial and coronal post-Eovist T1 VIBE images (18–20 min delay) showing large well-demarcated ablation zone adequately encompassing the treated lesion without evidence of residual tumor.

Results

MCT, similar to other thermal ablation techniques, has emerged as an effective minimally invasive method of treatment for HCC in patients with surgically unresectable disease or underlying medical comorbidities that preclude safe operation.[112,113,115–123] A single internally cooled microwave antenna is capable of inducing a field of coagulation necrosis measuring between 2.0 and 2.5 cm in diameter; however in clinical practice, arrays of multiple antennae or multiple sequential insertions of a single antenna are necessary to treat lesions > 2 cm in diameter.[7,112,113]

Complete tumor response rates to MCT are reported to range from 84% to 98% based on posttreatment imaging assessments, and the results appear to be dependent on tumor size.[116–124] Histopathologic analysis in a small number of patients has shown complete necrosis rates of approximately 95% in primary HCC measuring up to 5 cm in size.[125] With placement of multiple microwave antennae in cluster formation, there have been reports of complete treatment of liver tumors up to 6 cm in diameter.[122] Similar to RFA, however, the majority studies published in the literature regarding MCT treatment of HCC demonstrate greatest initial response and lowest recurrence rates for smaller tumors <4 cm in diameter.[116–124] This is likely due to the presence of inherent electrode edge effects and variable electric fields at tissue interfaces which can result in heterogeneous heat distribution within the target tissue, thereby reducing treatment efficacy.[7] This limitation, however, has been partially overcome by improvements in microwave antenna design. Use of spherical triple-loop antenna configurations for intraoperative sonographically guided treatment of HCC has been shown to achieve coagulation necrosis diameters of up to 6.4 cm on histopathologic specimens.[113]

Long-term outcome data for patients with HCC treated by MCT demonstrates one-, three-, and five-year survival rates of 93%–96%, 63%–73%, and 38%–52%, respectively.[117,122,124] Results are significantly better for patients with maximum tumor size < 4 cm, and the highest probability of long-term survival is noted in patients with Child-Pugh class A cirrhosis.[117] Overall survival data appears to be comparable with that of surgical resection for tumors measuring 4 cm or less in size.

Overall effectiveness of percutaneous MCT appears to be comparable with that of PEI and RFA for treatment of solitary small HCC. A retrospective analysis comparing MCT and PEI treatment of solitary nodular HCC ≤ 2 cm showed no significant difference in overall five-year survival or rate of local recurrence after treatment.[126] This study did show a statistically significant improvement in overall five-year survival rate for patients with moderately or poorly differentiated HCC subtypes that were treated with MCT versus PEI, however (78% vs. 35%, respectively). A prospective randomized controlled trial analyzing the efficacy of MCT versus RFA for treatment of small early-stage HCC demonstrated that these two modalities have equivalent therapeutic effects, with no significant difference in rate of residual disease following treatment. RFA treatment, however, was achieved with fewer individual electrode placements/treatments than MCT.[127] A subsequent similarly designed randomized controlled trial by other authors yielded statistically significant results in favor of RFA, demonstrating lower rates of local recurrence and improved overall survival when compared to MCT. This study also noted larger areas of tissue necrosis associated with RFA as opposed to MCT treatments.[128,129] Further analysis is warranted to establish clear benefit of one of these thermal ablation techniques over the other in this patient population.

Complications and contraindications

Although complication rates for MCT in the liver are lower than those reported for surgical resection, multiple clinical studies examining its applications in the treatment of HCC have demonstrated higher complication rates when compared with other thermal ablation techniques.[7,128,129] Overall rate of complication is reported to reach 12% in some series, and similar to RFA, appears to be highest with tumors >4 cm in size.[7,118,128,129] The potential complications and relative contraindications for MCT of HCC are similar to those previously discussed for RFA treatment in the liver. The incidence of pain and fever in the posttreatment period is noted to be higher in patients treated with MCT when compared with RFA, but symptoms are easily managed with anti-inflammatory medications. Risk of bile duct injury, pleural effusion, and reactive ascites also appears to be slightly higher in tumors treated with MCT when compared with RFA.[128,129]

Cryoablation

Basic principles

Cryoablation achieves tissue necrosis through the induction of extremely cold local temperatures to freeze tissue, ultimately leading to destruction of cellular membranes and subsequent cell death. This technology is based on the thermodynamic principle referred to as the *Joule–Thompson effect*. When a well-insulated high pressure gas at a constant temperature is allowed to pass through a narrow aperture into a contained area of lower pressure, the gas will undergo isenthalpic expansion and its temperature will decrease. As a gas expands, the average distance between its molecules will increase. Due to the presence of intermolecular attractive forces ("Van der Waals force"), expansion causes an increase in the potential energy of the gas. If the gas undergoes free expansion (no external work is performed in the process) and no heat is transferred, the total energy of the gas remains constant according to the law of conservation of energy. The increase in potential energy therefore equates to a decrease in kinetic energy of the gas, which manifests as a decrease in its temperature.[82]

A real gas may experience an increase or decrease in temperature via isenthalpic expansion according to the principles of the Joule–Thompson effect. Each real gas has a Joule–Thompson inversion temperature above which expansion at constant enthalpy causes the temperature to rise and below which such expansion causes cooling. This inversion temperature depends on the ambient pressure of the gas. For most gases at atmospheric pressure, the inversion temperature is above room temperature, so most gases can be cooled at room temperature by isenthalpic expansion. Other gases such as helium, hydrogen, and neon whose inversion temperatures are below room temperature undergo warming during expansion. This process can also be explained by the laws of thermodynamics. During gas molecule collisions, kinetic energy is temporarily converted into potential energy. As the average intermolecular distance increases with increasing volume of a gas, there is a drop in the number of collisions that occur per unit time, which results in an overall decrease in average potential energy of the gas. Since total energy of the gas is conserved during isenthalpic expansion, this leads to an increase in kinetic energy and thus temperature of the gas. Thus, for a given real gas, the former effect dominates below the Joule–Thompson inversion temperature, and free expansion causes a decrease in temperature. Above the inversion temperature, the latter effect dominates, and isenthalpic free expansion of the gas causes a temperature increase.[130]

Cryoablation achieves ultra-cold temperatures on the order of −160°C in tissue by allowing argon gas to expand from high pressure to low pressure through a constricted orifice (J–T port) within a cryoprobe. Helium gas has the opposite J–T effect and is used to warm the probe to facilitate its removal at the end of the procedure. The technique itself uses a cycle of subsequent freezing, thawing, and re-freezing tissue to induce osmotic shifts that result in cellular membrane rupture and eventual cell death within target tissue.

The cell killing effects of cryoablation may be the result of any of a number of proposed pathways. Proposed mechanisms include direct cytolysis via intracellular and extracellular ice crystal formation causing protein denaturation, intracellular dehydration and pH changes, ischemic necrosis via vascular injury, cellular edema and vessel disruption incurred during the thaw phase, or activation of anti-tumor immune responses and induction of cellular apoptosis. In addition, endothelial damage resulting from cryoablation leads to platelet aggregation and microthrombosis.[131,132]

Cryoablation technique

The preprocedural workup, patient preparation, and planning of an appropriate image-guided approach to cryoablation in the liver is the same as that which has been previously described for RFA. Percutaneous cryoablation may be performed under CT, ultrasound, or MRI guidance. However, CT is most commonly used due to its superior ability to visualized changes in density of tissue during the freezing process, allowing for more precise localization of the margins of the ablation zone. Frozen tissue is visualized as a well-defined, expanding "ice-ball" that is lower in density than normal surrounding tissue. Although ultrasound can also depict the effects of freezing in real time, complete visualization of the ablation zone is limited due to echogenic shadowing from the proximal edge of the ice-ball as it forms during treatment. MRI demonstrates excellent contrast resolution between frozen tissue and normal liver on T2-weighted imaging; however, the use of MRI in real-time guidance is technically challenging in comparison to US or CT imaging.

Percutaneous cryoablation is performed using an argon-based cryoablation system (Endocare, Irvine, CA; Galil Medical Plymouth Meeting, PA) and 1.5–2.4 mm diameter percutaneous cryotherapy applicators. Each cryoprobe is designed to produce a predictable freeze radius (up to about 4.5 cm); however, diameter may vary slightly according to tissue type and surrounding vascular structures that may cause local warming effects from inflowing blood.[112] As with any ablation procedure, initial placement of the cryotherapy applicators is planned according to the site and size of the target tumor, the shape of its margins, and its relationship to adjacent vital structures within or immediately adjacent to the liver.

During the cryoablation procedure, target tissue typically undergoes an initial 10-minute freeze, followed by a 5–8-minute active helium thaw, which is then followed by another 10-minute freeze. The number of freeze-thaw-freeze cycles may vary according to tissue type as well as limiting factors such as location to adjacent structures that may cause undesired thermal heating at the margins of the ablation zone. A CT scan is typically performed after treatment, and low density changes within the target tissue can be measured and approximated to the size of the ablated region. Visualized margins of the treatment zone may vary slightly from pathologic results, however, and a margin of 3–5 mm is therefore subtracted from the measured diameter of the treatment region on CT in order to more accurately approximate the true volume of tissue necrosis.

Cryoablation has the ability to achieve large ablation volumes through the summative use of multiple applicators and is associated with less procedural pain than both MCT and RFA, which may be due to a thermal analgesic effect on adjacent sensory nerves. Cryoablation also has the ability to preserve the collagen network and overall cellular architecture of treated tissue, thereby eliminating extensive scarring within the target organ. It is therefore less likely to cause nontarget tissue damage in structures immediately adjacent to the treatment zone. Visualization of the "ice ball" within treated tissue at the time of ablation enables more effective monitoring of the expanding margins of the ablation zone and minimizes inadvertent damage to adjacent nontarget tissues. Unlike with heat ablation, treated tissue is not denatured, so the cells of the body are able to reabsorb dead tissue and there is no residual ablation "cavity."[112,133–136]

Results

Overall efficacy data for cryoablation treatment of HCC is derived from a series of small prospective or retrospective observational studies.[137–140] These early studies analyzed initial treatment success rates and survival outcomes for percutaneous cryoablation treatment of small unresectable HCC < 5 cm in size. Although results of these early studies are limited by relatively small patient populations and variation in follow-up assessment, initial treatment response as determined by postprocedure imaging appears to lie within the range of 92%–100%.[137–140] Overall one-, two-, and three-year survival rates are reported at 92%–94%, 79%–82%, and 64%–80%, respectively. Recurrence-free survival is reported to range between 43% and 80% at three years after treatment.[139,140] Multivariate analysis in one study showed that advanced Child-Pugh class and higher levels of expression of VEGF in HCC tumor tissue are associated with a higher risk of local recurrence in tumors < 5 cm in diameter treated by cryoablation.[140]

Percutaneous cryoablation has two theoretical advantages in treatment of HCC when compared with other thermal ablation techniques: (1) more accurate intraprocedural monitoring of the size of the ablation zone ("ice ball") with CT fluoroscopy to ascertain appropriate tumor kill and minimize collateral damage to adjacent tissues and (2) the ability to treat larger tumors through simultaneous placement of multiple cryoprobes with a summative effect on freezing target tissue.[141] Although cryoablation has a potential application in treating HCC > 5 cm within the liver, there are currently no studies that establish its effectiveness in doing so.

At the time of this publication, there have been no randomized controlled trials conducted to establish the overall efficacy of cryoablation in comparison to either surgical resection or other thermal ablation therapies for treatment of early-stage unresectable HCC. A retrospective study of 64 patients with unresectable liver tumors treated with either RFA or cryoablation was performed, and results for a subset of 34 patients with HCC showed similar initial treatment success for both modalities by early follow-up imaging. Although the rate of local recurrence for metastatic disease in this study was higher in the cryotherapy group (73%) than in the RFA group (19%), there was no statistically significant difference in local recurrence rates for patients with primary HCC.[142] There is currently no scientific evidence to recommend or refute cryotherapy as an effective treatment for patients with unresectable HCC. Further analysis of this technique by way of carefully designed randomized controlled trials is necessary to establish its efficacy relative to other more thoroughly studied thermal ablation modalities.[143]

Complications and contraindications

Complications associated with cryotherapy treatment of liver tumors are not well published in the liver, likely owing to the infrequent use of this locoregional treatment relative to other thermal ablation techniques. Theoretical risks for bleeding and collateral damage to adjacent nontarget tissues exist, but risk of occurrence is unknown. Small observational studies published to date demonstrate low rates of major complications, comparable with other thermal ablation techniques. Risks for significant bleeding and damage to nontarget organs such as the colon may be minimized through use of laparoscopic or open surgical approaches, given the ability to mobilize adjacent critical organs and control bleeding if it occurs.[141]

Laser Ablation

Basic principles

Percutaneous laser ablation, or "laser interstitial tumor therapy" (LITT), is another method of inducing focal tissue coagulation necrosis via thermally mediated cell death, and it currently has practical use as a treatment modality for small unresectable HCC. The technique involves percutaneous placement of multiple small needles under imaging guidance into the target tissue lesion, through which a series of thin flexible optic fibers are inserted. A low-power laser energy source is then coupled to these optic fibers to deliver light energy to the target tissue, which in turn causes local heat deposition around the tips of the implanted optic fibers. Very high local tissue temperatures can be achieved, resulting in protein denaturation and cell death.[144–146]

Laser ablation is capable of creating well-defined regions of coagulative necrosis locally around the fiberoptic tip of the applicator with minimal damage to surrounding tissues. Similar to RFA, thermal profiles have been shown to correlate well with extent of coagulation necrosis on histopathologic analysis.[147] Most currently available systems that operate percutaneously in deep soft tissues use a standard laser source such as neodymium-yttrium-aluminum-garnet (Nd:YAG), erbium, or holmium capable of producing laser light with wavelengths ranging from 680 to 1060 nm. Special diffusing applicators are mounted on the ends of optic fibers which are surrounded by protective glass domes. The applicators serve to spread laser light evenly within target tissue to effective distances of 12–15mm from the applicator tip. Manufacturers have developed applicators that use optic fibers of varying composition, length, and diameter to alter the size of the heated volume of tissue during the ablation procedure. Modifications to the applicator tip can also influence the distribution of scattered light within target tissue, thus altering the shape of the ablation zone. Similar to application of RF energy, various algorithms for pulsed application of laser energy and use of internally cooled applicator tips can establish more uniform distribution of heat and avoid tissue charring that would otherwise limit effectiveness of the ablation procedure.[145,146,148]

Laser ablation technique

The preprocedural workup, patient preparation, and planning of an appropriate image-guided approach to laser ablation in the liver is the same as that which has been previously described for other thermal ablation modalities. This technique may be performed under CT, ultrasound, or MRI guidance for localization and accurate placement of applicator fibers within the target tumor. MRI is the preferred imaging modality due to its superior ability to visualize changes in temperature of tissue during the ablation process through the use of specialized MR-thermometry gradient-echo images. Since the presence of cytotoxic tissue temperatures closely correlate with the extent of coagulation necrosis for laser ablation, MR-thermometric techniques allow for the most precise localization of the margins of the ablation zone.[146–148]

Use of lasers in ablation treatment is associated with a number of unique safety concerns for both the patient and the operator. Protective eyewear is recommended at all times for both patients and operating staff within the treatment room to prevent exposure of the cornea and conjunctiva to potentially injurious laser scatter. The patient's exposed skin surfaces should be protected as well, and moist or nonflammable drapes should be used during the procedure to avoid contact burns and fire during accidental exposure. Use of potentially flammable antiseptics, anesthetics, and medical gases should be avoided during the procedure.[149]

Percutaneous laser ablation is performed with the patient under conscious sedation. While sedated, patients undergo continuous monitoring with pulse oximetry and electrocardiography and blood pressure measurements are obtained at five-minute intervals during the ablation procedure. The procedure is performed under sterile technique, and the skin entry site must be appropriately cleansed and draped prior to intervention. Local anesthesia is achieved with injection of 1% lidocaine hydrochloride solution both intradermally and into the deeper tissues through which the applicator needles will pass on their trajectory to the target lesion. Preliminary scout imaging confirms the size and location of the tumor to be ablated, and the optimal number and configuration of fiberoptic applicators to be placed is determined so as to achieve adequate coverage of the target lesion during ablation. Using imaging guidance, single or multiple thin cannulated puncture needles are percutaneously positioned within the target tissue lesion along a safe, pre-planned trajectory.

Once appropriately positioned, the inner stylet of each needle is removed and exchanged for a 600-micron-diameter laser optic fiber. The needle is then partially withdrawn to expose the optic fiber tip within the target tissue. Each optic fiber is then connected to a laser unit (usually Nd:YAG). Laser energy of approximately 1060 nm in wavelength is then applied at each location utilizing anywhere from 1–15 W of power for up to 10 minutes, depending on the type and location of tissue being treated. Similar to other thermal ablation modalities, internally cooled laser applicators are available to maximize the extent of heat deposition and coagulation necrosis within the ablation zone.

During the procedure, temperatures within the ablation zone are either monitored by a separately placed thermocouple sensor (when using CT or ultrasound guidance) or via specialized MR-thermometry imaging sequences that are sensitive to alterations in temperature within target tissues. The use of MRI guidance and MR-thermometry imaging is feasible with LITT because it uses a completely metal free system and does not produce any radiofrequency interference. These T1-weighted gradient echo FLASH sequences (TR/TE/NSA/FA: 93/12.7/3/60°) are repeatedly acquired during and after (60s, 180s) laser application to monitor the extent of coagulation necrosis in real time. Following the ablation procedure, the full extent of coagulation necrosis may be performed by comparing pre- and posttherapy unenhanced and contrast-enhanced dynamic MR images.[146,148]

Results

Although several studies evaluating the efficacy of LITT for treatment of HCC have been published in the literature, interpretation of overall efficacy and complication rates is difficult, as these studies utilize different laser fiber systems with differing energy delivery levels. In addition, lack of standardization regarding follow-up criteria by which to determine treatment success also makes interpretation of overall efficacy data difficult.[150]

Primary effectiveness rates of LITT for complete tumor ablation in the treatment of small HCC ≤ 4 cm in size are reported within the range of 78%–97% when assessed by either CT or MRI in the early postprocedure period.[151–154] Local recurrence rates ranged from 1.6% to 6.0% over the course of one to five years of follow-up. Reported range for overall survival rates at one-, three-, and five-year posttreatment are 92%–99%, 61%–68%, and 15%–34%, respectively.[153] One particular study noted improved five-year cumulative survival rate in a subset of younger patients with Child-Pugh class A cirrhosis and tumors ≤ 2.0 cm as compared to those with tumors 2.0 cm–4.0 cm in size. These investigators therefore concluded that ideal candidates for LITT of HCC are younger patients with normal serum albumin levels and tumor size ≤ 2 cm.[154]

There is only a single published prospective randomized controlled study to date that compares LITT to RFA in treatment of early-stage HCC. This study examined 95 tumors < 4 cm in size in 81 cirrhotic patients that were treated percutaneously with either LITT or RFA. Treatment effectiveness was assessed by CT in the early posttreatment period and thereafter for follow-up evaluation. Initial complete tumor ablation was noted in 78% of tumors treated by LITT and 94% or tumors treated by RFA. Cumulative overall survival rates were 91.8%, 59.0%, and 28.4% at one, three, and five years, respectively. Although patients treated with RFA demonstrated a slightly better overall survival rate at up to five years, these results were not statistically significant. Of note however, univariate analysis showed that survival outcomes were significantly improved in the RFA treatment group for tumor size < 2.5 cm, and in patients with a single vs. multiple tumors or Child-Pugh class A versus class B or C cirrhosis.[155]

Complications and contraindications

Overall complication rates for LITT are significantly lower than those for surgical resection of HCC.[150,156,157] Treatment-related mortality has been reported to range from 0.1% to 0.8%, with major complication rates of 1.5%–1.8%.[156,157] In a large study of 2520 liver tumors (both HCC and metastatic disease to the liver) treated with percutaneous LITT, reported major complications were similar to those associated with RFA or MCT in the liver, and included liver failure/segmental infarction, hepatic abscess/cholangitis, bile duct injury, and hemorrhage. Minor complications were more common and included asymptomatic pleural effusion, postprocedural fever, and severe pain in the immediate posttreatment period. Tumor seeding of the percutaneous laser fiber tracts is a very rare occurrence, and there were no reported cases in this study.[157]

Combination Therapies

In clinical practice, treatment of HCC involves a multimodality approach involving surgeons, interventional radiologists, and medical oncologists to specifically tailor therapy to each patient's disease status and degree of underlying liver dysfunction. Locoregional catheter-based and ablation therapies now play an important role in management of surgically unresectable disease; however, each technique is limited in its therapeutic effect due to limitations in treating multifocal disease, large tumors, and tumors with complete anatomy. Percutaneous ablation therapies have been shown to be most effective in treating solitary hepatomas < 3 cm in size, with significant rates of incomplete ablation and local tumor recurrence in larger tumors. Despite advancements in the design of thermal applicators, treatments are still inherently limited by heterogeneous heat convection profiles in hypervascular liver tissue. Use of transcatheter arterial chemoembolization (TACE) has been traditionally reserved for patients with more diffuse disease or tumors larger than 5 cm in size. The potential therapeutic benefits that can be achieved through synergistic use of these therapies, however, cannot be understated. Several investigators have explored the role of combination therapies in improving treatment success in patients with surgically unresectable HCC, including various combinations of PEI, thermal ablation, transarterial chemotherapy, vascular occlusive strategies, and chemoembolization.

Combination of TACE and PEI

Although the therapeutic efficacy and relative safety of PEI treatment of small solitary HCC are well established in the literature, it is known that the effectiveness of this technique alone is limited by the extent of local ethanol diffusion within the target tumor. Histologic examination of treated lesions often reveals residual viable tumor cells adjacent to areas of fibrous septation, and it is felt that intralesional structural barriers to diffusion and early washout of ethanol due to the hypervascular nature of HCC limit treatment efficacy, particularly in tumors > 3 cm in size.[21–24,158,159] Combined TACE and PEI is a therapeutic option that has recently been proposed to overcome the limitations of either therapy alone in treating larger hepatomas.[159–167]

The rational for combined PEI and TACE therapy in HCC is based on the theory that pretreatment with TACE will induce partial tumor necrosis, thereby disrupting intratumoral fibrous septa that may serve as barriers to homogeneous ethanol diffusion within the lesion. Additionally, the embolic effects of TACE decrease tumor vascularity and promote better retention of ethanol within the tumor. Ethanol distribution throughout the target tissue and the duration of its cytotoxic effect are subsequently improved using this combined technique.[161–163]

Several studies have investigated the combined effects of PEI and TACE, and the data suggest that initial rates of complete tumor necrosis and overall survival rates are improved in patients with HCC up to 7 cm in size treated with combination therapy as compared to treatment with either therapy alone.[160–167] Increases in rates of initial complete tumor necrosis and one to three years survival rates have also been noted for PEI combined with bland arterial embolization over bland arterial embolization alone.[159] Favorable outcomes with combined therapy appear to be more associated with solitary and encapsulated HCC with compensated cirrhosis and no portal vein thrombosis.[161]

Combination of TACE and RFA

RFA has been noted to effectively achieve complete tumor necrosis in small HCC ≤ 3.5 cm in diameter, achieving large volumes of tumor necrosis in a short period of time relative to other thermal ablation techniques. Despite the use of cluster electrodes to generate larger volumes of tumor necrosis, the efficacy of RFA in achieving initial complete tumor necrosis decreases with tumor diameter > 3 cm in size, which is likely due to innate heterogeneity of heat distribution within hypervascular HCC lesions, related to the "heat sink" effect of intratumoral vessels. Combination therapy with TACE and RFA has been used to induce larger areas of coagulation necrosis within tumor tissue by diminishing tumor vascularity through the embolic effects of TACE, thereby improving heat deposition within the target tissue.[168–171]

RFA performed after TACE has been shown to effectively treat HCC larger than those suitable for segmental TACE or RFA treatment alone.[167] Survival outcomes are also improved with combination TACE and RFA therapy when compared with TACE alone.[168–172] A recent randomized controlled trial assessing efficacy of TACE in combination with RFA therapy versus TACE or RFA therapy alone in treatment of 291 patients with HCC > 3 cm in size (range: 3.0–7.5 cm) found that patients in the TACE-RFA group had better overall survival and prolonged time to recurrence than those treated with TACE or RFA alone. An overall survival benefit was also noted in the TACE-RFA group than in the RFA group for patients with uninodular HCC, and in the TACE-RFA group than the TACE group for patients with multinodular HCC. These authors therefore concluded that combination therapy with TACE and RFA was superior to treatment with either TACE or RFA alone in HCC > 3 cm in size.[170] Combined RFA and TACE therapy does not appear to have any therapeutic benefit over RFA alone for HCC ≤ 3 cm in size, however.[171]

Combination of TACE and MCT

MCT has been shown to be effective in treating small HCC < 4 cm in size through use of multiple antennae. The advantage of MCT over other thermal ablation techniques appears to be its greater success rates in treating moderate to poorly differentiated subtypes of HCC. Nevertheless, MCT is subject to the same limitations of heat distribution within larger lesions, and treatment efficacy diminishes with increasing tumor size.

Combination therapy with TACE and MCT has been reported to limited extent within the literature. In a small observational study of 18 patients with cirrhosis and small HCC between 2.0 and 3.0 cm in diameter, MCT therapy within one to two days of TACE treatment yielded complete initial tumor necrosis by CT imaging in 94% of patients. Overall survival rate was 100% at short-interval follow-up of 12–31 months in this patient population.[172] Although these observational data is promising, larger scale clinical trials are required to define the role of combined TACE and MCT for treatment of HCC (Figure 14-7).

Combination of TACE and cryoablation

Percutaneous cryoablation has been reliably used to treat surgically unresectable HCC < 5 cm in size; however, the long-term efficacy of this technique diminishes with tumors > 3 cm in diameter. Combination therapy involving pretreatment of larger tumors with TACE in attempt to decrease tumor volume has evolved in attempt to improve the efficacy of cryoablation in this setting.[173–175]

A large retrospective study analyzed 429 patients with surgically unresectable HCC treated by either cryoablation alone or TACE followed by cryoablation for treatment efficacy. The study results demonstrated initial effectiveness rates of 77% in the group treated by cryoablation alone and 89% in patients undergoing sequential TACE and cryoablation treatment. Although the overall one- and two-year survival rates were similar for both treatment groups, long-term four- and five-year survival was significantly better in patients treated with sequential

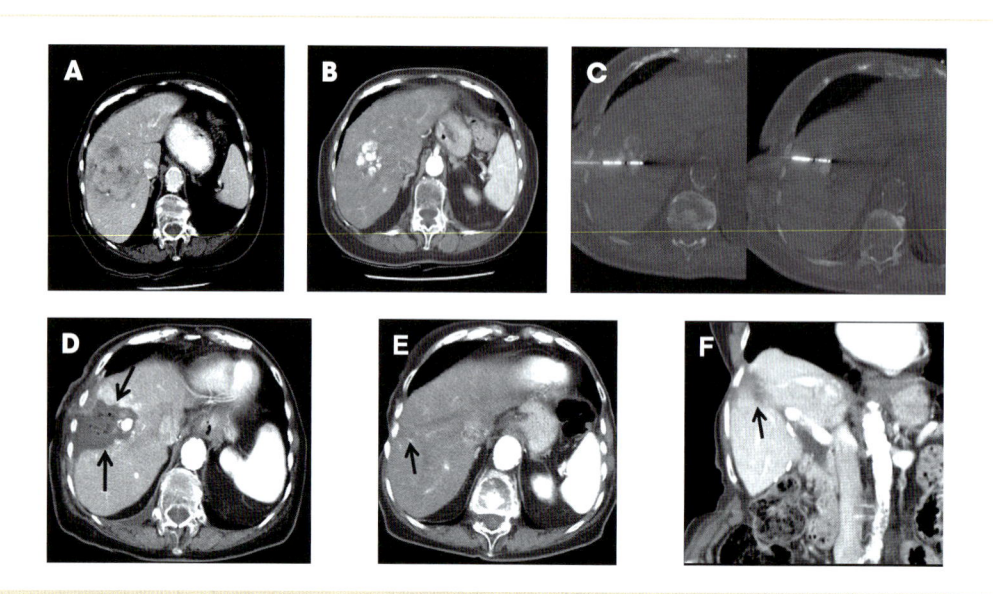

Figure 14-7: 86-year old woman with 7 cm right lobe HCC. (A) Contrast CT before treatment shows the large heterogeneously enhancing mass in the right lobe of the liver. (B) Two months after two TACE treatments contrast CT shows shrinkage of the mass with internal high-density lipiodol. (C) CT fluoroscopy images from MWA using three antennas. (D). Two week post-MWA contrast CT shows large thermocoagulation defect (arrows) with no residual enhancing tumor. (E, F) Two years posttreatment CT in the arterial phase axially (E) and coronal portal venous phase (F) shows thermal scar (arrow).

combination therapy. Sequential therapy with TACE followed by cryoablation was specifically shown to improve the long-term five-year survival in patients with tumors >5 cm in size. The authors, therefore, concluded that the sequential therapy with TACE followed by cryoablation was more effective than treatment with cryoablation alone in patients with surgically unresectable HCC > 5 cm in size.[173] Additional smaller retrospective studies report similar results, concluding that combination therapy with TACE and cryoablation improves treatment efficacy in patients with large unresectable HCC.[174,175]

Combination of TACE and laser ablation

Combination therapy with TACE and percutaneous laser ablation has also been investigated as a potential more-effective treatment for large or multifocal unresectable HCC (> 3.5 cm in size) compared to treatment with laser ablation alone. One retrospective study found that multiple TACE treatments (mean of 3.5 treatments per patient) performed on 48 patients with unresectable HCC measuring up to 8.0 cm in size was effective in reducing tumor size to <5.0 cm in 66.7% of patients prior to planned MR-guided LITT.[176] A small prospective randomized study of 89 patients with cirrhosis and HCC ≥ 4 cm demonstrated that combined therapy with TACE and LITT was more efficacious and resulted in greater overall survival rates for tumors ≥ 5 cm in size compared to therapy with LITT alone.[177]

Observational data derived from a study of 30 large HCCs ranging from 3.5 to 9.6 cm in diameter (mean diameter of 5.2 cm) that underwent palliative treatment with US-guided LITT followed by TACE showed complete tumor necrosis in 90% of the treated lesions by early CT follow-up imaging. Local recurrence rate was 7% over a three-year period, and overall survival rates at one, two, and three years were 92%, 68%, and 40%, respectively. The authors, therefore, concluded that LITT followed by TACE is an effective palliative therapy for large surgically unresectable HCC.[178]

Follow-Up Assessment

Immediate imaging assessment of ablation treatment efficacy

Adequacy of therapy during thermal ablation procedures is established by two specific endpoints: (1) intraprocedural monitoring of tissue temperature within the treated lesion and (2) defining the extent of coagulation necrosis by its imaging appearance.[52] Thermal monitoring is accomplished via a temperature sensing tip on the implanted electrode, which gives accurate temperature readings at the center of the ablation zone during the procedure. Following adequate ablation, the electrode tip is then repositioned at various locations within the target lesion to obtain temperature readings at the ablation zone periphery. Regions within the ablation zone that register temperatures lower than 50°C–55°C are then retreated to achieve cytotoxic temperature levels and confirm adequate coagulation necrosis.

Use of diagnostic imaging during RF, microwave, and laser ablation to assess real-time therapeutic efficacy is not as accurate in establishing the extent of cell death as intratumoral temperature monitoring.[52] Gray-scale and color-Doppler sonographic findings of coagulative necrosis in soft tissue are not sufficiently accurate in predicting the extent of the ablation zone. The most commonly reported sonographic finding is that of increasing tissue echogenicity that spreads in a radial fashion from the electrode tip during treatment. This hyperechogenicity typically resolves within one hour after treatment and is felt to represent artifact from the formation of microbubbles during tissue vaporization rather than actual coagulation necrosis (Figure 14-4).[17]

Although the appearance of tissue coagulation necrosis on CT, ultrasound, and MR imaging has been described, all are relatively unreliable in their ability to discriminate between necrotic and viable tissue in real time during treatment, owing to a lack of inherent tissue contrast and to limitations in spatial resolution.[17] Unenhanced CT images acquired during CT fluoroscopy may show increased density at the center of the treatment zone, surrounded by a region of relative hypoattenuation, but often do not provide enough tissue contrast to reliably discern real-time margins of the ablation zone during the procedure. Furthermore, the use of conjunctive therapy such as chemotherapy or embolization can expand the extent of the ablation zone, and these changes may not become evident on imaging studies until days after treatment.

Although real-time monitoring of tissue changes during thermal ablation is limited in its ability to accurately define the margins of coagulation necrosis, certain imaging modalities do provide useful information for intraprocedural monitoring of the ablation front. MRI shows some degree of promise as an effective and sensitive imaging modality when used in real-time monitoring of laser ablation therapy. Through the use of specialized diffusion-weighted and thermometric gradient-echo sequences, MRI is capable of demonstrating early reversible and irreversible thermal changes due to laser effects in tissue.[179] Likewise, CT demonstrates superior ability to visualize changes in density of frozen tissue during cryoablation, allowing for more precise localization of the margins of the ablation zone and minimizing the risk of inadvertent damage to adjacent structures during the ablation process. Frozen tissue is visualized as a well-defined, expanding "ice-ball" that is lower in density than normal surrounding liver tissue.[114]

Posttreatment imaging assessment of ablation efficacy

Efficacy of nonsurgical treatment for malignant tumors is usually evaluated with RECIST criteria, which involve comparative measurements of tumor size before and after treatment. By this system, decrease in tumor size is compatible with treatment success. Strict measurement criteria alone, however, do not take into account the extent of tumor necrosis that results in HCC following locoregional ablation therapy, and it is the extent of tumor necrosis, rather than overall tumor size that serves as a more appropriate measure of treatment response. For this reason, the European Association for Study of the Liver (EASL) has suggested that estimated reduction in viable tumor burden (unenhanced areas of tissue within tumor on dynamic contrast-enhanced imaging) be incorporated into the evaluation of response to locoregional therapy for HCC.[180] By this imaging-based system of follow-up evaluation, tumor response may be defined as follows:

> *Complete response* (*CR*): absence of enhanced tumor areas, reflecting complete necrosis

Partial response (PR): >50% decrease in tumor enhancement, reflecting partial tissue necrosis
Progressive disease (PD): >25% increase in the size of 1 or more measurable lesions, or the appearance of a new lesion
Stable disease (SD): any tumor response between PR and PD

Evaluation for the presence or absence of tissue enhancement within treated tumor lesions is of fundamental importance in assessing response to locoregional therapy for HCC in the liver. Assessment of treatment response is usually performed with contrast-enhanced CT or MRI either immediately following or several days after treatment to establish a new baseline imaging appearance. Treated tissue within this period is avascular and shows no enhancement, compared with normal tissue or residual tumor that shows variable enhancement. The nonenhancing treatment zone should be larger than and encompass the original tumor as seen on preprocedural imaging to ensure an adequate (>5 mm) ablative margin around the tumor itself. In small tumors (<3 cm in diameter), the absence of an ablative margin of at least 5 mm has the highest predictive value for local recurrence.[181] An adequate ablative margin is necessary not only to ensure adequate cell death at the tumor margin but also to prevent recurrence from occult satellite lesions.

On dynamic contrast-enhanced imaging, there are several pitfalls that may be encountered in assessing for residual or recurrent disease. On immediate follow-up CT or MRI, it is typical to see a thin (<1 mm), concentric, uniform enhancing rim of hyperemic tissue at the margin of the ablation zone (often referred to as "benign periablational enhancement"), which demarcates the interface between necrotic and viable tissue. This appearance is felt to be due to a physiologic inflammatory response to thermal injury within normal liver tissue, and it typically resolves within six months on follow-up imaging.[17] In addition, transient arterial-venous shunting may occur within the ablation zone, which may appear as small wedge-shaped areas of enhancement that mimic residual hypervascular tumor. These areas also typically resolve by 30 days posttreatment.[182] Although thick, nodular, or irregular marginal enhancement is useful in establishing the presence of residual tumor, it cannot be excluded in the absence of this finding, as normal marginal hyperemia can mask small foci of residual tumor at the edge of the treatment zone. The importance of follow-up imaging assessment therefore cannot be understated.

MRI may have distinct advantages over CT in detecting early local recurrence, largely owing to its superior contrast resolution. Alteration in T1- and T2-weighted signal intensity within successfully treated liver tumors has been reported on MRI immediately following RF ablation. Most lesions demonstrate heterogeneous T1 signal due to varying stages of necrosis over time (Figure 14-2). Adequately treated lesions are typically uniformly hypointense on T2-weighted images, which is likely due to tissue dehydration that accompanies coagulative necrosis. Foci of residual tumor tend to be T2-hyperintense, similar to the pretreatment appearance of HCC. Although it is not uncommon to see small T2-bright foci of liquifactive necrosis or hemorrhage within the treatment zone, these foci can be distinguished from residual tumor as they will not enhance on dynamic images.[17,183–186] Despite inherent improvements in tissue contrast with follow-up MRI, current imaging modalities remain limited by spatial resolution in their ability to detect residual or recurrent tumor. Studies have shown that radiologic–pathologic correlation in detecting margins of coagulative necrosis in soft tissue after locoregional ablation therapy lies somewhere within the realm of 2–3 mm for both CT and MRI.[184]

Conclusions and Future Directions

Locoregional ablation therapies now play an integral part in treatment of patients with surgically unresectable HCC; however, the overall success of these treatments remains limited by the size of the target tumor. Larger lesions require greater regions of tissue heating to achieve an adequate kill zone that encompasses both the tumor and an appropriate ablative margin to reduce the likelihood of local recurrence. Current technology, however, is limited by the extent of tissue heating that can be achieved with a single applicator. Although this problem can be partially overcome by the strategic placement of multiple applicators to expand the effective zone of tissue heating, these larger treatment zones often cannot be accurately shaped to specifically fit the anatomic distribution of the target tumor, resulting in nontarget tissue damage. Undertreatment in attempt to avoid collateral damage often leads to local recurrence due to inadequate treatment of tissue at the tumor margins. Although development of more advanced applicator devices capable of achieving treatment zones of various shapes may help to solve this problem, synergistic use of catheter-based therapies also shows promise in improving treatment efficacy for large or irregularly shaped tumors when compared to that which can be achieved by thermal or chemical ablation alone. Use of synergistic therapies for treatment of HCC in this manner will require a coordinated effort on the part of interventional radiologists, medical oncologists, oncologic surgeons, and radiation oncologists to decide the most appropriate course of treatment for each patient based on the overall size and location of the underlying tumor.

References

1. Parkin DM, Bray F, Ferlay J, Pisani P. Global cancer statistics, 2002. *CA Cancer J Clin*. 2005;55:74–108.
2. Skolnick AA. Armed with epidemiologic research, China launches programs to prevent liver cancer (news). *JAMA*. 1996;276:1458.
3. Tanaka H, Imai Y, Hiramatsu N, et al. Declining incidence of hepatocellular carcinoma in Osaka, Japan, from 1990 to 2003. *Ann Intern Med*. 2008;148:820.
4. El-Serag H. Hepatocellular carcinoma: recent trends in the United States. *Gastroenterology*. 2004;127:S27.
5. Lang K, Danchenko N, Gondek K, et al. The burden of illness associated with hepatocellular carcinoma in the United States. *J Hepatol*. 2009;50:89.
6. Llovet JM, Bru C, Bruix J, et al. Prognosis of hepatocellular carcinoma: the BCLC staging classification. *Semin Liver Dis*. 1999;19:329.
7. Goldberg SN, Ahmed M. Minimally invasive image-guided therapies for hepatocellular carcinoma. *J Clin Gastroenterol*. 2002;35:S115–S129.
8. Lau WY, Lai EC. The current role of radiofrequency ablation in the management of hepatocellular carcinoma: a systematic review. *Ann Surg*. 2009;249(1):20–25.
9. Zheng YB, Zheng Y. Research advance-ment in local ablation therapy for liver cancer. *Chin J Cancer*. 2009;28(11):1219–1224.
10. Vilgrain V. Advancement in HCC imaging: diagnosis, staging and treatment efficacy assessments: hepatocellular carcinoma: imaging in assessing treatment efficacy [Epub ahead of print November 19 2009]. *J Hepatobiliary Pancreat Surg*. 2010 Jul;17(4):374–9.
11. Gervais DA, Goldberg SN, Brown DB, et al. Society of Interventional Radiology position statement on percutaneous radiofrequency ablation for the treatment of liver tumors. *J Vasc Interv Radiol*. 2009;20:S342–S347.
12. Pawlik TM, Tseng JF, Vauthey JN. Controversies in staging of hepatocellular carcinoma. *Cancer Rev: Asia-Pacific*. 2003;1:179–189.
13. Vauthey JN, Lauwers GY, Esnaola NF, et al. Simplified staging for hepatocellular carcinoma. *J Clin Oncol*. 2002;20:1527–1536.
14. Henderson J, Sherman M, Tavill A, et al. AHPBA/AJCC consensus conference on staging of hepatocellular carcinoma: consensus statement. *HPB (Oxford)*. 2003;5:243.
15. Cillo U, Vitale A, Grigoletto F, et al. Prospective validation of the Barcelona Clinic Liver Cancer staging system. *J Hepatol*. 2006;44(4):723–731.
16. Bruix J, Sherman M. Management of hepatocellular carcinoma. *Hepatology*. 2005;42:1208–1236.
17. Goldberg SN, Gazelle GS, Mueller PR. Thermal ablation therapy for focal malignancy: a unified approach to underlying principles, techniques, and diagnostic imaging guidance. *AJR Am J Roentgenol*. 2000;174:323–331.
18. Goldberg SN. Radiofrequency tumor ablation: principles and techniques. *Eur J Ultrasound*. 2001;13(2):129–147.
19. Uflacker R, Paolini RM, Nobrega M. Ablation of tumor and inflammatory tissue with absolute ethanol. *Acta Radiol*. 1986;27:131–138.
20. Lencioni R, Pinto F, Armillotta N, et al. Long-term results of percutaneous ethanol injection therapy for hepatocellular carcinoma in cirrhosis: a European experience. *Eur Radiol*. 1997;7:514–519.
21. Hasegawa S, Yamasaki N, Hiwaki T, et al. Factors that predict intrahepatic recurrence of hepatocellular carcinoma in 81 patients initially treated by percutaneous ethanol injection. *Cancer*. 1999;86:1682.
22. Livraghi T, Benedini V, Lazzaroni S, et al. Long term results of single session percutaneous ethanol injection in patients with large hepatocellular carcinoma. *Cancer*. 1998;83:48.
23. Arii S, Yamaoka Y, Futagawa S, et al. Results of surgical and nonsurgical treatment for small-sized hepatocellular carcinomas: a retrospective and nationwide survey in Japan. The Liver Cancer Study Group of Japan. *Hepatology*. 2000;32:1224.

24. Pompili M, Rapaccini GL, Covino M, et al. Prognostic factors for survival in patients with compensated cirrhosis and small hepatocellular carcinoma after percutaneous ethanol injection therapy. *Cancer*. 2001;92:126.

25. Kuang M, Lu M, Xie X, et al. Ethanol ablation of hepatocellular carcinoma up to 5.0 cm by using a multi-pronged injection needle with high-dose strategy. *Radiology*. 2009;253(2):552–561.

26. Livraghi T, Goldberg SN, Lazzaroni S, et al. Small hepatocellular carcinoma: treatment with radiofrequency ablation versus ethanol injection. *Radiology*. 1999;210:655–661.

27. Lencioni R, Bartolozzi C, Caramella D, et al. Treatment of small hepatocellular carcinoma with percutaneous ethanol injection: analysis of prognositic factors in 105 Western patients. *Cancer*. 1995;76:1737–1746.

28. Livraghi T, Giorgio A, Marin G, et al. Hepatocellular carcinoma and cirrhosis in 746 patients: long-term results of percutaneous ethanol injection. *Radiology*. 1995;197:101–108.

29. Ryu M, Shimamura Y, Kinoshita T, et al. Therapeutic results of resection, transcatheter arterial embolization and percutaneous transhepatic ethanol injection in 3225 patients with hepatocellular carcinoma: a retrospective multicenter study. *Jpn J Clin Oncol*. 1997;27:251–257.

30. Teratani T, Ishikawa T, Shiratori Y, et al. Hepatocellular carcinoma in elderly patients: beneficial therapeutic efficacy using percutaneous ethanol injection therapy. *Cancer*. 2002;95:816–823.

31. Ebara M, Okabe S, Kita K, et al. Percutaneous ethanol injection for small hepatocellular carcinoma: therapeutic efficacy based on 20-year observation. *J Hepatol*. 2005;43:458–464.

32. Sung YM, Choi D, Lim HK, et al. Long-term results of percutaneous ethanol injection for the treatment of hepatocellular carcinoma in Korea. *Korean J Radiol*. 2006;7(3):187–192.

33. Taniguchi M, Kim SR, Imoto S, et al. Long-term outcome of percutaneous ethanol injection therapy for minimum-sized hepatocellular carcinoma. *World J Gastroenterol*. 2008;14(13):1997–2002.

34. Yoshio Y, Shigeki A, Kyoichi I, et al. Survey and follow-up study of primary liver cancer in Japan: report 14. *Liver Cancer Study Group Jpn*. 2000;20:9–27.

35. Shiina S, Teratani T, Obi S, et al. Nonsurgical treatment of hepatocellular carcinoma: from percutaneous ethanol injection therapy and percutaneous microwave coagulation therapy to radiofrequency ablation. *Oncology*. 2002;62:64–68.

36. Shiina S, Tagawa K, Unuma T, et al. Percutaneous ethanol injection therapy of hepatocellular carcinoma: analysis of 77 patients. *AJR Am J Roentgenol*. 1990;155:1221–1226.

37. Shiina S, Tagawa K, Niwa Y, et al. Percutaneous ethanol injection therapy for hepatocellular carcinoma: results in 146 patients. *AJR Am J Roentgenol*. 1993;160:1023–1028.

38. Huang GT, Lee PH, Tsang YM, et al. Percutaneous ethanol injection versus surgical resection for the treatment of small hepatocellular carcinoma: a prospective study. *Ann Surg*. 2005;242(1):36–42.

39. Jansen MC, van Hillegersberg R, Chamuleau RA, et al. Outcome of regional and local ablative therapies for hepatocellular carcinoma: a collective review. *Eur J Surg Oncol*. 2005;31(4):331–347.

40. Dettmer A, Kirchoff TD, Gebel M, et al. Combination of repeated single-session percutaneous ethanol injection and transarterial chemoembolisation compared to repeated singe-session percutaneous ethanol injection in patients with non-resectable hepatocellular carcinoma. *World J Gastroenterol*. 2006;12(23):3707–3715.

41. Seki T, Wakabayashi M, Nakagawa T, et al. Hepatic infarction following percutaneous ethanol injection therapy for hepatocellular carcinoma. *Eur J Gastroenterol Hepatol*. 1998;11:915–918.

42. Casella G, Cacopardo E, Rovere G, et al. Cutaneous seeding after ultrasound-guided percutaneous ethanol injection for treatment of hepatocellular carcinoma. *J Clin Ultrasound*. 2001;29:354–358.

43. Ishii H, Okada S, Okusaka T, et al. Needle tract implantation of hepatocellular carcinoma after percutaneous ethanol injection. *Cancer*. 1998;82:1638–1642.

44. Fujimoto T. The experimental and clinical studies of percutaneous ethanol injection therapy (PEIT) under ultrasonography for small hepatocellular carcinoma. *Acta Hepato Jpn*. 1988;29:52.

45. Lin SM, Kuo SH, Lin DY, et al. Cytologic changes in hepatocellular carcinoma after percutaneous acetic acid injection. Correlation with helical computed tomography findings. *Acta Cytol*. 2000;44:1–6.

46. Ohnishi K, Ohyama N, Ito S, Fujiwara K. Small hepatocellular carcinoma: treatment with US-guided intratumoral injection of acetic acid. *Radiology*. 1994;193:747–752.

47. Ohnishi K, Yoshioka H, Ito S, Fujiwara K. Treatment of nodular hepatocellular carcinoma larger than 3 cm with ultrasound-guided percutaneous acetic acid injection. *Hepatology*. 1996;24:1379–1385.

48. Ohnishi K, Nomura F, Ito S, Fujiwara K. Prognosis of small hepatocellular carcinoma (less than 3 cm) after percutaneous acetic acid injection: study of 91 cases. *Hepatology*. 1996;23:994–1002.
49. Ohnishi K, Yoshioka H, Ito S, Fujiwara K. Prospective randomized controlled trial comparing percutaneous acetic acid injection and percutaneous ethanol injection for small hepatocellular carcinoma. *Hepatology*. 1998;27:67–72.
50. Schoppmeyer K, Weis S, Mossner J, Fleig WE. Percutaneous ethanol injection or percutaneous acetic acid injection for early hepatocellular carcinoma. *Cochrane Database Syst Rev*. 2009;3:CD006745.
51. Gazelle GS, Goldberg SN, Solbiati L, Livraghi T. Tumor ablation with radio-frequency energy. *Radiology*. 2000;217:633–646.
52. Goldberg SN, Dupuy DE. Image-guided radiofrequency tumor ablation: challenges and opportunities—part I. *J Vasc Interv Radiol*. September 2001;12(9):1021–1032.
53. Dupuy DE, Goldberg SN. Image-guided radiofrequency tumor ablation: challenges and opportunities-part II. *J Vasc Interv Radiol*. 2001;12(10):1021, 1135–1148.
54. Cho YK, Kim JK, Kim MY, et al. Systematic review of randomized trials for hepatocellular carcinoma treated with percutaneous ablation therapies. *Hepatology*. 2009;49(2).453–459.
55. Chen MS, Li JQ, Zheng Y, et al. A prospective randomized trial comparing percutaneous local ablative therapy and partial hepatectomy for small hepatocellular carcinoma. *Ann Surg*. 2006;243(3):321–328.
56. Mazzaferro V, Regalia E, Doci R, et al. Liver transplantation for the treatment of small hepatocellular carcinomas in patients with cirrhosis. *N Engl J Med*. 1996;334:693–699.
57. Goldberg SN, Gazelle GS, Dawson SL, et al. Tissue ablation with radiofrequency: effect of probe size, gauge, duration, and temperature on lesion volume. *Acad Radiol*. 1995;2:399–404.
58. McGahan JP, Wei-Zhong G, Brock JM, et al. Hepatic ablation using bipolar radiofrequency electrocautery. *Acad Radiol*. 1996;3:418–422.
59. Lorentzen T. A cooled needle electrode for radiofrequency tissue ablation: thermodynamic aspects of improved performance compared with conventional needle design. *Acad Radiol*. 1996;3:556–563.
60. Solbiati L, Goldberg SN, Ierace T, et al. Hepatic metastases: percutaneous radiofrequency ablation with cooled-tip electrodes. *Radiology*. 1997;205:367–374.
61. Goldberg SN, Stein M, Gazelle GS, et al. Percutaneous radiofrequency tissue ablation: optimization of pulsed-RF technique to increase coagulation necrosis. *J Vasc Interv Radiol*. 1999;10:907–916.
62. Goldberg SN, Ahmed M, Gazelle GS, et al. Radiofrequency thermal ablation with adjuvant saline injection: effect of electrical conductivity on tissue heating and coagulation. *Radiology*. 2001;219:157–165.
63. Goldberg SN, Hahn PF, Tanabe KK, et al. Percutaneous radiofrequency tissue ablation: does perfusion-mediated tissue cooling limit coagulation necrosis? *J Vasc Interv Radiol*. 1998;9:101–111.
64. Goldberg SN, Hahn PF, Halpern E, et al. Radiofrequency tissue ablation: effect of pharmacologic modulation of blood flow on coagulation diameter. *Radiology*. 1998;209:761–769.
65. Ito S, Morita K, Ueda S, et al. Long-term results of hepatic resection combined with intra-operative local ablation therapy for patients with multinodular hepatocellular carcinomas. *Ann Surg Oncol*. 2009;16:3299–3307.
66. Livraghi T, Goldberg SN, Lazzaroni S, et al. Hepatocellular carcinoma: radiofrequency ablation of medium and large lesions. *Radiology*. 2000;214:761–768.
67. Lencioni R, Cioni D, Crocetti L, et al. Early-stage hepatocellular carcinoma in patients with cirrhosis: long-term results of percutaneous image-guided radiofrequency ablation. *Radiology*. 2005;234:961–967.
68. Buscarini L, Buscarini E, Di Stasi M, et al. Percutaneous radiofrequency ablation of small hepatocellular carcinoma: long-term results. *Eur Radiol*. 2001;11:914–921.
69. Tateishi R, Shiina S, Teratani T, et al. Percutaneous radiofrequency ablation for hepatocellular carcinoma: an analysis of 1000 cases. *Cancer*. 2005;103:1201–1209.
70. Lencioni R, Allgaier HP, Cioni D, et al. Small hepatocellular carcinoma in cirrhosis: randomized comparison of radiofrequency thermal ablation versus percutaneous ethanol injection. *Radiology*. 2003;228:235–240.
71. Lin SM, Lin CJ, Lin CC, et al. Radiofrequency ablation improves prognosis compared with ethanol injection for hepatocellular carcinoma ≤ 4 cm. *Gastroenterology*. 2004; 127:1714–1723.
72. Shiina S, Teratani T, Obi S, et al. A randomized controlled trial of radio-frequency ablation versus

ethanol injection for small hepatocellular carcinoma. *Gastroenterology*. 2005;129:122–130.

73. Lin SM, Lin CJ, Lin CC, et al. Randomized controlled trial comparing percutaneous radiofrequency thermal ablation, percutaneous ethanol injection, and percutaneous acetic acid injection to treat hepatocellular carcinoma of 3 cm or less. *Gut*. 2005;54:1151–1156.

74. Brunello F, Veltri A, Carucci P, et al. Radiofrequency ablation versus ethanol injection for early hepatocellular carcinoma: a randomized controlled trial. *Scand J Gastroenterol*. 2008;43:727–735.

75. Lu DS, Yu NC, Raman SS, et al. Radiofrequency ablation of hepatocellular carcinoma: treatment success as defined by histologic examination of the explanted liver. *Radiology*. 2005;234:954–960.

76. Lu DS, Raman SS, Limanond P, et al. Influence of large peritumoral vessels on outcome of radiofrequency ablation of liver tumors. *J Vasc Interv Radiol*. 2003;14:1267–1274.

77. Raut CP, Izzo F, Marra P, et al. Significant long-term survival after radiofrequency ablation of unresectable hepatocellular carcinoma in patients with cirrhosis. *Ann Surg Oncol*. 2005;12:616–628.

78. Machi J, Bueno RS, Wong LL. Long-term follow-up outcome of patients undergoing radiofrequency ablation for unresectable hepatocellular carcinoma. *World J Surg*. 2005;29:1364–1373.

79. Cabassa P, Donato F, Simeone F, et al. Radiofrequency ablation of hepatocellular carcinoma: long-term experience with expandable needle electrodes. *Am J Roentgenol*. 2006;186:S316–S321.

80. Choi D, Lim HK, Rhim H, et al. Percutaneous radiofrequency ablation for early-stage hepatocellular carcinoma as a first-line treatment: long-term results and prognostic factors in a large single-institution series. *Eur Radiol*. 2007;17:684–692.

81. Lu MD, Kuang M, Liang LJ, et al. Surgical resection versus percutaneous thermal ablation for early-stage hepatocellular carcinoma: a randomized clinical trial. *Chin Med J*. 2006;86:801–805.

82. Montorsi M, Santambrogio R, Bianchi P, et al. Survival and recurrences after hepatic resection or radiofrequency for hepatocellular carcinoma in cirrhotic patients: a multivariate analysis. *J Gastrointest Surg*. 2005;9:62–67.

83. Hong SN, Lee SY, Choi MS, et al. Comparing the outcomes of radiofrequency ablation and surgery in patients with a single small hepatocellular carcinoma and well-preserved liver function. *J Clin Gastroenterol*. 2005; 39:247–252.

84. Lupo L, Panzera P, Giannelli G, et al. Single hepatocellular carcinoma ranging from 3 to 5 cm: radiofrequency ablation or resection? *HPB (Oxford)*. 2007;9:429–434.

85. Guglielmi A, Ruzzenente A, Valdegamberi A, et al. Radiofrequency ablation versus surgical resection for the treatment of hepatocellular carcinoma in cirrhosis. *J Gastrointest Surg*. 2008;12:192–198.

86. Bouza C, Lopez-Cuadrado T, Alcazar R, et al. Meta-analysis of percutaneous radiofrequency ablation versus ethanol injection in hepatocellular carcinoma. *BMC Gastroenterol*. 2009;9:31.

87. Orlando A, Leandro G, Olivo M, et al. Radiofrequency thermal ablation vs. percutaneous ethanol injection for small hepatocellular carcinoma in cirrhosis: meta-analysis of randomized controlled trials. *Am J Gastroenterol*. 2009;104(2):514–524.

88. Hsieh CB, Chang HM, Chen TW, et al. Comparison of transcatheter arterial chemoembolization, laparoscopic radiofrequency ablation, and conservative treatment for decompensated cirrhotic patients with hepatocellular carcinoma. *World J Gastroenterol*. 2004;10(4):505–508.

89. Chok KS, Ng KK, Poon RT, et al. Comparable survival in patients with unresectable hepatocellular carcinoma treated by radiofrequency ablation or transarterial chemoembolization. *Arch Surg*. 2006;141:1231–1236.

90. Akahane M, Koga H, Kato N, et al. Complications of percutaneous radiofrequency ablation for hepatocellular carcinoma: imaging spectrum and management. *Radiographics*. 2005;25(suppl 1):S57–S68.

91. Livraghi T, Solbiati L, Meloni MF, et al. Treatment of focal liver tumors with percutaneous radiofrequency ablation: complications encountered in a multicenter study. *Radiology*. 2003;226:441–451.

92. De Baere T, Risse O, Kuoch V, et al. Adverse events during radiofrequency treatment of 582 hepatictumors. *Am J Roentgenol*. 2003;181:695–700.

93. Laspas F, Sotiropoulou E, Mylona S, et al. Computed tomography-guided radiofrequency ablation of hepatocellular carcinoma: treatment efficacy and complications. *J Gastrointestin Liver Dis*. 2009;18(3):323–328.

94. Perkins JD. Seeding risk following percutaneous approach to hepatocellular carcinoma. *Liver Transpl*. 2007;13:1603.

95. Chen TM, Huang PT, Lin LF, Tung JN. Major complications of ultrasound-guided percutaneous radiofrequency ablations for liver malignancies: single center

96. Rhim H. Complications of radio-frequency ablation in hepatocellular carcinoma. *Abdom Imaging.* 2005;30:409–418.
97. Mulier S, Mulier P, Ni Y, et al. Complications of radiofrequency coagulation of liver tumours. *Br J Surg.* 2002;89:1206–1222.
98. Kong W, Zhang W, Qiu Y, et al. Major complications after radiofrequency ablation for liver tumors: analysis of 255 patients. *World J Gastroenterol.* 2009;15(21):2651–2656.
99. Dodd GD, Napier D, Schoolfield JD, Hubbard L. Percutaneous radiofrequency ablation of hepatic tumors: postablation syndrome. *AJR Am J Roentgenol.* 2005;185:51–57.
100. Llovet JM, Vilana R, Bru C, et al. Increased risk of tumor seeding after percutaneous radiofrequency ablation for single hepatocellular carcinoma. *Hepatology.* 2001;33:1124–1129.
101. Jaskolka JD, Asch MR, Kachura JR, et al. Needle tract seeding after radiofrequency ablation of hepatic tumors. *J Vasc Interv Radiol.* 2005;16:485–491.
102. Livraghi T, Lazzaroni S, Meloni F, Solbiati L. Risk of tumor seeding after percutaneous radiofrequency ablation for hepatocellular carcinoma. *Br J Surg.* 2005;92:856–858.
103. Crocetti L, de Baere T, Lencioni R. Quality improvement guidelines for radiofrequency ablation of liver tumours [Epub ahead of print]. *Cardiovasc Intervent Radiol.* 2009 February;33(1):11–17. doi: 10.1007/s00270-009-9736-y.
104. Kim SH, Lim HK, Choi D, et al. Changes in bile ducts after radiofrequency ablation of hepatocellular carcinoma: frequency and clinical significance. *AJR Am J Roentgenol.* 2004;183:1611–1617.
105. Cha J, Rhim H, Lee JY, et al. Percutaneous radiofrequency ablation of hepatocellular carcinoma: assessment of safety in patients with ascites. *AJR Am J Roentgenol.* 2009;193:W424–W429.
106. Fiek M, Dorwarth U, Durchlaub I, et al. Application of radiofrequency energy in surgical and interventional procedures: are there interactions with ICDs? *Pacing Clin Electrophysiol.* 2004;27:293–298.
107. Tong NY, Ru HJ, Ling HY, et al. Extracardiac radiofrequency ablation interferes with pacemaker function but does not damage the device. *Anesthesiology.* 2004;100:1041.
108. Skonieczki BD, Wells C, Wasser EJ, Dupuy DE. Radiofrequency and microwave tumor ablation in patients with implanted cardiac devices: is it safe? *Eur J Radiol.* 2011;79:343–346.
109. King RWP, Shen LC, Wu TT. Embedded insulated antenna for communication and heating. *Electromagnetics.* 1981;4:51–72.
110. Foster KR, Schepps JL. Dielectric properties of tumor and noramal tissues at radio through microwave frequencies. *J Microw Power.* 1981;16:107–119.
111. Skinner MG, Iizuka MN, Kolios MC, Sherar MD. A theoretical comparison of energy sources—microwave, ultrasound and laser—for interstitial thermal therapy. *Phys Med Biol.* 1998;43:3535–3547.
112. Simon CJ, Dupuy DE, Mayo-Smith WW. Microwave ablation: principles and applications. *Radiographics.* 2005;25(suppl 1):S69–S83.
113. Yu NC, Lu DS, Raman SS, et al. Hepatocellular carcinoma: microwave ablation with multiple straight and loop antenna clusters—pilot comparison with pathologic findings. *Radiology.* 2006;239(1):269–275.
114. Organ LW. Electrophysiologic principles of radiofrequency lesion making. *Appl Neurophysiol.* 1976;39(2):69–76.
115. Liang P, Dong B, Yu X, et al. Prognostic factors for survival in patients with hepatocellular carcinoma after percutaneous microwave ablation. *Radiology.* 2005;235(1):299–307.
116. Liang P, Wang Y. Microwave ablation of hepatocellular carcinoma. *Oncology.* 2007;72(suppl 1):124–131.
117. Zhang X, Chen B, Hu S, et al. Microwave ablation with cooled-tip electrode for liver cancer: an analysis of 160 cases. *Hepatogastroenterolgy.* 2008;55(88):2184–2187.
118. Martin R, Scoggins C, McMasters K. Safety and efficacy of microwave ablation of hepatic tumors: a prospective review of a 5-year experience *Ann Surg Oncol.* 2010 Jan;17 (1):171-8. doi: 10.1245/s10434-009-0686-z.
119. Abe T, Shinzawa H, Wakabayashi H, et al. Value of laparoscopic microwave coagulation therapy for hepatocellular carcinoma in relation to tumor size and location. *Endoscopy.* 2000;32:598–603.
120. Aramaki M, Kawano K, Ohno T, et al. Microwave coagulation therapy for unresectable hepatocellular carcinoma. *Hepatogastroenterology.* 2004;51:1784–1787.
121. Dong BW, Liang P, Yu XL, et al. Sonographically-guided microwave coagulation treatment of liver cancer: an experimental and clinical study. *AJR Am J Roentgenol.* 1998;171:449–454.

122. Lu MD, Chen JW, Xie XY, et al. Hepatocellular carcinoma: US-guided percutaneous microwave coagulation therapy. *Radiology*. 2001;221:167–172.
123. Seki T, Wakabayashi M, Nakagawa T, et al. Ultrasonically guided percutaneous microwave coagulation therapy for small hepatocellular carcinoma. *Cancer*. 1994;74:817–825.
124. Dong BW, Liang P, Yu XL, et al. Long-term results of percutaneous sonographically-guided microwave ablation therapy of early-stage hepatocellular carcinoma. *Chin Med J*. 2008;86(12):797–800.
125. Yamashiki N, Kato T, Bejarano PA, et al. Histopathological changes after microwave coagulation therapy for patients with hepatocellular carcinoma: review of 15 explanted livers. *Am J Gastroenterol*. 2003;98(9):2052–2059.
126. Seki T, Wakabayashi M, Nakagawa T, et al. Percutaneous microwave coagulation therapy for patients with small hepatocellular carcinoma: comparison with percutaneous ethanol injection therapy. *Cancer*. 1999;85:1694–1702.
127. Shibata T, Limuro Y, Yamamoto Y, et al. Small hepatocellular carcinoma: comparison of radiofrequency ablation and percutaneous microwave coagulation therapy. *Radiology*. 2002;223(2):331–337.
128. Ohmoto K, Yoshioka N, Tomiyama Y, et al. Comparison of therapeutic effects between radiofrequency ablation and percutaneous microwave coagulation therapy for small hepatocellular carcinomas. *J Gastroenterol Hepatol*. 2009;24(2):223–227.
129. Ohmoto K, Yoshioka N, Tomiyama Y, et al. Thermal ablation therapy for hepatocellular carcinoma: comparison between radiofrequency ablation and percutaneous microwave coagulation therapy. *Hepatogastroenterology*. 2006;53(71):651–654.
130. Schroeder DV. *An Introduction to Thermal Physics*. Reading, MA: Addison Wesley Longman; 2000:142.
131. Hoffmann NE, Bischof JC. The cryobiology of cryosurgical injury. *Urology*. 2002:60:40–49.
132. Mazur P. Freezing of living cells: mechanisms and implications. *Am J Physiol*. 1984;143:C125–C142.
133. Maiwand MO. The role of cryosurgery in palliation of tracheo-bronchial carcinoma. *Eur J Cardiothorac Surg*. 1999;15(6):764–768.
134. Maiwand MO, Homasson JP. Cryotherapy for tracheobronchial disorders. *Clin Chest Med*. 1995;16(3):427–443.
135. Mala T, Edwin B, Samset E, et al. Magnetic-resonance-guided percutaneous cryoablation of hepatic tumors. *Eur J Surg*. 2001;167(8):610–617.
136. Silverman SG, Tuncali K, Adams DF, et al. MR imaging-guided percutaneous cryotherapy of liver tumors: initial experience. *Radiology*. 2000;217(3):657–664.
137. Zhou L, Yang YP, Feng YY, et al. Efficacy of argon-helium cryosurgical ablation on primary hepatocellular carcinoma: a pilot clinical study. *Chin J Cancer*. 2009;1:45–48.
138. Shimizu T, Sakuhara Y, Abo D, et al. Outcome of MR-guided percutaneous cryoablation for hepatocellular carcinoma. *J Hepatobiliary Pancreat Surg*. 2009;16(6):816–823.
139. Kerkar S, Carlin AM, Sohn RL, et al. Long-term follow up and prognostic factors for cryotherapy of malignant liver tumors. *Surgery*. 2004;136(4):770–779.
140. Wang C, Lu Y, Chen Y, et al. Prognostic factors and recurrence of hepatitis B-related hepatocellular carcinoma after argon-helium cryoablation: a prospective study. *Clin Exp Metastasis*. 2009;26(7):839–848.
141. Orlacchio A, Bazzocchi G, Pastorelli D, et al. Percutaneous cryoablation of small hepatocellular carcinoma with US guidance and CT monitoring: initial experience. *Cardiovasc Intervent Radiol*. 2008;31:587–594.
142. Adam R, Hagopian EJ, Linhares M, et al. A comparison of percutaneous cryosurgery and percutaneous radiofrequency for unresectable hepatic malignancies. *Arch Surg*. 2002;137(12):1332–1339.
143. Awad T, Thorlund K, Gluud C. Cryotherapy for hepatocellular carcinoma. *Cochrane Database Syst Rev*. 2009;4:CD007611.
144. Castren-Persons M, Lipasti J, Puolakkainen P, Schroder T. Laser-induced hyperthermia: comparison of two different methods. *Lasers Surg Med*. 1992;12:665–668.
145. Schwarzmaier HJ, Goldbach T, Kaufmann R, et al. New applicators for laser induced interstitial thermotherapy. *Minimal Invasive Med*. 1994;5:32–35.
146. Tranberg KG, Moller PH, Lindberg L, et al. Energy delivery and monitoring in interstitial laser thermotherapy. *Minimal Invasive Med*. 1994;5:36–41.
147. Dachman AH, McGehee JA, Beam TE, et al. US-guided percutaneous laser ablation of liver tissue in a chronic pig model. *Radiology*. 1990;176:129–133.
148. Vogl TJ, Mack MG, Muller P, et al. Recurrent nasopharyngeal tumors: preliminary clinical results with interventional MR imaging-controlled laser-induced thermotherapy. *Radiology*. 1995;196:725–733.
149. Dougherty TJ. An update on photodynamic therapy applications. *J Clin Laser Med Surg*. 2002;20(1):3–7.

150. Gough-Palmer AL, Gedroyc WMW. Laser ablation of hepatocellular carcinoma—a review. *World J Gastroenterol.* 2008;14(47):7170–7174.
151. Pacella CM, Bizzarri G, Francica G, et al. Analysis of factors predicting survival in patients with hepatocellular carcinoma treated with percutaneous laser ablation. *J Hepatol.* 2006;44:902–909.
152. Eichler K, Mack MG, Straub R, et al. Oligonodular hepatocellular carcinoma: MR-controlled laser-induced thermotherapy. *Radiologe.* 2001;41: 915–922.
153. Pacella CM, Bizzarri G, Magnolfi F, et al. Laser thermal ablation in the treatment of small hepatocellular carcinoma: results in 74 patients. *Radiology.* 2001;221(3):712–720.
154. Pacella CM, Francica G, Di Lascio FM, et al. Long-term outcome of cirrhotic patients with early hepatocellular carcinoma treated with ultrasound-guided percutaneous laser ablation: a retrospective analysis. *J Clin Oncol.* 2009;27(16):2615–2621.
155. Ferrari FS, Megliola A, Scorzelli A, et al. Treatment of small HCC through radiofrequency ablation and laser ablation: comparison of techniques and long-term results. *Radiol Med.* 2007;112:377–393.
156. Arienti V, Pretolani S, Pacella CM, et al. Complications of laser ablation for hepatocellular carcinoma: a multicenter study. *Radiology.* 2008;246:947–955.
157. Vogl TJ, Straub R, Eichler K, et al. Malignant liver tumors treated with MR imaging-guided laser-induced thermotherapy: experience with complications in 899 patients (2,520 lesions). *Radiology.* 2002;225:367–377.
158. Qian J, Feng GS, Vogl T. Combined interventional therapies for hepatocellular carcinoma. *World J Gastroenterol.* 2003;9(9):1885–1891.
159. Tanaka K, Nakamura S, Numata K, et al. The long-term efficacy of combined transcatheter arterial embolization and percutaneous ethanol injection in the treatment of patients with large hepatocellular carcinoma and cirrhosis. *Cancer.* 1998;8(2):78–85.
160. Koda M, Murawaki Y, Mitsuda A, et al. Combination therapy with transcatheter arterial chemoembolization and percutaneous ethanol injection compared with percutaneous ethanol injection alone for patients with small hepatocellular carcinoma: a randomized control study. *Cancer.* 2001;92:1516–1524.
161. Lencioni R, Paolicchi A, Moretti M, et al. Combined transcatheter arterial chemoembolization and percutaneous ethanol injection for the treatment of large hepatocellular carcinoma: local therapeutic effect and long-term survival rate. *Eur Radiol.* 1998;8: 439–444.
162. Kirchhoff T, Chavan A, Galanski M. Transarterial chemoembolization and percutaneous ethanol injection therapy in patients with hepatocellular carcinoma. *Eur J Gastroenterol Hepatol.* 1998;10: 907–909.
163. Kamada K, Kitamoto M, Aikata H, et al. Combination of transcatheter arterial chemoembolization using cisplatin-lipiodol suspension and percutaneous ethanol injection for treatment of advanced small hepatocellular carcinoma. *Am J Surg.* 2002;184: 284–290.
164. Allgaier HP, Deibert P, Olschewski M, et al. Survival benefit of patients with inoperable hepatocellular carcinoma treated by a combination of transarterial chemoembolization and percutaneous ethanol injection: a single-center analysis including 132 patients. *Int J Cancer.* 1998;79:601–605.
165. Bartolozzi C, Lencioni R, Armillotta N. Combined treatment of hepatocellular carcinoma with chemoembolization and alcohol administration: long-term results. *Radiol Med.* 1997;94:19–23.
166. Ishii H, Okada S, Sato T, et al. Effect of percutaneous ethanol injection for post-operative recurrence of hepatocellular carcinoma in combination with transcatheter arterial embolization. *Hepatogastroenterology.* 1996;43:644–650.
167. Dohmen K, Shirahama M, Shigematsu H, et al. Transcatheter arterial chemoembolization therapy combined with percutaneous ethanol injection for unresectable large hepatocellular carcinoma: an evaluation of the local therapeutic effect and survival rate. *Hepatogastroenterology.* 2001;48:1409–1415.
168. Buscarini L, Buscarini E, Di Stasi M, et al. Percutaneous radiofrequency thermal ablation combined with transcatheter arterial embolization in the treatment of large hepatocellular carcinoma. *Ultraschall Med.* 1999;20:47–53.
169. Bloomston M, Binitie O, Fraiji E, et al. Transcatheter arterial chemoembolization with or without radiofrequency ablation in the management of patients with advanced hepatic malignancy. *Am Surg.* 2002;68:827–831.
170. Cheng BQ, Jia CQ, Liu CT, et al. Chemoembolization combined with radiofrequency ablation for patients with hepatocellular carcinoma larger than 3 cm: a randomized controlled trial. *JAMA.* 2008;299(14): 1669–1677.
171. Shibata T, Isoda H, Hirokawa Y, et al. Small hepatocellular carcinoma: is radiofrequency ablation combined

with transcatheter arterial chemoembolization more effective than radiofrequency ablation alone for treatment? *Radiology*. 2009;252(3):905–913.
172. Seki T, Tamai T, Nakagawa T, et al. Combination therapy with transcatheter arterial chemoembolization and percutaneous microwave coagulation therapy for hepatocellular carcinoma. *Cancer*. 2000;89:1245–1251.
173. Xu KC, Niu LZ, Zhou Q, et al. Sequential use of transarterial chemoembolization and percutaneous cryosurgery for hepatocellular carcinoma. *World J Gastroenterol*. 2009;15(29):3664–3669.
174. Qian GJ, Chen H, Wu MC. Percutaneous cryoablation after chemoembolization of liver carcinoma: report of 34 cases. *Hepatobiliary Pancreat Dis Int*. 2003;2(4):520–524.
175. Clavien PA, Kang KJ, Selzner N, et al. Cryosurgery after chemoembolization for hepatocellular carcinoma in patients with cirrhosis. *J Gastrointest Surg*. 2002;6(1):95–101.
176. Zangos S, Eichler K, Balzer JO, et al. Large-sized hepatocellular carcinoma (HCC): a neoadjuvant treatment protocol with repetitive transarterial chemoembolization (TACE) before percutaneous MR-guided laser-induced thermotherapy (LITT). *Eur Radiol*. 2007;17(2):553–563.
177. Ferrari FS, Stella A, Gambacorta D, et al. Treatment of large hepatocellular carcinoma: comparison between techniques and long term results. *Radiol Med*. 2004;108:356–371.
178. Pacella CM, Bizzarri G, Cecconi P, et al. Hepatocellular carcinoma: long-term results of combined treatment with laser thermal ablation and transcatheter arterial chemoembolization. *Radiology*. 2001;219:669–678.
179. Aschoff AJ, Rafie N, Jesberger JA, et al. Thermal lesion conspicuity following interstitial radiofrequency thermal tumor ablation in humans: a comparison of STIR, turbo spin-echo T2-weighted, and contrast-enhanced T1-weighted MR images at 0.2 T. *J Magn Reson Imaging*. 2000;12:584–589.
180. Goldberg SN, Grassi CJ, Cardella JF, et al. Image-guided tumor ablation: standardization of terminology and reporting criteria. *Radiology*. 2005;235:728–739.
181. Nakazawa T, Kokubu S, Ono K, et al. Radiofrequency ablation of hepatocellular carcinoma: correlation between local tumor progression after ablation and ablative margin. *AJR*. 2007;188:480–488.
182. Vossen JA, Buijs M, Kamel IR. Assessment of tumor response on MR imaging after locoregional therapy. *Tech Vasc Interv Radiol*. 2006;9:125–132.
183. Anzai Y, Desalles A, Black KL, et al. Interventional MR imaging. *Radiographics*. 1993;13:897–904.
184. Boaz TL, Lewin JS, Chung YC, et al. MR monitoring of MR-guided radiofrequency thermal ablation of normal liver in an animal model. *J Magn Reson Imaging*. 1998;8:64–69.
185. Dromain C, de Baere T, Elias D, et al. Hepatic tumors treated with percutaneous radio-frequency ablation: CT and MR imaging follow-up. *Radiology*. 2002;223(1):255–262.
186. Ozkavukcu E, Haliloglu N, Erden A. Post-treatment MRI findings of hepatocellular carcinoma. *Diagn Interv Radiol*. 2009;15:111–120.

CHAPTER 15

Transcatheter Ablative Therapy for Liver Tumors

Karen T. Brown & Anne M. Covey

Hepatocellular carcinoma (HCC) is the fifth most common cancer worldwide,[1] and the incidence of this disease is rising in the western hemisphere[2,3] due to nonalcoholic steatohepatitis, and the increased incidence of hepatitis C, since most patients with HCC harbor either the hepatitis B or C virus.[4] More than 80% of patients present with advanced or unresectable disease, and the recurrence rate after surgical resection is as high as 50%.[5,6] Population-based studies show that the incidence rate continues to approximate the death rate, suggesting that the vast majority of patients who develop this disease succumb to it.[7]

While surgery remains the best hope for cure in patients with primary liver cancer[8,9] as well as metastatic disease[10] to the liver, most patients are not candidates for resection or transplantation at the time of their presentation due to the extent or distribution of disease, underlying liver function, or their general medical condition.[11] In the case of HCC, although transplantation may be curative, patients will spend time on a transplant list awaiting a donor organ and during this period are at risk for progression.[12] Effective therapies for advanced HCC remain an immediate need. In the realm of regional therapy for locally advanced disease, extensive work has been done in regard to the feasibility and effectiveness of different transcatheter ablative modalities, with many issues still hotly debated.

The presence of a dual blood supply to the liver prompted development of hepatic arterial therapies. The portal vein provides over 75% of the blood flow to the hepatic parenchyma, and is the primary trophic blood supply, although in cirrhotic patients with portal hypertension there is a shift toward more dependence upon arterial blood flow. In contrast to the liver parenchyma, studies performed in the early 1950s established that the primary blood supply to liver tumors was from the hepatic artery.[13] Following this observation, therapeutic surgical ligation of the hepatic artery was performed in the 1960s and early 1970s[14,15] to treat HCC. This technique was limited by the invasive nature of the surgery, the transient effect, and, more importantly, the limited ability to retreat recurrent or progressive disease. This is particularly true in the case of metastatic neuroendocrine tumor (NET) and HCC, where the quality of life[16] and survival[17–19] is directly related to the ability to control the disease in the liver. In such cases, the ability to re-treat recurrent or progressive disease is critical.

As angiographic methods became more sophisticated, it became clear that malignant tumors may be preferentially targeted by delivering treatments intra-arterially[20]; theoretically, agents administered in this fashion would have little effect on the hepatic parenchyma, and enhanced effect on the liver tumor. Since the treatment is administered directly into the hepatic artery, the hope was that there would be fewer systemic side effects as well.

The rational for regional hepatic therapy is that treatment of the liver tumor (primary or metastases) will positively impact quality of life and/or prolong survival. Historically, the group of patients most likely to benefit from regional therapy has been patients with one of three tumor types: NET, HCC, and colon cancer. Patients with neuroendocrine metastases to liver commonly present with symptoms related to the production of hormones by tumor. Any hormonal syndrome, whether related to production of vasoactive compounds, insulin, gastrin, or any other hormone, usually signifies liver metastases because hormones produced by the liver drain into the systemic circulation bypassing the first-pass hepatic metabolism than those produced by pancreatic or bowel tumors encounter. Transcatheter therapy is very effective at controlling debilitating symptoms ranging from hypoglycemia in the case of insulin-producing tumors to diarrhea and flushing from tumors that secrete 5-hydroxyindoleacetic acid or vasoactive intestinal peptide.[21]

For most other malignant tumors treated with transcatheter therapy, the aim of treatment is to prolong survival. Although many tumors involve the liver at the later stages of disease, the liver is not the sole site of metastases or the ultimate cause of mortality in most patients. This includes many common primary tumors such as breast and lung cancer, and therefore the rational for regional therapy including transcatheter therapy in these patients is limited.

There are currently three main categories of percutaneously administered transcatheter intra-arterial therapy: transarterial chemoembolization (TACE), bland hepatic arterial embolization (HAE), and radioembolization (RAE). RAE will be covered in Chapter 17. Recently drug-eluting beads (DEB) that can be loaded with chemotherapeutic agents have been used for treating primary and secondary hepatic malignancies. Use of these loaded embolic agents is considered a form of chemoembolization. Intra-arterial infusion therapies are usually carried out using permanently implanted ports or pumps, relying in part on first-pass hepatic extraction of the agents used, and are beyond the scope of this chapter.

In the last 30 years, many different techniques for performing transcatheter hepatic embolotherapy have been described to treat a variety of tumor types. Many practitioners used chemotherapeutic agents and lipiodol, despite the lack of pharmacokinetic data that convincingly demonstrated high local concentration of the chemotherapeutic agent in the tumor with little in the systemic circulation. Studies clearly demonstrating an increased concentration within tumors using either mitomycin C, doxorubicin, and aclarubicin dissolved in hydrocarbon solvents and then in lipiodol,[22] or a lipophilic chemotherapeutic agent,[23] methods which are not used in clinical practice. When a traditional chemotherapeutic agent dissolved in an aqueous solution is then mixed with lipiodol, it is administered as an emulsion; concentration of drug in the tumor is high immediately, but low at six hours, one day, and seven days.[22] In a study by Raoul et al.,[24] doxorubicin was administered to patients intra-arterially in three different ways: as an infusion, emulsified with lipiodol, or with lipiodol and gelatin sponge. There was no significant difference in total amount of doxorubicin released into the circulating blood; patients in whom gelatin sponge was used had less released within the first hour of treatment. A prospective randomized clinical trial evaluating the effect of lipiodol when added to intra-arterial *cis*-platinum and doxorubicin found no difference in response between the groups given only intra-arterial chemotherapy compared to those who received chemotherapy emulsified with lipiodol.[25] Another study evaluated intra-arterial doxorubicin versus doxorubicin with lipiodol, and found no difference in the area under the concentration time curve, or terminal half life, and no difference in pharmacokinetic or systemic toxicity using the same dose schedule compared with patients who received intravenous doxorubicin.[26] Pharmacokinetic data supporting the use of intra-arterial chemotherapy, or chemotherapy plus lipiodol, at least when mixed with hydrophilic chemotherapeutic agents commonly used today and administered as an emulsion, are not robust.

What has been demonstrated in both pharmacokinetic and clinical studies[24,27,28] is the benefit derived from the addition of an embolic agent, even a nonpermanent agent, such as Gelfoam, for chemoembolization. Some authors have suggested that the primary effect of chemoembolization may be primarily from the embolic agent and not the chemotherapy or lipiodol.[27,28] If the primary effect of chemoembolization is indeed from ischemia-induced cell death, then the goal must be to induce terminal vessel blockade, as we know that more proximal vessel occlusion within the liver leads to the almost immediate development of flow distal to the occluded artery via myriad collateral vessels, demonstrated by Michels in 1953.[29]

Conventional Transarterial Chemoembolization

The bland embolization/chemoembolization debate in the treatment of HCC has been going on for quite some time now. Proponents of TACE assert that this treatment results in deposition of high concentrations of chemotherapy within the tumor that stays there for a prolonged period of time and, rightly, point out that this method is the only one for which level I evidence of a survival benefit has been demonstrated in randomized trials published by Llovett and Lo in 2002.[17,18] Excellent results (level IIa evidence) following chemoembolization have also been reported from Japan in 8510 patients treated between 1994 and 2001, with one, three, and five year survival of 82%, 47% and 26%.[30] Seventy-four percent of the patients had positive hepatitis C serology. Patients were excluded if they had evidence of nodal disease or distant metastases, and only 4% of patients had more than second-order portal vein branch involvement; however almost half of the patients were Child class B or C. Llovett et al.[17] reported the probability of survival following chemoembolization in their group of 40 patients, the majority of whom had positive hepatitis C serology, to be 82%, 63%, and 29% at one, two, and three years, while Lo et al. reported survivals of 57%, 31% and 26% at one, two, and three years in their study of 40 patients, 90% of whom were hepatitis B serology positive.[18] These studies by Llovett and Lo are considered pivotal in establishing the superiority of conventional TACE over best supportive care for patients with unresectable HCC. The cumulative survival rate at one, two, and three years in a recent report on triple drug chemoembolization by Buijs et al.[31] who treated 190 patients was 58%, 39% and 29%. In this level IIb evidence study, 40% of patients were hepatitis C serology positive whereas 21% had positive hepatitis B serology.

What seems clear from this data is that arterial embolotherapy is an effective method of treating HCC in an effort to prolong the patient's survival. Comparable, or better, survival results have been demonstrated with bland embolization.[19]

Bland Embolization

Hepatic arterial embolization (HAE) with small particles intended to cause terminal vessel blockade is an effective method of intra-arterial treatment for hypervascular primary and metastatic tumors to the liver.[19,32,33] HAE avoids the added expense of chemotherapeutic agents and also spares the patient the potential systemic toxicities of chemotherapy. In a large series of patients with HCC treated with bland embolization by Maluccio et al.,[19] a subgroup of 159 patients who were without extrahepatic disease or portal vein involvement by tumor, similar to those treated in the studies by Llovet and Lo,[17,18] had one, two, and three year survival of 84%, 66%, and 51%; all of these patients were treated without the addition of chemotherapy or lipiodol to the embolic agent. HAE using small particles known to cause terminal vessel blockade is the primary method of intra-arterial therapy at some institutions, and level IIb evidence supporting this practice is provided by this data of Maluccio et al.[19] The results of HAE are essentially immediate, and the beginning of radiologic tumor necrosis can be demonstrated by imaging within hours of the procedure (Figure 15-1A–C). This is a particularly useful feature in patients who present with significant tumor burden where further progression may render them untreatable. Bland embolization is also effective for treating tumor thrombus within the portal vein (Figure 15-2A and B). Bland particle embolization can provide prompt control of disease. Little is written about the response time line in patients treated with TACE. TACE is not performed to "stasis" and the primary effect is considered to be chemotherapy related. Proponents of this method of treatment often point out that the intent is not to induce necrosis. These facts lead one to suspect that maximum response to treatment might not be seen immediately postembolization.

Drug-eluting Beads

Currently available DEB are preformed microspheres available in diameters ranging from 100 to 1200 μ. These spheresare deformable and made from a macromere derived from polyvinyl alcohol(PVA). They are typically loaded with doxorubicin when used to treat HCC, using up to 150 mg per treatment. The pharmacokinetic profile of the DEB is significantly different from that seen with conventional TACE, with level IIb evidence that the peak drug concentration in the serum is an order of magnitude lower for DEBs, and the area under the curve of drug concentration is significantly lower as well.[34] Objective response by the European Association for the Study of the Liver (EASL) criteria has been reported in 70%–80% of patients[34–36] and one and two year survival of 92.5% and 88.9% have been reported in a level IIa study of 27 patients with large/multifocal tumors.[34] More recent data demonstrate a better response to DEB

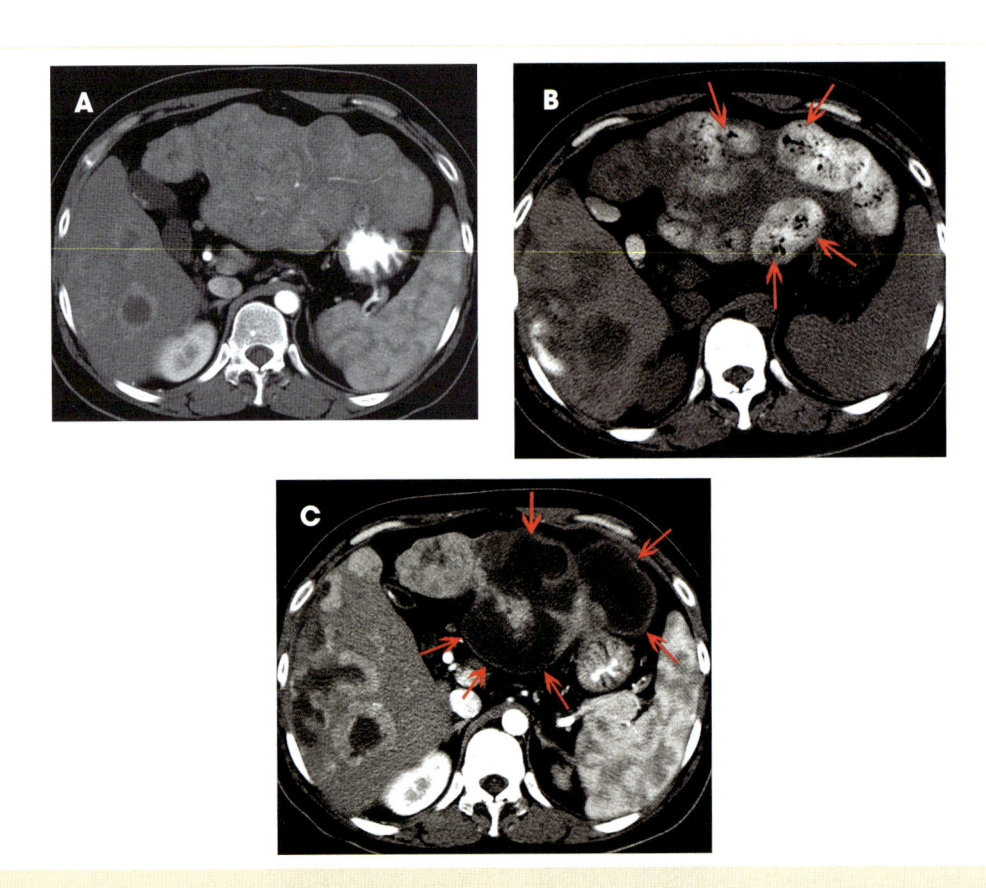

Figure 15-1: Images showing typical findings of tumor necrosis following bland embolization of multifocal HCC. At 12 hours postembolization, gas bubbles (arrows) and retained contrast are evident. At 1 month, the treated area is uniformly low density consistent with necrosis (arrows). Preembolization computed tomography (CT) (A), 12 hours after left hepatic arterial embolization (B), and 1 month after left hepatic arterial embolization (C).

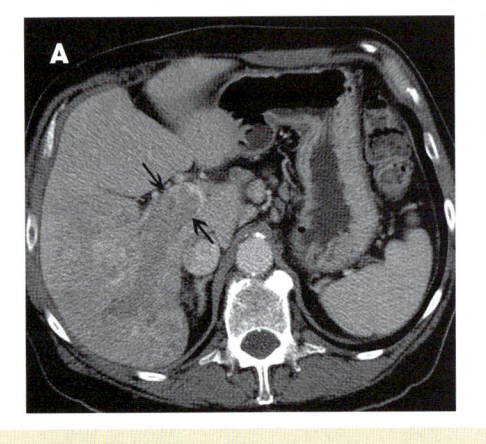

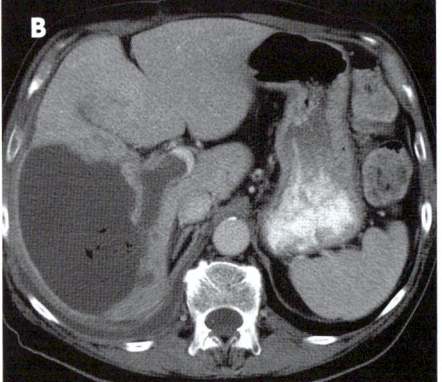

Figure 15-2: Images showing large HCC in right liver extending into portal vein (arrows) and 6 week follow-up CT. Pretreatment CT (A), and CT 6 weeks later (B).

compared to embolization with particles alone[37] or conventional TACE[38] but without demonstration of a survival benefit or proof of superiority. When compared to conventional TACE, treatment with DEB is better tolerated with a significant reduction in serious liver toxicity and significantly fewer doxorubicin-related side effects.[38]

Since Lee et al.[39] have demonstrated that microspheres larger than 100–300 μ do not penetrate into the tumor, if the purpose of using drug-eluting microspheres is to deliver drug to the tumor the 100–300 μ size would appear to offer an advantage over the larger sizes. When embolization is performed with these 100–300 μ spheres, and embolization is performed to stasis, the effect on the tumor can be seen very shortly after embolization. Immediately after embolization to stasis, the tumors retain contrast/particles in the targeted region, as is seen after bland HAE. On subsequent scans, successfully treated tumors become nonenhancing and then gradually decrease in size over weeks to months (Figure 15-3A–C).

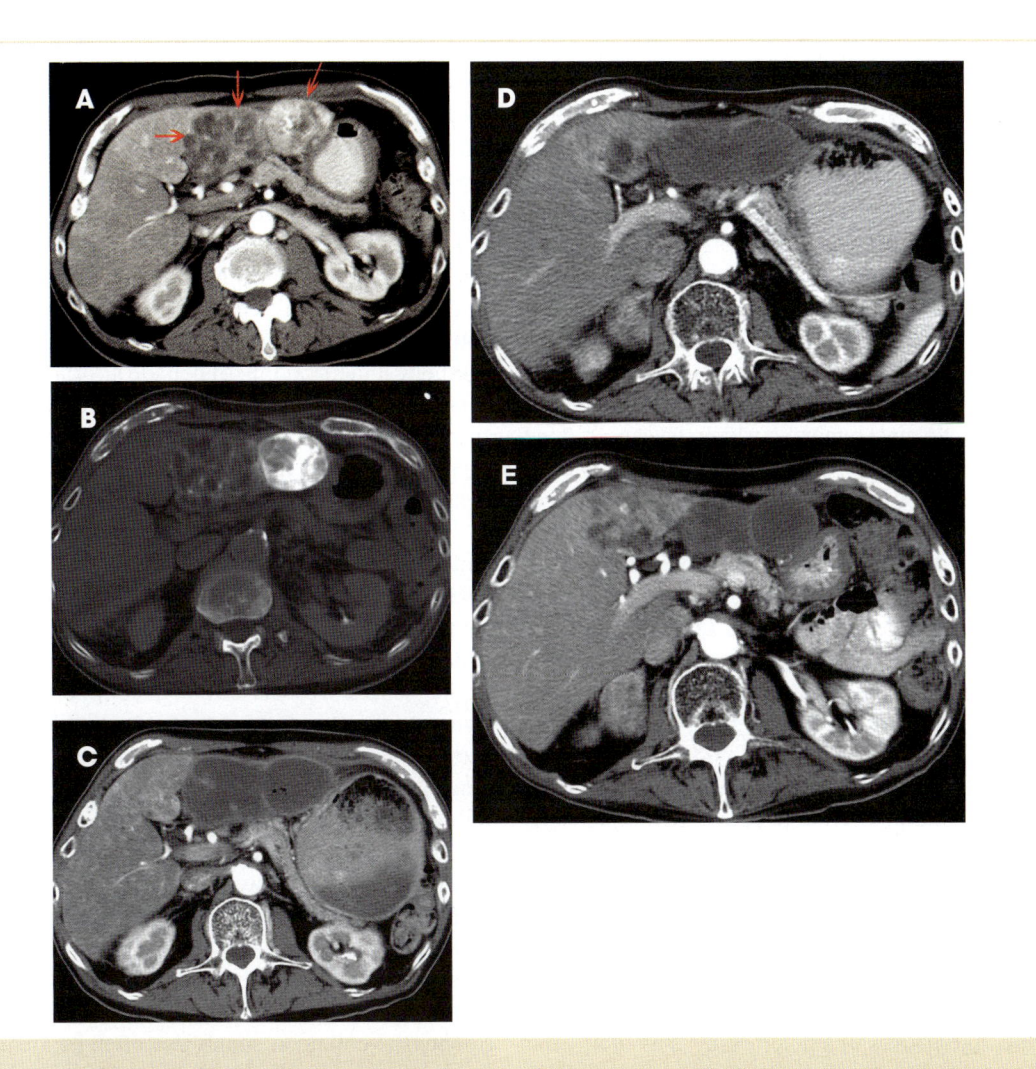

Figure 15-3: Images demonstrate progressive imaging changes in treated HCC. Pretreatment scan in patient with dominant HCC at tip of lateral segment and multiple satellite nodules (arrows) (A), scan immediately after left hepatic arterial embolization with drug-eluting beads (B), scan obtained 3 weeks following treatment (C), 3 months after treatment (D), and 9 months after treatment (E).

Patient Selection

The indications and contraindications for embolic therapies continue to evolve as tools improve and our understanding of the risks for different patients broadens. Inclusion criteria for transcatheter therapy vary by practitioner, institution, region, and country. Criteria to consider when selecting patients for transcatheter embolization include performance status, liver function (Child-Pugh, Okuda, Barcelona-Clinic Liver Cancer staging, etc.), volume of liver replaced by tumor, and the condition of the portal venous system. In our practice, we use the Child-Pugh staging system as a measure of liver function, and treat almost exclusively patients with Child-Pugh A or B cirrhosis who most commonly have tumor involving less than 50% of the hepatic parenchyma.

Performance status and underlying liver disease are important considerations for several reasons. Although minimally invasive, following embolization patients commonly experience a postembolization syndrome of pain, fever, and nausea that may last for several days to a week or two. It often takes four to six weeks to recover to baseline performance status. Unlike most tumors in which the cancer alone predicts prognosis, patients with HCC typically have a second, independent life-threatening disease: cirrhosis.[17] In poorly compensated cirrhosis (Child-Pugh B, C), life expectancy is more often determined by the underlying liver disease than the tumor itself. While embolization in patients with normal liver, or well-compensated cirrhosis, has a low risk of liver failure, the risk of further compromising liver function and hastening death in poorly compensated cirrhosis is significant.

Until recently portal vein occlusion has been seen as a contraindication to both TACE[40] and HAE because of the risk of liver failure. Portal vein tumor thrombus is uncommon in patients with NET or colorectal cancer metastases, but is seen in up to 40% of patients with HCC. The median survival in this group is 2.7–4 months with supportive therapy alone.[41-43] Because these patients have few therapeutic alternatives, embolotherapy has not been completely abandoned and retrospective studies have shown improved survival in comparison with historic controls.[44-46]

Anatomic Considerations

In standard, or classic, visceral anatomy the celiac axis gives rise to three branches.[47] The first branch is the left gastric, after which the vessel divides into the splenic artery and common hepatic artery (CHA). The CHA then bifurcates into the gastroduodenal and proper hepatic (PH) arteries, and the PH artery gives rise to the right and left hepatic arteries (Figure 15-4). Standard hepatic arterial anatomy has been reported in approximately 50% of patients on the basis of cadaveric[29] and angiographic reports.[48] The most common variants include an accessory or replaced right hepatic artery arising from the superior mesenteric artery or an accessory or replaced left hepatic artery arising from the left gastric artery. In 1969, Redman and Reuter[47] reported, in a frequently referenced article, that "most of the variations of the other 50% have little surgical significance." This may have been true at the time, but with the meteoric rise in the complexity of interventional techniques to treat both primary and metastatic liver tumors, a more complete understanding of hepatic arterial anatomy is critical. Failure to recognize the presence of an aberrant vessel or the presence of extrahepatic supply to a given tumor will result in incomplete treatment.

Because of the high risk of persistent or recurrent tumor after embolization and the frequent development of new lesions, long-term local control of disease is rarely achieved with a single embolization. Following TACE, arterial injury to the hepatic vessels is not uncommon and can result in the development of intra- and extrahepatic collateral supply to recurrent or residual tumor mass.[49] This appears to be less common following HAE.[50,51]

Injury to native vessels can result in difficulty catheterizing target vessels during subsequent procedures, or inability to deliver the embolic agent to the tumor through native vasculature. The spectrum of arterial injury is broad and ranges from distal vessel narrowing to proximal vessel occlusion or aneurysm. Nonhepatic collateral supply can often be identified on pretreatment arterial phase computed tomography (CT) and commonly arises from the phrenic, internal mammary, and gastroduodenal arteries

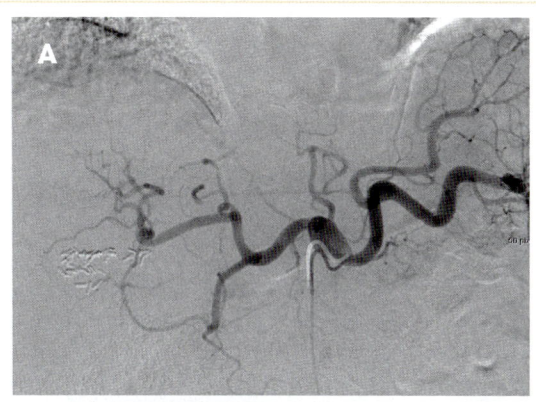

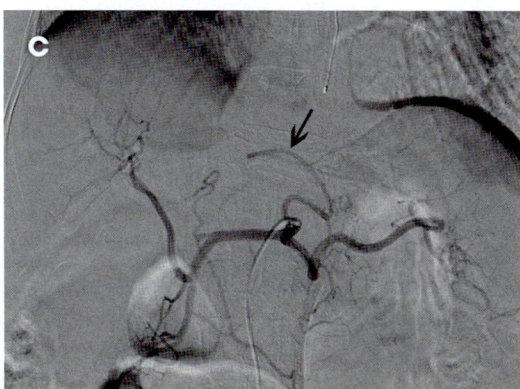

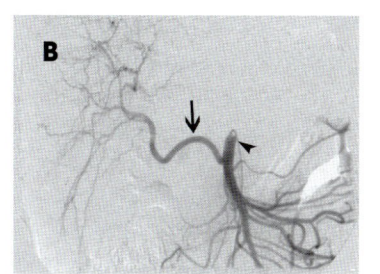

Figure 15-4: Standard hepatic arterial anatomy is seen in 55% of patients (A). Common variants include a replaced or accessory right hepatic artery (arrow) arising from the superior mesenteric artery (arrowhead) (B) and replaced or accessory left hepatic artery (arrow) arising from the left gastric artery (C).

(Figure 15-5). Less common is tumor supply from renal, adrenal, or colonic branches.[49] Intraprocedural CT or careful evaluation of the late phase angiographic images is helpful in determining whether the entire tumor has been treated during TACE or HAE (Figure 15-6). If there are defects in contrast deposition within the tumor, additional feeding vessels should be sought.

It is important to consider that embolization of nonhepatic arteries can result in complications related to the parent vessel. For example, embolization of phrenic or intercostal arteries can result in skin changes (Figure 15-7) that are typically clinically insignificant but could be worrisome to the patient if they are not forewarned. Similar changes can be seen when the internal mammary vessels are treated. It is possible that the use of chemotherapeutic agents for embolization of these nonhepatic vessels might result in clinically significant skin changes, and the use of chemotherapy in nonhepatic vessels is not recommended.

Another potential difficulty with embolizing nonhepatic vessels is the possibility of nontarget embolization of distal branches that supply nontumor bearing viscera. Coil embolization of the nontarget branches may be performed to protect the nontarget territory from distal embolization before administering the embolic agent(s). Nontarget embolization can occur when embolizing native hepatic arteries as well. The cystic artery and gastroduodenal artery are frequently at risk, and reflux into these vessels should be avoided. With improved resolution of modern imaging equipment, distal branches of the left hepatic artery can be seen to communicate with gastric branches. In this case, embolic agent administered to the left hepatic artery can cause injury to

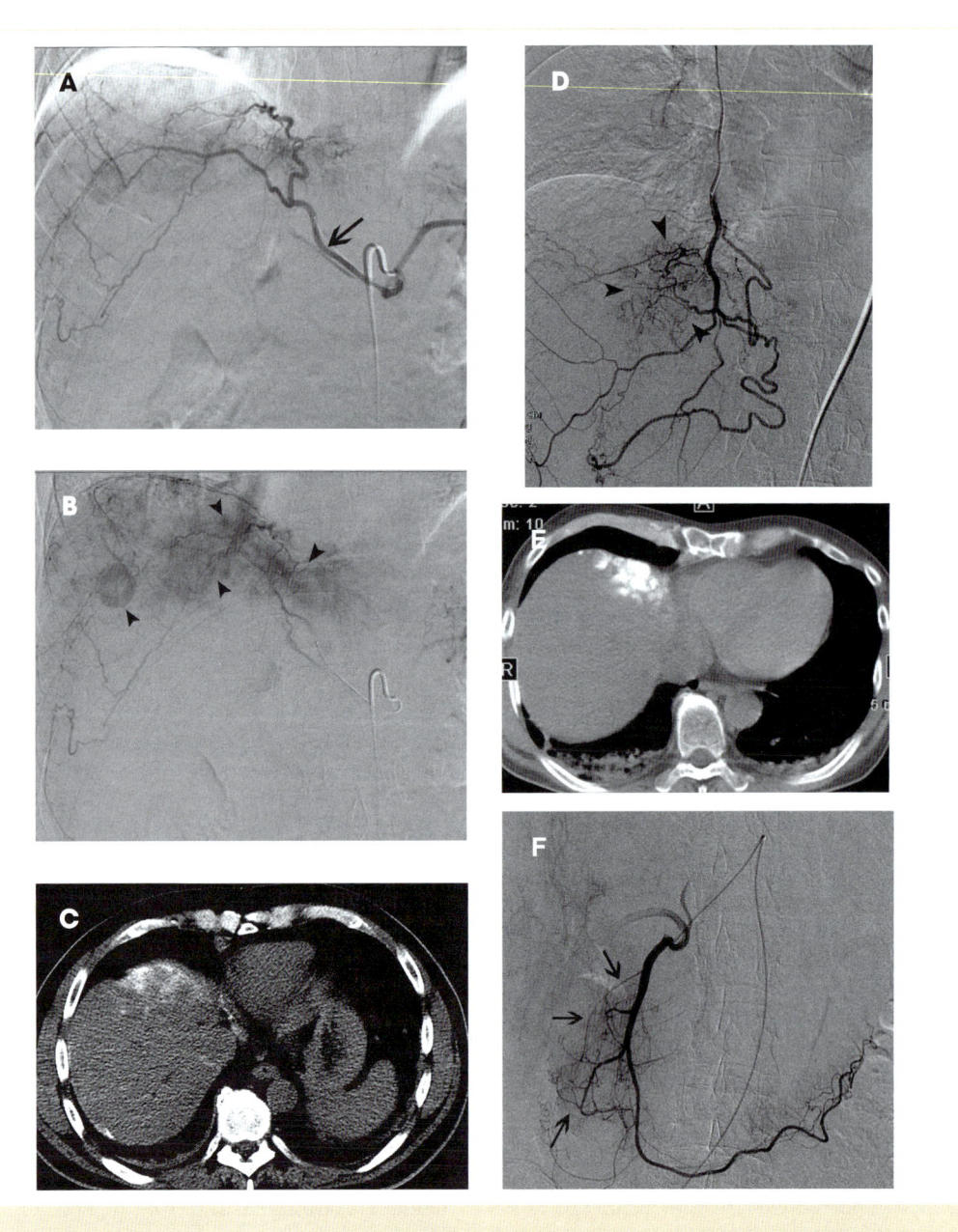

Figure 15-5: Extrahepatic collateral supply. Early and later phase angiogram of the right phrenic artery (arrow) show hypervascular HCC involving segments IV and VIII (arrowheads) (A and B). Noncontrast CT after embolization of this vessel shows retention of contrast/particles within tumor (C). In a different patient, selective embolization of right internal mammary artery branches supplying hypervascular tumor (arrowheads) was performed (D) and was followed by noncontrast CT showing the territory supplied by this vessel (E). Finally, tumor supply is seen originating from branches of the gastroduodenal artery (arrow) (F).

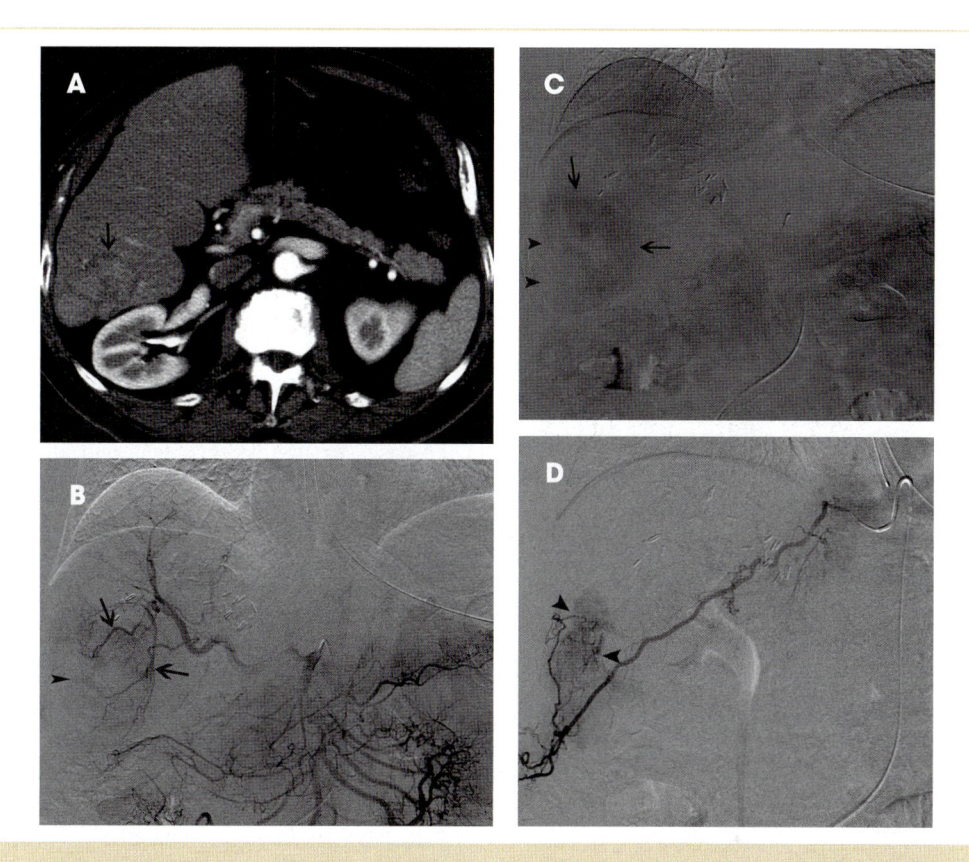

Transcatheter Ablative Therapy for Liver Tumors   363

Figure 15-6: Recurrent HCC in a patient who previously underwent right posterior hepatic resection (A). Early and late phase arteriogram of the replaced right hepatic artery (B and C) show partial enhancement of the tumor (arrow) with a defect in the lateral caudal aspect of the tumor (arrowheads) prompting a search for extrahepatic collateral supply. Selective angiography of the inferior intercostal (D) shows tumor enhancement complementary to that seen from the right hepatic artery (arrowheads). Embolization of this vessel was performed to complete the treatment of this lesion.

the fundus of the stomach. Inclusion of the stomach in the field of preembolization angiograms is necessary to alert the operator to this anomaly.

Postembolization Imaging

The ability to assess response to treatment is important prognostically and to determine when additional intervention is indicated. It has been shown with several different tumors including HCC that radiographic response to embolization correlates with survival.[33]

The typical CT findings after bland embolization and DEB are to see contrast-laden particles within the tumor immediately following embolization. This finding can last several days. Within 12 hours previously enhancing tumor is replaced by low-density necrotic material that often contains air (Figure 15-1). Air may remain within treated tumors for several weeks following embolization (Figure 15-2). Absence of enhancing tissue in the treated area is considered a sign of successful treatment.

Lipiodol used as a carrier in TACE is retained within tumor indefinitely, and because lipiodol

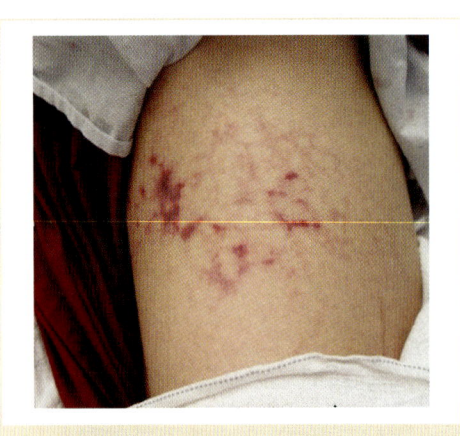

Figure 15-7: Photograph of the flank following embolization of the right phrenic artery to treat HCC. After embolization of the phrenic artery, nonblanching skin changes are common.

contains iodine, CT is not as useful in evaluating response to treatment after TACE. Lipiodol is not detected on magnetic resonance (MR), however, and gadolinium-enhanced MR is used to look for contrast enhancement suggesting persistent viable tumor. Recently, there has been interest in diffusion-weighted MR to evaluate response to embolotherapy. Diffusion weighting is an MR technique that maps the diffusion coefficient of water within cells. Because water molecules are bound in densely cellular tumors and more "free" in areas of necrosis, restricted diffusion is a marker of cellular viability. This technique has been used as a marker of response to systemic chemotherapy, radiation therapy, and, more recently, TACE.[52]

The most important outcome following treatment is survival or, in the case of NET, resolution of hormone-related symptoms. Because survival can only be calculated retrospectively, imaging has been used as surrogate marker to evaluate response. The most common classifications for evaluating response to therapy are the response evaluation criteria in solid tumors (RECIST)[53] and World Health Organization (WHO)[54] criteria, which have been used since 2001 and 1981, respectively to evaluate response to systemic chemotherapy. As the preceding paragraphs describe, however, following transcatheter embolization it is most common to see a change in the character of a target lesion, and less common to see a change in size (Figure 15-8). RECIST uses the sum of target tumor diameters and WHO the bidimensional measurement of target lesion(s), and both are therefore suboptimal in the evaluation of regional therapies that induce necrosis rather than shrinkage of tumor. Criteria were developed in 2000 by EASL,[55] and in 2008 a modification of RECIST (mRECIST)[55] was proposed by the American Association for the Study of Liver Diseases to address this issue and allow a more accurate evaluation of response to regional therapies (Table 15-1).

Summary

Several methods of transcatheter treatment for primary and secondary liver tumors exist including TACE, DEB, HAE, and RAE. None of these methods have been proven superior to any of the others in terms of survival. RAE is the most expensive of the four methods by a significant margin and unless a significant improvement in survival or progression-free survival is demonstrated, less expensive therapy might be tried first. There remains no convincing evidence that the therapeutic effectiveness of TACE is related to high concentration of chemotherapy within tumor for prolonged periods. Given the lack of convincing pharmacokinetic support for TACE, coupled with the excellent pharmacologic profile for DEB, TACE should probably be abandoned in favor of DEB for those who are convinced that inclusion of a chemotherapeutic agent is important. For those of us who believe that ischemia is the proximate cause of tumor cell death and response to treatment, and who are concerned with maintaining native hepatic branch vessel patency, as well as avoiding the potential for chemotherapy side effects as well as the expense, HAE will remain the mainstay of treatment for HCC and other hypervascular tumors.

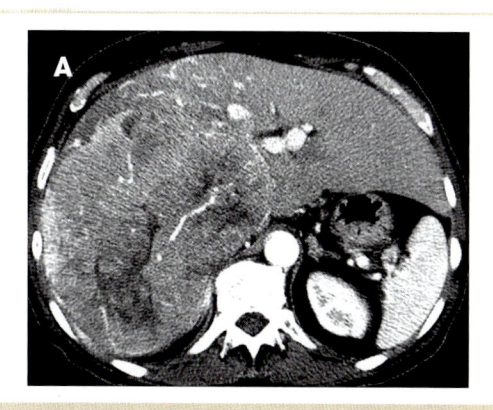

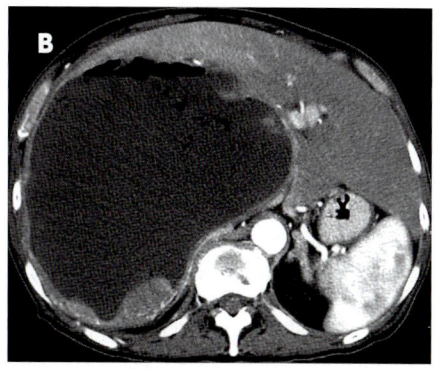

Figure 15-8: Massive HCC in a patient with profound right upper quadrant pain and early satiety (A). After bland embolization with PVA (B) there is marked change in the vascularity of the tumor which is largely necrotic. By response evaluation criteria in solid tumors (RECIST) or World Health Organization criteria, this is stable disease, whereas using modification of RECIST or European Association for the Study of the Liver this is more appropriately classified as a partial response.

TABLE 15-1: Comparison of the Methods Used to Assess Response to Treatment Following Regional Therapy

	RECIST	WHO	EASL	mRECIST
CR	Disappearance of all target lesions	Disappearance of all target lesions	Disappearance of all target lesions	Disappearance of intratumoral arterial enhancement in target lesions
PR	>30% decrease in sum of diameters of target lesions	>50% reduction of cross product of target lesion	>50% reduction of cross product of target lesion arterial enhancement	>30% decrease in sum of diameters of intratumoral arterial enhancement of target lesions
SD	Neither PD nor PR	Neither PD nor PR	Neither PD nor PR	Neither PD nor PR
PD	>20% increase in sum of diameters of target lesions	>25% increase in cross product of target lesion	>25% increase in cross product of target lesion arterial enhancement	>20% increase in sum of diameters of intratumoral arterial enhancement

Abbreviations: CR = Complete response; EASL, European Association for the Study of the Liver; mRECIST, modification of RECIST; PD = progressive disease; PR = partial response; RECIST, response evaluation criteria in solid tumors; SD = stable disease; WHO, World Health Organization.

References

1. Parkin DM, Bray F, Ferlay J, Pisani P. Estimating the world cancer burden: Globocan 2000. *Int J Cancer.* 2001;94:153–156.
2. El-Serag HB, Mason AC. Rising incidence of hepatocellular carcinoma in the United States. *N Engl J Med.* 1999;340(10):745–750.
3. Altekruse SF, McGlynn KA, Reichman ME. Hepatocellular carcinoma incidence, mortality, and survival trends in the United States from 1975 to 2005. *J Clin Oncol.* 2009;27(9):1485–1491. Epub 2009 Feb 17.
4. Ikeda K, Saitoh S, Koida I, et al. A multivariate analysis of risk factors for hepatocellular carcinogenesis: a prospective observation of 795 patients with viral and alcoholic cirrhosis. *Hepatology.* 1993;18(1):47–53.
5. Poon RT-P, Fan S-T, Lo C-M, et al. Intrahepatic recurrence after curative resection of Hepatocellular carcinoma: long-term results of treatment & prognostic factors. *Ann Surg.* 1999;229(2):216–222.
6. Cha C, Fong Y, Jarnagin WR, et al. Predictors and patterns of recurrence after resection of hepatocellular. *J Am Coll Surg.* 2003;197(5):753–758.
7. American Cancer Society. *Cancer Facts and Figures 2010.* Atlanta, GA: ACS; 2010.
8. Colombo M, Sangiovanni A. Etiology, natural history and treatment of hepatocellular carcinoma. *Antiviral Res.* 2004;60(2):145–150.
9. Llovet JM, Schwartz M, Mazzaferro V. Resection and liver transplantation for hepatocellular carcinoma. *Semin Liver Dis.* 2005;25(2):181–200.
10. Kemeny N. The management of resectable and unresectable liver metastases from colorectal cancer. Curr Opin Oncol. 2010;22(4):364–373.
11. Bruix J, Llovet JM. Prognostic prediction and treatment strategy in hepatocellular carcinoma. *Hepatology.* 2002;35(3):519–524.
12. Okuda K, Ohtsuki T, Obata H, et al. Natural history of hepatocellular carcinoma and prognosis in relation to treatment: study of 850 patients. *Cancer.* 1985;56:918–928.
13. Breedis C, Young G. Blood supply of neoplasms of the liver. *Am J Pathol.* 1954;30:969–985.
14. Nilsson LA. Therapeutic hepatic artery ligation in patients with secondary liver tumors. Rev Surg. 1966;23(5):374–376.
15. Madding GF, Kennedy PA, Sogemeier E. Hepatic artery ligation for metastatic tumor in the liver. Am J Surg. 1970;120(1):95–96.
16. Knox CD, Feurer ID, Wise PE, et al. Survival and functional quality of life after resection for hepatic carcinoid metastasis. J Gastrointest Surg. 2004;8(6):653–659.
17. Llovet JM, Real MI, Montana X, et al. Arterial embolization or chemoembolization versus symptomatic treatment in patients with unresectable hepatocellular carcinoma: a randomized controlled trial. *Lancet.* 2002;359:1734–1739.
18. Lo C-M, Ngan H, Tso W-K, et al. Randomized controlled trial of transarterial lipiodol chemoembolization for unresectable hepatocellular carcinoma. *Hepatology.* 2002;35(5):1164–1171.
19. Maluccio MA, Covey AM, Porat LB, et al. Transcatheter arterial embolization using particles only for the treatment of unresectable hepatocellular carcinoma. *JVIR.* 2008;19(6):862–869.
20. Doyon D, Mouson A, Jourde AM, et al. Hepatic, arterial embolization in patients with malignant liver tumors. *Ann Radiol.* 1974;17(6):593–603.
21. Chamberlain RS, Canes D, Brown KT, et al. Hepatic neuroendocrine metas-tases: does intervention alter-outcomes?. J Am Coll Surg. 2000;190(4):432–445.
22. Konno T. Targeting cancer chemotherapeutic agents by use of lipiodol contrast medium. *Cancer.* 1990;66:1897–1903.
23. Egawa H, Maki A, Mori K, et al. Effects of intraarterial chemotherapy with a new lipophilic anti-cancer agent, estradiol-chlorambucil (KM2210), dissolved in lipiodol on experimental liver tumors in rats. *J Surg Oncol.* 1990;44:109–114.
24. Raoul JL, Heresbach D, Bretagne JF, et al. Chemoembolization of hepatocellular carcinomas. A study of biodistribution and pharmacokinetics of doxorubicin. *Cancer.* 1992;70(3):585–590.
25. Carr B, Iwatsuki S, Baron R, et al. Intrahepatic arterial cis-platinum and doxorubicin with or without lipiodol for advanced hepatocellular carcinoma (HCC): a prospective randomized study (abstr). *Proc Am Soc Clin Oncol.* ASCO Annual meeting 1993.
26. Johnson PJ, Kalayci C, Dobbs N, et al. Pharmacokinetics and toxicity of intraarterial adriamycin for hepatocellular carcinoma: effect of coadministration of lipiodol. *Hepatology.* 1991;13:120–127.
27. Nakao N, Kamino K, Miura K, et al. Recurrent hepatocellular carcinoma after partial hepatectomy: value of treatment with transcatheter chemoembolization. *AJR.* 1991;156:1177–1179.
28. Ngan H, Lai C, Fan S, et al. Transcatheter arterial chemoembolization in inoperable hepatocellular carcinoma: Four year follow-up. *J Vasc Interv Radiol.* 1996;7:419–425.

29. Michels NA. Collateral arterial pathways to the liver after ligation of the hepatic artery and removal of the coeliac axis. *Cancer.* 1953;6:708.

30. Takayasu K, Arii S, Ikai I, et al. Prospective cohort study of transarterial chemoembolization for unresectable hepatocellular carcinoma in 8510 patients. *Gastroent.* 2006;131:461–469.

31. Buijs M, Vossen JA, Frangakis C, et al. Nonresectable hepatocellular carcinoma: Long-term toxicity in patients treated with transarterial chemoembolization—single-center experience. *Radiology.* 2008;249(1):346–354.

32. Brown KT, Koh BY, Brody LA, et al. Particle embolization of hepatic neuroendocrine metastases for control of pain and hormonal symptoms. *JVIR.* 1999;10:397–403.

33. Maluccio MA, Covey AM, Schubert J, et al. Treatment of metastatic sarcoma to the liver with bland embolization. *Cancer.* 1, 2006;107(7):1617–1623.

34. Varela M, Real MI, Burrel M, et al. Chemoembolization of heptocellular carcinoma with drug eluting beads: Efficacy and doxorubicin pharmacokinetics. *J Hepatol.* 2007;46:474–481.

35. Poon RTP, Tso WK, Pang RWC, et al. A phase I/II trial of chemoembolization for hepatocellular carcinoma using a novel intra-arterial drug-eluting bead. *Clin Gastroenterol Hepatol.* 2007;5:1100–1108.

36. Malagari K, Chatzimichael K, Alexopoulou E, et al. Transarterial chemoembolization of unresectable hepatocellular carcinoma with drug eluting beads: results of an open-label study of 62 patients. *Cardiovasc Intervent Radiol.* 2008;31:269–280.

37. Malagari K, Pomoni M, Kelekis A, et al. Prospective randomized comparison of chemoembolization with doxorubicin-eluting beads and bland embolization with Bead Block for hepatocellular carcinoma. *Cardiovasc Intervent Radiol.* 2010;33:541–551.

38. Lammer J, Malagari M, Vogl T, et al (On behalf of Precision V investigators). Prospective randomized study of doxorubicin-eluting-bead embolization in the treatment of hepatocellular carcinoma: results of the PRECISION V study. *Cardiovasc Intervent Radiol.* 2010;33:41–52.

39. Lee K-H, Liapi E, Vossen JA, et al. Distribution of iron oxide-containing embosphere particles after transcatheter arterial embolization in an animal model of liver cancer: evaluation with MR imaging and implication for therapy. *J Vasc Interv Radiol.* 2008;19:1490–1496.

40. Yamada R, Sato M, Kawabata M, et al. Hepatic arterial embolization in 120 patients with unresectable hepatoma. *Radiology.* 1983;148: 397–401.

41. Kiely JM, Rilling WS, Touzios JG, et al. Chemoembolization in patients at high risk: results and complications. *J Vasc Interv Radiol.* 2006;17:47–53.

42. Minagawa M, Makuuchi M. Treatment of hepatocellular carcinoma accompanied by portal vein tumor thrombus. *World J Gastroenterol.* 2006;12:7561–7567.

43. Giannelli G, Pierri F, Trerotoli P, et al. Occurrence of portal vein tumor thrombus in hepatocellular carcinoma affects prognosis and survival. A retrospective clinical study of 150 cases. *Hepatol Res.* 2002;24:50.

44. Georgiades CS, Hong K, D'Angelo M, Geshwind JF. Safety and efficacy of transarterial chemoembolization in patients with unresectable hepatocellular carcinoma and portal vein thrombosis. J Vasc Interv Radiol. 2005;16(12):1653–1659.

45. Deohodar A, Covey AM, Thornton R, et al. Safety and efficacy of transcatheter arterial embolization with particles only in the treatment of hepatocellular carcinoma with portal vein tumor. *J Interv Oncol.* 2010;3(1):3–11.

46. Lee HS, Kim JS, Choi IJ, et al. The safety and efficacy of transcatheter arterial chemoembolization in the treatment of patients with hepatocellular carcinoma and main portal vein obstruction. A prospective controlled study. *Cancer.* 1997;79:2087–2094.

47. Redman HC, Reuter SR. Angiographic demonstration of surgically important vascular variations. *Surg Gynecol Obstet.* 1969;129(1):33–39.

48. Covey AM, Brody LA, Maluccio MA, et al. Variant hepatic arterial anatomy revisited: digital subtraction angiography performed in 600 patients. *Radiology.* 2002;224(2):542–547.

49. Kim HC, Chung JW, Lee W, et al. Recognizing extrahepatic collateral vessels that supply hepatocellular carcinoma to avoid complicationsof transcatheter arterial chemoembolization. *RadioGraphics.* 2005;25(suppl 1):S25–S393.

50. Erinjeri JP, Salhab HM, Covey AM, et al. Arterial patency after repeated hepatic artery bland particle embolization. *J Vasc Interv Radiol.* 2010;21(4):522–526.

51. Geschwind JF, Ramsey DE, Cleffken B. Transcatheter arterial chemoembolization of liver tumors: effects of embolization protocol on injectable volume of chemotherapy and subsequent arterial patency. Cardiovasc Intervent Radiol. 2003;26(2):111–117. Epub 2003 Mar 6.

52. Kamel IR, Bluemke DA, Eng J, et al. The role of functional MR imaging in the assessment of tumor response after chemoembolization in patients with

hepatocellular carcinoma. J Vasc Interv Radiol. 2006;17(3):505–512.

53. Bruix J, Sherman M, Llovet JM, et al. Clinical management of hepatocellular carcinoma. Conclusions of the Barcelona-2000 EASL conference. European Association for the Study of the Liver. *J Hepatol.* 2001;35:421–430.

54. Therasse P, Arbuck SG, Eisenhauer EA, et al. New guidelines to evaluate the response to treatment in solid tumors. European Organization for Research and Treatment of Cancer, NCI (US and Canada). *J Natl Cancer Inst.* 2000;92(3):205–216.

55. Lencioni R, Llovet JM. Modified RECIST (mRECIST) assessment for hepatocellular carcinoma. Semin Liver Dis. 2010;30(1):52–60. Epub 2010 Feb 19.

CHAPTER 16

High Intensity Focused Ultrasound for Liver Tumors

Kelvin K. Ng

Hepatocellular carcinoma (HCC) is the most common primary liver cancer in the world, with a high prevalence in Asia and an increasing incidence in Western countries.[1] Meanwhile, the liver is also a frequent site for secondary tumors, in particular colorectal liver metastasis. Partial hepatectomy and liver transplantation are the potentially curative treatments for HCC. However, the applicability of these treatments is limited since a high proportion of patients have advanced tumor stages on presentation and there is a global problem of the shortage of donor livers. Even after surgery, there is a high tendency of tumor recurrence in HCC patients due to the intrahepatic metastasis or multicentric tumor occurrence in the background of liver cirrhosis.[2] For patients with colorectal cancer, between 35% and 55% of patients will develop liver metastasis. Following curative hepatectomy, about 65% of patients had tumor recurrence.[3] Hence, the current management of liver cancer is challenging and its difficulties lead to the development of less invasive techniques for liver cancer. With the advancement in technologies, local ablation therapies have emerged as effective treatment options for unresectable HCC. These include cryoablation therapy, interstitial laser therapy, microwave coagulation, radiofrequency ablation (RFA), and high-intensity focused ultrasound (HIFU). These methods aim to minimize tissue trauma in the setting of high tumor ablation rate. Therefore, the number of patients who can receive therapy can be increased. Among these treatment options, HIFU is the only treatment modality that is completely extracorporeal.[4] Theoretically, it is the ideal treatment for cirrhotic patients with advanced HCC and severe portal hypertension, which renders percutaneous puncture of ablation needle with an increased risk of bleeding. Furthermore, puncture of liver tumor by ablation needle of RFA is associated with a small but definite risk of tumor cell seeding along the needle track, which may convert a local tumor to disseminated disease.

Mechanisms of HIFU

HIFU is based on the unique characteristics of ultrasound beams (0.8–3.5 MHz), which can be focused at a distance from the radiating transducer. The ability of inducing immediate cell death at a distance from the ultrasound source makes HIFU an attractive treatment option for liver cancer without the need of surgery or insertion of ablation instruments. In theory, ultrasound is an acoustic pressure wave that propagates through the living tissue without deposition of significant energy. However, if the ultrasound beams from multiple directions are focused into a focal point where all the acoustic energy is concentrated, the cumulative energy will lead to significant thermal change. This can induce tissue necrosis of the targeted lesion, without causing damage to the surrounding vital structures. The goal of HIFU treatment is to induce a local temperature change (up to 50°C–60°C) in a small focus (a few millimeters) for a short time (within a minute). The smaller the focus and the shorter the time, the more accurate is the ablation zone. Normally, intrahepatic blood flow might cause some heat-sink effect on the ablation zone of HIFU, but the short exposure time may counteract this negative effect resulting in a homogenous ablation zone with sharp margins.[5] With the high acoustic intensities (up to 10,000 W/cm^2), HIFU can induce instantaneous cell death by two major mechanisms, namely thermal effect and mechanical effect.[6] The thermal effect of HIFU involves heat generation due to absorption of acoustic energy by the target tissue. A lethal temperature of up to 60°C causes immediate coagulative necrosis (Figure 16-1). Since high-intensity energy is focused at a small volume, the damage to the tissue between the transducer and target lesion can be minimized. On the other hand, the mechanical effects involve cavitation,[7] microstreaming,[8] and radiation forces.[9] Cavitation is related to the process of alternating compression and expansion of tissue in the region where the ultrasound waves propagate. With sufficient magnitude of tissue expansion, intracellular gas will be extracted out, resulting in bubble formation. The violent oscillation of gas bubble within the ultrasound field causes mechanical damage to the cell (Figure 16-2). Microstreaming is the phenomenon in which rapid movement of fluid near gas bubbles occurs due to its oscillating motion. The resulting high shearing forces close to the bubble can disrupt cell membranes within the target lesion.

Radiation forces are the energy that develops when the ultrasound waves are either absorbed or reflected in a nonliquid medium like human tissue. These forces press against the medium, producing radiation pressure and subsequent mechanical cell damage. With all these destructive mechanisms, irreversible cell death occurs through coagulative necrosis and apoptosis. Coagulative necrosis is the primary mechanism for tumor cell destruction in HIFU treatment, in which there is denaturation of protein and lipid bilayers of tumor cells. In the process of apoptosis, there is evidence of cell self-destruction and rapid degradation of DNA by endonucleases. It is

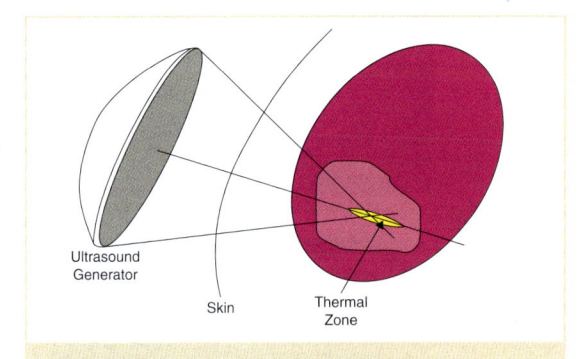

Figure 16-1: Accumulation of acoustic energy from different ultrasound beams leads to lethal thermal changes within the target lesion.

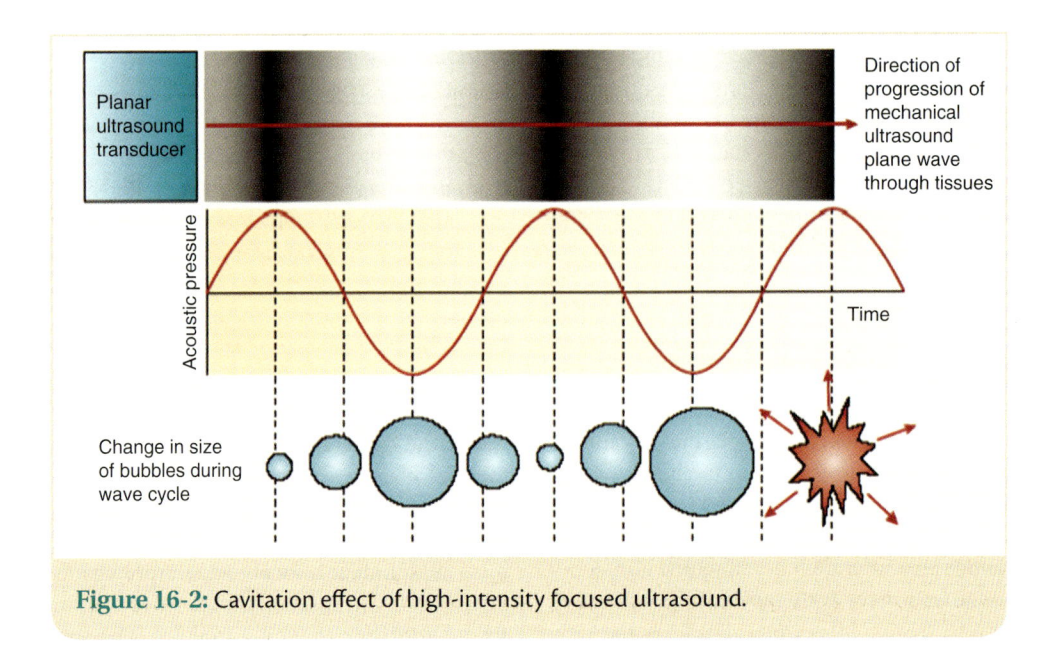

Figure 16-2: Cavitation effect of high-intensity focused ultrasound.

postulated that apoptosis may be an important delayed bioeffect in the tissue exposed to HIFU, especially in poorly regenerating cells.

The JC HIFU system (Chongqing Haifu Technology, Chongqing, China) is an ultrasound-guided system (Figure 16-3). The ablation process is guided by real-time ultrasound imaging. This system is composed of a real-time diagnostic ultrasound device, integrated ultrasound therapy transducer (12 cm in diameter), a six-directional therapeutic planning system, an ultrasound generator, a degassed water circulation unit, and a computer unit for automated master control. The focused ultrasound is produced by the transducer operating at 0.8 MHz (aperture 120 mm, focal length 150 mm). The target lesion is identified using an integral central 3.5 MHz diagnostic ultrasound probe, which is integrated in the center of the therapeutic transducer. Both diagnostic and therapeutic ultrasound beams are emitted simultaneously in the same direction (Figure 16-4). The degassed water provides optimal acoustic environment between the transducer and the patient. The focal region of the HIFU transducer is ellipsoid in shape, with dimensions of 9.8 mm along the beam axis and 1.3 mm in the transverse direction. Treatment by HIFU is performed under general anesthesia. Prior to treatment, the patient's skin is shaved and degassed in the area of treatment. The patient is then anesthetized and endotracheal intubation is carried out. General anesthesia is necessary to alleviate deep visceral pain caused by HIFU and to ensure immobilization. Temporary inspiratory or expiratory control by the anesthesiologist helps to minimize the liver movement caused by ventilation during HIFU treatment. In patients with tumors at the dome of liver, an artificial right pleural effusion is induced before HIFU treatment. A 12 gauge pinal is inserted at the ninth intercostal space along the mid-axillary line into the right pleural cavity under ultrasound guidance. Eight-hundred milliliters of normal saline is infused into the right pleural cavity. The patient is then put in the prone or right lateral position and immobilized. Detailed treatment planning is carried out according to the tumor size and location as detected by the diagnostic ultrasound transducer. The target tumor is then divided into parallel slides separated by 5 mm. Using provisional therapeutic parameters based on the depth and vascular supply of the target tumor, the tumor on each slide is completely ablated from the deep to superficial regions by successful sweeps of the HIFU treatment head. The ablation process is repeated region by region to achieve coverage of the entire tumor ablation (Figure 16-5). During the

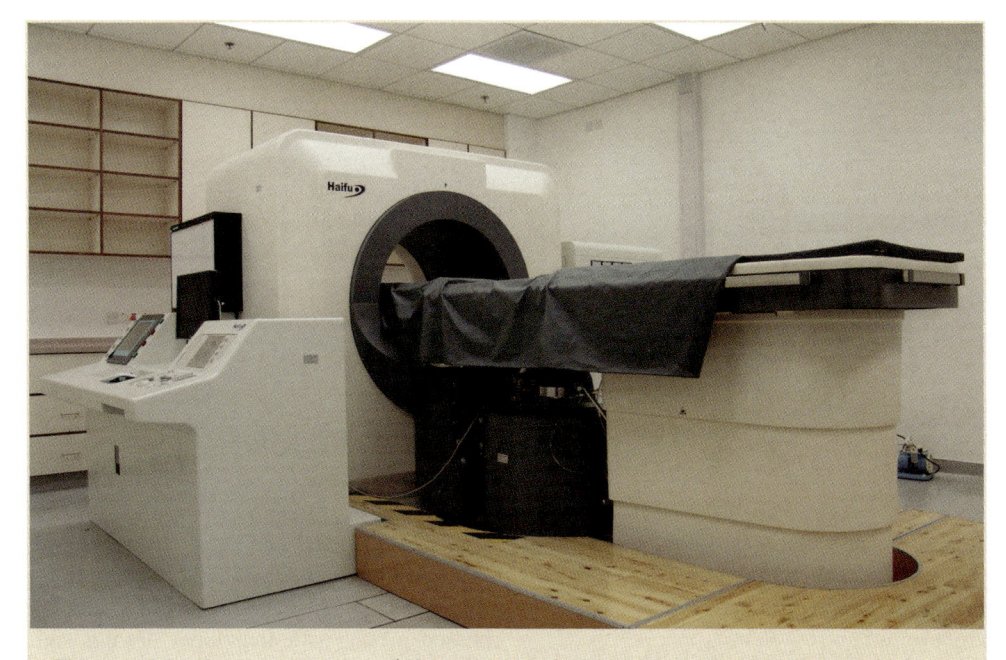

Figure 16-3: The JC HIFU system (Chongqing Haifu Technology, Chongqing, China).

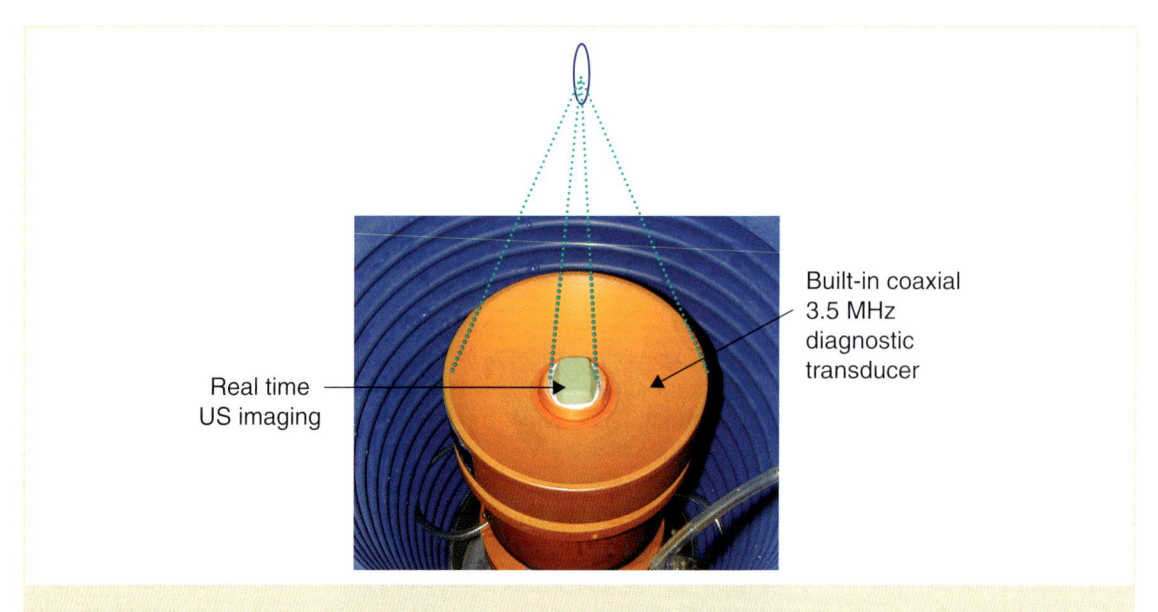

Figure 16-4: Diagnostic and therapeutic ultrasound of JC HIFU system (Chongqing Haifu Technology, Chongqing, China).

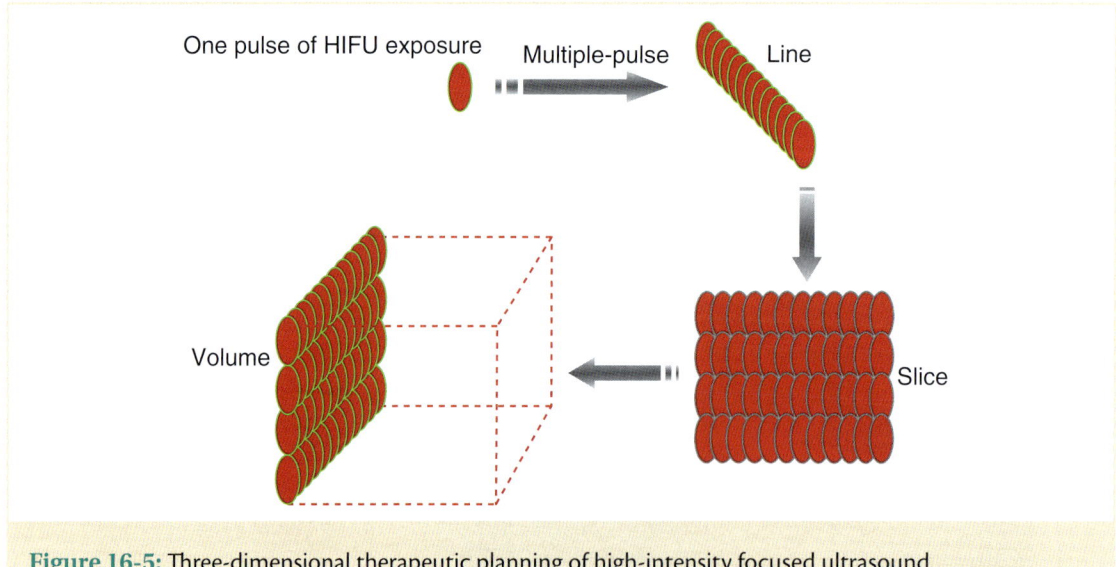

Figure 16-5: Three-dimensional therapeutic planning of high-intensity focused ultrasound.

procedure, gray-scale changes on the ultrasound images following each therapeutic exposure are used to evaluate the extent of coagulative necrosis of the target tumor.

The magnetic resonance image (MRI)-guided HIFU is another system based on MRI as the guiding imaging study. The latest developed transducers (ExAblate 2000, 3000, 4000, InSightec, Haifa, Israel) consist of increasing numbers of multiple-element phased arrays with individual driving signals and the ability to electronically steer the focus within a limited zone.[10] Using this system, numerous focal points can be applied in the target area. Thus, it can reduce the treatment time and increase the accuracy of the targeting power. When a moving organ like liver is treated with this system, the focal point can be steered in real time to further improve the targeting of HIFU. Another advantage of the phased array is its potential use in correcting or compensating for bone-caused phase distortion. Since the liver is covered by the right lower rib cage, it is possible to block and activate elements of the multiple-element phased arrays that are overlapping the ribs in order to avoid the unnecessary skin complications. Practically, MRI enables the accurate definition of liver tumor margins and the detection of ablation volume. The ability of MRI to perform temperature mapping is also critical for monitoring and controlling the HIFU treatment.[11] With temperature monitoring, various sonications can be tailored to achieve the desired temperature within the target lesion. The temperature/time curves at each location allows for the prediction of what tissue has been successfully ablated, resulting in a closed-loop feedback.

Initial Development of HIFU

Wood and Loomis first described the biologic and chemical effects of acoustic energy in 1927. By 1942, Lynn et al. studied the application of HIFU for liver tumors using animal models. However, the success of these studies was hindered by the fact that the ribs acted as an obstacle in the way of the merging ultrasound beams. In 1950, Fry et al. started to use HIFU for brain diseases including tumors. This pioneering work had initiated extensive further research for HIFU as an effective treatment for abdominal tumors.[5] Two major obstacles had to be overcome in the development of HIFU for liver tumors. First, the liver moves with respiration and the monitoring HIFU procedure and precise control of energy deposition within the target volume is essential for treatment success. Hence, a temperature-sensitive and motion-insensitive imaging method is necessary. Second, the obstructing bony ribcage can represent a seemingly impenetrable acoustic window. Currently, MRI has emerged as the image guidance method for HIFU because of its ability to detect tumors with high sensitivity and to monitor and quantify temperature changes. On the other hand, ultrasound imaging has the advantages of wide availability, portability, and low cost. Combined with ultrasound contrast agents, its diagnostic power is similar as that of MRI. Nevertheless, the ability of the accurate assessment of tissue ablation by ultrasound is inferior to that of MRI.

Clinical Applications of HIFU for Liver Cancer

The application of HIFU technology in the management of patients with advanced liver cancer is still in its infancy period. The feasibility and safety of HIFU for liver tumors were demonstrated in early 1990. Following the success of animal studies, the first human treatment was performed in 1993, demonstrating that HIFU was feasible to treat liver tumors under minimal sedation. To avoid problems with organ motion, patients were trained to hold breath repeatedly during sonications.[12] However, this technology has not gained much enthusiasm, primarily due to the difficulties in targeting and monitoring of the ablation process. With the recent advance in ultrasound technology, the accuracy of targeting power of HIFU has much improved. The initial experience of HIFU for HCC was obtained from researchers in China using the JC HIFU system. In a study by Wu et al.,[13] 55 patients with large HCC (mean diameter of 8.14 cm) and cirrhosis received HIFU treatment. There was no major complication. Completeness of ablation was assessed in 26 patients and complete ablation rate was only 69.2%. The overall survival rates were 61.5% at 12 months and 35.3% at 18 months. In another study by the same group,[14] the efficacy of HIFU combined with transcatheter arterial chemoembolization (TACE) was compared with that of TACE alone in 50 patients with advanced HCC. Patients who had undergone combined treatment had significantly better survival than those who received TACE alone. In that study, only eight patients had MRI assessment for the completeness of HIFU ablation and the complete ablation rate was 88%. The efficacy of this HIFU system for the treatment of liver tumors was also validated in a Western population.[15]

Although the treatment efficacy and survival benefits of HIFU for patients with liver cancer were documented in the previous studies,[13,14,16–20] clinicopathologic factors influencing the completeness of tumor ablation and patient survival were not studied in detail. A study on 49 patients with unresectable HCC treated by HIFU was carried out in the authors' center from October 2006 to December 2008.[21] The selection criteria for HIFU were as follows: (1) The maximal tumor diameter was less than 8 cm. (2) The number of tumor nodules was less than three. (3) The tumor could be detected by ultrasound imaging and there was no bowel adjacent to the tumor. Each selected patient underwent a single session of HIFU aiming at complete ablation of all detected tumors. A total of 57 tumors were ablated. During the initial phase of the study period (from October 2006 to May 2007), 21 patients had transarterial injection of iodized poppy seed oil (lipiodol) into their tumors about two weeks before HIFU treatment because previous research suggested that lipiodol could reduce tumor blood supply and increase the deposition of ultrasonic energy in the tumor.[13,14] In the later phase of the study (from June 2007 to December 2008), 28 patients received HIFU only. Tumor response to HIFU was assessed by MRI, which was performed one month after the procedure. Successful tumor ablation was defined as complete absence of hyperintensity signal in T2W images and absence of contrast enhancement within the original tumor region (Figure 16-6). Any contrast-enhancing area within the original tumor region on postablation MRI scan indicated residual tumor. RFA or chemoembolization was performed in selected patients to treat residual tumors. All patients had monitoring of serum α-fetoprotein concentration, chest radiographs, and MRI scan every three months to detect tumor recurrence.

One patient in the early part of the series died of myocardial infarction one day after HIFU treatment. This patient had underlying ischemic heart disease, which was not diagnosed before the HIFU treatment. The hospital mortality rate was 2%. The treatment-related complication rate was 8.1% ($n = 4$). The complications included a first-degree burn in one patient and second-degree skin burn around the treatment zone in two patients. These complications were due to an error of higher acoustic power administration. One patient developed bruising over the right chest wall which extended to the right flank region. This was caused by bleeding from intercostal vessels that were injured during induction of the artificial pleural effusion. The median hospital stay was 4 days (range: 2–16 days).

Ten patients (20.4%) had residual tumors detected by MRI one month after the treatment. The primary technique effectiveness rate was 79.5% (39 of 49 patients). Taking into consideration the total number of ablated tumor nodules, the primary technique effectiveness rate was 82.4% (47 out of 57 nodules). Four patients received percutaneous RFA treatment

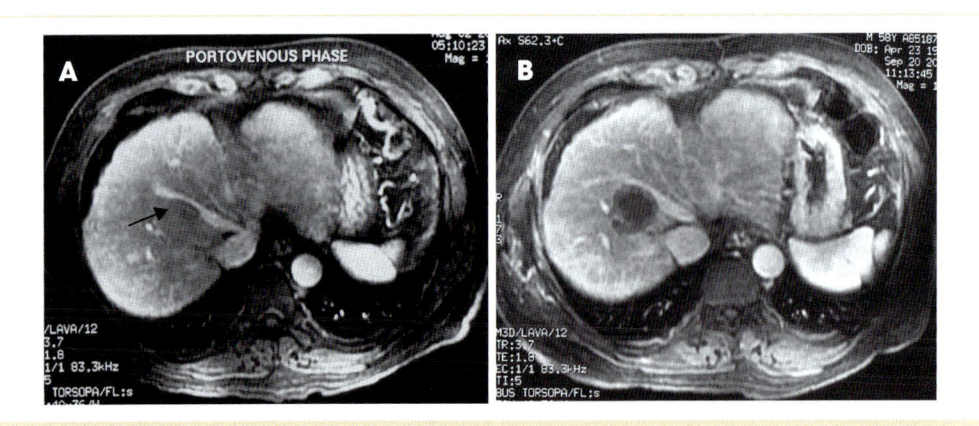

Figure 16-6: Magnetic resonance imaging scan shows a 2.7-cm segment VIII hepatocellular carcinoma before (A) and after (B) high-intensity focused ultrasound (HIFU) treatment. Arrow indicates the tumor impinging on the middle hepatic vein before HIFU treatment. Complete ablation was achieved after a single session of HIFU treatment without pretreatment lipiodol deposition. Thin rim of contrast enhancement surrounding the ablation zone represents benign peritumoral enhancement.

for residual tumor and three of them were rendered tumor-free after RFA. Another four patients having residual tumors underwent transarterial chemoembolization but tumor control was incomplete. The overall secondary technique effectiveness rate after HIFU and RFA was 85.7% (42 out of 49 patients). Tumor size was the only significant risk factor affecting the primary technique effectiveness rate of HIFU. Patients with primary technique effectiveness had significantly smaller tumors than those with residual tumors after HIFU treatment (median tumor size: 2.29 cm vs. 3.75 cm, $P = 0.013$). The cut-off value of tumor size as the significant risk factor for incomplete ablation by HIFU was 3.0 cm. The primary technique effectiveness for tumors <3.0 cm was 90.6% (29 out of 32 patients), whereas that for tumors ≥3.0 cm was 58.8% (10 out of 17 patients). The primary technique effectiveness rate of patients with HIFU alone (89.2%) was higher than that of those with HIFU and pretreatment lipiodol deposition (66.6%), although the difference was not statistically significant.

The median follow-up period was 24 months (range: 3–38 months). Among the 42 patients with tumors completely ablated by primary and secondary techniques, nine patients (21.4%) developed local recurrence at the HIFU treatment zone. All of these nine patients belonged to the group in which HIFU treatment was preceded by lipiodol deposition. On the other hand, all patients treated by HFIU alone did not develop local tumor recurrence at HIFU treatment site. Seventeen patients (40.4%) had intrahepatic tumor recurrence (away from the ablation site). Four patients (9.5%) developed extrahepatic metastasis. The overall recurrence rate was 61.9% (26 out of 42 patients). The one- and three-year overall survival rates were 87.7% and 62.4%, respectively. The one- and three-year disease-free survival rates were 40.7% and 0%, respectively. Among the clinicopathologic factors, Child-Pugh grade was the only significant prognostic factors influencing overall survival. The overall one- and three-year survival rates of the patients with Child-Pugh class A were 90.2% and 68.5%, respectively, whereas those of the patients with Child-Pugh class B were 75% and 33.3%, respectively ($P = 0.028$). The overall survival rates of patients with secondary technique effectiveness (one-year survival rate: 92.9%; three-year survival rate: 66.8%) were better than patients with residual tumors after sequential local ablation (one-year survival rate: 53.6%; three-year survival rate: 35.7%) ($P = 0.06$).

Conclusion

HIFU has emerged as a promising "ideal" noninvasive treatment for liver cancer. Recently, advancements in MRI and ultrasound imaging technologies have overcome the problem of tumor targeting and procedure monitoring and there is a new role of HIFU in the management of advanced liver cancer. Nevertheless, accurate respiratory motion compensation is yet to be resolved to ensure precise targeting and temperature monitoring. Future development in ultrasound transducer is still crucial for effective tumor ablation by HIFU.

References

1. El Serag HB, Mason AC. Rising incidence of hepatocellular carcinoma in the United States. *N Engl J Med.* 1999;340:745–750.
2. Poon RT, Fan ST, Wong J. Risk factors, prevention, and management of postoperative recurrence after resection of hepatocellular carcinoma. *Ann Surg.* 2000;232:10–24.
3. Mayo SC, Pawlik TM. Current management of colorectal hepatic metastasis. *Expert Rev Gastroenterol Hepatol.* 2009;3:131–144.
4. Kennedy JE. High-intensity focused ultrasound in the treatment of solid tumours. *Nat Rev Cancer.* 2005;5:321–327.
5. Fischer K, Gedroyc W, Jolesz FA. Focused ultrasound as a local therapy for liver cancer. *Cancer J.* 2010;16:118–124.
6. Dubinsky TJ, Cuevas C, Dighe MK, et al. High-intensity focused ultrasound: current potential and oncologic applications. *AJR Am J Roentgenol.* 2008;190:191–199.
7. Yang R, Reilly CR, Rescorla FJ, et al. High-intensity focused ultrasound in the treatment of experimental liver cancer. *Arch Surg.* 1991;126:1002–1009.
8. Holland CK, Apfel RE. Thresholds for transient cavitation produced by pulsed ultrasound in a controlled nuclei environment. *J Acoust Soc Am.* 1990;88:2059–2069.
9. Vaezy S, Shi X, Martin RW, et al. Real-time visualization of high-intensity focused ultrasound treatment using ultrasound imaging. *Ultrasound Med Biol.* 2001;27:33–42.
10. Hynynen K, Clement GT, McDannold N, et al. 500-element ultrasound phased array system for

noninvasive focal surgery of the brain: a preliminary rabbit study with ex vivo human skulls. *Magn Reson Med.* 2004;52:100–107.
11. McDannold NJ, Jolesz FA. Magnetic resonance image-guided thermal ablations. *Top Magn Reson Imaging.* 2000;11:191–202.
12. Vallancien G, Chartier-Kastler E, Harouni M, et al. Focused extracorporeal pyrotherapy: experimental study and feasibility in man. *Semin Urol.* 1993;11:7–9.
13. Wu F, Wang ZB, Chen WZ, et al. Extracorporeal high intensity focused ultrasound ablation in the treatment of patients with large hepatocellular carcinoma. *Ann Surg Oncol.* 2004;11:1061–1069.
14. Wu F, Wang ZB, Chen WZ, et al. Advanced hepatocellular carcinoma: treatment with high-intensity focused ultrasound ablation combined with transcatheter arterial embolization. *Radiology.* 2005;235:659–667.
15. Illing RO, Kennedy JE, Wu F, et al. The safety and feasibility of extracorporeal high-intensity focused ultrasound (HIFU) for the treatment of liver and kidney tumours in a Western population. *Br J Cancer.* 2005;93:890–895.
16. Li CX, Xu GL, Jiang ZY, et al. Analysis of clinical effect of high-intensity focused ultrasound on liver cancer. *World J Gastroenterol.* 2004;10:2201–2204.
17. Li YY, Sha WH, Zhou YJ, Nie YQ. Short and long term efficacy of high intensity focused ultrasound therapy for advanced hepatocellular carcinoma. *J Gastroenterol Hepatol.* 2007;22:2148–2154.
18. Wu F, Wang ZB, Chen WZ, et al. Extracorporeal high intensity focused ultrasound ablation in the treatment of 1038 patients with solid carcinomas in China: an overview. *Ultrason Sonochem.* 2004;11:149–154.
19. Wu F, Wang ZB, Chen WZ, et al. Extracorporeal focused ultrasound surgery for treatment of human solid carcinomas: early Chinese clinical experience. *Ultrasound Med Biol.* 2004;30:245–260.
20. Zhang L, Zhu H, Jin C, et al. High-intensity focused ultrasound (HIFU): effective and safe therapy for hepatocellular carcinoma adjacent to major hepatic veins. *Eur Radiol.* 2009;19:437–445.
21. Ng KK, Poon RT, Chan SC, et al. High intensity focused ultrasound for hepatocellular carcinoma: a single-center experience. *Ann Surg.* 2011;253:981–987.

CHAPTER 17

Radiotherapy for Liver Cancers

Guo-Liang Jiang & Jian-Dong Zhao

Historically, radiation therapy (RT) had not had a role in the treatment of hepatic malignancies due to the poor treatment platforms in radiation technology and poor radiation tolerance of the liver. Today, in the era of modern radiotherapy technology and increased understanding of partial liver tolerance to radiation radiotherapy, it is being used more frequently.[1,2] Early trials using modern techniques have resulted in encouraging outcomes for liver cancers, especial hepatocellular carcinoma (HCC), and prompted radiation oncologists to reconsider the role of radiotherapy for liver cancers. Modern RT technology, including 3-dimensional (3-D) conformal RT, intensity-modulated RT, image-guided RT, and the breathing motion control technique, has allowed escalation of irradiation dose to liver cancers with tolerable toxicity (Figure 17-1). In Korea, a recent multicenter retrospective cohort study of practice patterns and clinical outcomes on radiotherapy for HCC, included 398 patients with HCC over two years, and the predominant radiotherapy technique used was 3-D conformal RT (81.9%) with a total dose of ≥ 45 Gy. Both 3-D conformal RT and image-guided RT yielded three-year overall survivals of 30% by conventional fractionation. Although many of those studies were retrospective, it indicated that RT was quite effective in controlling HCC progression.[6] Recently more data have been published on stereotactic body radiotherapy demonstrating the feasibility of this technique and a better local control and lower morbidity, especially for small-sized HCC, when compared with the conventional fractionation.[7] With the most advanced technology of proton and heavy ion RT has showed an even more promising future with three-year local control rates of 80%–90% comparable with that treated by surgery.[4,5] Although at the present time, RT has been mostly considered as a palliative treatment for locally advanced HCC, it has increasingly been recognized as a potentially curative option for some liver cancer patients, especially for small-sized HCC (Figure 17-2).[3] For metastatic liver cancers, radiotherapy has also been a palliative treatment choice, but for selected patients, it could be curative (Figure 17-3).

Radiosensitivity of HCC

In the past, HCC has been misunderstood as a radioresistant tumor. This concept resulted from poor clinical outcomes of the early clinical studies, which used total liver radiation and insufficient radiation doses so as to avoid radiation-induced liver disease (RILD). Through the accumulated experiences using substantial doses with conformal radiotherapy, the radiosensitivity of HCC has been regarded as moderate similar to epithelium carcinomas.[8–10]

Hepatic Cirrhosis

It should be noted that HCC is a complex disease with cancer and chronic liver disease. Asia has a disproportionately large share of the world's HCC, mainly because of the endemic status of chronic hepatitis B virus infection, which leads

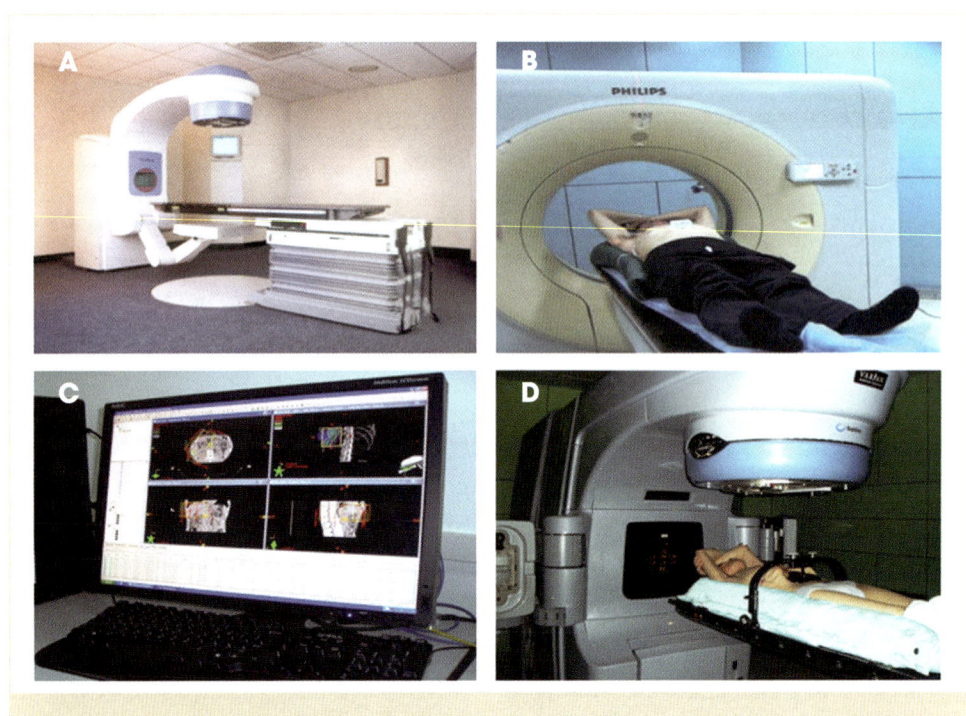

Figure 17-1: Radiotherapy platforms. Conventional simulator (A) (courtesy of Varian) and computerized tomography simulator (B); radiation treatment planning system (C); linear accelerator (D).

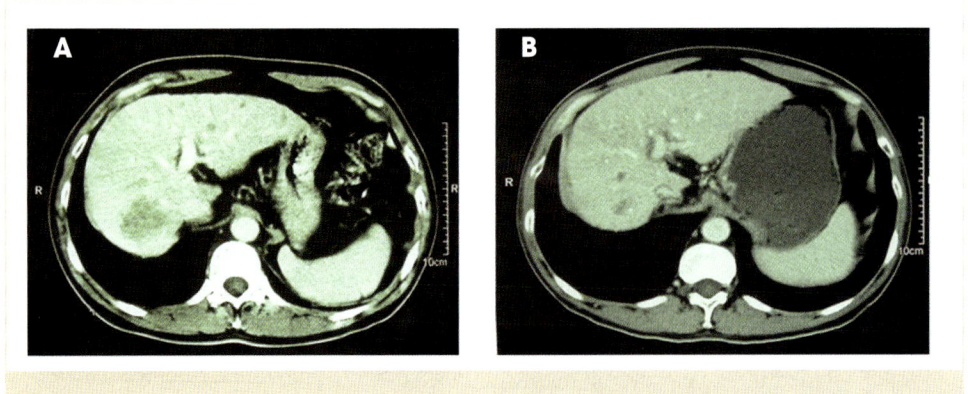

Figure 17-2: (A) Computed tomography image of a patient with HCC before RT; (B) five months after RT with 54 Gy in 27 fractions, showing a remarkably reduction in lesion size.

to liver cirrhosis and an increased risk of HCC. Other risk factors leading to liver cirrhosis include heavy exposure to aflatoxin, algal hepatotoxins, betel nut chewing, diabetes mellitus, and alcohol abuse.[11] Several clinical studies have demonstrated that the severity of hepatic cirrhosis was an independent predictor of RILD.[12,13] Therefore, prescribed radiation dose should be tailored according to severity of hepatic cirrhosis and liver function reservation.

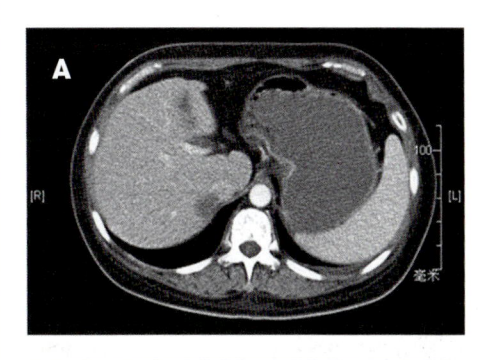

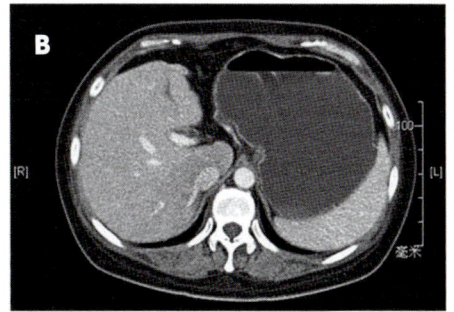

Figure 17-3: (A) Pre-RT computed tomography image of a segment six liver metastasis from breast cancer treated with 40 Gy in 10 fractions using active breathing control. (B) Post-RT complete response at three months.

Liver Regeneration

The liver is a unique organ that has a strong potential to regenerate after physical, biological, or chemical injury. An experiment on rats showed partial liver irradiation could stimulate the unirradiated liver to regenerate[14] Ren and colleagues did a series of studies to investigate liver proliferation after partial liver irradiation. For healthy rats, 25 Gy partial liver irradiation could stimulate regeneration in the protected liver and low-dose irradiated liver. In livers receiving 2.5–7.5 Gy, the potential to regenerate was stronger than in higher dose-irradiated livers. However, irradiation delayed hepatocyte mitosis. For rats associated with thioacetamide induced hepatic cirrhosis, both unirradiated and low dose—irradiated cirrhotic livers were able to regenerate triggered by partial liver irradiation.[19] Higher doses and irradiation to larger areas of the liver triggered a more enhanced regeneration. In clinical practice, several authors have also found unirradiated liver regions regenerating about one year after liver cancer radiotherapy.[10,15,16] For HCC patients with hepatic cirrhosis after proton radiation, the untreated liver portion also showed compensatory hypertrophy following radiotherapy.[17] Those findings hint that if enough normal liver tissue is protected or irradiated to a threshold dose (which was mean liver segment doses less than 23.9 Gy reported by Pan et al.[18]), the spared liver could regenerate to compensate for the radiation deteriorated liver function.

The classic critical volume model classifies liver as the parallel organ, and radiation damage to a portion of liver may not impair the entire liver function. As long as the volume irradiated is limited and enough liver tissue is spared, radiation dose can be escalated to the tumoricidal level without deteriorating liver function. In a recent (2009) radiotherapy clinical trial of Chinese HCC associated with hepatic cirrhosis, results showed the radiation dose could be safely escalated to 62 Gy for tumor diameters of 5–10 cm and 52 Gy for those bigger than or equal to 10 cm.[19] In another phase I/II trial of stereotactic body radiation therapy (SBRT) for liver metastases, 700 mL of normal liver was required to be spared, which had to receive <15 Gy, and the total dose was safely escalated from 36 to 60 Gy in three fractions.[20]

Liver regeneration after partial liver irradiation could be explored in liver irradiation to reduce hepatic toxicity and to prevent hepatic failure due to liver irradiation injury. When a liver irradiation plan is designed, protection of a part of normal liver tissue from being irradiated and keeping irradiation dose to the normal liver as low as possible should be always kept in mind.

Radiation-induced Lung Disease (RILD)

The most severe complication in liver irradiation is RILD, which is an almost fatal late complication.[21–23] The definition of RILD was proposed by

Lawrence and colleagues.[22] It occurs two weeks to several months after the completion of irradiation and manifests as either (1) classic RILD with anicteric elevation of alkaline phosphatase level of at least twofold the upper limit of normal level and nonmalignant ascites or (2) nonclassic RILD with elevated transaminases of at least fivefold the upper normal limit or of pretreatment levels (grade 3 or 4 hepatic toxicity of CTC). However, progression of liver cancer should be ruled out for the diagnosis of RILD. Histopathologically, RILD is characterized by a pathologic change of venous occlusive disease, which is irreversible and refractory to treatment. Once RILD occurs, steroids could be used to relieve symptoms, but the mortality rate is over 80%. Therefore, prevention of RILD is critical.

Liver Irradiation Tolerance and Lyman Model in Predicting RILD

Since the high mortality of RILD has been recognized, prevention of RILD should be of paramount importance when a hepatic irradiation plan is designed and optimized. The dose to the normal liver should be kept at a tolerable level. For livers without cirrhosis, the tolerable doses are 50, 45, and 30 Gy, respectively, for one-third volume, two-third volume, and whole liver irradiation when conventional fractionation is used (2 Gy/fraction, 5 fractions per week).[70] For a cirrhotic liver, the tolerance doses are much less than normal livers because of the jeopardized liver potential for repair and repopulation. From the experience in HCC irradiation, which included 109 patients, using the Child-Pugh grading scale for liver cirrhosis, 93 cases (85%) were Child-Pugh grade A and 16 cases (15%) were Child-Pugh grade B irradiated by hypofractionation (5 Gy/fraction, 3 fractions per week). The tolerance dose was mean dose to normal liver of 23 Gy. A dose volume histogram was proposed to illustrate the tolerance dose in a homogenously irradiated liver.[1]

For irradiation plan optimization, a few dosimetric models that make use of dose–volume histograms have been generated to quantify the probability of RILD.[22,24] The Lyman model was one of the models widely used to predict the normal-tissue complication probability (NTCP). This model assumed a sigmoid relationship between a uniform radiation dose given to a part of the volume in an organ and the probability of a complication.[25] The parameters of the Lyman model reported by Michigan University for patients who were treated with hyperfractionated 3D conformal RT and fluorodeoxyuridine were n = 0.97, m = 0.12, tolerance dose for 50% complication risk for whole organ irradiated uniformly (TD50(1)) = 45.8 Gy for patients with liver metastases and TD50(1) = 39.8 Gy for patients with primary hepatobiliary cancer.[28] However, the patients with HCC are more susceptible to RILD because of underlying cirrhosis.[26,27] Liang and colleagues retrospectively analyzed 109 HCC patients with hepatic cirrhosis treated by hypofractionated irradiation and reported modifications of n = 1.1, m = 0.28, and TD50 (1) = 40.5 Gy and n = 0.7, m = 0.43, and TD50 (1) = 23 Gy for patients with liver function of Child-Pugh A and B, respectively.[13]

The differences of liver irradiation tolerance in the Lyman NTCP model between North America and Asia were predominantly attributed to liver background difference. The North American data were mostly derived from irradiation of metastatic liver cancers which were not associated with hepatic cirrhosis. In addition in the Liang series, hypofractionation with 5 Gy/fraction, 3 fractions per week, and TACE used in one-third of patients rendered poor irradiation tolerance.

One should be aware of the hepatic background when liver irradiation tolerance is discussed. When irradiating a liver with intact liver function, the Michigan Lyman model is appropriate for the prediction of RILD, but the liver with impaired liver function, the modified Lyman model should be applied.[29]

The fractionation is another issue to be considered in liver tolerance. Tai and colleagues proposed a new expression of normalized total dose (NTD) to convert NTCP data between different treatment schemes. This new form of NTD may be used to predict NTCP for treatment planning of innovative liver irradiation with different fractionations, such as hypofractioned stereotactic body RT.[30]

Fraction Size of Radiation Dose

Tai and colleagues have developed a radiobiologic model for primary liver tumors. Through analyzing three published clinical series of primary liver cancer treated with different dose fractionation. The radiobiologic parameters for liver tumors were estimated to be: α/β = 15.0 Gy +/− 2.0 Gy, α = 0.010 +/− 0.001 Gy (−1), T(d) = 128 +/− 12 day.[31] From radiobiology studies, the liver is considered as a late-responding normal organ with a low value of α/β.[32] Theoretically, hepatic tolerance doses would be lesser as the fraction size is increased, but with small size fraction by hyperfractionation, the liver tolerance would be improved, as shown by the Michigan group.

Determination of Total Radiation Dose

One of the guidelines for determining radiation dose was based on the portion of nontumorous liver volume and indocyanine green (ICG) retention rate at 15 minutes, which was proposed by Cheng and colleagues.[33] Radiation dose to the target volume ranged from 40 to 60 Gy depending on the tolerance and the functional reserve of the liver. It could be useful to prescribe a radiation dose to a patient with HCC, but clinical settings are much more complicated. For example, smaller tumors adjacent to stomach or duodenum with treatment doses more than 50 Gy may lead to gastrointestinal ulcer or bleeding. The ICG retention test needs to be combined with other variables (serum bilirubin level, serum albumin level, prothrombin activity, and ascites) to assess residual liver function more accurately.[34] Some authors suggested that post-treatment, not the pretreatment ICG retention rate of 15 could be a useful indicator for predicting RILD. Other authors only used the fraction of the nontumor liver receiving >50% of the isocenter dose to determine the total dose.[35] Thus the significance of the ICG retention rate of 15 as a guideline for radiotherapy requires further investigation. We advocate that patients with Child-Pugh B liver function should not be treated with RT.[13] According to the non-tumor liver portion and ICG retention rate guideline, some Child-Pugh B patients will have a high risk of developing RILD.

Another dose prescription policy came from a NTCP model for intrahepatic malignancy developed by Lawrence and colleagues.[22] Individualized doses were prescribed on the basis of the effective liver volume irradiated (Veff) and NTCPs of RILD of 10%–15%.[24,36] The parameters of the model mostly derived from irradiation of metastatic liver cancers.

In clinical practice, the situation looks more complex with several intercepting factors, such as presence of concurrent chronic liver disease in a majority of patients and frequent usage of combination treatment. Concurrent chronic liver diseases, which are more frequent in Asian patients, might deteriorate hepatic functional reserve. Combination treatment might also alter the hepatic functional reserve.[33]

Seong and colleagues retrospectively investigated the national practice processes of care and outcomes of radiotherapy for HCC in South Korea.[37] Three hundred ninety-eight patients with HCC from 10 institutes were selected for more detailed analysis. They had not found a consensus on the optimum radiation dose and fractionation schedule in radiotherapy of HCC. In the authors' experience,[38,39] the total tumor dose was decided by the physicians' own judgments according to the comprehensive consideration of patients' general conditions, hepatic function, and tumor size. In a dose-escalation clinical trial,[19] the maximum tolerated dose of 3-D conformal RT/image-guided RT combined with transcatheter arterial chemoembolization (TACE) for locally advanced HCC was studied. The patients with a solitary lesion and liver function of Child-Pugh A were included. The irradiation dose was safely escalated in patients with HCC by using 3-D conformal RT/image-guided RT with active breathing coordinator. The maximum tolerated dose was 62 Gy for patients with tumor diameter of <10 cm and 52 Gy for patients with tumor diameter of ≥10 cm.

Since HCC radiosensitivity is moderate, high doses to tumor is needed for sterilization, especially for larger tumors. It would be appropriate to deliver doses to HCC as high as possible as long as the liver and adjacent critical organs could tolerate it.

Management of Breathing Motion

One of the most pertinent issues during liver radiation is the target motion due to breathing, and it has been proven that breathing induced motion is mainly at cranio-caudal direction with a range of 1–3 cm.[40–42] To mitigate the motion, an extra margin is usually added to ensure sufficient coverage of the clinical target volume traditionally. As such, larger volume of normal liver would be irradiated, and the doses to liver parenchyma would be increased. Such planning strategy is usually associated with increased RILD.

Techniques including active breathing coordinator,[43,44] respiratory gating system,[45] and real-time tumor tracking system[46] have been tested to reduce the negative impact of organ motion due to respiration in liver cancer irradiation.

The optimal technique described above for a specific patient varies due to several considerations, including comfort, compatibility with the device, and regularity of breathing. It should be noted that despite those interventions, interfraction and intrafraction reproducibility and residual set-up errors of liver tumor position still exist due to the physiologic and pathologic changes in breathing pattern and changes in liver tumor shape and size during the radiation course. The reproducibility issue should be considered during the expansion of clinical target volume to internal target volume. It is advisable to verify the location of liver tumor at the time of simulation and before each treatment fraction through image-guided RT techniques.

Another method to alleviate the respiratory motion problems is to use 4-dimensional (4-D) radiotherapy, which would make determination of internal target volume more accurate. Its application and benefit are under investigation.[47,48]

Transcatheter Arterial Chemoembolization before RT

TACE has been widely used for unresectable HCC and metastatic liver cancers with relatively good outcome. Combination of RT and TACE is strongly recommended for the following considerations:

1. *To assist in the RT planning design:* Because the margin of HCC is not very sharp on computed tomography in many cases, the delineation of the gross tumor volume becomes inaccurate and difficult. However, after TACE, the gross tumor volume delineation would be easier than that without TACE due to the deposit of iodine in the tumor. Before implementation of the RT plan, it should be verified. The deposited iodine in the tumor makes the gross tumor volume visible under simulation fluoroscope, thus the RT plan verification becomes an easier job.
2. *Potential to reduce or delay the intrahepatic spread of HCC:* Although there are no prospective trials of direct comparison of TACE and TACE plus irradiation, Zeng and colleagues reported a retrospective comparison of patients treated with TACE alone and those treated with TACE plus irradiation. The three-year overall survival rates were 11% (54 patients) for TACE alone and 24% (149 patients) for TACE plus RT suggesting more effectiveness of TACE plus irradiation.[53]

Clinical Experience

Three-Dimensional Conformal RT and Intensity-Modulated Conformal RT

Computed tomography-based planning allows greater confidence in ascertaining the tumor target volume to be irradiated and surrounding organs at risk to be protected. The 3-D conformal RT technique uses multiple beams from different angles, including coplanar or noncoplanar beams, which focuses at the target with conformal shape of the beams aided by cerrobend blocks or multiple leave collimator. The shape of the high dose is conformal to the shape of the tumor in three dimensions, and on the other hand, the adjacent normal structures or organs at risk receive very low doses, but in large volumes. Thus, 3-D conformal RT could deliver very high irradiation doses to tumors, meanwhile sparing the adjacent critical organs.

Image-guided RT is another technologic advancement that can produce a modulated flounce pattern for each beam, thus facilitating the delivery of even more highly conformal RT, which can achieve the best target coverage and spare organs at risk. Dosimetric parameter comparison between image-guided RT and 3-D conformal RT has found the potential superiority of image-guided RT over 3-D conformal RT in HCC. Thomas and colleagues analyzed the planning computed tomography data of 15 intrahepatic tumor patients irradiated with 3-D conformal RT. Eight of 15 patients' planning target volumes were overlapped with stomach and/or duodenum. Because of the planning target volume dose homogeneity varies, the generalized version of the equivalent uniform dose was used to do the optimization. They concluded that image-guided RT has the capacity to improve the maximal dose achievable across the planning target volumes, expressed in terms of the *equivalent uniform dose*[55] Cheng and colleagues[56] redid image-guided RT plans for 12 patients with HCC who had previously experienced RILD after 3-D conformal RT. They found image-guided RT was capable of preserving acceptable target coverage and improving or at least maintaining nonhepatic organ sparing in HCC. However for the normal liver, they noted a reduction in NTCP with image-guided RT, despite a significant increase in the mean liver dose. The authors recognized that the true impact of image-guided RT on the liver might depend on the exact volume effect of this organ.

As early as 1993, the University of Michigan reported the safety and efficacy of combined treatment of primary hepatobiliary cancers with conformal RT and regional chemotherapy.[49] The final results from 128 patients of this series showed an objective response rate of 56% in patients with HCC, a median survival of 15.2 months, and one-year survival rates of 57% and five-year survival rates of 11%.[3]

Although the fractionation and total doses of RT for HCC varied considerably in a series of publications, clinical studies have indicated the effects of radiotherapy on liver cancer. Liang and colleagues reported a local response rate of 55% and a three-year overall survival rate of 33% for locally advanced HCC irradiated by 3-D conformal RT with hypofractionation by 5 Gy/fraction given every other day.[39] Another clinical trial with conventional fractionated radiotherapy for HCC yielded a median survival of 17 months and three-year survival of 28%.[38] In the literature, for locally advanced HCC response rates ranged from 20% to ~90% and one-year and three-year survival rates, 40% to ~70% and 15% to ~30%, respectively, after 3-D conformal RT (Table 17-1).

Stereotactic Body RT for Liver Cancer

SBRT requires extremely conformal dose distributions with high dose volumes that falloff very rapidly in all directions out of the target. This requires the use of multiple-shaped beams utilized by a variety of radiotherapeutic innovations including 3-D conformal RT, intensity-modulated RT, and image-guided RT. The other approach would be to use smaller nonshaped beams and reposition the beam to treat successive regions within a tumor target as is used with the Gamma Knife and Cyberknife.

Characteristics of SBRT include:

1. secure immobilization of patients and rigorous accounting of organ motion;
2. accurate repositioning from simulation to treatment and stereotactic registration between the target and a system of external coordinates before treatment delivery;
3. ablative dose fractionation delivered to tumor with subcentimeter accuracy and minimization of normal tissue exposure.

The use of ablative dose fractionation is the most critical characteristic, which disrupts both clonogenicity and cellular function.

SBRT studies have shown promising crude local control rates of 61%–95% with a low incidence of complications.[57] In general for liver cancer, the indications for SBRT are (1) the maximum lesion diameter should not exceed 5 cm in diameter and (2) the number of liver lesions less than or equal to three. However, the optimal dose fraction size and fractionation scheme for SBRT in treating liver lesions remains undefined.

In the early 1990s, SBRT started in Sweden for liver cancers. The first clinical trials of SBRT for HCC and liver metastasis showed its effectiveness. The doses of 15–45 Gy were delivered in 1 to 3 fractions. Tumor remission and growth delay occurred in most patients, and acute toxicity was not severe. All patients with HCC reached local control, and 18 of 19 metastatic liver cancers had tumors locally controlled. Hemorrhagic gastritis and duodenal ulcer occurred in two cases.[58]

Since then different dose fractionations of SBRT have been published. Herfarth and colleagues[59] used single dose of SBRT to treat 37 liver cancer patients with 60 unresectable lesions (the maximum diameter no >6 cm). The dose was escalated from 14 to 26 Gy, which was the maximum dose at a reference point with 80% isodose volume covering clinical target volume. Overall actuarial local tumor control rates were 75%, 71%, and 67% at 6-month, 12-month, and 18-months of follow-up, respectively. In the Mendez's study of eight patients with HCC and 17 liver metastases with total 45 lesions, different dose fractionations

TABLE 17-1: Outcomes after Conformal Radiotherapy for Liver Cancer

Author (y)	N	Treatment	Radiotherapy Dose (dose/F)	Response Rate	Median Survival (mo)	Overall Survival (y and %)
Robertson JM (1997)[50]	22	RT + HAC	48 or 66 Gy/(1.5–1.65 Gy/F bid)	90.9%	16	4 y: 20.0%
Seong J (1999)[51]	30	RT + TACE	44.0 +/− 9.3 Gy (1.8/F)	63.3%	17	1, 2, and 3 y: 67, 33.3 a
Seong J (2000)[52]	27	RT	51.8 +/− 7.9 Gy/(1.8/F)	66.7%	14	1, 2, and 3 y: 55.9, 35.7% and 21.4%
Park HC (2002)[8]	158	RT	48.2 +/− 7.9 Gy/(1.8/F)	67.1%	10	1 and 2 y: 41.8% and 19.9%
Zeng ZC (2004)[53]	54	RT + TACE	Median: 50 Gy/(2Gy/F)	76%	NA	1, 2, and 3 y: 71.5%, 42.3%, and 24.0%
Park W (2005)[54]	59	RT	30.0–55 Gy/(2–3 Gy/F)	66.1%	10	1, 2, and 3 y: 51.0%, 27.4%, and 14.6%
Ben-Josef E (2005)[36]	128	RT + HAC	40–90 Gy (1.5/F bid)	42%	15.8	3 y: 17%
Liang SX (2005)[39]	128	RT +/− TACE	53.6 +/− 6.6 Gy (4.88 +/− 0.47 Gy/F)	55%	20	1, 2, and 3 y: 65%, 43%, and 33%
Zhou ZH (2007)[38]	50	RT + TACE	43 +/− 6.3 Gy (2 Gy/F)	18%	17	1, 2, and 3 y: 60%, 38%, and 28%

Abbreviations: F, fraction; HAC, hepatic artery chemotherapy; N, patients; NA, not available; TACE, transcatheter arterial chemoembolization.

of SBRT were investigated based on different tumor size, which included 12.5 Gy/fraction for three fractions, 10 Gy/fraction for three fractions, and 5 Gy/fraction for five fractions. The dose was prescribed at 65% isodose volume. Local control rates were 94% at one year and and 82% at two year. The better local control rate (94% vs. 82%) and survival rate (85% vs. 75%) were seen in liver metastasis patients than that in patients with HCC. All tumors in the Mendez's study irradiated with 12.5 Gy/fraction for three fractions remained locally controlled, which suggests better local control with higher doses. RILD occurred in one patient and grade 3 toxicity in four cases.[60]

Lee and colleagues studied 68 patients with inoperable liver metastases treated at Princess Margaret Hospital, Hong Kong.[61] Individualized radiation doses were chosen to keep the same risk of RILD for three estimated risk levels (5%, 10%, and 20%). The median SBRT dose was 41.8 Gy (27.7–60 Gy) in six fractions over two weeks. The doses at the highest RILD risk level were safe and associated with no dose-limiting toxicity. Hepatic toxicity of grade 3 occurred in two cases, but no RILD was seen. The one-year local control rate was 71%. The median overall survival was 17.6 months.

Cardenes and colleagues at Indiana University[62] conducted a phase I individualized trial of SBRT for patients with HCC enrolling 17 patients. Dose escalation started at 36 Gy in three fractions (12 Gy per fraction) with a 2 Gy per fraction increment. The rates of complete response, partial response, and stable disease were 25%, 56%, and 19%, respectively. At a median follow-up of 24 months, the local control rate was 100%, and survival rates were 75% at one year and 60% at two years.

Wulf and colleagues[63] from University of Wuerzburg treated 24 hepatic lesions with 10 Gy/fraction for three fractions using SBRT. Their actuarial local control was 76% at one year and 61% at two years with no grade 3 or higher toxicities. Schefter and colleagues[64] completed a phase I dose-escalation study of SBRT for 18 patients with liver metastases. Dose-escalation began with 36 Gy and until 60 Gy in three fractions and did not find any dose-limiting toxicity. Recently, this same group reported a phase II study at their highest dose of 60 Gy in 47 patients with 63 metastatic lesions. One-year and two-year actuarial in-field local control rates were 95% and 92%, respectively, with a median follow-up of 16 months. Overall survival at two years was 30%, and only one patient experienced grade 3 toxicity.[20]

Goodman and colleagues recently published a phase I study of single-fraction dose-escalation study SBRT for liver metastases.[65] In this study, 26 patients were treated for 40 identifiable lesions from intrahepatic cholangiocarcinomas and HCC. The prescribed radiation dose was escalated from 18 to 30 Gy at 4-Gy increments with a planned maximum dose of 30 Gy. All patients tolerated the single-fraction SBRT well without a dose-limiting toxicity. After a median of 17 months follow-up, the cumulative risk of local failure at 12 months was 23%, the median survival was 28.6 months, and the two-year actuarial overall survival was 50.4%.

Proton and Carbon Ion Radiotherapy for Liver Cancer

Although particle therapy was started over 50 years ago, it was not commonly used until 2000. Because of modern technology in the manufacture of cychrotron and synchrotron combined with advanced techniques in diagnostic and therapeutic radiology, the dedicated facilities of particle therapy, mainly proton and carbon ions, have been available for cancer treatments. The clinical data including over 50,000 cases treated by proton and over 5000 cases treated by carbon ion demonstrates an excellent outcome which is much superior to RT methods utilizing photons. The predominant advantage of proton and carbon ion therapy is the sparing of normal organs adjacent to the tumor. In addition, carbon is three time stronger than photons for hypoxic tumor cell sterilization.

The clinical experience of particle therapy so far is very promising. Kato and colleagues[66] reported a phase I to II trial on 24 patients with HCC. Patients were irradiated by a carbon beam with total doses of 49.5–79.5 GyE at 15 fractions in 5 weeks. The local control rates were 92% and 81%, respectively, at one year and five years, and overall survival rate were 25% at five years. Tokuuye[67] treated 22 patients with HCC larger than 10 cm in diameter using proton beam radiation. Median total delivered dose was 72.6 GyE in 22 fractions. With a median follow-up period of 13.4 months, two-year overall, and progression-free survival rates were 36% and 24%, respectively. Kawashima[68] used the same fractionation scheme to treat 30 patients with HCC. A total of 24 patients achieved complete disappearance of the primary tumor. The local progression-free rate was 96% at two years and overall survival, 89% and 27% at one year and three years, respectively. Hepatic insufficiency was observed in eight patients within 4 months after radiotherapy. Bush[69] provided more evidence to support the role of proton radiotherapy from a phase II trial of 34 patients with HCC. They assessed six patients receiving liver transplantation 6 months to 18 months after proton radiotherapy (63GyE/15FX) and found that no tumor cells were detected in two patients by biopsy. The two-year actuarial local control rate was 75% and the overall survival was 55%.

Summary

Screening programs for HCC in China and Asia have not been widely carried out. Thus, once patients are diagnosed, only one-fourth are good candidates for surgery, and surgery is the only modality for cure at the present time. Unfortunately, none of the available modalities are very effective for the majority of medically inoperable and unresectable HCC. Because of this modern RT technology, including 3-D conformal RT, intensity-modulated RT, image-guided RT, stereotactic body RT and particle therapy, combined with a new understanding of HCC radiosensitivity, liver tolerance and RILD, RT has been reconsidered in its role in treating HCC. The clinical experience in utilizing these modern irradiation techniques has demonstrated sufficient evidence to change our practice in the management of HCC. Today, RT should be considered as a treatment choice for medically inoperable and unresectable HCC not only as palliative care but also a curative one for highly selected patients. These indications are single lesion, Child-Pugh A liver function and good performance status (EORTC 0-1 or KPS >=70). Portal vein tumor thrombosis is also an indication for palliation.

Regarding RT techniques, 3-D conformal RT is one of the choice, but intensity-modulated RT could be used for large sized lesions, with less normal liver tissue left affected and/or poor hepatic function. Particle therapy would be the best if facilities are available.

For RT fractionation, including fraction size, total dose, and total treatment time, there has not been consensus in the RT society. In general, conventional fractionation has been more often applied owing to the consideration of liver tolerability in a cirrhotic liver. For small-sized lesions or portal vein thrombosis, large fraction (hypofractionation) is also recommended. Prevention of RILD should be a priority and is critical for a successful RT plan. Intrahepatic failure is the major failure pattern after RT. Therefore, combination of RT and TACE, or immunologic modulators, or target therapy, for example, Sorafinib should be primary topics for further study.

Metastatic liver cancers have become a growing problem because of the increase of colorectal cancers in China and Asia. More patients are presenting with liver metastases. In addition to TACE and systemic chemotherapy, RT should be one of the options for treatment of liver metastases. The indications for a favorable patient include:

1. solitary hepatic lesion or lesions less than or equal to 3;
2. lesion size for each less than or equal to 5 cm in diameter; and
3. the interval between surgery for primary tumor and liver metastasis of longer than two years.

Hypofractionation by 3-D conformal RT or stereotactic body RT has been recommended. However, the optimum fractionation is unknown. For widely disseminated hepatic tumor with severe pain, whole liver irradiation could also be tried, but only for palliation.

References

1. Liang SX, Zhu XD, Xu ZY, et al. Radiation-induced liver disease in three-dimensional conformal radiation therapy for primary liver carcinoma: the risk factors and hepatic radiation tolerance. *Int J Radiat Oncol Biol Phys*. 2006;65(2):426–434.
2. Dawson LA, Ten HRK. Partial volume tolerance of the liver to radiation. *Semin Radiat Oncol*. 2005;15(4):279–283.
3. Hawkins MA, Dawson LA. Radiation therapy for hepatocellular carcinoma: from palliation to cure. *Cancer*. 2006;106(8):1653–1663.
4. Sugahara S, Oshiro Y, Nakayama H, et al. Proton beam therapy for large hepatocellular carcinoma. *Int J Radiat Oncol Biol Phys*. 2010;76(2):460–466.
5. Kato H, Tsujii H, Miyamoto T, et al. Results of the first prospective study of carbon ion radiotherapy for hepatocellular carcinoma with liver cirrhosis. *Int J Radiat Oncol Biol Phys*. 2004;59(5): 1468–1476.
6. Seong J, Lee IJ, Shim SJ, et al. A multicenter retrospective cohort study of practice patterns and clinical outcome on radiotherapy for hepatocellular carcinoma in Korea. *Liver Int*. 2009;29(2):147–152.
7. Greco C, Catalano G, Di GA, Orecchia R. Radiotherapy of liver malignancies. From whole liver irradiation to stereotactic hypofractionated radiotherapy. *Tumor*. 2004;90(1):73–79.
8. Park HC, Seong J, Han KH, et al. Dose-response relationship in local radiotherapy for hepatocellular carcinoma. *Int J Radiat Oncol Biol Phys*. 2002;54(1):150–155.
9. Cheng JC, Chuang VP, Cheng SH, et al. Local radiotherapy with or without transcatheter arterial chemoembolization for patients with unresectable hepatocellular carcinoma. *Int J Radiat Oncol Biol Phys*. 2000;47(2):435–442.
10. Dawson LA, McGinn CJ, Normolle D, et al. Escalated focal liver radiation and concurrent hepatic artery fluorodeoxyuridine for unresectable intrahepatic malignancies. *J Clin Oncol*. 2000;18(11): 2210–2218.
11. Poon D, Anderson BO, Chen LT, et al. Management of hepatocellular carcinoma in Asia: consensus statement from the Asian Oncology Summit 2009. *Lancet Oncol*. 2009;10(11):1111–1118.
12. Cheng JC, Wu JK, Lee PC, et al. Biologic susceptibility of hepatocellular carcinoma patients treated with radiotherapy to radiation-induced liver disease. *Int J Radiat Oncol Biol Phys*. 2004;60(5): 1502–1509.
13. Xu ZY, Liang SX, Zhu J, et al. Prediction of radiation-induced liver disease by Lyman normal-tissue complication probability model in three-dimensional conformal radiation therapy for primary

liver carcinoma. *Int J Radiat Oncol Biol Phys*. 2006;65(1):189–195.

14. Zhao JD, Jiang GL, Hu WG, et al. Hepatocyte regeneration after partial liver irradiation in rats. *Exp Toxicol Pathol*. 2009;61(5):511–518.

15. Andrews AE, Goff JB. Regeneration of the liver after radiation therapy demonstrated by liver scanning. *J Ark Med Soc*. 1973;70(3):109–110.

16. Tokuuye K, Sumi M, Kagami Y, et al. Radiotherapy for hepatocellular carcinoma. *Journal of Radiation Oncology, Biology, Physics*. 2000;176(9):406–410.

17. Ohara K, Okumura T, Tsuji H, et al. Radiation tolerance of cirrhotic livers in relation to the preserved functional capacity: analysis of patients with hepatocellular carcinoma treated by focused proton beam radiotherapy. *Int J Radiat Oncol Biol Phys*. 1997;38(2):367–372.

18. Pan CC, Krishnan U, Normolle D, et al. Liver regeneration in patients with intrahepatic malignancies treated with focal liver radiation therapy. *Int J Radiat Oncol Biol Phys*. 2007;69(3)(suppl 1):S81.

19. Ren ZG, Zhao JD, Gu K, et al. Three-dimensional conformal radiation therapy and intensity modulated radiation therapy combined with transcatheter arterial chemoembolization for locally advanced hepatocellular carcinoma: an irradiation dose escalation study. *Int J Radiat Oncol Biol Phys*. 2010;79(2):496–502.

20. Rusthoven KE, Kavanagh BD, Cardenes H, et al. Multi-institutional phase I/II trial of stereotactic body radiation therapy for liver metastases. *J Clin Oncol*. 2009;27(10):1572–1578.

21. Lawrence TS, Robertson JM, Anscher MS, et al. Hepatic toxicity resulting from cancer treatment. *Int J Radiat Oncol Biol Phys*. 1995;31(5):1237–1248.

22. Lawrence TS, Ten HRK, Kessler ML, et al. The use of 3-D dose volume analysis to predict radiation hepatitis. *Int J Radiat Oncol Biol Phys*. 1992;23(4):781–788.

23. Cheng JC, Wu JK, Huang CM, et al. Radiation-induced liver disease after radiotherapy for hepatocellular carcinoma: clinical manifestation and dosimetric description. *Radiother Oncol*. 2002;63(1):41–45.

24. McGinn CJ, Ten HRK, Ensminger WD, et al. Treatment of intrahepatic cancers with radiation doses based on a normal tissue complication probability model. *J Clin Oncol*. 1998;16(6):2246–2252.

25. Lyman JT. Complication probability as assessed from dose-volume histograms. *Radiat Res Suppl*. 1985;8:S13–S19.

26. Kim JH, Park JW, Kim TH, et al. Hepatitis B virus reactivation after three-dimensional conformal radiotherapy in patients with hepatitis B virus-related hepatocellular carcinoma. *Int J Radiat Oncol Biol Phys*. 2007;69(3):813–819.

27. Liang SX, Zhu XD, Xu ZY, et al. Radiation-induced liver disease in three-dimensional conformal radiation therapy for primary liver carcinoma: the risk factors and hepatic radiation tolerance. *Int J Radiat Oncol Biol Phys*. 2006;65(2):426–434.

28. Dawson LA, Normolle D, Balter JM, et al. Analysis of radiation-induced liver disease using the Lyman NTCP model. *Int J Radiat Oncol Biol Phys*. 2002;53(4):810–821.

29. Jiang GL. In response to Dr. Ten Haken et al. *Int J Radiat Oncol Biol Phys*. 2006;66(4):1272–1273.

30. Tai A, Erickson B, Li XA. Extrapolation of normal tissue complication probability for different fractionations in liver irradiation. *Int J Radiat Oncol Biol Phys*. 2009;74(1):283–289.

31. Tai A, Erickson B, Khater KA, et al. Estimate of radiobiologic parameters from clinical data for biologically based treatment planning for liver irradiation. *Int J Radiat Oncol Biol Phys*. 2008;70(3):900–907.

32. Fisher DR, Hendry JH. Dose fractionation and hepatocyte clonogens: alpha/beta congruent to 1-2 Gy, and beta decreases with increasing delay before assay. *Radiat Res*. 1988;113(1):51–57.

33. Cheng SH, Lin YM, Chuang VP, et al. A pilot study of three-dimensional conformal radiotherapy in unresectable hepatocellular carcinoma. *J Gastroenterol Hepatol*. 1999;14(10):1025–1033.

34. Chung H, Kudo M, Haji S, et al. A proposal of the modified liver damage classification for hepatocellular carcinoma. *Hepatol Res*. 2006;34(2):124–129.

35. Seong J, Park HC, Han KH, et al. Clinical results of 3-dimensional conformal radiotherapy combined with transarterial chemoembolization for hepatocellular carcinoma in the cirrhotic patients. *Hepatol Res*. 2003;27(1):30–35.

36. Ben-Josef E, Normolle D, Ensminger WD, et al. Phase II trial of high-dose conformal radiation therapy with concurrent hepatic artery floxuridine for unresectable intrahepatic malignancies. *J Clin Oncol*. 2005;23(34):8739–8747.

37. Seong J, Lee IJ, Shim SJ, et al. A multicenter retrospective cohort study of practice patterns and clinical outcome on radiotherapy for hepatocellular carcinoma in Korea. *Liver Int*. 2009;29:147–52

38. Zhou ZH, Liu LM, Chen WW, et al. Combined therapy of transcatheter arterial chemoembolization

and three-dimensional conformal radiotherapy for hepatocellular carcinoma. *Br J Radiol.* 2007;80(951):194–201.

39. Liang SX, Zhu XD, Lu HJ, et al. Hypofractionated three-dimensional conformal radiation therapy for primary liver carcinoma. *Cancer.* 2005;103(10):2181–2188.

40. Shimizu S, Shirato H, Xo B, et al. Three-dimensional movement of a liver tumor detected by high-speed magnetic resonance imaging. *Radiother Oncol.* 1999;50(3):367–370.

41. Davies SC, Hill AL, Holmes RB, et al. Ultrasound quantitation of respiratory organ motion in the upper abdomen. *Br J Radiol.* 1994;67(803):1096–1102.

42. Kubo HD, Hill BC. Respiration gated radiotherapy treatment: a technical study. *Phys Med Biol.* 1996;41(1):83–91.

43. Eccles C, Brock KK, Bissonnette JP, et al. Reproducibility of liver position using active breathing coordinator for liver cancer radiotherapy. *Int J Radiat Oncol Biol Phys.* 2006;64(3):751–759.

44. Zhao JD, Xu ZY, Zhu J, et al. Application of active breathing control in 3-dimensional conformal radiation therapy for hepatocellular carcinoma: the feasibility and benefit. *Radiother Oncol.* 2008;87(3):439–444.

45. Wagman R, Yorke E, Ford E, et al. Respiratory gating for liver tumors: use in dose escalation. *Int J Radiat Oncol Biol Phys.* 2003;55(3):659–668.

46. Kitamura K, Shirato H, Shimizu S, et al. Registration accuracy and possible migration of internal fiducial gold marker implanted in prostate and liver treated with real-time tumor-tracking radiation therapy (RTRT). *Radiother Oncol.* 2002;62(3):275–281.

47. Guckenberger M, Sweeney RA, Wilbert J, et al. Image-guided radiotherapy for liver cancer using respiratory-correlated computed tomography and cone-beam computed tomography. *Int J Radiat Oncol Biol Phys.* 2008;71(1):297–304.

48. Beddar AS, Kainz K, Briere TM, et al. Correlation between internal fiducial tumor motion and external marker motion for liver tumors imaged with 4D-CT. *Int J Radiat Oncol Biol Phys.* 2007;67(2):630–638.

49. Robertson JM, Lawrence TS, Dworzanin LM, et al. Treatment of primary hepatobiliary cancers with conformal radiation therapy and regional chemotherapy. *J Clin Oncol.* 1993;11(7):1286–1293.

50. Robertson JM, Lawrence TS, Andrews JC, et al. Long-term results of hepatic artery fluorodeoxyuridine and conformal radiation therapy for primary hepatobiliary cancers. *Int J Radiat Oncol Biol Phys.* 1997;37(2):325–330.

51. Seong J, Keum KC, Han KH, et al. Combined transcatheter arterial chemoembolization and local radiotherapy of unresectable hepatocellular carcinoma. *Int J Radiat Oncol Biol Phys.* 1999;43(2):393–397.

52. Seong J, Park HC, Han KH, et al. Local radiotherapy for unresectable hepatocellular carcinoma patients who failed with transcatheter arterial chemoembolization. *Int J Radiat Oncol Biol Phys.* 2000;47(5):1331–1335.

53. Zeng ZC, Tang ZY, Fan J, et al. A comparison of chemoembolization combination with and without radiotherapy for unresectable hepatocellular carcinoma. *Cancer J.* 2004;10(5):307–316.

54. Park W, Lim DH, Paik SW, et al. Local radiotherapy for patients with unresectable hepatocellular carcinoma. *Int J Radiat Oncol Biol Phys.* 2005;61(4):1143–1150.

55. Thomas E, Chapet O, Kessler ML, et al. Benefit of using biologic parameters (EUD and NTCP) in IMAGE-GUIDED RT optimization for treatment of intrahepatic tumors. *Int J Radiat Oncol Biol Phys.* 2005;62(2):571–578.

56. Cheng JC, Wu JK, Huang CM, et al. Dosimetric analysis and comparison of three-dimensional conformal radiotherapy and intensity-modulated radiation therapy for patients with hepatocellular carcinoma and radiation-induced liver disease. *Int J Radiat Oncol Biol Phys.* 2003;56(1):229–234.

57. Kavanagh BD, Schefter TE, Cardenes HR, et al. Interim analysis of a prospective phase I/II trial of SBRT for liver metastases. *Acta Oncol.* 2006;45(7):848–855.

58. Blomgren H, Lax L, Naslund L, et al. Stereotactic high dose fraction radiation therapy of extracranial tumors using an accelerator. Clinical experience of the first thirty-one patients. *Acta Oncol.* 1995;34(6):861–870.

59. Herfarth KK, Debus J, Wannenmacher M. Stereotactic radiation therapy of liver metastases: update of the initial phase-I/II trial. *Front Radiat Ther Oncol.* 2004;38:100–105.

60. Mendez RA, Wunderink W, Hussain SM, et al. Stereotactic body radiation therapy for primary and metastatic liver tumors: a single institution phase i-ii study. *Acta Oncol.* 2006;45(7):831–837.

61. Lee MT, Kim JJ, Dinniwell R, et al. Phase I study of individualized stereotactic body radiotherapy of liver metastases. *J Clin Oncol.* 2009;27(10):1585–1591.

62. Cardenes HR, Price TR, Perkins SM, et al. Phase I feasibility trial of stereotactic body radiation therapy for primary hepatocellular carcinoma. *Clin Transl Oncol.* 2010;12(3):218–225.
63. Wulf J, Hadinger U, Oppitz U, et al. Stereotactic radiotherapy of targets in the lung and liver. *Journal of Radiation Oncology, Biology, Physics.* 2001;177(12):645–655.
64. Schefter TE, Kavanagh BD, Timmerman RD, et al. A phase I trial of stereotactic body radiation therapy (SBRT) for liver metastases. *Int J Radiat Oncol Biol Phys.* 2005;62(5):1371–1378.
65. Goodman KA, Wiegner EA, Maturen KE, et al. Dose-escalation study of single-fraction stereotactic body radiotherapy for liver malignancies. *Int J Radiat Oncol Biol Phys.* 2010;78(2):486–493.
66. Kato H, Tsujii H, Miyamoto T, et al. Results of the first prospective study of carbon ion radiotherapy for hepatocellular carcinoma with liver cirrhosis. *Int J Radiat Oncol Biol Phys.* 2004;59(5):1468–1476.
67. Sugahara S, Oshiro Y, Nakayama H, et al. Proton beam therapy for large hepatocellular carcinoma. *Int J Radiat Oncol Biol Phys.* 2010;76(2):460–466.
68. Kawashima M, Furuse J, Nishio T, et al. Phase II study of radiotherapy employing proton beam for hepatocellular carcinoma. *J Clin Oncol.* 2005;23(9):1839–1846.
69. Bush DA, Hillebrand DJ, Slater JM, et al. High-dose proton beam radiotherapy of hepatocellular carcinoma: preliminary results of a phase II trial. *Gastroenterology.* 2004;127(5)(suppl 1):S189–S193.
70. Emami B, Lyman J, Brown A, et al. Tolerance of normal tissue to therapeutic irradiation. *Int J Radiat Oncol Biol Phys.* 1991;21(1):109–122.

CHAPTER 18

Yttrium-90 Microsphere Radiomicrosphere Therapy of Hepatic Malignancies

Seza A. Gulec, Tushar C. Barot & Yuman Fong

Introduction

Radiomicrosphere therapy (RMT) refers to an intraarterial administration of microspheres of *any chemical composition* labeled with *any radioisotope*. The first clinical applications of the technique date back to early 1960s.[1] Currently, the β-particle–emitting yttrium-90 (Y-90) is the radioisotope of choice for the commercially available resin and glass microspheres. The radioisotope Y-90 is a high-energy β-particle, which is incorporated in biocompatible microspheres measuring 30–40 µ. These preparations are approved for use in the treatment of primary and metastatic liver cancers, and many other uses are currently under investigation.

The intellectual basis of Y-90 microsphere treatment is the superior distribution of microspheres in the tumor compartment than the normal hepatocellular parenchyma. Tumor blood supply is mostly derived from the hepatic artery, as the neovasculature resulting from tumor angiogenesis is mainly based on hepatic arterial branches. Therefore, therapies infused into the hepatic artery would preferentially target tumor, proportional to the tumor to liver blood flow to perfusion ratio. Y-90 microspheres infused into the hepatic artery are entrapped in the microvasculature with a high tumor to liver concentration ratio. The result is delivery of a tumoricidal dose of radiation with limited radiation injury to the normal hepatocellular parenchyma (Figure 18-1).

RMT differs from nonradioactive transarterial particle therapies directed at tumor in one important aspect: namely that the goal is nonocclusive delivery of particles. In bland embolization or chemoembolization, the goal is to achieve occlusion of the tumor vasculature to produce tumor killing by hypoxia. In RMT, the therapeutic effectiveness requires continued blood flow to enhance free radical–dependent cell death.[2] Radiation combined with embolization-induced hypoxia is undesirable because the biologic response is optimized by preservation of blood flow, and hence oxygenation, to the target area.

Y-90 Microspheres Products in Clinical Use

Currently, there are two commercially available Y-90 microsphere products: Glass microspheres (Thera-Sphere; MDS Nordion, Ottawa, Ontario, Canada) and resin microspheres (SIR-Spheres; Sirtex Medical, Sydney, Australia). Both microspheres have relatively consistent sizes ranging from 20 to 40 µ. Neither product is metabolized or excreted and remains in the liver permanently. The main differences are in the density (gram/cubic centimeter) and specific activity (activity/sphere). The glass micro-spheres are three times heavier per

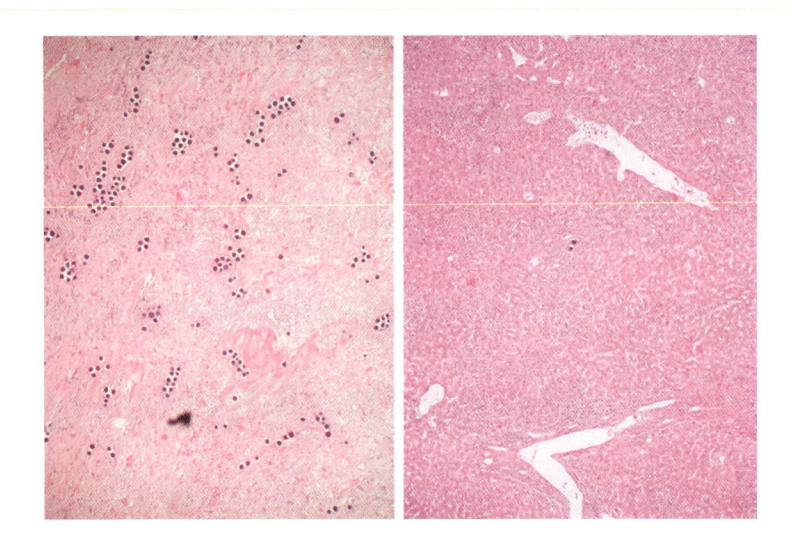

Figure 18-1: Distribution of microspheres infused by transarterial route into the liver. Note the arterial position of the microspheres within the tumor (left panel). The right panel shows the rare deposit of microsphere within the normal liver parenchyma.

volume and carry 50 times more activity per weight than resin microspheres.

Clinical Data for Hepatic Colorectal Metastases

There have been numerous studies testing the use of RMT using Y-90 microspheres as treatment for unresectable metastatic colorectal cancer (CRC). There have been a retrospective studies from New Zealand and the United States. More recently, encouraging data from phase I and II trials have led to two phase III trials.[3-7]

Retrospective data from New Zealand: The RMT technique adapted by Stubbs et al. involved administration of 2–3 GBq Y-90 microspheres into the hepatic artery through a subcutaneous port followed at four-week intervals by regional chemotherapy with 5-fluorouracil. An early report on 50 patients with advanced, unresectable colorectal liver metastases who were treated with RMT demonstrated that RMT was well tolerated with no treatment-related mortality. However, morbidity including duodenal ulceration was noted in 12 of 50 patients (24%). Median carcinoembryonic antigen (CEA) values one and two months after RMT (expressed as percent of initial CEA) were 19% and 13%, respectively. Median survival for patients who developed extrahepatic disease within six months of RMT ($n = 26$) was 6.9 months (range: 1.3–18.8 months). In those who did not develop extrahepatic disease ($n = 24$), the median survival was 17.5 months (range: 1.0–30.3 months).[8]

Retrospective data from the United States in the salvage setting: Cumu-lative data analyzed by Kennedy et al. on 208 patients who were treated at seven institutions with a median follow-up of 13 months (1–42 months) indicated a median survival of 10.5 months for responders and 4.5 months for nonresponders. No treatment-related procedure deaths or radiation-related liver failures were encountered. Response rates defined by computed tomography (CT), CEA, and 18-fluorodeoxyglucose positron emission tomography (FDG-PET) were 35%, 70%, and 91%, respectively.[9]

Phase I/II dose-escalation study in combination with oxaliplatin: Twenty patients were studied in a phase I/II dose escalation trial of systemic chemotherapy using FOLFOX 4 plus RMT. The study population consisted of patients with non-resectable, liver-dominant met-astatic colorectal adenocarcinoma, who had not previously been treated with chemotherapy. The investigators were successful at achieving safe delivery of standard doses of oxaliplatin (85 mg/m^2). The toxicity profile of combined FOLFOX and RMT was very similar to that observed in other phase III trials of FOLFOX 4 alone. The only difference was the presence of abdominal pain, which was reported at grade 1–3 levels in 50% of patients within 48 hours of RMT administration. These episodes of abdominal pain were self-limiting. The overall response as measured by Response Evaluation Criteria in Solid Tumors (RECIST) was 90% (complete response [CR] + partial response [PR]), with the remaining patients (10%) having stable disease. Of note, 2 of 20 patients in this study had their disease sufficiently downstaged to allow subsequently surgically resection.[5]

Phase I/II dose escalation study in combination with irinotecan: A phase I/II dose escalation trial of systemic chemotherapy using irinotecan plus RMT was also performed. Twenty-five patients who had failed previous chemotherapy, but were naive to irinotecan, were included in the study. Irinotecan was given, starting the day before RMT, for a maximum of nine cycles. The irinotecan dose was escalated from 50 to 100 mg/m^2. Early stage acute and self-limiting nausea, vomiting, and liver pain were experienced by most patients. Mild lethargy and anorexia were also common. Grade 3/4 toxic events were seen in 4 of 6 patients at 50 mg/m^2, 5 of 13 patients at 75 mg/m^2, and 2 of 6 patients at 100 mg/m^2. Of evaluable patients, partial responses were seen in 9 of 17 patients. Median time to liver progression was 7.5 months, and median survival was 12 months.[6]

Randomized phase II comparison of chemotherapy versus chemotherapy plus Selective Internal Radiation Treatment (SIRT) as first-line treatment (Chemo-SIRT Trial): A phase II clinical trial using resin micro-spheres concomitantly with modern chemo-therapy regimens as a front-line application was completed at the Center for Cancer Care in Goshen, India.[7] Patients with disease limited predominantly to the liver were eligible for the study. SIRT was administered to either one lobe or the whole liver on day 2 of the first chemotherapy course. Chemotherapy (FOLFOX or FOLFIRI) was repeated on a biweekly schedule. CEA levels, RECIST, and metabolic response by PET/CT were used to determine tumor response at 4, 8, and 12 weeks after therapy. Fifteen patients have been enrolled. Mean tumor-absorbed dose was 137 Gy (range: 50–285 Gy). Mean liver-absorbed dose was 39 Gy (range: 6–93 Gy). All tumors in chemo-RMT–treated lobes showed a response by PET criteria (functional volume [VF]) (Figure 18-2). Mean percent decreases in functional volume for chemo-RMT– and chemo-alone–treated fields were 86% and 35%, respectively. Mean percent decreases in anatomic volume for chemo-RMT– and chemo-alone–treated fields were 59% and 22%, respectively. A functional volume decrease of >90% (complete metabolic response) was observed in 73% of chemo-RMT and 40% of chemo-alone treatment fields. No disease progression was observed in the chemo-RMT–treated fields, whereas 27% of the chemo-alone–treated fields showed disease progression during the course of therapy. The changes in functional volume preceded the changes in cross-sectional scanning and can be documented as early as four weeks (Figure 18-3). The mean decrease in Total Lesion Glycolysis (TLG) values in the tumors receiving chemo-SIRT and chemo-only treatment were 86.26% ± 18.57% and 31.74% ± 80.99% ($P < 0.01$), 93.13% ± 11.81% and 40.80% ± 73.32% ($P = 0.01$), and 90.55% ± 19.75% and 54.91% ± 38.55% ($P < 0.01$) at four weeks, two to four months, and six to eight months posttreatment, respectively. Func-tional tumor volume changes were in concordance with the Total Lesion Glycolysis (TLG) changes (Figures 18-4 and 18-5).

Randomized phase III regional chemotherapy versus RMT plus regional chemotherapy: A randomized phase III trial was performed comparing hepatic arterial chemotherapy

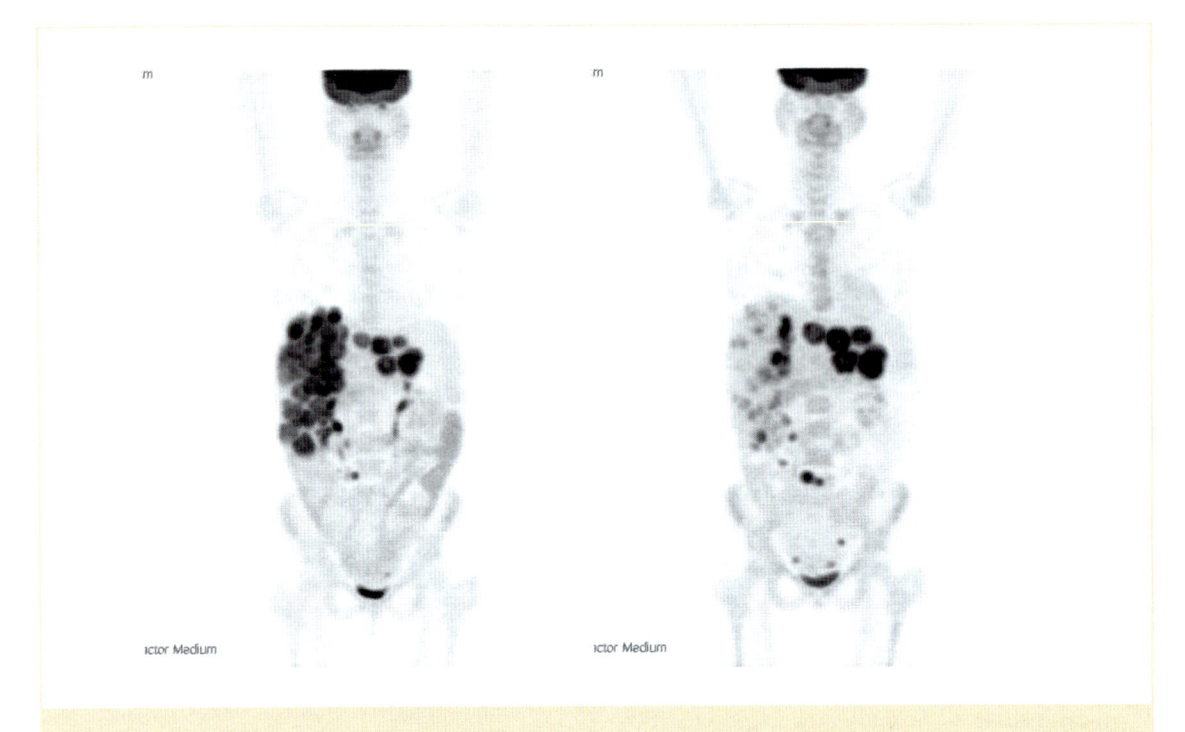

Figure 18-2: Positron emission tomography demonstrating response of tumor in the right lobe of liver to combined radiomicrosphere therapy and chemotherapy.

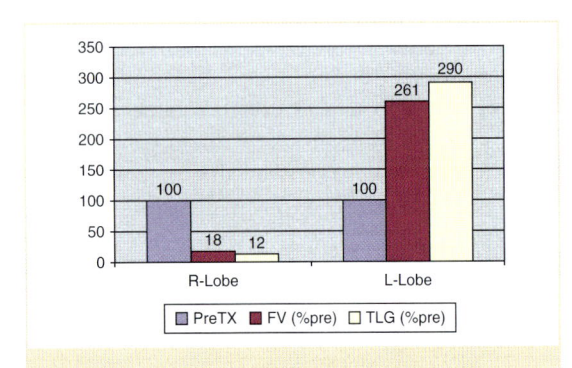

Figure 18-3: 18-Flourodeoxyglucose uptake before (Pre-transplantation (TX)) and after combined radiomicrosphere therapy (delivered to right lobe) and chemotherapy. Results are shown for right (R-lobe) and left lobe (L-Lobe) of the liver.

(Flurodeoxyuridine [FUDR] 0.3 mg/kg/d for 12 days and repeated every four weeks for 18 months) alone versus combined RMT (2–3 GBq of Y-90 activity) plus hepatic arterial chemotherapy with Flurodeoxyuridine. The outcome documented in this 74 patient trial showed significant improvement resulting from the addition of RMT to systemic chemotherapy.

Toxicity data showed no difference in grade 3 or 4 toxicity between the two treatment arms. There was a significant increase in the CR and PR rate (CR + PR = 17.6%–44%, $P = 0.01$) and prolongation of time-to-disease progression in the liver (9.7–15.9 months, $P = 0.001$) for patients receiving the combination treatment. Although the trial design was not of sufficient statistical power to detect a survival difference, there was a trend observed toward improved survival for the combination treatment arm (Figure 18-6). Exploratory subset regression analysis suggested improved survival for those patients who survived at least 15 months ($P = 0.06$).[3] Despite the high response rate from regional treatment of the liver metastases, failure to control the disease at extrahepatic sites was problematic among the

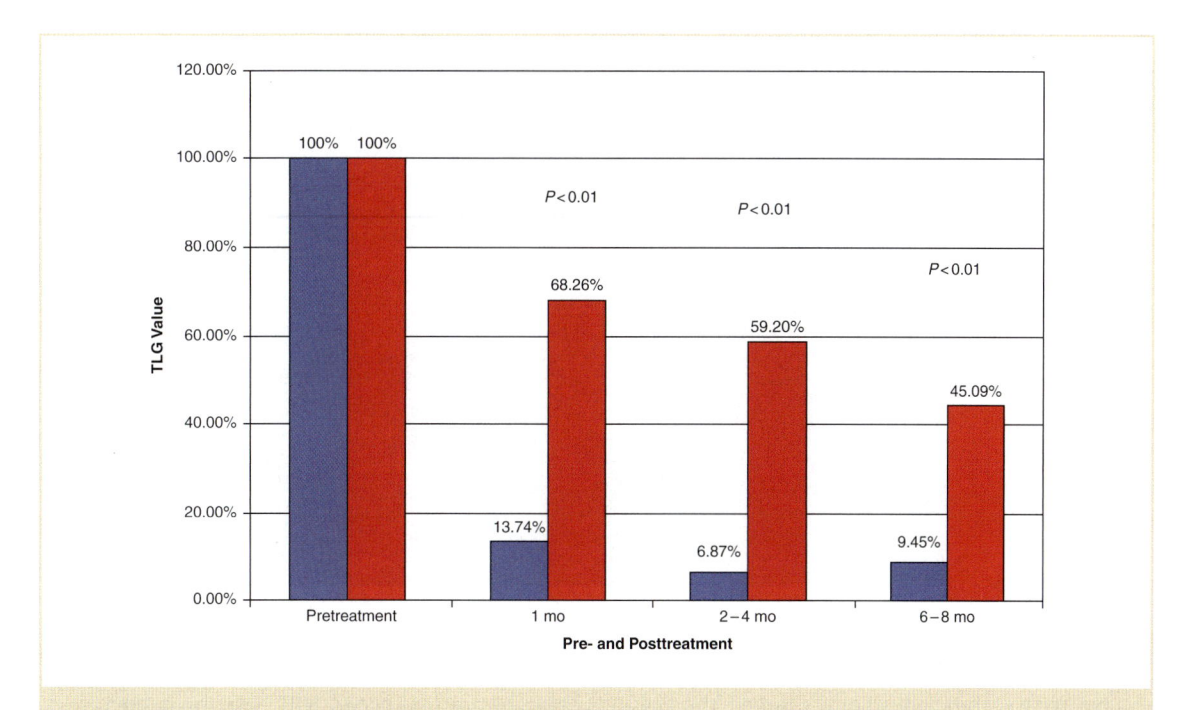

Figure 18-4: Total Lesion Glycolysis (TLG) values (%) in the tumor: pretreatment and posttreatment at 4 weeks, 2–4 months, and 6–8 months.

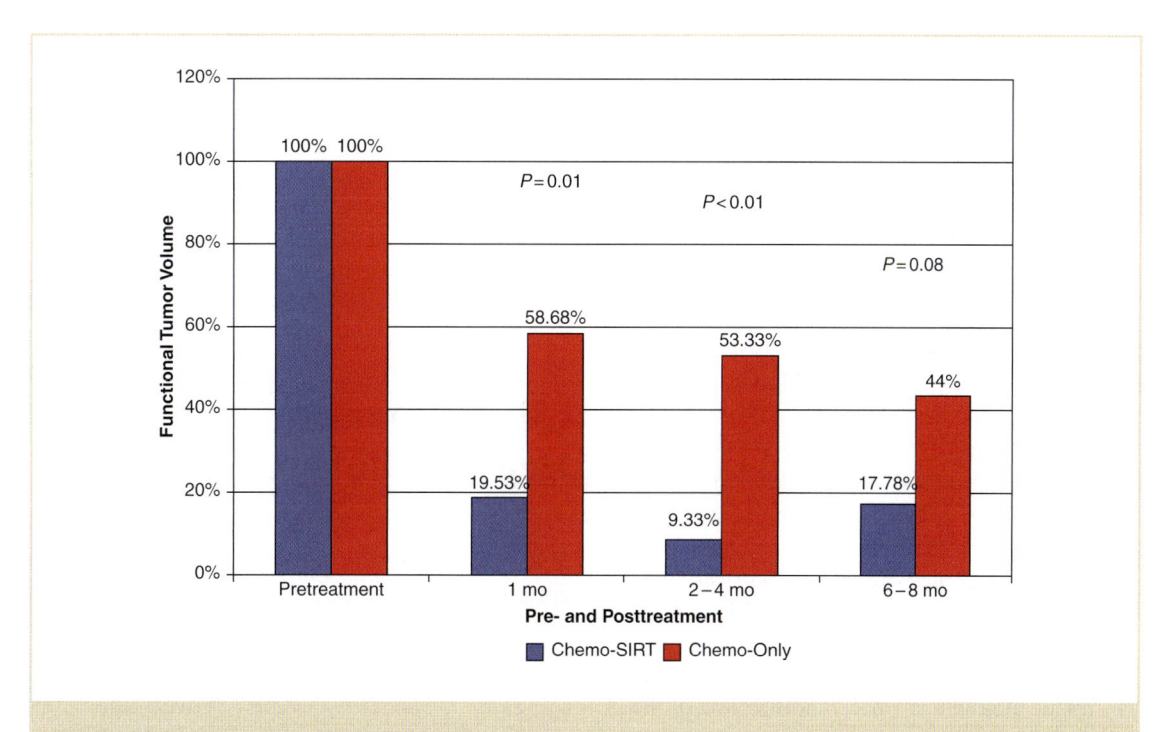

Figure 18-5: Functional tumor volume (%): pretreatment and posttreatment at 4 weeks, 2–4 months, and 6–8 months. SIRT, Selective Internal Radiation Treatment.

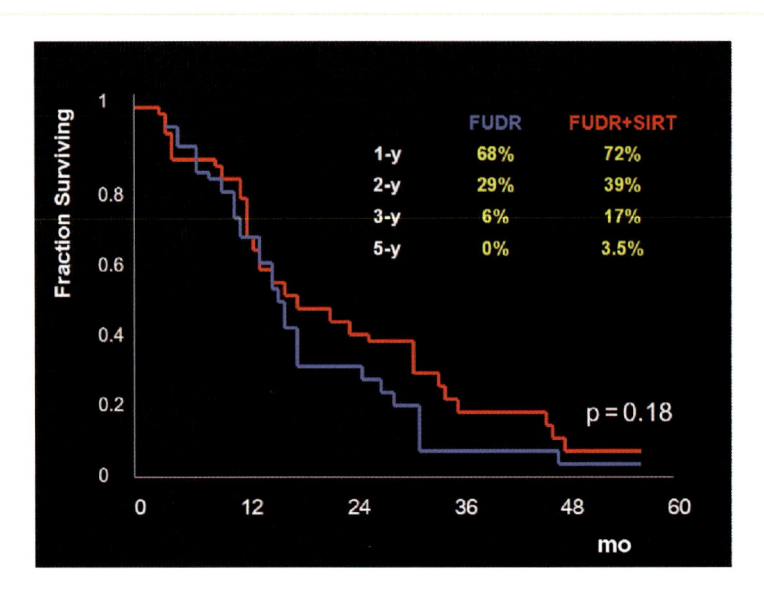

Figure 18-6: Overall survival of patients subjected to regional chemotherapy alone (blue curve) vs. those subjected to combined radiomicrosphere therapy and chemotherapy (red curve). SIRT, Selective Internal Radiation Treatment.

patients in this phase III trial. This is consistent with findings from the meta-analysis of hepatic arterial chemotherapy and indicates the need to add systemic treatment to this management strategy.

Randomized trial of systemic chemotherapy versus RMT plus chemotherapy: A study combining RMT with systemic chemotherapy (5-fluorouracil/Leucovorin) was designed as a randomized phase II/III trial. One arm was RMT in combination with systemic chemotherapy and the other arm was chemotherapy alone. The hypothesis tested in this study was that systemic chemotherapy potentiates RMT and results in better response rates in the liver. In addition, a beneficial effect of systemic chemotherapy on extrahepatic metastases was sought.

This trial accrued only 21 patients because of the impressive response to combined therapy (Figure 18-7). The toxicity profile was higher in patients receiving the combination treatment, although a dose modification of RMT decreased the toxicity profile to an acceptable level. Progression-free survival in the combination therapy arm was 18.6 months compared with 3.4 months in the chemotherapy alone arm ($P < 0.0005$). Overall median survival was 29.4 months in the combination therapy arm, compared with 12.8 months in the chemotherapy alone arm ($P = 0.02$). There was no difference in quality of life over a three-month period between the two treatments when rated by patients ($P = 0.96$) or physicians ($P = 0.98$).[4]

Clinical Data for Hepatocellular Carcinoma

There have been no randomized clinical trials with Y-90 microsphere treatment in hepatocellular carcinoma (HCC). However, an extensive worldwide clinical experience in this patient population has been reported.

Data from Hong Kong: Given the high prevalence of HCC in the region, Hong Kong has been a pivotal site for early (and ongoing)

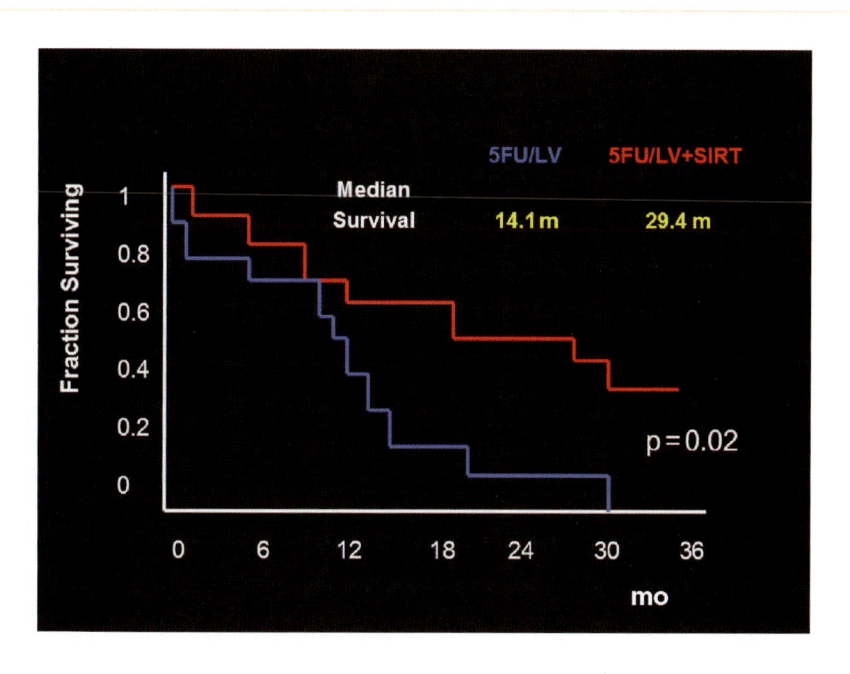

Figure 18-7: Overall survival of patients subjected to systemic chemotherapy alone (5-fluorouracil/Leucovorin) (blue curve) vs. those subjected to radiomicrosphere therapy and systemic chemotherapy (red curve).

experience with Y-90 microsphere safety and efficacy studies. Early Y-90 microsphere trials by Hong Kong investigators concentrated on issues of safety and efficacy. In 1998, Lau et al. reported that the objective response with respect to changes in α-fetoprotein level was 89% (PR 67% and CR 22%). Of additional importance, this study reported that nontumorous liver appears more tolerant to internal radiation than external beam radiation.[10] These investigators also correlated treatment efficacy with yttrium dose.[11] In a series of 18 patients treated with Y-90 microspheres for inoperable HCC, tumor regression was found to be dose related with statistically improved survival for those patients treated with tumor dose exceeding 120 Gy. In 2001, Lau et al. reported, in a series of 82 patients, variables that may predict a more favorable outcome (improved survival) following Y-90 microsphere therapy: lower pretreatment level of α-fetoprotein and higher tumor to normal Y-90 microsphere uptake ratio. This study was also important in suggesting that Y-90 microsphere treatment is effective for large tumors and tumor recurrence following surgical resection.[12]

Data from the United States: Most early clinical work in the United States has focused on patient selection criteria. In a series of 121 patients, Goin et al. reported poor prognostic indicators: infiltrative or bulky disease, increase in liver enzyme levels, tumor volume at least 50% in combination with decreased serum albumin, elevated bilirubin, or predicted lung dose of >30 Gy.[13] Patients with any of these risk factors were at a greater risk for early death (<3 months) and were at an increased risk of adverse events related to therapy. In the absence of these risk factors, patients demonstrated improved survival (median: 466 days) relative to patients in the high-risk group (median: 108 days).

Salem et al., who has published extensively on Y-90 microsphere therapy, has further stressed the importance of patient selection to optimize treatment outcomes and avoid unnecessary morbidity and mortality. One study with 43 patients reported a median survival of 24.4 months for early stage disease and 12.5 months for later stage disease.[14] The factors found to be associated with decreased survival included those reported by Goin et al.: presence of ascites, Eastern Cooperative Oncology Group performance status >0, presence of extrahepatic disease, >25% tumor burden, infiltrative disease, main portal vein thrombosis, and α-fetoprotein > 400 ng/mL. Salem et al. has also shown that, using appropriate selection and technique, Y-90 microsphere therapy can be administered to patients with compromised portal venous flow in the presence of portal vein thrombosis.[15] This report helped expand the patient population who can be treated safely with Y-90 microspheres.

Clinical Data for Neuroendocrine Metastases to the Liver

To date there have been no randomized clinical trials with Y-90 microsphere SIRT in carcinoid or other neuroendocrine tumors (NETs). In a retrospective analysis by Kennedy et al., both glass and resin Y-90 microspheres were evaluated in the treatment of 40 patients with NET. Radiographic response was demonstrated (CR and PR) in 93% (n = 34). There was low toxicity, and a subset of patients was able to discontinue palliative somatostatin therapy.[16] A recent report by Rhee et al. evaluated 42 patients treated with ceramic and resin microspheres. Greater radiotherapeutic activity was administered with ceramic microspheres without a significant difference in radiographic response (92% in the case of ceramic microspheres and 94% in the case of resin microspheres) with overall medial survival of 25 months.[17] Kennedy et al. has reported median survival of 70 months in a 148 patient cohort undergoing resin microsphere therapy for metastatic NET.[18] Therapy was well tolerated with only 13% of patients reporting toxicities of 3 or higher (nausea, fatigue, pain, or ascites).

Radiographic response reported as complete in 3% (n = 5), partial in 60.5% (n = 112), stable in 22.7% (n = 42), and progressive in 4.9% (n = 9).

An earlier retrospective study of 20 patients by Gulec et al. providing dosimetric data demonstrated that Y-90 microsphere therapy produced a significant objective response rate with no significant toxicity.[19] This study reviewed liver and tumor radiation doses using the medical internal radiation dosimetry technique. Liver toxicity was assessed clinically and by liver function tests, and the response to treatment was evaluated by octreoscan, CT, and tumor markers. All patients had unresectable liver disease. Fifteen of 20 patients (75%) were symptomatic despite maximal medical treatment, and 2 of 20 patients had extrahepatic disease. The average administered activity was 1.6 GBq (0.6–3.2 GBq). Liver-absorbed doses ranged from 0.3 Gy to 99.5 Gy (mean: 28.9 Gy). Tumor-absorbed doses ranged from 19.2 Gy to 262.7 Gy (mean: 128.5 Gy). No treatment-related mortality, clinical radiation hepatitis, or veno-occlusive liver failure was seen. An objective response by CT and/or octreoscan was observed in 18 of 20 patients (90%), and symptom control was achieved in 11 of 15 (73%) patients. Figure 18-8 demonstrates an excellent radiologic response with RMT in a case in which the treatment was given in a segmental fashion.

Clinical Data for Other Primary and Metastatic Cancers

Much of the Y-90 microsphere research to date has concentrated on primary HCC and CRC liver metastases. Many other tumors also demonstrate liver metastases, and those patients with liver dominant disease have been considered potential candidates for Y-90 microsphere therapy. Successful RMT in small series has been reported in a number of other primary and metastatic liver cancers. These include cholangiocarcinoma,[20] breast cancer,[21] pancreatic cancer,[22] and other.[23] All series have demonstrated a therapeutic profile similar to more definitively studied liver cancers.

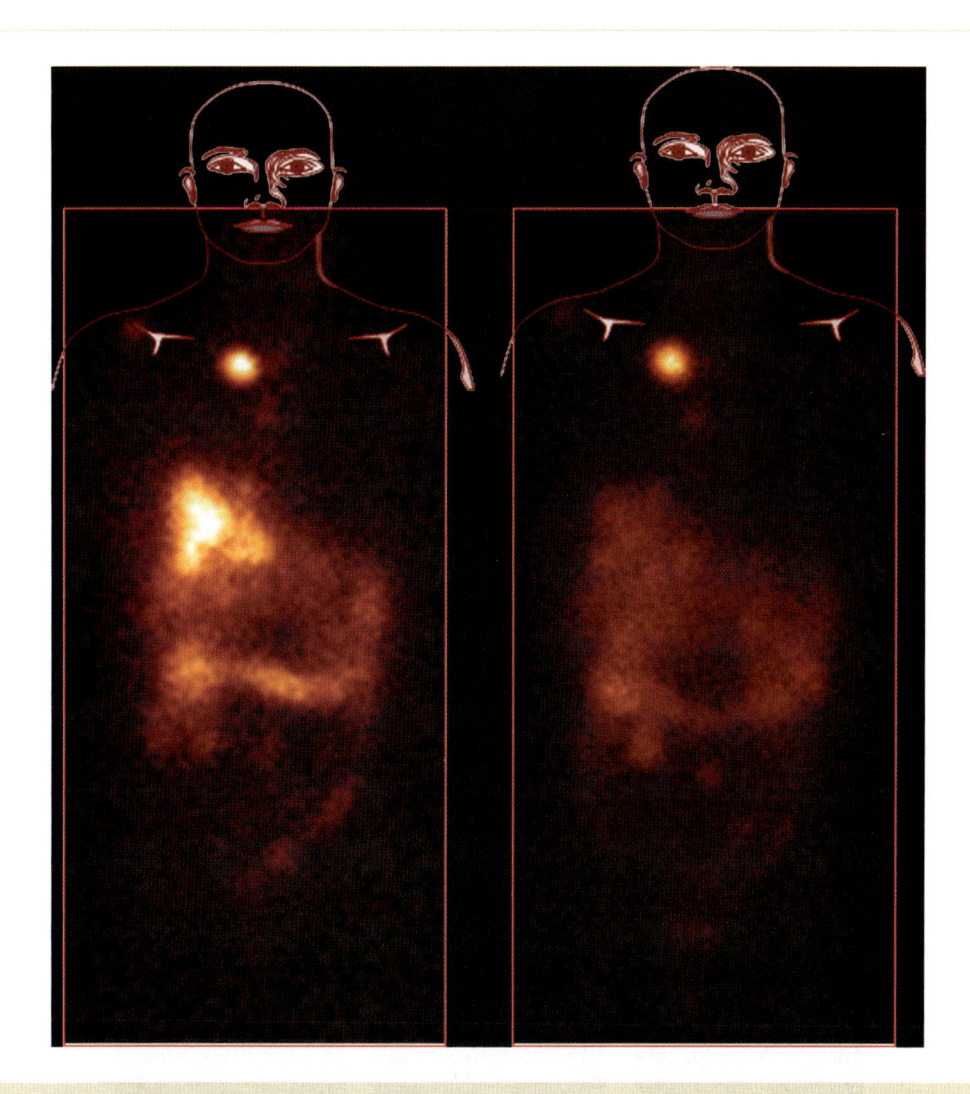

Figure 18-8: Demonstration of an excellent radiologic response with radiomicrosphere therapy in a case where the treatment was given in a segmental fashion.

Clinical Practice of RMT

Pretreatment Evaluation/Patient Selection

Evaluation of liver function: Liver reserve is affected by eoplastic replacement and prior hepatotoxic treatments. Alanineamino tranferease/aspartate aminotransferase and alkaline phosphatase/GGT are the markers for acute and subacute hepatocellular and bilio-canalicular injury, respectively. More difficult to evaluate is the real "functional volume" in the anatomically intact appearing liver regions. Bilirubin is a composite marker of liver reserve and has been widely used in many classification systems as a predictive measure. In practical terms, a bilirubin level >2 mg/dL in the absence of correctable obstructive etiology precludes RMT.

Cross-sectional radiologic evaluation of tumor: Standard imaging for detection and characterization of liver lesions is a multiphase liver scan.

A good triphasic helical CT is the standard for assessing liver tumors.[24] This will provide the portal venous phase imaging important in showing CRC liver metastases, as well as the arterial phase imaging essential for depicting tumors such as HCC and carcinoid/NET. Arterial phase imaging also offers a fairly detailed overview of the arterial anatomy to the liver and dominant arteries contributing to tumor vascularity. A good quality examination will also allow for facile and reliable evaluation of response to therapy.

Functional imaging: FDG PET scanning clearly improves diagnostic yield in patients with CRC liver metastases.[25–27] FDG-PET is also superior in detection of extrahepatic metastases and may assist in patient selection. Most recently, FDG-PET has also been found useful in evaluation of response to Y-90 microsphere treatment[28,29] (Figure 18-9).

Angiography: Angiography has a paramount importance in the planning and administration of RMT. Angiography depicts the vascular anatomy, identifies variant blood vessels, and allows exclusion of gastrointestinal (GI) branches with coil embolization. A methodical interrogation of the hepatic and visceral vasculature should be performed in all patients using digital subtraction imaging and power injection technique to define tumor vascularity and discover variant anatomy. Major complications of RMT are due to nontarget Y-90 microsphere localization (Figure 18-10).

It is critical to identify and investigate any and all potentially extrahepatic branches. These extrahepatic branches may contribute to the tumor volume in question or supply visceral structures at risk for nontargeted embolization. These branches typically include the gastroduodenal artery, right and left gastric, phrenic, supraduodenal, and retroduodenal arteries. It is typically a standard practice to identify and coil embolize any enteric branches that may be a source for nontarget embolization. Aside from the gastroduodenal artery, the right gastric is the extrahepatic artery that is most commonly encountered. An active search for this vessel should be routine as this is a potential source of morbidity. The right gastric artery most commonly originates from the left hepatic artery but may also arise from the common/proper hepatic artery, the right hepatic artery, or the

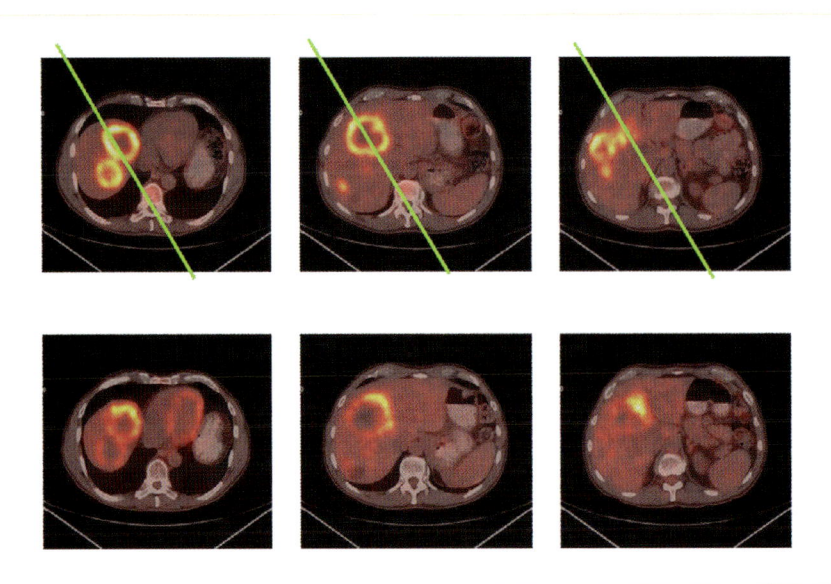

Figure 18-9: Response evaluation using 18-fluorodeoxyglucose positron emission tomography/Computed tomography. Differential visual response in chemo-SIRT treated lobe vs. chemo-only lobe. The line delineates right and lobe border.

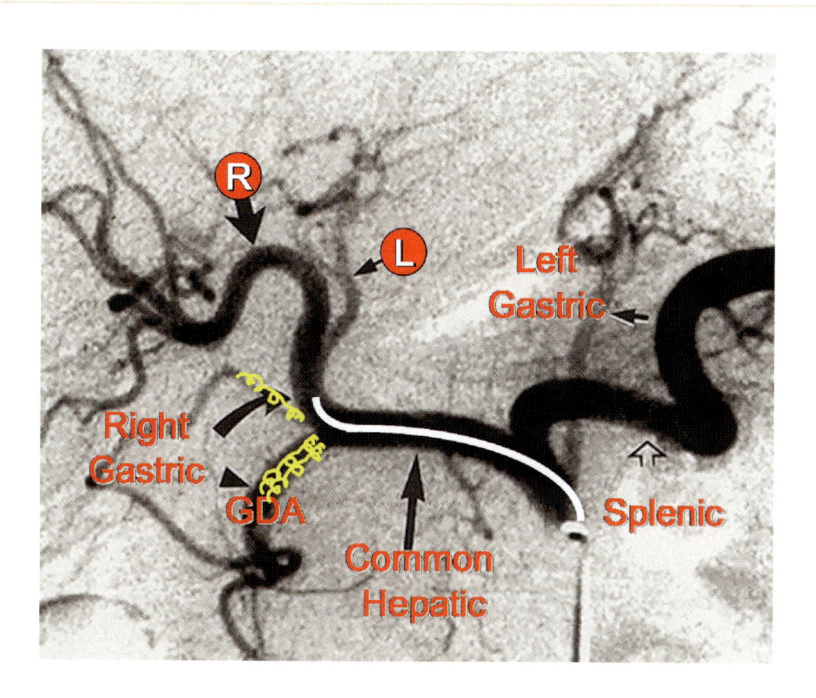

Figure 18-10: Hepatic angiogram performed prior to Y-90 microsphere treatment. Gastroduodenal artery and right gastric artery are coiled to prevent reflux into the gastrointestinal (GI) tract. Other identifiable GI branches are also coiled if their takeoff is close to the planned administration site of Y-90 microspheres.

gastroduodenal artery. Liu et al. have published a comprehensive review detailing angiographic technique and visceral anatomy pertinent to delivery of Y90 microspheres.[30] These authors have reported a GI toxicity rate <1%. This angiographic diligence is crucial as the deposition of Y-90 microspheres into gastroenteropancreatic vessels can result in significant morbidity (GI inflammation/ulceration, pancreatitis, dermal pain/ulceration) if proper angiographic technique is not followed.

Detailed understanding of patient-specific vascular anatomy also allows for accurate lobar volume calculations to prescribe the optimal Y-90 microsphere dose. To maximize tumor response and conserve normal liver function, it is extremely important that dosimetry calculations be based on the liver volume supplied by the arterial distribution that is to be catheterized at the time of treatment.

Technetium-99m macroaggregated albumin scanning: Macroaggregate albumin (MAA) is a particulate form of albumin with an average size of 20–40 μ. Its density is close to that of resin microspheres, and the number of particles per unit volume can be adjusted to a desirable range. Tc-99m MAA injection into the hepatic artery serves as a reasonable surrogate diagnostic radiopharmaceutical to simulate Y-90 microsphere distribution.

The Tc-99m MAA unit dose is injected through the hepatic arterial catheter at the completion of visceral angiography. Shortly after the administration, anterior–posterior planar images of the chest and abdomen and Single Positron Emission Computed Tomography (SPECT) images of the liver are obtained. Three objectives of the Tc-99m MAA study are as follows:

1. Detection and quantitation of hepatic shunting that could result in exaggerated doses of radioactive particles in the lungs (Figure 18-11A). The hypervascular primary

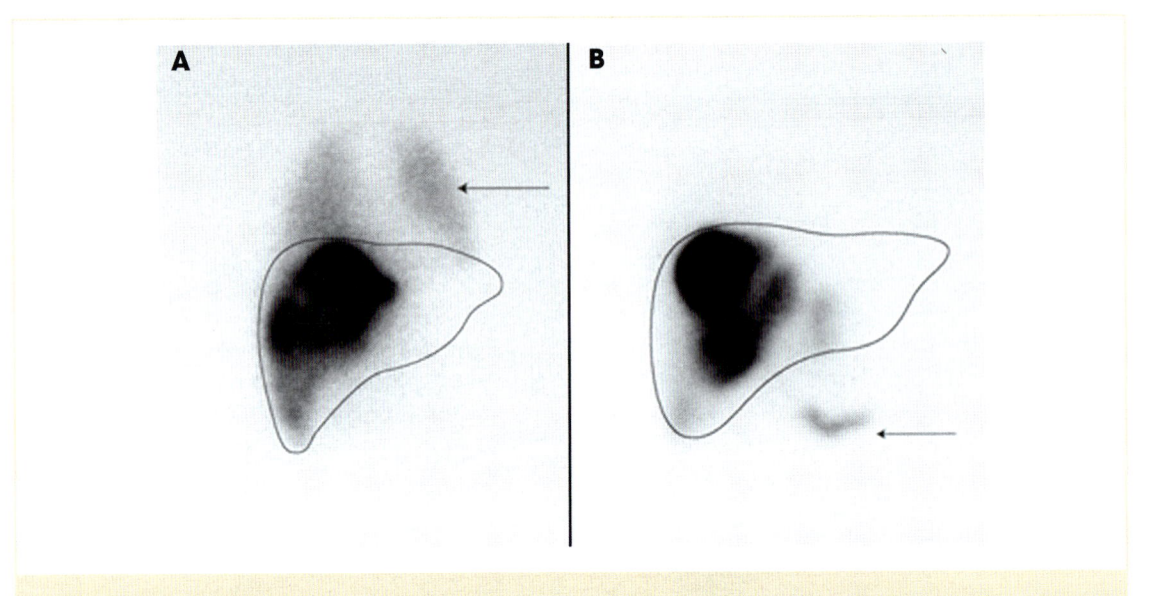

Figure 18-11: Technitium-99m macroaggregated albumin scanning demonstrating extrahepatic perfusion. (A) Radioactive particles in the lungs on left pane; (B) duodenal perfusion on the right pane.

intrahepatic arteriovenous shunting. This phenomenon somewhat correlates with the degree of tumor vascularity and is most prominent with HCC and metastatic NETs. Clinically significant arteriovenous shunting may also be observed in CRC liver metastases. Lung shunt fraction (LSF) is determined by regions of interest analysis on Tc-99m MAA planar images using the following formula.

$$LSF = \sqrt{\frac{(Counts_{Lung\langle Anterior\rangle} \times Counts_{Lung\langle Posterior\rangle})}{(Counts_{Lung+Liver\langle Anterior\rangle} \times Counts_{Lung+Liver\langle Posterior\rangle})}}$$

2. Tc-99m MAA imaging helps to identify extrahepatic GI uptake that might be caused by unrecognized hepatofugal vascular run off (Figure 18-11B). Scintigraphically detectable extrahepatic uptake is invariably associated with symptomatic GI complications such as ulceration. This finding, depending on its size, might preclude further treatment with Y-90 microspheres unless a safe interventional plan for prevention of extrahepatic flux can be made.

3. Tc-99m MAA hepatic scintigraphy allows differentiation of the blood flow ratio between the tumor and normal liver compartments, which is the major determinant of the effectiveness of tumor targeting. Tumor to liver uptake ratio (TLR) is best determined from SPECT images using the following formula. Utilization of dedicated acquisition and processing protocols improve accuracy of quantitation, which is a prerequisite for reliable dosimetry.

$$TLR = \frac{Counts/Pixel_{Tumor}}{Counts/Pixel_{liver}}$$

Y-90 Microsphere Dosimetry and Treatment Planning: The strict definition of dosimetry is the calculation of radiation-absorbed dose in target lesions and organs. However, the term is used rather loosely in the clinical practice of Y-90 microsphere treatment where the decision regarding a reasonably safe or acceptable amount of administered activity is referred to as dosimetry. In actuality, this is merely an activity prescription or written directive.

Currently, a written directive for Y-90 microsphere therapy is based on the four methods (see Appendix for detailed description):

1. Body surface area method
2. Empiric method[31,32]
3. Medical internal radiation dosimetry, noncompartmental macrodosimetry method
4. Medical internal radiation dosimetry, compartmental macrodosimetry method (partition method). This approach was used for resin microsphere therapy of HCC cases by Ho et al.[33–35]

Treatment and Follow-up Procedures

The administration of Y-90 microspheres is performed in an angiography suite, by an interventional radiologist and the authorized user. The catheter is usually positioned at a location determined by the desired treatment mode (whole liver, lobar, or segmental). Both Y-90 microsphere products have their own dedicated delivery device designed to facilitate the administration. Because the resin microspheres have a much higher number of microspheres per unit dose, there is an embolic tendency especially toward the last stages of administration, which is performed in a manually controlled manner with fluoroscopic monitoring. Observation of increasing reflux is a sign of increased embolic effect and risk for hepatofugal flux and therefore might be an indication to discontinue the administration. Strict adherence to radiation safety guidelines is critically important in patient and personnel safety.

Y-90 microsphere treatment is usually an outpatient treatment. Patients who experience moderate embolic syndrome can be admitted for <24 hours. Symptomatic treatment might be indicated for pain or nausea. Routine prophylactic use of antibiotics, proton pump inhibitors, or steroids is not indicated. Patients are provided with radiation safety instructions upon discharge.

Bremsstrahlung Imaging

Y-90 is a pure β-emitter, and therefore, standard γ imaging is not feasible. However, due to interactions between high-energy β-particles and atomic nuclei, secondary photons, known as Bremsstrahlung (breaking) radiation, are generated, which can be imaged. Bremsstrahlung imaging involves the use of medium or high-energy collimation and an empirically selected broad photon energy window to enhance camera sensitivity. Imaging the distribution of Y-90 could be helpful to confirm the localization of radioactivity in the tumor/liver compartments and is recommended by most users. Bremsstrahlung imaging can be performed any time during the first 24 hours of treatment (Figure 18-12).

Follow-up Studies

Routine follow-up after RMT involves monitoring for liver toxicity and assessing treatment response using multiphase liver scan with PET/CT and CEA levels. Determination of the frequency of follow-up studies is based on the clinical protocol (chemo-RMT vs. RMT-alone) and overall clinical assessment. FDG-PET imaging is very sensitive in early demonstration of response.

Complications of Y-90 Microsphere Therapy

Commonly Observed After-Effects

Post-Y-90 microsphere therapy lethargy and mild nausea are common symptoms lasting up to 10 days and may require medication. Most patients develop mild fever for several days following Y-90 microsphere therapy that does not require treatment.

Postembolization Syndrome

Postembolization syndrome (PES) refers to a clinical picture of acute abdominal pain, nausea, vomiting, and fever resulting from acute ischemic insult to the liver. PES in its most severe form is seen after chemoembolization. RMT is not (and should not be) a devascularization treatment. Never-theless, in approximately one-third of patients, administration of Y-90 microsphere

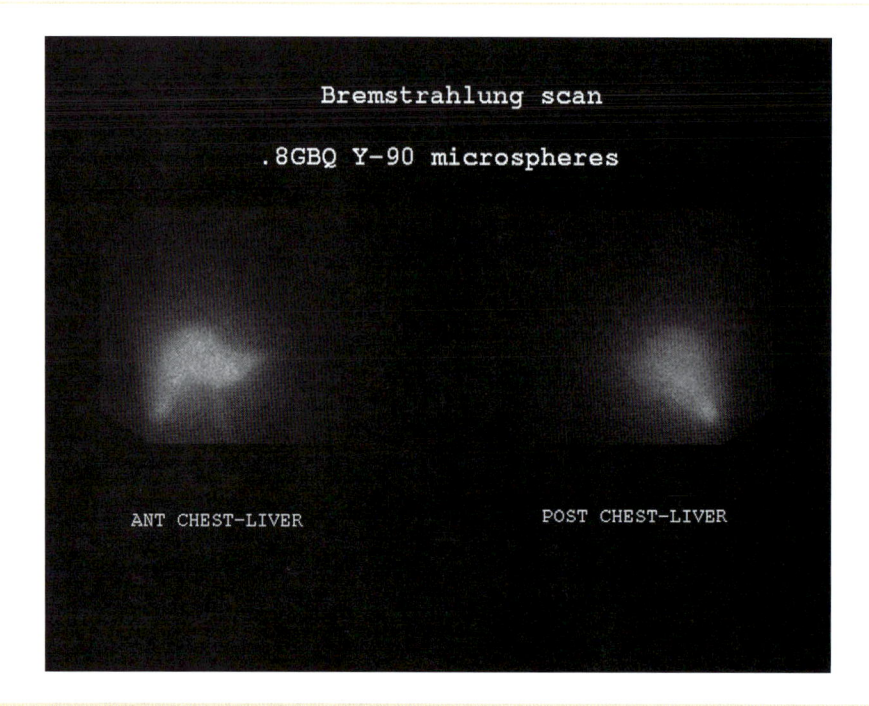

Figure 18-12: Bremsstrahlung imaging showing the radiopharmaceutical localization in the treatment field. It also demonstrates successful tumor localization without any discernible lung shunting or extrahepatic gastrointestinal uptake.

therapy causes early, short-term abdominal pain requiring narcotic analgesia. This side effect is more common with increasing number of microspheres administered. This can be avoided with slow, well-controlled administration of microspheres and has been uncommon in experienced hands. PES typically does not occur with glass microsphere treatment given the difference in embolic load.[36]

Hepatic Injury

The pathogenesis of radiation damage to the liver from conventional external beam radiation is dominated by vascular injury in the central vein region. Early alterations in the central vein caused by external beam radiation include intimal damage that leads to eccentric wall thickening. This process, when diffuse and progressive, results in clinical "veno-occlusive disease" characterized by development of postsinusoidal portal hypertension, ascites, and deterioration of liver function tests.[37]

Y-90 microsphere therapy–associated radiation injury has a different pattern. Radiation from microspheres is deposited primarily in the region of the portal triad away from the central vein and thus is distinct from the damage pattern seen in radiation hepatitis from external beam sources. Radiation-induced liver disease secondary to radioembolization is not common but has been reported and may be more common in patients also treated with systemic chemotherapy.[38] Chemo-SIRT patients' postresection specimens commonly demonstrate steatosis or steatohepatitis, which are not typically seen in SIRT-alone specimens. It is important to note that sinusoidal obstruction, perisinusoidal fibrosis, and veno-occlusive disease are not uncommon with chemotherapy-associated hepatic toxicity. Particularly in patients with CRC liver metastases who have received prior or concomitant chemotherapy, the hepatic toxicity picture may be a combination pattern.[39]

A review by Atassi et al. involving 569 Y-90 microsphere treatments in 327 patients reported a 10% incidence of grade 3 bilirubin toxicity.[40] Portal hypertension, as a sequela of Y-90 microsphere therapy, has been described in early studies and case reports.[41] Subclinical portal hypertension may manifest by splenomegaly.

Radiation Pneumonitis

A fraction of microspheres may shunt through the liver and into the lungs. Radiation pneumonitis has been reported to occur at estimated lung dose levels of 30 Gy.[33] Proper lung shunting studies and incorporation of this information in dosimetry models should be practiced universally. The risk of radiation pneumonitis is mitigated if the cumulative lung dose is limited to 50 Gy.[33]

GI Complications

The most commonly affected site in the GI tract is the gastroduodenal segment due to rich hepatofugal collaterals. Collateral vessels posing heightened risk for nontarget embolization should be coiled. The Y-90 microsphere therapy–induced GI ulceration rate is <5% and is close to minimal in experienced hands. However, when these ulcer occur, RMT-induced ulcers are more challenging than accustomed peptic ulcerations and might be refractory to standard treatment regimens (Figure 18-13). Y-90 microsphere therapy may cause radiation cholecystitis. Although clinically relevant radiation cholecystitis requiring cholecystectomy is rare, imaging findings of gallbladder injury (i.e., enhancing wall, mural rent) are quite common. Other possible biliary complications reported include biliary necrosis, biloma, and stricture.[40]

Summary of Complications

Therefore, the most common complications are the abdominal pain that occurs in one-third of patients. The most serious complications include nontarget radiation in the GI tract, cholecystitis, radiation pneumonitis, and radiation-induced liver disease (i.e., radiation hepatitis). Distant organs are not subjected to β-radiation due to the short

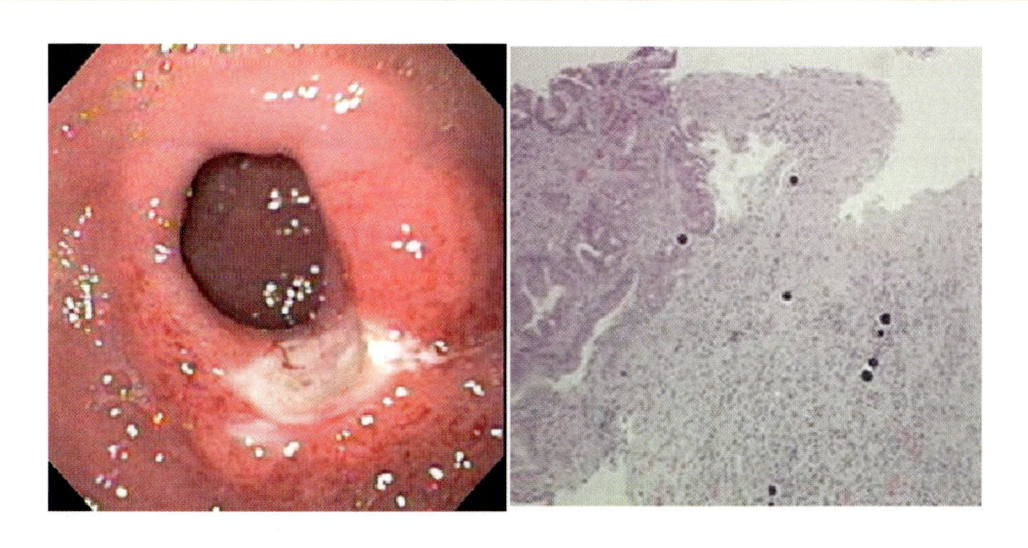

Figure 18-13: Gastric/duodenal ulcer resulting from reflux of Y-90 radiomicrospheres into the gastrointestinal vascular bed. (A) Endoscopic appearance of a gastric ulceration caused by Y-90 microspheres; (B) Hematoxylin and eosin microscopy of the ulcer showing microspheres in the necrotic (ulcerated) mucosa. The adjacent mucosa preserves its viability.

TABLE 18-1: Adverse Events/Complications Following Microsphere Therapy

Adverse Event/Complication	Incidence
Flu-like symptoms Fatigue Low-grade fever Nausea/vomiting Mild abdominal pain	50%
Postembolic syndrome	1%–2% with resin microspheres None with glass microspheres
Ulceration	0%–20% (median 5%)
Cholecystitis	<1%
Radiation-induced liver disease	Classic radiation-induced liver disease (characterized by veno-occlusive disease): <1% Radiomicrosphere-induced liver disease (characterized by portal triaditis): 0%–10% (median 5%)
Radiation pneumonitis	<1%

range of β-particles. Radiation doses to the gonads are unlikely, given the distance to the liver and very short range of the β-particles of Y-90. Similarly, radiation doses to the bone marrow are unlikely, and data have not demonstrated myelosuppression. Adverse events and complications following microsphere therapy are shown in Table 18-1.

Conclusion

Y-90 radiomicrosphere treatment for primary and metastatic liver cancer is no longer purely experimental or investigational. This treatment modality has been shown to be safe and efficacious and is approved for the treatment of metastatic CRC and HCC. Treatment paradigms have significantly evolved and continue to be refined. Based on the literature to date, this therapy is increasingly being utilized to treat primary and metastatic liver cancer. Y-90 RMT is increasingly considered earlier in the course of treatment as opposed to the salvage setting, and ongoing trials are currently accruing patients to support this role. However, there is a need for development of a clinically practical dosimetry technique and more unified patient selection criteria for treatment planning and execution.

References

1. Ariel IM, Pack GT. Treatment of inoperable cancer of the liver by intra-arterial radioactive isotopes and chemotherapy. *Cancer*. 1967;20(5):793–804.
2. Huang P, Feng L, Oldham EA, et al. Superoxide dismutase as a target for the selective killing of cancer cells. *Nature*. 2000;407(6802):390–395.
3. Gray B, Van Hazel G, Hope M, et al. Randomised trial of SIR-Spheres plus chemotherapy vs. chemotherapy alone for treating patients with liver metastases from primary large bowel cancer. *Ann Oncol*. 2001;12(12):1711–1720.
4. Van Hazel G, Blackwell A, Anderson J, et al. Randomised phase 2 trial of SIR-Spheres plus fluorouracil/leucovorin chemotherapy versus fluorouracil/leucovorin chemotherapy alone in advanced colorectal cancer. *J Surg Oncol*. 2004;88(2):78–85.
5. Sharma RA, Van Hazel GA, Morgan B, et al. Radioembolization of liver metastases from colorectal cancer using Yttrium-90 microspheres with concomitant systemic oxaliplatin, fluorouracil, and leucovorin chemotherapy. *J Clin Oncol*. 2007;25(9):1099–1106.
6. van Hazel GA, Pavlakis N, Goldstein D, et al. Treatment of fluorouracil-refractory patients with liver metastases from colorectal cancer by using Yttrium-90 resin microspheres plus concomitant

7. Gulec S, Hall M, Atkinson H, et al. Efficacy of 90Y radiomicrosphere and chemotherapy combination treatment in patients with colorectal cancer liver metastases. *J Nucl Med Meeting Abstracts*. 2008;49[abstracts]:103.

8. Stubbs RS, Cannan RJ, Mitchell AW. Selective internal radiation therapy with 90yttrium microspheres for extensive colorectal liver metastases. *J Gastrointest Surg*. 2001;5(3): 294–302.

9. Kennedy AS, Coldwell D, Nutting C, et al. Resin 90Y-microsphere brachytherapy for unresectable colorectal liver metastases: modern USA experience. *Int J Radiat Oncol Biol Phys*. 2006;65(2): 412–425.

10. Lau WY, Ho S, Leung TW, et al. Selective internal radiation therapy for nonresectable hepatocellular carcinoma with intraarterial infusion of 90yttrium microspheres. *Int J Radiat Oncol Biol Phys*. 1998;40(3):583–592.

11. Lau WY, Leung WT, Ho S, et al. Treatment of inoperable hepatocellular carcinoma with intrahepatic arterial Yttrium-90 microspheres: a phase I and II study. *Br J Cancer*. 1994;70(5):994–999.

12. Lau WY, Ho S, Leung WT, et al. What determines survival duration in hepatocellular carcinoma treated with intraarterial Yttrium-90 microspheres? *Hepatogastroenterology*. 2001; 48(38):338–340.

13. Goin JE, Salem R, Carr BI, et al. Treatment of unresectable hepatocellular carcinoma with intrahepatic Yttrium 90 microspheres: a risk-stratification analysis. *J Vasc Interv Radiol*. 2005;16(2 pt 1): 195–203.

14. Salem R, Lewandowski RJ, Atassi B, et al. Treatment of unresectable hepatocellular carcinoma with use of 90Y microspheres (TheraSphere): safety, tumor response, and survival. *J Vasc Interv Radiol*. 2005;16(12): 1627–1639.

15. Salem R, Lewandowski R, Roberts C, et al. Use of Yttrium-90 glass microspheres (TheraSphere) for the treatment of unresectable hepatocellular carcinoma in patients with portal vein thrombosis. *J Vasc Interv Radiol*. 2004;15(4):335–345.

16. Kennedy A, Coldwell D, Nutting C, et al. Hepatic brachytherapy for GI neuroendocrine tumors with 90y-microspheres: long term USA experience (abstract 285). Paper presented at: 16th International Conference on Anti-Cancer Treatment; February 1–4, 2005; Paris, France.

17. Rhee TK, Lewandowski RJ, Liu DM, et al. 90Y radioembolization for metastatic neuroendocrine liver tumors: preliminary results from a multi-institutional experience. *Ann Surg*. 2008;247(6): 1029–1035.

18. Kennedy A, Liu DM, Dezarn WA, et al. Resin 90y-microsphere brachytherapy for unresectable neuroendocrine hepatic metastases. Paper presented at: Liver Directed Radiotherapy With Microspheres: Second Annual Clinical Symposium; April 27–28, 2006; Scottsdale, AZ.

19. Gulec SA, Hostetter R, Schwartzentruber D, et al. Treatment of neuroendocrine tumor liver metastases with Y-90 microspheres: an effective cytoreduction for disease consolidation and symptom control. *Ann Surg Oncol*. 2007;14:93.

20. Ibrahim SM, Mulcahy MF, Lewandowski RJ, et al. Treatment of unresectable cholangiocarcinoma using Yttrium-90 microspheres: results from a pilot study. *Cancer*. 2008;113(8): 2119–2128.

21. Bangash AK, Atassi B, Kaklamani V, et al. 90Y radioembolization of metastatic breast cancer to the liver: toxicity, imaging response, survival. *J Vasc Interv Radiol*. 2007;18(5): 621–628.

22. Gulec SA, Hall MJ, Wheller J, et al. A phase II study of Selective Internal Radiation Treatment (SIRT) and Selective External Radiation Treatment (SERT) with chemotherapy in patients with recurrent/metastatic pancreatic cancer: preliminary results. Paper presented at: World Conference on Interventional Oncology; 2008; Los Angeles, CA.

23. Lewandowski RJ, Atassi BA, Wong CO, et al. Use of Yttrium-90 microspheres for the treatment of liver neoplasia: long-term follow-up. Paper presented at: The Annual Meeting of the Cardiovascular and Interventional Society of Europe; 2006; Rome, Italy.

24. Catalano O. Proper terminology for multiple-phase helical CT of the liver. *AJR Am J Roentgenol*. 2001;176(2):547–548.

25. Fong Y, Saldinger PF, Akhurst T, et al. Utility of 18F-FDG positron emission tomography scanning on selection of patients for resection of hepatic colorectal metastases. *Am J Surg*. 1999;178(4):282–287.

26. Arulampalam TH, Francis DL, Visvikis D, et al. FDG-PET for the pre-operative evaluation of colorectal liver metastases. *Eur J Surg Oncol*. 2004;30(3):286–291.

27. Bipat S, van Leeuwen MS, Comans EF, et al. Colorectal liver metastases: CT, MR imaging, and PET for diagnosis—meta-analysis. *Radiology*. 2005;237(1):123–131.

28. Bienert M, McCook B, Carr BI, et al. 90Y microsphere treatment of unresectable liver metastases: changes in 18F-FDG uptake and tumour size on PET/CT. *Eur J Nucl Med Mol Imaging*. 2005;32(7):778–787.

29. Wong CY, Salem R, Qing F, et al. Metabolic response after intraarterial 90Y-glass microsphere treatment for colorectal liver metastases: comparison of quantitative and visual analyses by 18F-FDG PET. *J Nucl Med*. 2004;45(11):1892–1897.

30. Liu DM, Salem R, Bui JT, et al. Angiographic considerations in patients undergoing liver-directed therapy. *J Vasc Interv Radiol*. 2005;16(7):911–935.

31. Kennedy AS, Dezarn WA, McNeillie P, et al. Fractionation, dose selection, and response of hepatic metastases of neuroendocrine tumors after 90Y-microsphere brachytherapy. *Brachytherapy*. 2006;5(2):103.

32. Kennedy AS, Dezarn WA, McNeillie P, et al. Dose selection of resin 90Y-microspheres for liver brachytherapy: a single center review. *Brachytherapy*. 2006;5(2):103–104.

33. Ho S, Lau WY, Leung TW, et al. Clinical evaluation of the partition model for estimating radiation doses from Yttrium-90 microspheres in the treatment of hepatic cancer. *Eur J Nucl Med*. 1997;24(3):293–298.

34. Gulec SA, Mesoloras G, Stabin M. Dosimetric techniques in 90Y-microsphere therapy of liver cancer: the MIRD equations for dose calculations. *J Nucl Med*. 2006;47(7):1209–1211.

35. Gulec SA, Mesoloras G, Dezarn WA, et al. Safety and efficacy of Y-90 microsphere treatment in patients with primary and metastatic liver cancer: the tumor selectivity of the treatment as a function of tumor to liver flow ratio. *J Transl Med*. 2007;5:15.

36. Sato K, Lewandowski RJ, Bui JT, et al. Treatment of unresectable primary and metastatic liver cancer with Yttrium-90 microspheres (TheraSphere): assessment of hepatic arterial embolization. *Cardiovasc Intervent Radiol*. 2006;29(4):522–529.

37. Cheng JC, Wu JK, Huang CM, et al. Radiation-induced liver disease after radiotherapy for hepatocellular carcinoma: clinical manifestation and dosimetric description. *Radiother Oncol*. 2002;63(1):41–45.

38. Sangro B, Gil-Alzugaray B, Rodriguez J, et al. Liver disease induced by radioembolization of liver tumors: description and possible risk factors. *Cancer*. 2008;112(7):1538–1546.

39. Schouten van der Velden AP, Punt CJ, Van Krieken JH, et al. Hepatic veno-occlusive disease after neo-adjuvant treatment of colorectal liver metastases with oxaliplatin: a lesson of the month. *Eur J Surg Oncol*. 2008;34(3):353–355.

40. Atassi B, Bangash AK, Lewandowski RJ, et al. Biliary sequelae following radioembolization with yttrium-90 microspheres. *J Vasc Interv Radiol*. 2008;19(5):691–697.

41. Jakobs TF, Saleem S, Atassi B, et al. Fibrosis, portal hypertension, and hepatic volume changes induced by intra-arterial radiotherapy with 90yttrium microspheres. *Dig Dis Sci*. 2008;53(9):2556–2563.

Appendix

Body Surface Area Method

The body surface area method is used for resin microsphere activity prescription. The user manual for the resin Y-90 microspheres recommends the following formula for determination of the activity to be administered.

$$\text{Activity (GBq)} = \frac{(\text{BSA} - 2) + \text{Tumor Volume}}{\text{Liver Volume}}$$

Empiric Method

The empiric method is also used for resin microsphere activity prescription. The user manual for resin Y-90 microspheres recommends the guidelines below for determination of the activity to be administered. In practice, it has been shown that if this method is employed, only 50% of the treatments will be complete due to vascular stasis.

Empirical model for written directive

Degree of Tumor Involvement (%)	Recommended Activity (GBq)
>50	3.0
25–50	2.5
<25	2.0

Dose modifiers for lung shunting and lobular treatment

% Lung Shunt	Dose Modifier	Part of Liver	Dose Modifier
10–15	0.8	Right lobe	0.7
15–20	0.6	Left lobe	0.3
>20	No treatment	—	—

Medical Internal Radiation Dosimetry, Noncompartmental Macrodosimetry Method

This method, essentially, is the calculation of the absorbed dose in the liver from an administered activity. This methodology has been recommended in dose calculations for glass microsphere treatment. The adopted methodology uses a simplistic method and does not consider tumor and liver compartments separately. The method assumes that the distribution of the microspheres is even in the tumor and the liver compartments, which leads to an overestimation of the absorbed dose in the liver. Safe liver dose estimates of 100–150 Gy have been reported in the literature. The activity required to achieve the "intended" dose in this approach is calculated with the following formula.

$$\text{Activity (GBq)} = \frac{\text{Desired Dose (Gy)} \times \text{Target Liver Mass (g)}}{50 \times (1 - \text{LSF})}$$

Lung shunt fraction (LSF) is determined by Tc-99m MAA imaging.

Medical Internal Radiation Dosimetry, Compartmental Macrodosimetry Method

Also known as the *partition method*, this technique is based on assessment of the tumor and liver volumes and activity distribution in these two compartments. This method is relatively easy to use when the tumor margins are well defined by anatomic and functional imaging modalities. It is highly challenging and perhaps impractical in routine clinical applications. This method can provide reasonably accurate and reproducible average radiation-absorbed dose estimates for liver and tumor compartments. Because of the labor-intensive nature of this methodology, the technique has been mostly used in selected cases with limited number of liver lesions.

A patient-specific administered activity determination involves a compartmental approach (partition model) in all cases regardless of the challenges encountered with increasing number of lesions in the tumor compartment. The microspheres are biocompatible but not biodegradable, and therefore, no biologic elimination occurs after they lodge in the terminal arterioles of the hepatic vasculature. Thus, the total radiation-absorbed dose that is delivered over a period of time is solely determined by the 64-hour physical half-life of Y-90. A detailed derivation of the formulas used in the compartmental model has been demonstrated by Gulec et al.[34] Use of this method requires three measurements: (1) volume of tumor and normal liver generally obtained from CT scans; (2) proportion of the total administered activity that lodges in tumor and normal liver as determined from a Tc-99m MAA SPECT scan; and (3) fraction of the total administered activity lodged in the lungs, LSF, as determined from a Tc-99m MAA planar scan. Thus, the TLR and the LSF are measured. The partition model can best be used when tumor mass is localized in a discrete area within the liver, and tumor regions of interest can be identified and reliably drawn. This is usually relatively easy to perform in patients with primary hepatocellular carcinoma where there is often a large single tumor mass. The technique would be more demanding for routine application in the presence of metastatic disease with multiple lesions. Despite the technical challenges, the compartmental model has been successfully adapted for clinical use in both primary and metastatic settings.[35]

Activity to be administered for a desired liver dose can be calculated using the following formula:

$$\text{Activity}_{\text{admin}} \text{(GBq)} = \frac{\text{Dose}_{\text{Liver}} \text{(Gy)} \times m_{\text{Liver}} \text{(g)}}{50 \times \text{Fractional Uptake}_{\text{Liver}}}$$

The dose to the liver delivered from a given administered activity is

$$\text{Dose}_{\text{Liver}} \text{(Gy)} = \frac{\text{Activity}_{\text{admin}} \text{(GBq)} \times 50 \times \text{Fractional Uptake}_{\text{Liver}}}{m_{\text{Liver}} \text{(g)}}$$

VI SECTION

Systemic and Regional Chemotherapies and Biologic Therapies

Ghassan K. Abou-Alfa

CHAPTER 19

Systemic Chemotherapy for Hepatocellular Carcinoma

Syed A. Hussain & Daniel H. Palmer

The prognosis of hepatocellular carcinoma (HCC) is generally poor, and treatment decisions are based on the stage of disease, comorbidities, and liver function, which is dependent on underlying liver disease. Cirrhosis limits therapeutic options, life expectancy, and tolerance to therapy. Potentially curative therapies such as hepatic resection, liver transplantation, or local ablation have led to improvement in the survival of carefully selected patients with HCC. However, these treatments are typically constrained by size and/or number of tumors. For other patients with well-compensated liver function and a patent portal venous system, chemo-embolization may afford a modest survival benefit. For the remainder, providing liver function and performance status permit, systemic therapies are often used with palliative intent. Traditionally, this has taken the form of cytotoxic chemotherapy or endocrine manipulation although more recently molecular-targeted therapies have been employed.

This chapter aims to summarize the current status of chemotherapy with reference to the limitations of these data and recommendations for future research directions.

Chemotherapy for Advanced Hepatocellular Carcinoma

A large number of studies using the major classes of chemotherapeutic drugs as single agents or in combination have been performed and are summarized in Tables 19-1 and 19-2.

Response rates for single-agent chemotherapy are low, and durable remission is rare. The anthracycline, doxorubicin, has been the most studied agent largely in small, uncontrolled phase II studies, the first study reporting a response rate of 79% in a cohort of patients in Uganda.[1] Subsequent studies failed to corroborate this apparent activity and in 15 other trials the response rate[2-14] ranged from 1% to 35%. The overall response rate for more than 700 patients treated in these studies was 18%. The method of response assessment, particularly in earlier studies often in the form of clinical examination, is likely to have contributed to an overestimation of response, and the true objective radiological response rate is likely to be lower, as reflected in more recent trials. The presence of liver cirrhosis, electrolyte imbalances, decreased liver synthetic reserve, and portal hypertension has made the design of systemic therapy trials for HCC challenging. Additionally staging of HCC using the tumor node metastases system, but ignoring the underlying liver disease, makes it extremely difficult to compare results of different trials as such effects of doxorubicin on overall survival cannot be elucidated. Only one small randomized trial has compared doxorubicin with symptom control. This study reported a statistically significant survival advantage in favor of doxorubicin. However, with median survival of 10.6 weeks versus 7.5 weeks, absolute difference in survival was modest with very short survival in both arms, suggesting inclusion of patients with very advanced disease and/or poor liver function. There was also significant doxorubicin-related toxicity, including cardiotoxicity, which may

TABLE 19-1: Phase II Trials of Single-Agent Chemotherapy in Hepatocellular Carcinoma

Drug	Dose (mg/m²)	N	Response Rate (%)	Reference
Cisplatin		28	15	22
Doxorubicin	75	14	79	1
	20–75	41	11	2
	60	44	32	3
	40–60	31	10	4
	75	74	30	5
	60	63	35	6
	60	28	28	7
	75	52	11	8
	70	45	25	9
	40–60	51	10	10
	40–60	29	11	11
	60	34	21	12
	60	109	1	13
	60	29	11	14
	60–75	60	3	15
	60	30	18	16
Epirubicin		18	17	19
		44	9	20
5-FU		25	28	23
Gemcitabine		28	18	34
Irinotecan		14	7	61
Mitoxantrone		17	23	21
Nolatrexed		28	7	27
T-136		34	9	25

be accounted for by many patients receiving a cumulative dose exceeding 500 mg/m².[15]

The main toxicity for doxorubicin is myelosuppression, and this correlates with serum bilirubin, which is particularly relevant to patients with HCC, who typically have underlying chronic liver disease. This was demonstrated in a study including patients with normal or with elevated bilirubin levels. The response rate in patients with normal bilirubin was 46% but was only 10% in those with elevated bilirubin. This is likely to be due to dose reductions to ameliorate toxicity in the elevated bilirubin group leading to suboptimal dosing and emphasizes the need for careful patient selection for trials involving doxorubicin and further confounds the interpretation of trials to date. Another study administered doxorubicin to patients with inoperable HCC, a proportion of which were hyperbilirubinemic. These patients experienced marked myelosuppression, with the degree of neutropenia being directly related to the serum bilirubin concentration, but not to any other standard liver test, or the presence or absence of cirrhosis. The area under the log concentration–time curve was significantly greater in patients who were hyperbilirubinemic implying a greater drug exposure leading to more myelosuppression.[16]

Pegylation of doxorubicin prolongs its circulating half-life, reduces systemic toxicity, and may

TABLE 19-2: Phase II Trials of Combination Chemotherapy in Hepatocellular Carcinoma

Drugs	Patient Number	Response Rate (%)	Reference
PIAF (Phase II)	50	26	30
(Phase III)	149	17	31
Epirubicin + etoposide	36	39	32
Cisplatin + 5-FU	38	47	33
Gemcitabine + oxaliplatin	32	18	35
Gemcitabine + oxaliplatin + Bevacizumab	33	20	45

promote drug accumulation in the liver. However, two trials indicate no advantage over regular doxorubicin in the setting of HCC. In one small study, 16 patients were evaluable for response. No objective response was achieved, and the median survival time was 140 days. Treatment toxicities grade 3 or higher composed of increased liver enzymes in patients with preexisting grade 1 or 2 elevation ($n = 6$), hematologic toxicity ($n = 5$), and hypersensitivity.[17] In another 40-patient phase II study of liposomal doxorubicin, toxicities were usually mild but unexpectedly, three cirrhotic patients died of infection without neutropenia. Four patients (10%) had a partial response with a median duration of response of 5.6 months. However, overall median time to tumor progression and median survival were only two and three months, respectively. Patients with advanced HCC had lower initial serum concentration, larger volume of distribution and more rapid clearance than patients with normal liver function. However, these pharmacokinetic parameters correlated with neither toxicity nor response.[18]

Another anthracycline epirubicin has been investigated in HCC as this is known to be less cardiotoxic at therapeutic dose as compared to doxorubicin. Eighteen patients, all without prior treatment, were treated with epirubicin every three weeks with dose escalation where possible. Five patients were treated by six-hour infusion and 13 by intravenous bolus injection, with a median dose of 90 mg/m². The patients were of diverse ethnic background and included some with underlying cirrhosis and hepatitis B surface antigenemia. Three patients had partial responses (6, 12, and 48 weeks) for a response rate of 17%. Four patients also had prolonged stable disease (14, 26, 27, and 38 weeks). Toxicity was mild, although cardiac toxicity developed in three patients at 685, 825, and 1460 mg/m² cumulative dose. The response to epirubicin in this study appears to be similar to the reported response rates for doxorubicin but with decreased toxicity.[19] In another study, 52 patients with nonresectable disease were treated with weekly epirubicin 20 mg/m² iv on days 1, 8, and 15 repeated every four weeks to a maximum dose of 1000 mg/m². Forty-four patients were eligible for analysis. One patient achieved a complete response, 3 (6.8%) had partial responses, and 16 (36%) had stable disease. For patients with successful disease control (complete and partial responders) and patients with stable disease, the median survival was 16.2 months; for nonresponders, it was 6.1 months ($p < 0.003$) indicating that epirubicin may be an active therapeutic option for patients with nonresectable HCC.[20] However, there are no randomized controlled trials to assess the impact on survival or quality of life.

In studies involving 118 patients treated with mitoxantrone, an anthracendione, the toxicity was mild and the response rate was 16%, and this became the first systemic agent to be licensed for use in HCC[21] although again there are no data to determine its effect on survival, and it has not been widely adopted as a standard treatment.

Many drugs (including oral 5-FU, ifosfamide, paclitaxel, and irinotecan) appear to be essentially inactive in the context of advanced HCC at least according to radiological response criteria. Other drugs have demonstrated some single agent activity (cisplatin response rate 5%–15%; etoposide 0%–24%; intravenous 5-FU 0%–28%; topotecan 14%) but few have been rigorously tested in randomized controlled trials[22,23] (summarized in Table 19-1).

A randomized trial has compared the oral fluoropyrimidine, UFT, with supportive care. UFT comprises tegafur, an orally active 5-FU prodrug metabolized by the liver to 5-FU, and uracil, a biochemical modulator of 5-FU through inhibition of dihydropyrimidine dehydrogenase (DPD, the rate limiting enzyme of 5-FU metabolism). HCC is reported to have high levels of DPD, which may explain resistance to 5-FU, and therefore, DPD inhibition may enhance 5-FU activity. Fifty-six consecutive patients with unresectable stage IV-A HCC were studied prospectively to examine the efficacy of enteric-coated tegafur/uracil in HCC and to determine the significant prognostic factors. Twenty-eight patients were treated with UFT. Another 20 patients were given conservative management only. The remaining eight patients withdrew from the study. Although radiological responses were uncommon, the group receiving UFT, the median survival was 12 months, and one and two year survival rates were 55.3% and 36.9%, respectively. In the control group, the median survival was 6.2 months, and one year survival rate was 5.5%. By both univariate analysis and multivariate analysis treatment with UFT was shown to be the factor most significantly associated with better prognosis. The side effects of UFT were minimal, and treatment was well tolerated. In particular, no problems with renal function were noted, a complication that has been reported in cirrhotic patients. These results suggest that UFT may improve survival time by inducing a cytostatic effect, rather than by tumor reduction, and suggests that radiological response may not correlate with survival.[24]

T-138067 (Tularik Inc) is a novel inhibitor of tubulin polymerization, which therefore inhibits cell division. Preclinical studies indicated activity against the hepatoblastoma cell line HepG2 and in a phase I dose-escalation study, one of five HCC patients achieved a partial response.[25] In a 34-patient phase II study, there were three partial responses and 13 patients with disease stability, prompting the randomized phase III trial. Disappointingly, this early promise failed to translate into a survival benefit, with median survival of six months in both arms.[26] Of course it cannot be established whether this is a failure of both drugs and whether both are modestly active.

Nolatrexed is a novel thymidylate synthase inhibitor that unlike other antifolates, such as 5-FU, is lipophilic such that it does not require active uptake into cells and is orally available. Furthermore, it does not require polyglutamation for its activation. Both reduced cellular uptake and impaired glutamation can contribute to antifolate resistance. Nolatrexed has demonstrated in vitro activity even in HCC cells lines resistant to other antifolates. In a phase II trial of 28 patients with HCC, there were two partial responses and a further 16 minor responses/disease stabilisations,[27] prompting a 54-patient randomized phase II trial with doxorubicin as the comparator. Although there were no objective responses in either arm, there was a trend toward longer survival in those receiving nolatrexed (139 vs. 104 days).[28] Being a small, randomized phase II trial, statistical comparison of the two arms could not be made. Based on these data, a phase III trial comparing nolatrexed with doxorubicin recruiting 445 patients was conducted. The starting dose of nolatrexed was 800 mg/m^2 as a 24-hour continuous infusion for five days every three weeks. Doxorubicin was administered at a dose of 60 mg/m^2 intravenously every 21 days. Patients with a bilirubin of ≥1.2 mg/dL were initially treated with a dose of 30 mg/m^2. Left ventricular ejection fraction (LVEF) was performed before each dose above 240 mg/m^2, and doxorubicin was discontinued when there was a drop of ≥10% LVEF from the baseline value. Median overall survival was 22.3 weeks for nolatrexed and 32.3 weeks for doxorubicin ($P = 0.0068$). The hazard ratio was 0.753 in favor of doxorubicin. Objective response rate (complete response plus partial response) was 1.4% for nolatrexed and 4.0% for doxorubicin. Grade 3 and 4 stomatitis, vomiting, diarrhea, and thrombocytopenia were more common in the nolatrexed arm. Nolatrexed has a half-life of 11 hours and was thus given as a prolonged intravenous infusion. On the basis of the findings from the early phase I and II studies, an infusion period of 120 hours (five days) was chosen. In retrospect, this may have been too long and may have contributed to the high incidence of serious toxicities seen with this regimen. More patients were withdrawn from study for toxicity in the nolatrexed arm than in the doxorubicin arm. Despite the encouraging evidence of activity in the earlier trials, in fact patients receiving nolatrexed survived significantly less long than those in the control arm.[29] Although the statistical assumptions used in the design of this trial were based on demonstrating superiority for nolatrexed, because there were no obvious nolatrexed-related early deaths, some have argued that this study provides evidence that doxorubicin may, in fact, positively influence survival in appropriately selected patients. Nevertheless, although conventional cytotoxic therapy has undoubted activity against HCC, whether this translates into a survival advantage still requires appropriately designed and robustly statistically powered randomized controlled trials.

Combination Chemotherapy for Advanced Hepatocellular Carcinoma

On the basis of its modest activity as a single agent, doxorubicin has provided the backbone for combination studies in partnership with various other drugs. A phase II study of a four-drug combination of cisplatin, interferon-α2b, doxorubicin, and 5-fluorouracil (PIAF) reported a response rate of 26%. However, of 13 partial responders, 9 had their disease rendered resectable, and in some of these cases, there was a complete pathological response, again intimidating that radiological assessment may underestimate chemotherapy activity in HCC.[30] However, despite these encouraging findings, a prospective randomized study comparing PIAF to doxorubicin failed to demonstrate any improvement in survival with the combination. The median survival of the doxorubicin and PIAF groups was 6.83 and 8.67 months, respectively ($P = 0.83$). The hazard ratio for death from any cause in the PIAF compared with the doxorubicin groups was 0.97. Eighty-six of the 94 patients receiving doxorubicin and 91 of the 94 receiving PIAF were assessable for response. The overall response rates in the doxorubicin and PIAF groups were 10.5% and 20.9%, respectively. Neutropenia, thrombocytopenia, and hypokalemia were statistically significantly more common in patients treated with PIAF than in patients treated with doxorubicin. This study also conducted exploratory analysis of prognostic factors for response and survival. The only factor associated with better treatment response was high albumin level, whereas independent predictors for improved overall survival included high albumin level, low total bilirubin level, and low alanine transaminase level.[31]

Nondoxorubicin-based chemotherapy combinations have not demonstrated any consistently improved activity over single agents, with some notable exceptions. In a phase II study, the combination of etoposide plus epirubicin was well tolerated, and a response rate of 39% was reported.[32] A phase II study of infusional 5-FU with cisplatin reported objective response rate[33] of 47%.

A phase II study of gemcitabine reported an encouraging response rate. The therapy consisted of gemcitabine 1250 mg/m^2 intravenously over 30 minutes on days 1, 8, and 15 in a 28-day cycle for a total of six cycles.[34] A partial response was achieved in 5 of 28 patients, for an overall response rate of 17.8%. Seven patients had stable disease (25%). The median survival for all 28 patients was 18.7 weeks, and, for those patients who achieved a partial response, it was 34.7 weeks. Grade 3–4 toxicity consisted primarily of leucopenia (10.7%), anemia (14.3%), thrombocytopenia (10.7%), and hepatotoxicity (14.3%). Both hematologic and nonhematologic toxicity was mild, with thrombocytopenia constituting the dose-limiting side effect.[34] This good safety profile lends it to combination with other agents, and in particular, there is preclinical and clinical evidence for synergy with platinum compounds. The combination of gemcitabine and oxaliplatin is active and tolerated well in a number of cancers, and the lack of renal and liver toxicity is attractive in the context of HCC and underlying cirrhosis. Phase II studies have reported encouraging efficacy with good tolerance, although it is important to be mindful of gemcitabine-induced thrombocytopenia in patients with cirrhosis and hypersplenism and of oxaliplatin-induced neurotoxicity in patients with alcoholic liver disease who may have preexisting peripheral neuropathy. Thirty-four patients with previously untreated advanced-stage HCC were prospectively enrolled. The chemotherapy regimen consisted of gemcitabine 1000 mg/m^2 on day 1 and oxaliplatin 100 mg/m^2 on day 2. The treatment was repeated every 2 weeks until disease progression or limiting toxicity. In all, 323 treatment cycles were administered. Hematological grade 3–4 toxicity consisted of thrombocytopenia (27% of patients) and neutropenia (24%), including two febrile neutropenia. Grade 3 oxaliplatin-induced neurotoxicity was observed in three (9%) patients. The overall response rate was 18%, and disease stabilization was observed in 58% of patients giving a disease control rate of 76%. Median progression-free and overall survival times were 6.3 and 11.5 months, respectively. Treatment was more effective in patients with nonalcoholic cirrhosis than in those with alcoholic cirrhosis.[35] These studies again suggest that HCC can be chemosensitive and that chemotherapy can be administered safely and with manageable toxicity in appropriately selected patients. However, randomized trials of combination chemotherapy have been conducted rarely and those that have been mostly statistically underpowered to detect significant improvements in survival and have not stratified according to known prognostic factors so that, in general, meaningful conclusions cannot be drawn.

Chemotherapy in Combination with Novel Targeted Agents

Sorafenib is a small molecule that inhibits tumor-cell proliferation and tumor angiogenesis and induces apoptosis in a wide range of tumor models.[36,37] It acts by inhibiting the serine–threonine kinases Raf-1 and B-Raf and the receptor tyrosine kinase activity of vascular endothelial growth factor receptors 1, 2, and 3 and platelet-derived growth factor receptor-β.

Sorafenib is discussed at length in Chapter 21.[38–40] Pathways that are inhibited by novel targeted therapies including MAP Kinase signaling (raf/mek/erk) may also contribute to drug resistance such that combination of these agents with chemotherapy may reverse this. Indeed, there is preclinical evidence of synergy between doxorubicin and raf inhibition. In a vascular endothelial model, resistance to doxorubicin is, at least in part, mediated through fibroblast growth factor (FGF)-mediated raf-dependent survival signals providing rationale for combining doxorubicin with the raf inhibitor, sorafenib, or inhibitors of FGF receptor tyrosine kinase such as brivanib.[41] Furthermore, as there is preclinical evidence of synergy between doxorubicin and raf inhibition, a randomized phase II study has investigated the combination of sorafenib and doxorubicin compared to doxorubicin alone.[42] As expected given the addition of a chemotherapy agent, the adverse event profile in patients with advanced HCC who received combination therapy with sorafenib plus doxorubicin differed somewhat to that seen with sorafenib monotherapy in the SHARP trial. In patients receiving sorafenib plus doxorubicin, the most commonly occurring all-cause adverse events included fatigue, neutropenia, diarrhea, elevated bilirubin levels, abdominal pain, hand–foot skin reaction, left ventricular dysfunction, hypertension, and febrile neutropenia. The overall survival in the combination arm was more than double the control arm (13.7 months compared to 6.5 months, HR 0.45). However, this being a randomized phase II study, the aim was to determine whether the combination should be taken into a phase III setting rather than to allow statistically robust comparisons between treatment arms. To establish whether this benefit is attributable to synergy between the two agents or to sorafenib alone requires a further randomized trial of the combination using sorafenib as the control arm. The combination of antiangiogenic agents with conventional chemotherapy in other tumor types has shown clinical evidence of benefit. In patients with metastatic colorectal cancer, the anti-VEGF monoclonal antibody, bevacizumab, significantly prolongs survival when added to chemotherapy.[43] The central mechanism of action of bevacizumab is postulated to be antiangiogenic, but laboratory studies suggest that it may act through normalization of highly permeable tumor vessels, reducing interstitial pressure in the tumor, thereby increasing blood flow and improving chemotherapy delivery to the tumour.[44] A single arm phase II study in hepatocellular cancer has investigated the addition of bevacizumab to combination chemotherapy comprising gemcitabine and oxaliplatin, demonstrating some activity with a response rate of 20% and median survival of 9.5 months.[45] The significance of these results within the context of a single arm phase II study is difficult to interpret, but they do not appear to be significantly better than other phase II studies using chemotherapy alone.

Bortezomib is a selective proteosome inhibitor, which inhibits NFκB signaling.[46] Antitumor activity of bortezomib as a single agent and in combination with chemotherapeutic agents has been demonstrated in preclinical models[46,47] and a phase I/II trial demonstrated good tolerance in HCC patients, with 7 of 15 evaluable patients achieving disease stability.[48] As proteosome inhibition attenuates pathways implicated in anthracycline and other cytotoxic drug resistance, combination studies are of interest. However, results from a phase II study of doxorubicin plus bortezomib were disappointing with a response rate of 2.3% and median survival of 5.7 months.[49]

Adjuvant Systemic Therapy for Hepatocellular Carcinoma

Following surgical resection or local ablation, tumor recurrence and/or new tumor formation occurs commonly, and adjuvant therapy has been investigated in the form of systemic chemotherapy, hepatic arterial treatment, radiopharmaceuticals, and immunotherapy. Clinical trials of hepatic arterial chemotherapy with or without embolization in the adjuvant or neoadjuvant setting have not shown any survival benefit. Studies using adjuvant systemic chemotherapy have also failed to demonstrate a survival advantage. These studies have been small and not powered to detect modest differences.[50–56] As the benefit in the setting of curative treatment options are going to be small, clinical trials have to be adequately powered to detect a small but meaningful difference in the treatment versus no treatment arms. Novel approaches have shown promise in small trials, but larger trials with sufficient follow-up are required. Design of such studies raises interesting questions regarding the nature of HCC recurrence, being either due to micrometastases from the original tumor or de novo cancer formation in the remaining cirrhotic liver. Thus, the duration of adjuvant therapy may be difficult to determine, and the agents that may eradicate micrometastases may not prevent new tumor formation.

α-Fetoprotein as a Biomarker of Response to Chemotherapy

α-Fetoprotein (AFP) is a glycoprotein that is secreted by approximately 70% of HCC. Serum AFP is frequently measured in clinical practice during the course of treatment of HCC based on the hypothesis that AFP is continuously reflective of tumor activity and burden. Clinical trials have shown the cytostatic effects of systemic therapies with stable disease as the best radiological response but still translating into improved survival, indicating that radiological response may not be a good surrogate for clinical benefit from systemic therapy.

Evaluation of serial AFP measurements was undertaken in patients participating in the phase III trial comparing PIAF with doxorubicin.[57] The objectives of the study were to assess the significance of AFP decrease in relation to response to chemotherapy, to evaluate the role of serial AFP decrease in prediction of survival, and to assess the clinical significance of AFP decrease in a subgroup of patients who achieved stable disease based on radiologic assessment. AFP response was defined as a greater than 20% fall following at least two cycles of chemotherapy. Of 188 patients, 117 patients with elevated serum AFP (>20 μg/L) and documented radiologic evaluation had received at least two cycles of chemotherapy. A total of 47 AFP responders were identified. AFP responders had better survival than nonresponders (13.5 vs. 5.6 months, respectively; $P < 0.0001$), and AFP response was strongly associated with radiologic response ($P < 0.0001$). Multivariate analysis suggested that AFP response was significantly associated with survival (hazard ratio, 0.413; $P < .0001$). AFP responses were commonly observed in patients with radiologically stable disease and tended to identify a subgroup of stable disease patients with better survival, indicating that objective radiological response rate may tend to underestimate chemotherapy effect. Another retrospective study was performed on 107 patients with advanced HCC enrolled in five phase II clinical trials. Patients were separated into three groups based on a 50% change in serum AFP from baseline.[58] Eighteen patients experienced a >50% AFP decline, 57 patients had a >50% AFP increase, and 32 patients had a <50% change in serum AFP in either direction. Compared with patients with a <50% change in serum AFP (median PFS, 5.6 months), patients with a >50% AFP decrease had a longer PFS time (median, 16.9 months; $p = 0.029$), whereas those with a >50% increase had a shorter PFS time (median, 2.3 months; $p = 0.038$).[58] Patients with a >50% rise in AFP had a shorter OS time than those with a <50% change (median, 6.3 months vs. 11.1 months, respectively; $p = 0.004$), whereas a >50% AFP decrease was not associated with a significant difference in OS (median, 13.0 months; $p = 0.87$). Further studies are required to investigate AFP response and its significance in other treatment modalities. As most of the targeted therapies currently in use in HCC are cytostatic, serial measurement of AFP response to evaluate treatment outcome appears to be crucial for clinical trials.

Hepatitis B Virus Reactivation in Patients Undergoing Chemotherapy

Cancer patients who are hepatitis B virus (HBV) carriers and undergo chemotherapy are at risk of HBV reactivation, and globally, this is particularly pertinent to HCC, given the importance of HBV as a risk factor for this tumor. In a prospective study of 102 HBsAg-positive patients with inoperable HCC underwent systemic chemotherapy with PIAF or single-agent doxorubicin. They were followed during and for eight weeks after chemotherapy. In 102 patients, 59 (58%) developed hepatitis among whom 37 (36%) were attributable to HBV reactivation of whom twelve (30%) died of HBV reactivation. Elevated baseline alanine aminotransferase was found to be a risk factor.[59] Reactivation can be reduced by anti-viral therapy such as lamivudine. A study was done assessing the efficacy of lamivudine in reducing the incidence of HBV reactivation and diminishing morbidity and mortality of cancer patients with chronic HBV infection during chemotherapy has been conducted.[60] Two groups were compared in a nonrandomized manner. The prophylactic lamivudine group consisted of 65 patients who participated in phase II studies in which they were treated with lamivudine before and until 8 weeks after discontinuing chemotherapy. The historical controls consisted of 193 consecutive patients who underwent chemotherapy without prophylactic lamivudine. There was significantly less HBV reactivation (4.6% vs. 24.4% in the controls; $P < 0.001$), fewer incidences of hepatitis (17.5% vs. 44.6%; $P < 0.0001$) that were less severe (4.8% vs. 18.7%; $P = 0.0005$), and less disruption of chemotherapy (15.4% vs. 34.6%; $P = 0.0029$) in patients receiving lamivudine or not respectively.[59] Thus prophylactic lamivudine significantly reduced the incidence of HBV reactivation and the overall morbidity of cancer patients undergoing chemotherapy. As lamivudine prophylaxis was not routinely used prior to this, it is quite possible that HBV reactivation contributed to apparent toxicity in earlier chemotherapy studies, especially those conducted in HBV-endemic regions.

Discussion

In phase I studies of cytotoxic drugs for HCC, impaired drug metabolism due to underlying cirrhosis may affect the toxicity profile and dose intensity such that a suboptimal doses may be selected for further study. Conversely, using patients with well-preserved liver function may select a dose which might be poorly tolerated by patients with deranged liver functions. The issue of application of trial data derived from fit and well patients to a more general population is important to understand. It is encouraging to see more pragmatically designed phase I studies that incorporates patient liver functions in trial designs with two groups of patents being recruited in parallel, one with normal liver functions and the other with deranged liver functions to find the relevant dose limiting toxicity for the two groups separately.

The next step in the development of anticancer drugs is the phase II trial. This is the point where a decision must be taken to move a treatment further in large randomized and costly phase III trials or to abandon the compound. Traditionally, radiological response rate has been used as the primary endpoint. Clinical trials have questioned the wisdom in the setting of HCC with evidence from studies suggesting that changes in tumor size are not necessarily a good surrogate for clinical benefit. The recent sorafenib trials, showed a radiological response rate of just 2%, but these studies did report significantly prolonged survival.[38,39,40] Progression-free survival or time to progression may be more pragmatic endpoints for phase II trials. The two sorafenib trials clearly demonstrates the difficulty of predicting the natural history of HCC with a median survival in the control group of the Asian study and the European studies at 4.2 months and 7.9 months, respectively, despite similar eligibility criteria thus reflecting the patient heterogeneity as an important determinant of the clinical outcome irrespective of the treatments offered. The diversity within most disease categories is reflected by diversity in response to treatment. This clinical heterogeneity reflects underlying clinical and molecular characteristics and is not captured by the current staging system and that need to be understood and accounted for when designing new studies. This challenge to an extent may be met by using a randomized phase II trial design with a contemporary comparator.

Careful clinical trial design is required in multicenter settings where patients are utilized as a huge resource in well-designed randomized phase II studies with particular reference to patient characteristics (notably performance status and liver function), the choice of endpoint, and randomization to an appropriate control arm. This will help in taking the best systemic therapies forward in large randomized phase III trials.

For phase III trials, overall survival remains the appropriate end point, with a measure of quality of life that should be incorporated. However, patients with HCC develop symptoms due to underlying liver disease and due to the cancer and these are highly interrelated and difficult for currently available quality of life tools to differentiate.

The increasing understanding of the molecular biology of HCC will increase the possibilities of targeted therapy, and there are promising agents on the horizon. VEGF inhibitors, EGFR inhibitors, and mTOR inhibitors in combination with chemotherapy are potentially interesting combinations. Alteration of Wnt pathway, inhibition of the cell cycle as well as the proteosome, and epigenetic therapy may be other promising targets in HCC. The HCC clinical research agenda has recently moved on with advent of novel targeted therapies. However, conventional chemotherapy should not be disregarded and there is strong rationale for its combination with targeted agents. The main challenge over this decade is to establish randomized and adequately powered clinical trials combining novel therapies with chemotherapy treatments based on synergy. Such clinical trials will improve outcomes for patients with HCC and will help in eliminating mythology generated by anecdotes and hence reduce the variation in clinical practice.

References

1. Olweny CL, Toya T, Katongole-Mbidde E, et al. Treatment of hepatocellular carcinoma with adriamycin. Preliminary communication. *Cancer*. 1975;36(4):1250–1257.
2. Vogel CL, Bayley AC, Brooker RJ, et al. A phase II study of adriamycin (NSC 123127) in patients with hepatocellular carcinoma from Zambia and the United States. *Cancer*. 1977;39(5):1923–1929.
3. Johnson PJ, Williams R, Thomas H, et al. Induction of remission in hepatocellular carcinoma with doxorubicin. *Lancet*. 1978;1(8072):1006–1009.
4. Falkson G, Moertel CG, Lavin P, et al. Chemotherapy studies in primary liver cancer: a prospective randomized clinical trial. *Cancer*. 1978;42(5):2149–2156.
5. Olweny CL, Katongole-Mbidde E, Bahendeka S, et al. Further experience in treating patients with hepatocellular carcinoma in Uganda. *Cancer*. 1980;46(12):2717–2722.
6. Williams R, Melia WM. Liver tumours and their management. *Clin Radiol*. 1980;31(1):1–11.
7. Melia WM, Johnson PJ, Williams R. Induction of remission in hepatocellular carcinoma. A comparison of VP 16 with adriamycin. *Cancer*. 1983;51(2):206–210.
8. Chlebowski RT, Tong M, Weissman J, et al. Hepatocellular carcinoma. Diagnostic and prognostic features in North American patients. *Cancer*. 1984;53(12):2701–2706.
9. Choi TK, Lee NW, Wong J. Chem-otherapy for advanced hepatocellular carcinoma. Adriamycin versus quadruple chemotherapy. *Cancer*. 1984;53(3):401–405.
10. Falkson G, MacIntyre JM, Schutt AJ, et al. Neocarzinostatin versus m-AMSA or doxorubicin in hepatocellular carcinoma. *J Clin Oncol*. 1984;2(6):581–584.
11. Falkson G, MacIntyre JM, Moertel CG, et al. Primary liver cancer. An Eastern Cooperative Oncology Group Trial. *Cancer*. 1984;54(6):970–977.
12. Colombo M, Tommasini MA, Del Ninno E, et al. Hepatocellular carcinoma in Italy: report of a clinical trial with intravenous doxorubicin. *Liver*. 1985;5(6):336–341.
13. Sciarrino E, Simonetti RG, Le Moli S, Pagliaro L. Adriamycin treatment for hepatocellular carcinoma. Experience with 109 patients. *Cancer*. 1985;56(12):2751–2755.
14. Melia WM, Johnson PJ, Williams R. Controlled clinical trial of doxorubicin and tamoxifen versus doxorubicin alone in hepatocellular carcinoma. *Cancer Treat Rep*. 1987;71(12):1213–1216.
15. Lai CL, Wu PC, Chan GC, et al. Doxorubicin versus no antitumor therapy in inoperable hepatocellular carcinoma. A prospective randomized trial. *Cancer*. 1988;62(3):479–483.

16. Johnson PJ, Dobbs N, Kalayci C, et al. Clinical efficacy and toxicity of standard dose adriamycin in hyperbilirubinaemic patients with hepatocellular carcinoma: relation to liver tests and pharmacokinetic parameters. *Br J Cancer*. 1992;65(5):751–755.

17. Halm U, Etzrodt G, Schiefke I, et al. A phase II study of pegylated liposomal doxorubicin for treatment of advanced hepatocellular carcinoma. *Ann Oncol*. 2000;11(1):113–114.

18. Hong RL, Tseng YL. A phase II and pharmacokinetic study of pegylated liposomal doxorubicin in patients with advanced hepatocellular carcinoma. *Cancer Chemother Pharmacol*. 2003;51(5):433–438.

19. Hochster HS, Green MD, Speyer J, et al. 4'Epidoxorubicin (epirubicin): activity in hepatocellular carcinoma. *J Clin Oncol*. 1985;3(11):1535–1540.

20. Pohl J, Zuna I, Stremmel W, Rudi J. Systemic chemotherapy with epirubicin for treatment of advanced or multifocal hepatocellular carcinoma. *Chemotherapy*. 2001;47(5):359–365.

21. Lai KH, Tsai YT, Lee SD, et al. Phase II study of mitoxantrone in unresectable primary hepatocellular carcinoma following hepatitis B infection. *Cancer Chemother Pharmacol*. 1989;23(1):54–56.

22. Ravry MJ, Omura GA, Bartolucci AA, et al. Phase II evaluation of cisplatin in advanced hepatocellular carcinoma and cholangiocarcinoma: a Southeastern Cancer Study Group Trial. *Cancer Treat Rep*. 1986;70(2):311–312.

23. Zaniboni A, Simoncini E, Marpicati P, Marini G. Phase II study of 5-fluorouracil (5-FU) and high dose folinic acid (HDFA) in hepatocellular carcinoma. *Br J Cancer*. 1988;57(3):319.

24. Ishikawa T, Ichida T, Sugitani S, et al. Improved survival with oral administration of enteric-coated tegafur/uracil for advanced stage IV-A hepatocellular carcinoma. *J Gastroenterol Hepatol*. 2001;16(4):452–459.

25. Leung TW, Feun L, Posey J, et al. A phase II study of T138067-sodium in patients (pts) with unresectable hepatocellular carcinoma (HCC). *Proc Am Soc Clin Oncol*. 2002;21. abstr 572.

26. Posey J, Johnson P, Mok T, et al. Results of a phase 2/3 open-label, randomized trial of T138067 versus doxorubicin (DOX) in chemotherapy-naïve, unresectable hepatocellular carcinoma (HCC). *J Clin Oncol*. 2005;23(16S). ASCO Annual Meeting Proceedings. Part I of II (June 1 Supplement), 2005:4035.

27. Stuart K, Tessitore J, Rudy J, et al. A Phase II trial of nolatrexed dihydrochloride in patients with advanced hepatocellular carcinoma. *Cancer*. 1999;86(3):410–414.

28. Mok TS, Leung TW, Lee SD, et al. A multi-centre randomized phase II study of nolatrexed versus doxorubicin in treatment of Chinese patients with advanced hepatocellular carcinoma. *Cancer Chemother Pharmacol*. 1999;44(4):307–311.

29. Gish RG, Porta C, Lazar L, et al. Phase III randomized controlled trial comparing the survival of patients with unresectable hepatocellular carcinoma treated with nolatrexed or doxorubicin. *J Clin Oncol*. 2007;25(21):3069–3075.

30. Leung TW, Patt YZ, Lau WY, et al. Complete pathological remission is possible with systemic combination chemotherapy for inoperable hepatocellular carcinoma. *Clin Cancer Res*. 1999;5(7):1676–1681.

31. Yeo W, Mok TS, Zee B, et al. A randomized phase III study of doxorubicin versus cisplatin/interferon alpha-2b/doxorubicin/fluorouracil (PIAF) combination chemotherapy for unresectable hepatocellular carcinoma. *J Natl Cancer Inst*. 2005;97(20):1532–1538.

32. Bobbio-Pallavicini E, Porta C, Moroni M, et al. Epirubicin and etoposide combination chemotherapy to treat hepatocellular carcinoma patients: a phase II study. *Eur J Cancer*. 1997;33(11):1784–1788.

33. Tanioka H, Tsuji A, Morita S, et al. Combination chemotherapy with continuous 5-fluorouracil and low-dose cisplatin infusion for advanced hepatocellular carcinoma. *Anticancer Res*. 2003;23(2C):1891–1897.

34. Yang TS, Lin YC, Chen JS, et al. Phase II study of gemcitabine in patients with advanced hepatocellular carcinoma. *Cancer*. 2000;89(4):750–756.

35. Louafi S, Boige V, Ducreux M, et al. Gemcitabine plus oxaliplatin (GEMOX) in patients with advanced hepatocellular carcinoma (HCC): results of a phase II study. *Cancer*. 2007;109(7):1384–1390.

36. Wilhelm SM, Carter C, Tang L, et al. BAY 43-9006 exhibits broad spectrum oral antitumor activity and targets the RAF/MEK/ERK pathway and receptor tyrosine kinases involved in tumor progression and angiogenesis. *Cancer Res*. 2004;64:7099–7109.

37. Chang YS, Adnane J, Trail PA, et al. Sorafenib (BAY 43-9006) inhibits tumor growth and vascularization and induces tumor apoptosis and hypoxia in RCC xenograft models. *Cancer Chemother Pharmacol*. 2007;59:561–574.

38. Abou-Alfa GK, Schwartz L, Ricci S, et al. Phase II study of sorafenib in patients with advanced hepatocellular carcinoma. *J Clin Oncol*. 2006;24:4293–4300.

39. Llovet JM, Ricci S, Mazzaferro V, et al. Sorafenib in advanced hepatocellular carcinoma. *N Engl J Med.* 2008;359(4):378–390.

40. Cheng AL, Kang YK, Chen Z, et al. Efficacy and safety of sorafenib in patients in the Asia-Pacific region with advanced hepatocellular carcinoma: a phase III randomised, double-blind, placebo-controlled trial. *Lancet Oncol.* 2009;10(1):25–34.

41. Alavi A, Hood JD, Frausto R, et al. Role of Raf in vascular protection from distinct apoptotic stimuli. *Science.* 2003;301(5629):94–96.

42. Abou-Alfa G, Johnson P, Knox J, et al. Preliminary results from a Phase II, randomized, double-blind study of sorafenib plus doxorubicin versus placebo plus doxorubicin in patients with advanced hepatocellular carcinoma. Proceedings of the 2007 meeting of the European Cancer Organization. *Eur J Cancer Suppl.* 2007;5:259. abstr 3500.

43. Hurwitz H, Fehrenbacher L, Novotny W, et al. Bevacizumab plus irinotecan, fluorouracil, and leucovorin for metastatic colorectal cancer. *N Engl J Med.* 2004;350(23):2335–2342.

44. Jain RK. Normalization of tumor vasculature: an emerging concept in antiangiogenic therapy. *Science.* January 7, 2005;307(5706):58–62.

45. Zhu AX, Blaszkowsky LS, Ryan DP, et al. Phase II study of gemcitabine and oxaliplatin in combination with bevacizumab in patients with advanced hepatocellular carcinoma. *J Clin Oncol.* 2006;24(12):1898–1903.

46. Hideshima T, Richardson P, Chauhan D, et al. The proteasome inhibitor PS-341 inhibits growth, induces apoptosis, and overcomes drug resistance in human multiple myeloma cells. *Cancer Res.* 2001;61(7):3071–3076.

47. Cusack JC Jr, Liu R, Houston M, et al. Enhanced chemosensitivity to CPT-11 with proteasome inhibitor PS-341: implications for systemic nuclear factor-kappaB inhibition. *Cancer Res.* 2001;61(9):3535–3540.

48. Hegewisch-Becker S, Sterneck M, Schubert U, et al. Phase I/II trial of bortezomib in patients with unresectable hepatocellular carcinoma (HCC). *J Clin Oncol.* 2004;22(14S). ASCO Annual Meeting Proceedings (Post-Meeting Edition). (July 15 Supplement), 2004: 4089.

49. Berlin JD, Powell ME, Su Y, et al. Bortezomib (B) and doxorubicin (dox) in patients (pts) with hepatocellular cancer (HCC): a phase II trial of the Eastern Cooperative Oncology Group (ECOG 6202) with laboratory correlates. *Clin Oncol.* May 20, 2008;26(suppl). abstr 4592.

50. Lai EC, Lo CM, Fan ST, et al. Postoperative adjuvant chemotherapy after curative resection of hepatocellular carcinoma: a randomized controlled trial. *Arch Surg.* 1998;133(2):183–188.

51. Wu CC, Ho YZ, Ho WL, et al. Preoperative transcatheter arterial chemoembolization for resectable large hepatocellular carcinoma: a reappraisal. *Br J Surg.* 1995;82(1):122–126.

52. Izumi R, Shimizu K, Iyobe T, et al. Postoperative adjuvant hepatic arterial infusion of Lipiodol containing anticancer drugs in patients with hepatocellular carcinoma. *Hepatology.* 1994;20(2):295–301.

53. Yamasaki S, Hasegawa H, Kinoshita H, et al. A prospective randomized trial of the preventive effect of pre-operative transcatheter arterial embolization against recurrence of hepatocellular carcinoma. *Jpn J Cancer Res.* 1996;87(2):206–211.

54. Yamamoto M, Arii S, Sugahara K, Tobe T. Adjuvant oral chemotherapy to prevent recurrence after curative resection for hepatocellular carcinoma. *Br J Surg.* 1996;83(3):336–340.

55. Ono T, Nagasue N, Kohno H, et al. Adjuvant chemotherapy with epirubicin and carmofur after radical resection of hepatocellular carcinoma: a prospective randomized study. *Semin Oncol.* 1997;24(2 suppl 6):S6-18–S6-25.

56. Kohno H, Nagasue N, Hayashi T, et al. Postoperative adjuvant chemotherapy after radical hepatic resection for hepatocellular carcinoma (HCC). *Hepatogastroenterology.* 1996;43(12):1405–1409.

57. Chan SL, Mo FK, Johnson PJ, et al. New utility of an old marker: serial alpha-fetoprotein measurement in predicting radiologic response and survival of patients with hepatocellular carcinoma undergoing systemic chemotherapy. *J Clin Oncol.* 2009;27(3):446–452.

58. Vora SR, Zheng H, Stadler ZK, et al. Serum {alpha}-fetoprotein response as a surrogate for clinical outcome in patients receiving systemic therapy for advanced hepatocellular carcinoma. *Oncologist.* 2009;(7):717–725.

59. Yeo W, Lam KC, Zee B, et al. Hepatitis B reactivation in patients with hepatocellular carcinoma undergoing systemic chemotherapy. *Ann Oncol.* 2004;15(11):1661–1666.

60. Yeo W, Chan PK, Ho WM, et al. Lamivudine for the prevention of hepatitis B virus reactivation in hepatitis B s-antigen seropositive cancer patients undergoing cytotoxic chemotherapy. *J Clin Oncol.* 2004;22(5):927–934.

CHAPTER 20

Intraarterial Chemotherapy for Liver Tumors

Maeve Lowery & Nancy E. Kemeny

Hepatic arterial infusion (HAI) therapy refers to the delivery of chemotherapeutic agents directly into the liver through the hepatic artery. The technique for delivery of chemotherapy through the hepatic artery was first developed almost 40 years ago for the treatment of colorectal cancer liver metastases. Over the past several decades, the mode of delivery has been developed and refined to allow for safe and controlled administration by totally implantable pump. The rationale for the development of HAI therapy is based on the discovery that colorectal cancer metastases to the liver derive their blood supply from the hepatic artery.[1] Administration of chemotherapy through the hepatic artery therefore results in increased exposure of malignant cells to the drug, with relative sparing of the normal liver parenchyma. In parallel to advances in systemic therapy and surgical technique for colorectal liver metastases, the use of HAI has evolved from HAI therapy alone to treat hepatic metastases to include incorporation of modern systemic chemotherapy regimens. In this chapter, we review the principles of drug selection, mode of administration, and management of toxicities associated with HAI therapy and the evidence for use of HAI in colorectal liver metastases and in primary liver tumors.

Pharmacological Principles for Drug Selection in Hepatic Arterial Infusion

There are unique pharmacokinetic and pharmacodynamic properties of the drug used for HAI administration (Table 20-1). The aim of HAI therapy is to achieve a high concentration of the drug within the liver, with a low systemic concentration.[2] This is achieved by using the agents that have a high hepatic extraction ratio and have a short plasma half-life. The hepatic extraction ratio describes the extent of first-pass effect experienced by a drug; ideally drugs used for HAI have a high hepatic extraction ratio, which remains constant even at high drug doses. The drug should be cleared quickly from the body to avoid recirculation through the systemic circulation, thereby minimizing systemic toxicity, and the rate of clearance of the drug should remain constant even at high doses. CL_{TB} describes the total body clearance of a drug, reflecting the rate of elimination of a drug relative to its plasma concentration. In drugs that demonstrate first-order kinetics, this value remains constant regardless of the plasma concentration of the drug. Therefore, the ideal drug for HAI has a high CL_{TB} but exhibits first-order kinetics. The Collins formula describes the advantage of a regional administration over

TABLE 20-1: Ideal Drug Properties for HAI

Ideal Drug Properties for HAI
• High hepatic extraction ratio
• Short plasma half-life
• High CL_{TB}
• First-order kinetics
• Dose-dependent antitumor activity

Abbreviations: CL_{TB}, total body clearance of a drug; HAI, hepatic arterial infusion.

systemic administration for a given drug based on total body clearance, hepatic artery flow rate, and hepatic extraction.[3]

$$\text{Advantage} = \frac{1 + \text{Total body clearance of a drug}}{\text{Hepatic artery flow rate }*}$$

*1–fraction of drug extracted across the liver.

The selected agent should be effective against the tumor being treated and ideally should have dose-dependent activity, whereby increasing local concentration of drug leads to an increased therapeutic response rate. The therapeutic advantage of HAI arises from the ability to increase drug exposure to tumor cells above that which is obtainable by systemic administration alone.

5 Fluoro-2-Deoxyuridine

Multiple therapeutic agents have been studied in trials of HAI therapy, but 5 fluoro-2-deoxyuridine (FUDR) remains the drug of choice for HAI. FUDR is an antimetabolite that exerts its activity by inhibiting thymidylate synthase, thereby interfering with DNA replication and resulting in cell death. It has been shown to have a 94%–99% extraction rate within the liver, demonstrating extensive first-pass metabolism.[2] CL_{TB} is 15–25 mL/min for FUDR, and it exhibits first-order kinetics. Intrahepatic FUDR levels have been shown to have a 100- to 400-fold estimated increase in hepatic exposure compared to 5FU, which demonstrates a 10-fold increase in intrahepatic levels compared to systemic infusion.[4] These early studies established FUDR as the drug of choice for use in HAI; it has remained the backbone of HAI therapy in subsequent clinical trials over the past 30 years.

FUDR administration through the portal vein has been compared to HAI administration of FUDR. Intraoperative injection of radioactive FUDR into either the portal vein or the hepatic artery of patients with colorectal liver metastases was followed by tumor biopsy and measurement of tissue drug concentration.[5] Hepatic colorectal metastases were found to have a 15 times higher concentration of FUDR following administration through the hepatic artery when compared to levels obtained by portal vein infusion, effectively demonstrating the advantage of HAI FUDR administration over portal vein administration.

HAI with Nonfluoropyrimidine Drugs

Other agents evaluated for use in HAI include BCNU, 5FU, doxorubicin, mitomycin, and cisplatin. They all have some advantage when used by regional infusion but do not have all the advantages seen with FUDR.[6] More recently, trials of systemic administration of oxaliplatin and irinotecan have demonstrated significant benefit in patients with metastatic colorectal cancer, leading to their evaluation as HAI therapy. Preclinical studies comparing hepatic arterial to systemic administration of oxaliplatin have demonstrated a pharmacokinetic advantage to HAI administration, leading to the evaluation of HAI oxaliplatin in a number of phase II trials.[7] Irinotecan is metabolized to an active form SN38 by the carboxylesterases in the liver, serum, and small intestine. Pharmacokinetic studies of HAI administration of irinotecan compared to systemic administration showed no significant difference in systemic SN38 levels between the two methods of administration.[8] The lack of significant first-pass extraction of irinotecan limits the benefit of HAI administration.[9]

HAI Infusion Pump

Initial attempts at HAI utilized catheters connected to external infusion pumps. Despite encouraging response rates, these early trials were limited by a high incidence of catheter-related complications, including infection, bleeding, and thrombosis of the hepatic artery or catheter. The use of a totally implantable pump with no requirement for an external power source was first reported in 1980 and significantly improved the complication rate and overall quality of life for patients treated with HAI.[10] Although there are several implantable HAI pumps currently available, all utilize the same basic mechanism (Figure 20-1). The pump is composed of a hollow cylinder divided into two chambers.[11] One chamber contains charging fluid with fluorocarbon and is permanently sealed,

Intraarterial Chemotherapy for Liver Tumors

whereas the other contains the chemotherapy drug and connects to the catheter. The fluorocarbon liquid in the sealed chamber converts to gas when heated to body temperature. This causes a constant gaseous pressure on the drug chamber, resulting in a constant flow rate into the catheter at any given temperature. The drug chamber is refillable by accessing through a resealable septum; injection into the septum causes the drug chamber to expand and reduce the volume of the charging liquid chamber, thereby causing the vapor to condense to liquid.

Preoperative Evaluation

In order to be considered for HAI therapy, patients must have no evidence of extrahepatic disease. Preoperative investigations include thorough radiological assessment of disease status by imaging with computed tomography (CT), magnetic resonance imaging, or positron emission tomography. Arteriography is required presurgery to determine the presence of a variant arterial anatomy; conventional arteriography has now largely been replaced by CT arteriography. The presence of a patent portal vein must be determined preplacement of HAI catheter to avoid hepatic ischemia. After placement of the catheter, further imaging with injection of microaggregated albumin through the side port is performed to ensure perfusion of both lobes of the liver.

Technique for Insertion of HAI Catheter

The catheter tip is inserted into the gastroduodenal artery, as this has a lower rate of arterial thrombosis than placement directly into the hepatic artery. Ligation is performed of the right gastric artery and of the vascular structures that supply the superior border of the stomach and the duodenum. This prevents the occurrence of misperfusion of these

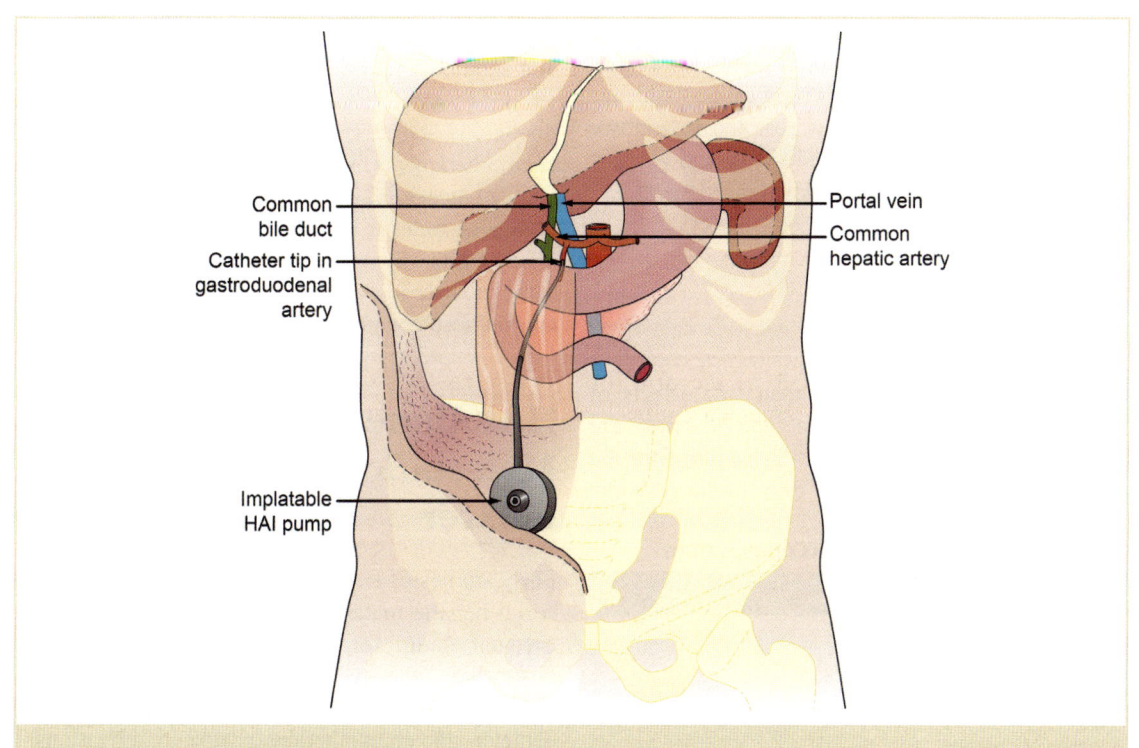

Figure 20-1: Implantable pump for hepatic arterial infusion (HAI) therapy.

structures with resulting gastritis, duodenitis, and ulceration. Cholecystectomy is usually performed at time of pump placement due to risk of chemical cholangitis secondary to HAI. The pump is placed in a subcutaneous pocket in either the left or right lower quadrant.

Catheter-related Complications

Complications reported related to HA catheter placement include pump malfunction, pocket infection, catheter thrombosis or displacement, catheter erosion, arterial thrombosis/dissection, extrahepatic perfusion, and incomplete perfusion (Table 20-2). Initial reports of catheter-related complications reported a wide variation in rates, with reported incidence approaching 40% in some centers.[12] The largest reported series of HAI catheter placement retrospectively evaluated 544 patients and found that lack of surgeon experience, presence of variant arterial anatomy, and cannulation of a vessel other that the gastroduodenal artery were significant factors associated with increased risk of complications.[13] Pump complications were seen in 22% of patients; however, early complications occurring in the first 30 days post placement were salvaged in 70% of cases. Incidence of pump failure were 9% at one year and 16% at two years, demonstrating the overall safety and efficacy of implantable HAI pumps in experienced hands.

Toxicity of HAI Chemotherapy

Classical chemotherapy-associated side effects of hematological toxicity, nausea, and diarrhea are generally not associated with HAI administration of FUDR due to low levels of drug in the systemic circulation. The most common side effect seen is hepatic toxicity secondary to perfusion of the bile ducts by HAI therapy. Approximately 15%–25% of patients undergoing HAI therapy will have an elevation of serum bilirubin.[14] The bile ducts derive their blood supply from the hepatic artery and so are exposed to high concentrations of chemotherapy[15]; this in combination with relative ischemia secondary to partial occlusion of the hepatic artery accounts for the biliary toxicity unique to HAI. Careful monitoring of patients liver function tests is required during treatment. Elevated aspartate aminotransferase (AST) is generally the first abnormality seen, followed by a rise in alkaline phosphatase and bilirubin. Withdrawal of treatment for a short time can usually reverse hepatic toxicity secondary to HAI, allowing subsequent resumption of therapy at a lower dose. A subset of patients however will develop biliary strictures with a sclerosing cholangitis-like appearance at ERCP and require biliary stenting. Cross-sectional imaging of the liver is needed before intervention to out rule obstruction from metastatic disease as a cause of jaundice. The addition of dexamethasone to hepatic infusion of FUDR has shown a trend to reduced bilirubin levels with increased response rate and overall survival and should be routinely used.[16]

Gastrointestinal complications of gastritis, duodenitis and ulcer formation occur as a result of chemotherapy perfusion of the structures and can be avoided by careful ligation of vessels perfusing these organs at time of catheter insertion. Similarly, the introduction of prophylactic cholecystectomy during catheter insertion eliminates the risk of chemotherapy-induced chemical cholecystitis.

HAI Alone for Unresectable Metastatic Colorectal Cancer to Liver

Early studies of HAI therapy for unresectable colorectal hepatic metastases were performed using an external pump for administration. Despite demonstrating unprecedented response rates up to 65%, these trials were limited by the high rates of catheter- and chemotherapy-related complications.[17] However with the advent of the totally implantable pump in 1980, and increasing experience with management and prophylaxis of toxicities, a series

TABLE 20-2: Catheter-related Complications

Catheter-Related Complications
• Pump malfunction
• Pocket infection
• Catheter thrombosis
• Catheter displacement/erosion
• Arterial thrombosis/dissection
• Extrahepatic/incomplete perfusion

of single-arm studies using HAI FUDR were successfully completed demonstrating acceptable toxicity and confirming the increased response rates previously reported.[18–23] This led to the evaluation of HAI FUDR in the management of unresectable colorectal hepatic metastases in several randomized trials of HAI compared to systemic chemotherapy. To date 10 randomized clinical trials and 3 meta-analyses have been published[24–33] (Table 20-3).

Early trials were evaluated in two separate meta-analyses published in 1996, both of which found an overall survival benefit to the use of HAI (Table 20-4). The first meta-analysis included six published trials and reported a statistically significant improvement in one-year survival of 10%.[34] The second included seven trials and demonstrated an overall survival hazard ratio of 0.73 in favor of HAI ($P = 0.0009$).[35] Both meta-analyses confirmed a statistically significant higher response rate for the HAI arm.

Three randomized trials have been published since 2000, two from European groups and one from the CALGB collaborative group. The German Cooperative group study evaluated 168 patients with unresectable colorectal liver metastases.[31] Patients were randomly assigned to treatment with 5FU/LV by HAI, systemic 5FU/LV, and HAI FUDR. Median survival was 18.7, 17.6, and 12.7 months, respectively, whereas response rates were 45%, 19.7%, and 43.2%, respectively. In this study however, 31% of patients did not receive HAI therapy as planned. HAI chemotherapy was administered predominantly by port, as use of implantable pump was optional. No FUDR dose reductions for toxicity were incorporated into the protocol, and dexamethasone was not administered with FUDR by HAI. The EORTC/MRC group randomized 290 patients with unresectable colorectal liver metastases to IV 5FU/LV versus HAI 5FU/LV.[32] HAI chemotherapy was administered through port

TABLE 20-3: Randomized Trials of Hepatic Arterial Infusion Therapy

Study	Treatment (HAI vs. SYS)	Number Enrolled	Percentage Receiving Assigned Therapy	Response Rate (%)	Overall Survival (months)
Chang (1987)[24]	HAI FUDR	64	66	62	17
	IV FUDR		92	17	12
Kemeny (1987)[25]	HAI FUDR	99	94	50	17
	IV FUDR[a]		94	20	12
Hohn (1989)[26]	HAI FUDR	143	75	42	16.5
	IV FUDR		86	9	15.8
Martin (1990)[27]	HAI FUDR	69	79	48	12.6
	IV 5FU		83	21	10.5
Wagman (1990)[28]	HAI FUDR	41	100	55	13.8
	IV 5FU		100	20	11.6
Rougier (1992)[29]	HAI FUDR	163	87	41	15
	IV 5FU		50	9	11
Allen-Mersh (1994)[30]	HAI FUDR	100	96	—	13.5
	IV 5FU		20		7.5
Lorenz (2000)[31]	HAI FUDR	168	69	43	12.7
	HAI 5FU		70	45	18.7
	IV 5FU[a]		91	27	17.6
Kerr (2003)[32]	HAI 5FU	290	66	22	14.7
	IV 5FU		87	19	14.8
Kemeny (2006)[33]	HAI FUDR	135	87	47	24.4
	IV 5FU		87	24	20

Abbreviations: FUDR, 5 fluoro-2-deoxyuridine; HAI, hepatic arterial infusion; SYS, systemic.
Note: Overall survival calculated based on intention to treat.
[a]Crossover from systemic to HAI allowed.

TABLE 20-4: Meta-analyses of Hepatic Arterial Infusion Therapy

Publication	Number of Trials	Response Rate (HAI vs. Systemic)	P	Overall Survival (HAI vs. Systemic)	P
Harmantas (1996)[34]	6	—	—	1-y survival benefit 12.9% vs 2-y survival benefit 7.5%	0.002 0.026
JNCI (1996)[35]	7	41% vs. 14%	<10–10	HR 0.73	0.0009
Mocellin (2007)[36]	10	49% vs. 18.4%	<0.001	Median survival 15.9 mo vs. 12.4 mo	0.24

Abbreviation: HAI, hepatic arterial infusion; HR, hazard ratio.

in all cases; 37% of patients assigned to the HAI arm did not receive treatment. Median overall survival was 14.7 months for the HAI group and 14.8 months for the IV group ($P = 0.79$), with no progression-free survival benefit seen.

Evaluation of treated patients was not done. In contrast to these studies, the CALBG 9481 study randomized 135 patients to receive HAI FUDR with dexamethasone versus systemic bolus 5FU/LV.[33] In this study, no crossover was permitted, and only 13.2% of patients in the HAI arm did not receive therapy as planned. Overall survival was significantly prolonged in the HAI arm; 24.4 versus 20 months ($P = 0.0034$), with a doubling of tumor response rate seen: 47% in the HAI group and 24% in the systemic group ($P = 0.012$).

The most recent meta-analysis published in 2008 concluded that although HAI results in a significantly higher response rate when compared to systemic fluoropyrimidine-based treatment, there is no evidence for an overall survival benefit to HAI.[36] Tumor response rates were 42.9% versus 18.4% for HAI and systemic therapy, respectively ($P < 0.001$), whereas median overall survival was 15.9% and 12.4% ($P = 0.24$). Significantly, this meta-analysis did not address the role of HAI in combination with systemic treatment, or the issue that cross-over of patients to HAI from systemic treatment was allowed in a number of included studies.

Interpretation of these data is limited by the size and quality of the randomized controlled trials conducted to date. A number of these studies were not adequately powered to evaluate overall survival. Four of the randomized trials utilized a crossover design, resulting in a significant number of patients in the systemic treatment arm ultimately receiving HAI and making determination of an overall survival benefit difficult. In three of the trials, patients with extrahepatic disease were included; it is now well established that patients with extrahepatic disease do not benefit from HAI therapy. Other confounding factors include inappropriate dosing of FUDR, use of ports instead of pumps for delivery and low numbers of patients actually receiving therapy on the HAI arms. As more effective systemic options for management of metastatic colorectal cancer have become available however, recent studies have moved away from the use of HAI FUDR alone and rather focused on evaluating the use of HAI in combination with modern systemic chemotherapy and biologic agents.

Response to HAI with Nonfluoropyrimidine Chemotherapy Agents

Several studies have evaluated irinotecan when administered by HAI, but response rates in phase II studies have not been shown to be superior to systemic administration, likely due its unsuitable pharmacokinetic properties discussed earlier in text.[37,38] Several phase II clinical trials have demonstrated safety and tolerability of HAI oxaliplatin, with response rates up to 64% when administered in combination with IV 5FU/LV for first line treatment of colorectal cancer liver metastases.[39,40] Abdominal pain was seen in a significant number of patients treated with HAI oxaliplatin, whereas the rate of neurotoxicity appeared lower than that seen with intravenous administration. HAI administration of oxaliplatin has not to date been evaluated in a randomized comparison with systemic infusion, so the benefit over systemic administration remains unclear.

HAI in Combination with Systemic Chemotherapy

Initial trials evaluating HAI FUDR in combination with systemic 5FU demonstrated a significant overall survival advantage with the addition of systemic therapy to HAI (Table 20-5). In a trial of 76 patients randomized to HAI versus HAI plus systemic bolus 5FU and leucovorin overall survival, response rate and time to progression were all significantly prolonged in the systemic chemotherapy plus HAI arm.[41]

Recent studies have focused on the evaluation of HAI in combination with newer systemic combination chemotherapy regimens. A phase I study of 46 patients with unresectable liver metastases, all of whom had previous treatment, reported a response rate of 74% with HAI FUDR combined with systemic irinotecan.[42] The combination was well tolerated with most common toxicities being diarrhea and neutropenia. A subsequent phase I trial evaluated 36 patients with unresectable liver metastases, randomized to HAI FUDR in combination with oxaliplatin/5FU or oxaliplatin/CPT11 systemic chemotherapy.[43] Response rates were 90% and 87%, respectively, with median survival time 36 and 22 months, respectively, although over 89% of these patients had received prior therapy. Overall the combination was well tolerated, with most common grade 3/4 toxicities being diarrhea, neutropenia, and neurotoxicity attributable to systemic treatment.

A retrospective analysis examined 39 patients with liver confined colorectal metastases, all of whom had progressed on systemic chemotherapy with oxaliplatin, treated with combination of HAI FUDR and Dex with concurrent systemic irinotecan. A response rate of 44% was seen in this heavily pretreated patient group, with median overall survival from time of initiation of HAI of 20.1 months.[44] Most recently, a phase I trial evaluated

TABLE 20-5: Trials of Hepatic Arterial Infusion in Combination with Systemic Chemotherapy

Trial	N	Trial	Treatment	Response Rate (%)	Overall Survival
Fiorentini (2006)[41]	76	Randomized	HAI FUDR vs. HAI FUDR and IV 5FU/LV	47.5 vs 41.7 $P = 0.09$	20 vs. 14 $P = 0.0033$
Kemeny (2001)[42]	46	Prospective	HAI FUDR and IV irinotecan	74%	—
Kemeny (2005)[43]	36	Prospective	HAI FUDR and IV oxaliplatin/5FU or HAI FUDR and IV oxaliplatin/irinotecan	90% vs. 87%	36 vs. 22
Gallagher (2007)[44]	39	Retrospective[a]	HAI FUDR and IV irinotecan	44%	20.1
Kemeny (2009)[45]	49	Phase 1	HAI FUDR and IV oxaliplatin and irinotecan	92%	50.8 (chemo naive) 35 (pretreated with chemo)

Abbreviations: FUDR, 5 fluoro-2-deoxyuridine; HAI, hepatic arterial infusion.
Note: Overall survival calculated from initiation of HAI therapy.
[a]Heavily pretreated patients.

49 patients with unresectable liver metastases, 53% of whom had previously received chemotherapy, treated with HAI FUDR and Dex in combination with systemic oxaliplatin and irinotecan.[45] A 92% response rate was seen, median survival in chemotherapy naïve and previously treated patients was 50.8 and 35 months, respectively.

HAI FUDR plus modern systemic chemotherapy has yet to be compared in a prospective randomized trial to modern systemic chemotherapy alone, however promising response rates and an acceptable toxicity profile makes this a treatment approach deserving of further investigation in larger clinical trials for first- or second-line treatment of unresectable colorectal liver metastases.

Conversion to Resectability

Surgical resection of liver metastases in colorectal cancer has been shown to result in long-term survival and even cure in multiple large case series. No randomized clinical trial has addressed the issue, however recently reported five-year survival rates post complete surgical resection (R0 resection) are in the order of 10%–30%.[46] The 5-year survival rates for patients converted to resectability by preoperative chemotherapy approaches that of patients who are candidates for hepatic resection at presentation.[47] Given that surgical resection provides the greatest likelihood of long-term survival, conversion to resectability has become a new endpoint in the evaluation of therapeutic strategies for unresectable hepatic metastases. For patients with initially unresectable disease, some studies have suggested that the rate of surgical resection correlates with response to chemotherapy.[48] However, a subsequent retrospective analysis of 111 patients who received neo-adjuvant chemotherapy followed by surgical resection for colorectal liver metastases did not find a correlation between response to neo-adjuvant chemotherapy and overall survival.[49]

The high response rates achieved by the use of HAI-based chemotherapy have also translated into a high rate of conversion to resectability in patients presenting with unresectable liver metastases. In the phase I trial described above of HAI FUDR in combination with oxaliplatin and irinotecan, a 47% rate of conversion to resectability was reported, with a higher rate of 57% seen in chemotherapy naïve patients.[50] Other phase I and retrospective studies have demonstrated rates of conversion to resectable disease of 18%–26% using HAI FUDR in combination with systemic oxaliplatin or irinotecan.[43,44]

Adjuvant HAI Posthepatic Resection

The majority of patients who undergo hepatic resection for metastatic colorectal cancer relapse and ultimately die of their disease. The liver itself is the most common first site of recurrence postsurgical resection of liver metastases. Without adjuvant chemotherapy, 60% of patients relapse at a median time to relapse of 9–12 months, 50% of these with new hepatic metastases. Systemic chemotherapy alone has shown an increase in progression-free survival, but not a significant benefit in overall survival.[51] Given the high incidence of intrahepatic relapse, likely secondary to microscopic residual disease, the use of HAI in combination with systemic chemotherapy posthepatic resection is especially attractive (Table 20-6).

Early trials compared HAI postsurgical resection to no adjuvant therapy. A German trial that evaluated 226 patients randomized patients to 5FU HAI versus no adjuvant therapy.[52] This trial was terminated early due to interim analysis showing no benefit to HAI over observation, however 33% of patients randomized to the HAI arm did not receive treatment.

A multicenter cooperative group study randomized 109 patients to surgery alone versus surgery with postoperative HAI FUDR combined with IV 5FU, the endpoint was recurrence-free survival.[53] The four-year recurrence-free survival was significantly better in the adjuvant therapy arm compared to the control at 45.7% versus 25.2%, respectively. Median overall survival was not significantly improved; however, this study was slow to accrue patients and was not powered to evaluate overall survival.

In 1999, a single-center randomized study was published comparing six cycles of HAI FUDR plus systemic 5FU/LV versus six weeks of systemic 5FU/LV alone.[54] About 156 patients were randomized at time of resection of colorectal hepatic metastases. At median follow-up of 10 years, a

TABLE 20-6: Randomized Trials of Adjuvant Hepatic Arterial Infusion Postresection of Liver Metastases

Trial	N	Treatment	Disease-Free Survival (Median or %)	P	Overall Survival	P
Lorenz (1998)[52]	226	HAI 5FU vs. observation	14.2 vs. 13.7	NS	34.5 vs. 40.8	0.1519
Kemeny (2002)[53]	109	HAI FUDR and IV 5FU vs. observation	46% vs. 25% (4-y DFS)	0.04	47 vs. 34	0.19
Kemeny (1999)[54]	156	HAI FUDR and IV 5FU vs. IV 5FU	31.3 vs. 17.2	0.02	68.4 vs. 58.8	0.10
Lygidakis (2001)[61]	122	HAI mitomycin C, 5FU, LV, IL2 vs. IV mitomycin C, 5FU, LV, IL2	60 vs. 35 (5-y DFS)	0.0002	79 vs. 66	0.04

Abbreviations: FUDR, 5 fluoro-2-deoxyuridine; HAI, hepatic arterial infusion; DFS, disease free survival.

significant benefit in progression-free survival was seen in the HAI + SYS arm. Ten year survival rates were 41% and 27% in the HAI + SYS and systemic alone arms, respectively. Results of a recently published phase I trial of systemic oxaliplatin in combination with HAI FUDR posthepatic resection for colorectal cancer metastases reported a four-year survival of 88%, with progression free survival of 50% at four years.[50] The regimen was well tolerated.

In a meta-analysis of 1067 patients undergoing liver resection for metastatic colorectal cancer at MSKCC over a 12-year period, postoperative HAI chemotherapy was associated with improved survival by multivariate analysis.[55] In a retrospective analysis of 125 patients who received adjuvant HAI FUDR in combination with systemic FOLFOX or FOLFIRI compared patients to matched controls who received adjuvant systemic FOLFOX or FOLFIRI alone,[56] at a 43 months median follow-up, the disease-free survival was 75% in the HAI plus systemic group versus 52% in the systemic chemotherapy alone group ($p = 0.004$). These retrospective studies provide a sound rationale for a prospective trial comparing FOLFOX alone to HAI FUDR plus FOLFOX as adjuvant therapy posthepatic resection of colorectal liver metastases.

HAI for Primary Liver Cancer

Hepatocellular carcinoma (HCC) and intrahepatic cholangiocarcinoma (ICC) frequently present at an advanced stage not amenable to surgical resection. Despite recent advances in systemic therapy for HCC and bile duct cancers, patients with unresectable tumors still have a poor prognosis.[57,58] Primary liver tumors, similar to liver metastases, derive their blood supply from the hepatic artery rather than the portal vein and frequently have prolonged periods of liver-confined disease, providing rationale for the use of HAI therapy for unresectable disease.

An early trial of HAI mitomycin in combination with FUDR in 10 patients with unresectable primary liver cancer (8 HCC and 2 cholangiocarcinoma) reported a median overall survival of 14.5 months from initiation of therapy, with a response rate of 40%.[59] Clavien et al. in 2002 reported down staging of inoperable HCC enabling surgical resection in three of five cases following treatment with HAI FUDR in combination with bolus cisplatin and doxorubicin.

Most recently, results of a phase II trial evaluating the use of HAI FUDR in 34 patients (26 ICC and 8 HCC) were published.[60] Median survival was 29.5 months, with 2-year survival of 67%. Response rate was 47.1% by RECIST criteria; 41.2% of patients had stable disease. A higher response rate of 53.8% was seen in patients with ICC compared to 25% for HCC. One patient with unresectable disease at presentation had sufficient response to therapy to enable surgical resection. The specimen had complete necrosis with no tumor found.

Conclusion

HAI chemotherapy can now be safely administered in the outpatient setting by the use of totally implantable pump, with low complication rates. HAI FUDR is well tolerated in combination with modern systemic chemotherapy regimens incorporating oxaliplatin or irinotecan and results in a high rate of conversion to resectability in patients presenting with initially unresectable metastases. This is especially relevant in the management of patients with a known K-RAS mutant tumor, as cetuximab and panitumumab are no longer therapeutic options for this subset of patients. In the adjuvant setting posthepatic resection, HAI has demonstrated improvement in both overall and hepatic disease-free survival. HAI has a role to play in the multidisciplinary management of metastatic colorectal cancer, in combination with surgery, radiofrequency ablation, systemic chemotherapy, and biologic agents. The use of HAI in the treatment of primary bile duct cancers appears promising and is currently under further investigation.

References

1. Ackerman NB. The blood supply of experimental liver metastases. IV. Changes in vascularity with increasing tumor growth. *Surgery*. 1974;75:589–596.
2. Ensminger W. Intrahepatic arterial infusion of chemotherapy: pharmacologic principles. *Semin Oncol*. 2002;29:119–125.
3. Collins J. Pharmacologic rationale for regional drug delivery. *J Clin Oncol*. 1984;2:498–504.
4. Ensminger WD, Rosowsky A, Raso V, et al. A clinical-pharmacological evaluation of hepatic arterial infusions of 5-fluoro-2'-deoxyuridine and 5-fluorouracil. *Cancer Res*. 1978;38:3784–3792.
5. Sigurdson ER, Ridge JA, Kemeny N, Daly JM. Tumor and liver drug uptake following hepatic artery and portal vein infusion. *J Clin Oncol*. 1987;5:1836–1840.
6. Ensminger WD, Gyves JW. Clinical pharmacology of hepatic arterial chemotherapy. *Semin Oncol*. 1983;10:176–182.
7. Dzodic R, Gomez-Abuin G, Rougier P, et al. Pharmacokinetic advantage of intra-arterial hepatic oxaliplatin administration: comparative results with cisplatin using a rabbit VX2 tumor model. *Anti-Cancer Drugs*. 2004;15:647–650.
8. Van Riel JMGH, Van Groeningen C, Kedde M, et al. Continuous administration of irinotecan by hepatic arterial infusion: a phase I and pharmacokinetic study. *Clin Cancer Res*. 2002;8:405–412.
9. De Jong FA, Mathijssen RH, Verweij J. Limited potential of hepatic arterial infusion of irinotecan. *J Chemother*. 2004;16(suppl 5):48–50.
10. Buchwald H, Grage TB, Vassilopoulos PP, et al. Intraarterial infusion chemotherapy for hepatic carcinoma using a totally implantable infusion pump. *Cancer*. 1980;45:866–869.
11. Skitzki J, Chang A. Hepatic artery chemotherapy for colorectal liver metastases: technical considerations and review of clinical trials. *Surg Oncol*. 2002;11:123–135.
12. Campbell KA, Burns RC, Sitzmann JV, et al. Regional chemotherapy devices: effect of experience and anatomy on complications. *J Clin Oncol*. 1993;11:822–826.
13. Allen P, Nissan A, Picon A, et al. Technical complications and durability of hepatic artery infusion pumps for unresectable colorectal liver metastases: an institutional experience of 544 consecutive cases. *J Am Coll Surg*. 2005;201:57–65.
14. Koea JB, Kemeny N. Hepatic artery infusion chemotherapy for metastatic colorectal carcinoma. *Semin Surg Oncol*. 2000;19:125–134.
15. Strazzabosco M, Fabris L. Functional anatomy of normal bile ducts. *Anat Rec*. 2008;291:653–660.
16. Kemeny N, Seiter K, Niedzwiecki D, et al. A randomized trial of intrahepatic infusion of fluorodeoxyuridine with dexamethasone versus fluorodeoxyuridine alone in the treatment of metastatic colorectal cancer. *Cancer*. 1992;69:327–334.
17. Tandon RN, Bunnell IL, Cooper RG. The treatment of metastatic carcinoma of the liver by the percutaneous selective hepatic artery infusion of 5-fluorouracil. *Surgery*. 1973;73:118–121.
18. Kemeny N, Daly J, Oderman P, et al. Hepatic artery pump infusion: toxicity and results in patients with metastatic colorectal carcinoma. *J Clin Oncol*. 1984;2:595–600.

19. Niederhuber JE, Ensminger W, Gyves J, et al. Regional chemotherapy of colorectal cancer metastatic to the liver. *Cancer*. 1984;53:1336–1343.
20. Balch C, Urist M. Intraarterial chemotherapy for colorectal liver metastases and hepatoma using a totally implantable drug infusion pump. *Recent Results Cancer Res*. 1986;100:234–247.
21. Shepard KV, Levin B, Karl RC, et al. Therapy for metastatic colorectal cancer with hepatic artery infusion chemotherapy using a subcutaneous implanted pump. *J Clin Oncol*. 1985;3:161–169.
22. Weiss GR, Garnick MB, Osteen RT, et al. Long-term hepatic arterial infusion of 5-fluorodeoxyuridine for liver metastases using an implantable infusion pump. *J Clin Oncol*. 1983;1:337–344.
23. Schwartz SI, Jones LS, McCune CS. Assessment of treatment of intrahepatic malignancies using chemotherapy via an implantable pump. *Ann Surg*. 1985;201:560–567.
24. Chang AE, Schneider PD, Sugarbaker PH, et al. A prospective randomized trial of regional versus systemic continuous 5-fluorodeoxyuridine chemotherapy in the treatment of colorectal liver metastases. *Ann Surg*. 1987;206:685–693.
25. Kemeny N, Daly J, Reichman B, et al. Intrahepatic or systemic infusion of fluorodeoxyuridine in patients with liver metastases from colorectal carcinoma. A randomized trial. *Ann Intern Med*. 1987;107:459–465.
26. Hohn DC, Stagg RJ, Friedman MA, et al. A randomized trial of continuous intravenous versus hepatic intraarterial floxuridine in patients with colorectal cancer metastatic to the liver: the Northern California Oncology Group trial. *J Clin Oncol*. 1989;7:1646–1654.
27. Martin JK, O'Connell MJ, Wieand HS, et al. Intra-arterial floxuridine vs systemic fluorouracil for hepatic metastases from colorectal cancer. A randomized trial. *Arch Surg*. 1990;125:1022–1027.
28. Wagman LD, Kemeny MM, Leong L, et al. A prospective, randomized evaluation of the treatment of colorectal cancer metastatic to the liver. *J Clin Oncol*. 1990;8:1885–1893.
29. Rougier P, Laplanche A, Huguier M, et al. Hepatic arterial infusion of floxuridine in patients with liver metastases from colorectal carcinoma: long-term results of a prospective randomized trial. *J Clin Oncol*. 1992;10:1112–1118.
30. Allen-Mersh TG, Earlam S, Fordy C, et al. Quality of life and survival with continuous hepatic-artery floxuridine infusion for colorectal liver metastases. *Lancet*. 1994;344:1255–1260.
31. Lorenz M, Mller HH. Randomized, multicenter trial of fluorouracil plus leucovorin administered either via hepatic arterial or intravenous infusion versus fluorodeoxyuridine administered via hepatic arterial infusion in patients with nonresectable liver metastases from colorectal carcinoma. *J Clin Oncol*. 2000;18:243–254.
32. Kerr D, McArdle C, Ledermann J, et al. Intrahepatic arterial versus intravenous fluorouracil and folinic acid for colorectal cancer liver metastases: a multicentre randomised trial. *Lancet*. 2003;361:368–373.
33. Kemeny N, Niedzwiecki D, Hollis D, et al. Hepatic arterial infusion versus systemic therapy for hepatic metastases from colorectal cancer: a randomized trial of efficacy, quality of life, and molecular markers (CALGB 9481). *J Clin Oncol*. 2006;24:1395–1403.
34. Harmantas A, Rotstein LE, Langer B. Regional versus systemic chemotherapy in the treatment of colorectal carcinoma metastatic to the liver. Is there a survival difference? Meta-analysis of the published literature. *Cancer*. 1996;78:1639–1645.
35. Meta-analysis group in cancer. Reappraisal of hepatic arterial infusion in the treatment of nonresectable liver metastases from colorectal cancer. *J Natl Cancer Inst*. 1996;88:252–258.
36. Mocellin S, Pilati P, Lise M, Nitti D. Meta-analysis of hepatic arterial infusion for unresectable liver metastases from colorectal cancer: the end of an era? *J Clin Oncol*. 2007;25:5649–5654.
37. Fiorentini G, Rossi S, Dentico P, et al. Irinotecan hepatic arterial infusion chemotherapy for hepatic metastases from colorectal cancer: a phase II clinical study. *Tumori*. 2003;89:382–384.
38. Van Riel JMGH, Van Groeningen CJ, De Greve J, et al. Continuous infusion of hepatic arterial irinotecan in pretreated patients with colorectal cancer metastatic to the liver. *Ann Oncol*. 2004;15:59–63.
39. Boige V, Malka D, Elias D, et al. Hepatic arterial infusion of oxaliplatin and intravenous LV5FU2 in unresectable liver metastases from colorectal cancer after systemic chemotherapy failure. *Ann Surg Oncol*. 2008;15:219–226.
40. Ducreux M, Ychou M, Laplanche A, et al. Hepatic arterial oxaliplatin infusion plus intravenous chemotherapy in colorectal cancer with inoperable hepatic metastases: a trial of the gastrointestinal group of the Federation Nationale des Centres de Lutte Contre le Cancer. *J Clin Oncol*. 2005;23:4881–4887.
41. Fiorentini G, Cantore M, Rossi S, et al. Hepatic arterial chemotherapy in combination with systemic

chemotherapy compared with hepatic arterial chemotherapy alone for liver metastases from colorectal cancer: results of a multi-centric randomized study. *In Vivo*. 2006;20:707–709.

42. Kemeny N, Gonen M, Sullivan D, et al. Phase I study of hepatic arterial infusion of floxuridine and dexamethasone with systemic irinotecan for unresectable hepatic metastases from colorectal cancer. *J Clin Oncol*. 2001;19:2687–2695.

43. Kemeny N, Jarnagin W, Paty P, et al. Phase I trial of systemic oxaliplatin combination chemotherapy with hepatic arterial infusion in patients with unresectable liver metastases from colorectal cancer. *J Clin Oncol*. 2005;23:4888–4896.

44. Gallagher DJ, Capanu M, Raggio G, Kemeny N. Hepatic arterial infusion plus systemic irinotecan in patients with unresectable hepatic metastases from colorectal cancer previously treated with systemic oxaliplatin: a retrospective analysis. *Ann Oncol*. 2007;18:1995–1999.

45. Kemeny N, Melendez FDH, Capanu M, et al. Conversion to resectability using hepatic artery infusion plus systemic chemotherapy for the treatment of unresectable liver metastases from colorectal carcinoma. *J Clin Oncol*. 2009;27: 3465–3471.

46. Abdalla E, Adam R, Bilchik A, et al. Improving resectability of hepatic colorectal metastases: expert consensus statement. *Ann Surg Oncol*. 2006;13:1271–1280.

47. Adam R, Wicherts DA, de Haas RJ, et al. Patients with initially unresectable colorectal liver metastases: is there a possibility of cure? *J Clin Oncol*. 2009;27:1829–1835.

48. Folprecht G, Grothey A, Alberts S, et al. Neoadjuvant treatment of unresectable colorectal liver metastases: correlation between tumour response and resection rates. *Ann Oncol*. 2005; 16:1311–1319.

49. Gallagher D, Zheng J, Capanu M, et al. Response to neoadjuvant chemotherapy does not predict overall survival for patients with synchronous colorectal hepatic metastases. *Ann Surg Oncol*. 2009; 16:1844–1851.

50. Kemeny N, Capanu M, D'Angelica M, et al. Phase I trial of adjuvant hepatic arterial infusion (HAI) with floxuridine (FUDR) and dexamethasone plus systemic oxaliplatin, 5-fluorouracil and leucovorin in patients with resected liver metastases from colorectal cancer. *Ann Oncol*. 2009;20:1236–1241.

51. Mitry E, Fields ALA, Bleiberg H, et al. Adjuvant chemotherapy after potentially curative resection of metastases from colorectal cancer: a pooled analysis of two randomized trials. *J Clin Oncol*. 2008;26:4906–4911.

52. Lorenz M, Mller HH, Schramm H, et al. Randomized trial of surgery versus surgery followed by adjuvant hepatic arterial infusion with 5-fluorouracil and folinic acid for liver metastases of colorectal cancer. German cooperative on liver metastases (Arbeitsgruppe Lebermetastasen). *Ann Surg*. 1998;228: 756–762.

53. Kemeny MM, Adak S, Gray B, et al. Combined-modality treatment for resectable metastatic colorectal carcinoma to the liver: surgical resection of hepatic metastases in combination with continuous infusion of chemotherapy–an intergroup study. *J Clin Oncol*. 2002;20:1499–1505.

54. Kemeny N, Huang Y, Cohen AM, et al. Hepatic arterial infusion of chemotherapy after resection of hepatic metastases from colorectal cancer. *N Engl J Med*. 1999;341:2039–2048.

55. Ito H, Are C, Gonen M, et al. Effect of postoperative morbidity on long-term survival after hepatic resection for metastatic colorectal cancer. *Ann Surg*. 2008;247:994–1002.

56. House MG, Kemeny N, Gonen M et al. Comparison of adjuvant systemic chemotherapy with or without hepatic arterial infusional chemotherapy after hepatic resection for metastatic colorectal cancer. *Ann Surg*. 2011 Dec;254(6):851-6.

57. Rimassa L, Santoro A. Sorafenib therapy in advanced hepatocellular carcinoma: the SHARP trial. *Expert Rev Anticancer Ther*. 2009;9: 739–745.

58. Yang J, Yan L-N. Current status of intrahepatic cholangiocarcinoma. *World Journal of Gastroenterology*. 2008;14:6289–6297.

59. Atiq OT, Kemeny N, Niedzwiecki D, Botet J. Treatment of unresectable primary liver cancer with intrahepatic fluorodeoxyuridine and mitomycin C through an implantable pump. *Cancer*. 1992;69:920–924.

60. Jarnagin WR, Schwartz LH, Gultekin DH, et al. Regional chemotherapy for unresectable primary liver cancer: results of a phase II clinical trial and assessment of DCE-MRI as a biomarker of survival. *Ann Oncol*. 2009;20:1589–1595.

61. Lygidakis NJ, Sgourakis G, Vlachos L, et al. Metastatic liver disease of colorectal origin: the value of locoregional immunochemotherapy combined with systemic chemotherapy following liver resection. Results of a prospective randomized study. *Hepatogastroenterology*. 2001;48:1685–1691.

CHAPTER 21

Novel Therapeutics for Liver Tumors

Ghassan K. Abou-Alfa, Celina Ang & Eileen M. O'Reilly

Introduction

Liver malignancies encompass several tumor types with either a primary liver origin, for example, hepatocellular carcinoma (HCC) or intrahepatic cholangiocarcinoma (ICC), or as a site of local extension, for example, extrahepatic cholangiocarcinoma and gallbladder cancer; or metastatic, including origin from the gastrointestinal tract, breast, lung, and multiple other sites.

HCC is the commonest primary liver malignancy. It is the fifth most common solid tumor cancer with respect to incidence and the third most common cause of cancer-related mortality globally.[1] It is commonly "two diseases in one," the cancer itself and the underlying cirrhosis responsible for the development of HCC, for example, hepatitis B, C viral infection, alcoholic cirrhosis, and nonalcoholic steatohepatitis.

Several chemotherapeutic agents have been tested as single agents or in combination in HCC, but none have shown an impact on survival. The advent of novel therapeutics and the recognition of important pathways at a molecular level involved in the development of HCC have led to identification of new treatments for this traditionally difficult-to-treat malignancy.

In the case of ICC, there have been parallel but more limited efforts in evaluating biologic therapies compared to HCC. Although the liver is a common site of metastatic disease for several solid tumors, systemic biologic therapies have been studied and approved without necessarily any specific reference to the liver disease. More focused efforts on liver metastases are discussed in Chapter 20.

Therapeutic Biologic Pathways

The complex network of growth factors, cell surface receptors, and their associated downstream signal transduction pathways that are responsible for normal cell development is highly regulated. In the malignant state, dysregulation of many of the components of these pathways network can occur (Figure 21-1).[2] A window of opportunity for targeted therapies for HCC has evolved, particularly given the lack of standard therapies for this disease.

Epidermal Growth Factor Receptor

The epidermal growth factor receptor (EGFR) is probably the most studied therapeutic target for cancer. At the cell surface, varying ligands bind to different cell receptors triggering receptor dimerization and auto-phosphorylation of several tyrosine residues. These now phosphorylated residues act as docking sites for cytoplasmic proteins that undergo conformational modifications that trigger intracellular signaling through varied pathways.[3] In cancer conditions, this "switched on" activity can go unchecked, leading to continued cell replication. EGFR expression in HCC is a subject of controversial data; some studies show no difference in EGFR expression compared

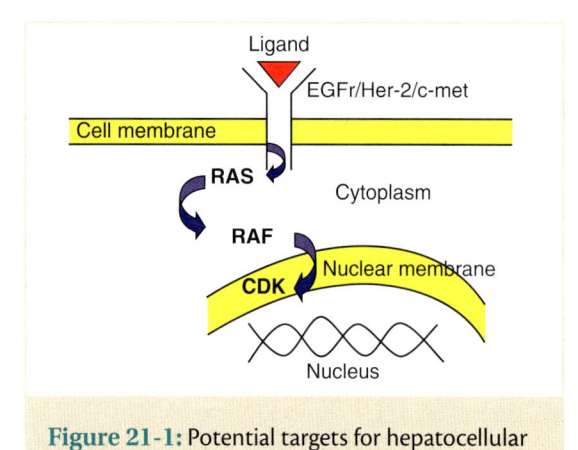

Figure 21-1: Potential targets for hepatocellular carcinoma therapy along the signal transduction pathway.

to normal cells counterparts, whereas others report over-expression in 17% of HCC cases.[4–6]

Despite this controversy, EGFR-specific receptor tyrosine kinase (RTK) inhibitors are being evaluated in advanced HCC. Erlotinib was studied in 38 patients with advanced HCC as part of a single-agent, single-arm phase II study.[7] Although 71% of all patients had Child–Pugh A limited cirrhosis, nearly 50% had not received prior therapy. The primary end-point—progression-free survival (Progression-free survival) at six months using RECIST criteria—was reached in 12 of 38 patients (32%), with a median Progression-free survival of 3.8 months and a median overall survival (Overall survival) of 13 months. Response was limited to three partial responses (8%). Similar to the experience with other tumors, high EGFR expression by immunohistochemical staining was not associated with improved outcome. The most frequent grade 3–4 toxicities were skin rash 13%, diarrhea 8%, and fatigue 8%. Erlotinib was also studied in combination with bevacizumab.[8] This is discussed in details in the combination therapy section.

Cetuximab was reported to have some preclinical activity in HCC.[9] In human HCC cell lines, cetuximab triggered a growth arrest with noted increased expression of the cyclin-dependent kinase inhibitors p21 and p27 and decreased expression of cyclin D1, resulting in G_0/G_1 cell-cycle arrest. The combination of cetuximab with tyrosine kinase inhibitors or with the well-studied anthracycline in HCC—doxorubicin— resulted in a synergistic effect. Nonetheless cetuximab remains to be tested clinically in HCC.

In contrast, and despite the rare expression of Her-2/Neu in human HCC tissues,[10] lapatinib, a dual inhibitor of EGFR and tyrosine kinase 1 and 2 (Her2/Neu), was studied as part of a phase II trial in advanced HCC.[11] In a group of 40 patients with advanced HCC treated with lapatinib at a starting dose of 1500 mg/d, the drug showed no efficacy. The primary endpoint, response rate, was 5%. Progression-free survival and median overall survival were 2.3 (95% CI: 1.7–5.6) and 6.2 (95% CI: 5.1 to infinity) months respectively; both did not compare favorably to historical data. EGFR genotyping indicated that HCC patients with <20 repeats have the worst progression-free survival.

Hepatocyte growth factor (HGF) and its receptor c-met are of interest in HCC, as both are overexpressed in 33% and 20% respectively of human HCC tissues.[6] The authors' group found c-met to be overexpressed preferentially in early stage resected HCC, with no association with outcome as measured by median overall survival.[12] Transgenic mouse models that over-expresses HGF or the c-met receptor in their germline were found to develop different types of cancer.[13] Transgenic mice over-expressing human wild-type met in hepatocytes and no over-expression of HGF were noted to develop HCC, through a mechanism dependent on cell adherence rather than any ligand attachment.[14] When the transgene was inactivated, tumors regressed, including those in advanced stages. This tumor regression occurred through apoptosis and cessation of proliferation. These observations suggest that genetic abnormalities leading to the development of HCC do not lose relevance once the neoplasm is established and may constitute potential therapeutic targets. Tivantinib has been evaluated in a phase study in a 2:1 randomization versus placebo. The study showed a notable improvement in median time to progression of 2.7 versus 1.4 months (HR=0·43; 95% CI, 0·19–0·97; p=0·03) and median overall survival of 7.2 versus 3.8 months (HR=0·38; 95% CI, 0·18-0·81; p=0·01) among patients with c-met positive tumors (defined as majority (≥50%) of tumor cells with moderate or strong (2+ or 3+) staining intensity).[15,16] Cabozantinib (XL184), was also evaluated in the second line setting in HCC as part of phase II randomized discontinuation study. Among 41 patients on study, median PFS was

4.4 months and median OS 15.1 months.[17] In vitro studies of gene therapy strategies to silence or downregulate c-met, including the use of antisense RNA,[18] vector-mediated expression of the HGF antagonist, NK4,[19] or manipulation of microRNA expression have been shown to diminish the migratory and invasive properties of HCC cell lines. In addition, the multitargeted tyrosine kinase inhibitor SU5416 exhibited a similar effect on HCC cells by blocking the phosphorylation of c-met and its downstream effectors in a dose-dependent fashion.[20,21]

Serum IGFBP-3 is a more effective predictor than IGF receptors and binding proteins and IGF-2 for the development of hepatocellular carcinoma in patients with chronic HCV infection.[22,23] The combination of AVE1642, an IGF-1R antibody, with gefitinib was shown to be synergistic in blocking downstream cell-signaling in preclinical studies, indicating the relevance of IGF1 and EGFR interactions.[24] Another IGF-1R inhibitor, IMC-A12 is being investigated in combination with sorafenib in an ongoing phase II study (www.clinicaltrials.gov, NCT00906373). A phase II study of IMC-A12 as a single agent was suspended early because of lack of efficacy.[25] BIIB022 is yet another IGF-1R antagonist, which acts in a similar fashion to AVE1642 and IMC-A12 to prevent downstream PI3K/Akt activation.[25] A phase Ib/II study of BIIB022 with or without sorafenib has also been suspended for unspecified reasons (www.clinicaltrials.gov, NCT00956436). A randomized phase II trial of OSI-906, inhibitor of both IGF-1R and the insulin receptor (IR) is expected to open (www.clinicaltrials.gov, NCT01101906).

To summarize so far regarding targeting the EGF pathway, the data thus far do not provide sufficient support for the routine use of any of the single-agent EGFR inhibitors in the management of HCC and results of several ongoing trials will further refine the utility of targeting this pathway.

Cytoplasmic Downstream Targets

Downstream of the cell membrane receptors, and on the cytoplasmic side lies Ras, an anchoring protein that is mutated approximately 20%–30% of all malignancies.[26] Its relevance in HCC has been controversial. Some reported no correlation between Ras mutational status and the development of HCC,[27] whereas others showed an average of 15% occurrence of Ras mutations in patients with HCC due to viral hepatitis and alcoholic liver cirrhosis,[28] with the highest percentage (42%) reported among patients with HCC with previous vinyl chloride exposure averaging 9942 ppm-years or approximately 250 months of exposure.[29] The rate-limiting step and potential therapeutic target for Ras processing and anchoring to the cell membrane is a posttranslational farnesylation of a cytosine residue located at its carboxyl terminal.[30] The farnesyltransferase inhibitor, ABT-100, has been shown to inhibit growth, cell-cycle progression and invasiveness of the HCC cell lines HepG2 and Huh7.[31] As yet, these concepts remain untested in a clinical setting. As HMG-CoA reductase is a regulator of farnesyltransferase, there has also been interest in evaluating the antitumor activity of simvastatin,[32] and pravastatin.[33,34] A randomized phase III trial of sorafenib with or without pravastatin is currently ongoing (www.clinicaltrials.gov, NCT01075555). In addition, a phase IB trial of neoadjuvant SCH 66336, a direct farnesyltransferase inhibitor, with or without gemcitabine in patients with resectable HCC has been completed with results pending (www.clinicaltrials.gov, NCT00020774).

Following downstream from Ras, the Raf/MEK/ERK signaling pathway plays a key role in the neoplastic transformation of hepatocytes. Activation of MEK1/2 and its downstream target, MAPK, has been reported in HCC tumors.[35] The virus core protein, hepatitis C virus 1(HCV-1), of hepatitis C can induce a high basal activity of Raf-1, which itself leads to a sustained response to EGF by hepatocytes, resulting in an increased possibility of neoplastic transformation.[36] The serine/threonine kinase Raf-1 inhibitor, sorafenib, has been studied extensively in HCC. Sorafenib, also an antiangiogenic [vascular endothelial growth factor receptor (VEGFR)-1, -2, -3; and platelet-derived growth factor receptor (PDGFR)-β] and tumorigenic (RET, Flt-3, and c-Kit) RTK inhibitor,[37] is discussed in extensive detail in the antiangiogenic section.

The mammalian target of rapamycin (mTOR) is a component of the PI3K/Akt pathway, which is normally antagonized by the phosphatase and tensin homolog deleted on chromosome 10 (PTEN) tumor suppressor gene.[38] mTOR activation has pro-angiogenic and pro-proliferative effects,[39,40] making it a key target in anticancer therapy. Aberrant mTOR activity was found in approximately 50% of human HCC tumors, in association with upregulated EGF and

IGF signaling and downregulation of PTEN. Patients with mTOR activated tumors had a poorer disease phenotype, most strikingly reflected by a 25-month reduction in time to recurrence compared to those without. Furthermore, in vitro and in vivo models of HCC demonstrated tumor regression with everolimus, as well as apoptosis when an EGFR/VEGFR inhibitor was added.[41] Experience with mTOR inhibition in the clinical domain thus far is primarily limited to retrospective series documenting significant improvements in survival among patients treated with sirolimus following transplantation for HCC.[42–46] A small prospective study including 21 patients with HCC not amenable to surgery or any locally ablative therapies reported a single partial response and stabilization of disease in five subjects treated with sirolimus.[47] Multiple phase I–II studies evaluate the safety and activity of various mTOR inhibitors as single agents including everolimus (www.clinicaltrials.gov, NCT00390195), temsirolimus (www.clinicaltrials.gov, NCT01079767), sirolimus (www.clinicaltrials.gov, NCT00467194), and AZD8055 (www.clinicaltrials.gov, NCT00999882). A phase I trial of temsirolimus and sorafenib is currently recruiting (www.clinicaltrials.gov, NCT01008917), and another phase I trial testing this combination in patients with liver dysfunction (www.clinicaltrials.gov, NCT01013519). The safety and efficacy of everolimus and sorafenib are also being investigated in phase I (www.clinicaltrials.gov, NCT00828594) and II studies (www.clinicaltrials.gov, NCT01005199). Two phase II studies are evaluating bevacizumab combined with everolimus (www.clinicaltrials.gov, NCT00775073)[48] and temsirolimus (www.clinicaltrials.gov,NCT01010126).

Inhibitors of the Proangiogenic Pathway

HCC is a highly vascular solid tumor, with high expression of VEGF, a major player in HCC development and its metastatic potential, along with PDGFR-β.[49]

Sorafenib remains the most studied antiangiogenic drug in HCC. An initial phase II trial evaluating response to sorafenib in 137 patients with advanced HCC did not meet its primary endpoint, showing a low response rate (2% response rate) by WHO bi-dimensional radiologic criteria.[50] The study however showed an improved median time-to-tumor progression (TTP) of 4.2 months and median overall survival of 9.2 months, both of which compare favorably to historical controls.[51] This was commensurate with stable disease of a minimum of four months duration, noted in a 34% of patients. This high rate of stable disease was associated with an observed phenomenon of central tumor necrosis (TN) noted on the arterial phase of triphasic CT scans (Figure 21-2). This central TN was quantifiable, and the volume of the tumor it is encompassed within, was measured using a computer algorithm for semiautomated delineation of tumors.[52] The ratio of the percentage of the described TN over the tumor volume (V) was found to correlate with disease control ($p = 0.02$).[53] TN/V ratio is pending validation, and its use is being

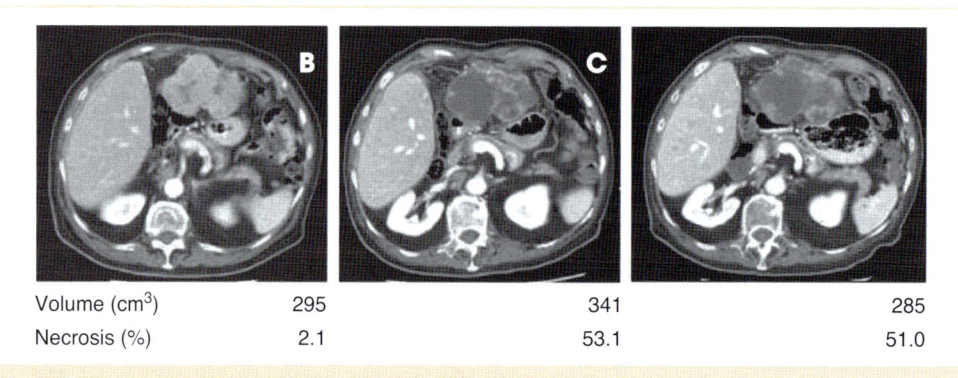

Volume (cm³)	295	341	285
Necrosis (%)	2.1	53.1	51.0

Figure 21-2: A representative example of baseline and serial follow-up scans demonstrating tumor necrosis in a hepatocellular carcinoma patient. Abou-Alfa, G. K. et al. *J Clin Oncol*; 24:4293–4300 2006.

assessed in several prospective HCC clinical trials. Triphasic CT scans in patients with HCC may also prove to be valuable in evaluating response to antiangiogenic therapies. Sorafenib had an acceptable adverse events profile in the aforementioned phase II study. The main grade 3–4 toxicities were fatigue (9.5%), diarrhea (8%), and hand-foot syndrome (5.1%), manifested by tingling that may evolve to erythema and ultimately skin desquamation if not managed optimally (see later in text).

The intriguing improved median TTP and overall survival noted in the phase II study evaluating sorafenib in HCC led to a large double-blinded, randomized phase III trial (SHARP) evaluating sorafenib versus placebo in patients with advanced HCC.[54] The study, with two primary endpoints of overall survival and time to symptomatic progression (TTSP), using the FHSI8-TSP instrument was limited to patients with Child–Pugh A cirrhosis. This phase III trial of 602 (524 male and 78 female) patients had approximately 300 patients per arm, the demographics of which were comparable, with a median age of 65 and 56 years on the sorafenib and placebo arms, respectively. Patients' risk factors for developing HCC in the combined study arms (experimental and placebo) were hepatitis C in approximately 30%, hepatitis B in 20%, alcohol in 26%, other causes in 10%, and unknown in 18%. This distribution is similar to that reported in a retrospective analysis of patients with HCC seen and evaluated for systemic therapy at Memorial Sloan-Kettering Cancer Center.[55] The study demonstrated an improvement in median survival of 10.7 months for patients who received sorafenib compared to 7.9 months for those randomized to placebo ($p < 0.001$, HR = 0.69). The second primary endpoint of TTSP showed no difference between the two treatment arms ($p = 0.77$). This latter observation is generally explained by the poor understanding of the validity of FHS18-TSP instrument in this setting add to the lack of symptoms among many of the accrued patients. The toxicity profile of sorafenib was similar to that noted in the phase II study, with 8% grade 3–4 diarrhea and hand-foot syndrome. There were rare bleeding events (<1%) that infer a note of caution considering the antiangiogenic nature of sorafenib, similar to other agents in its class, for example, bevacizumab and sunitinib, that may cause fatal bleeds.[56,57] Based on this phase III trial, sorafenib was approved by the Food and Drug Administration and other regulatory agencies worldwide as a standard therapy for unresectable HCC.

A second randomized phase III study evaluating sorafenib in patients with advanced HCC and Child–Pugh A cirrhosis was conducted in the Asia-Pacific region where HCC is mainly associated with a hepatitis B etiology.[58] The study had similar eligibility criteria compared to the SHARP trial, with two differences in the design; the study had a 2:1 randomization design presumably to assist accrual and did not have a predefined primary endpoint, but rather evaluated several endpoints. The Asia-Pacific study showed an improvement in median survival for patients who received sorafenib (6.5 months) compared to those who received placebo (4.2 months). This statistically significant improvement ($p = 0.014$), however, was not of the same magnitude as the SHARP trial, despite a similar hazard ratio of 0.68 and 0.69 in the Asia-Pacific and SHARP studies, respectively. In an attempt to explain the difference in magnitude of the median overall survival it was theorized that patients in the Asia-Pacific study had more advanced disease and were more ill at the time of study enrolment, compared to patients accrued on SHARP trial.[59] With similar hazard rations, the benefit for sorafenib may have been registered at two different times in the natural history of the disease—an earlier one in the SHARP trial and a later one or the Asia-Pacific study—on presumably the same survival curve.

A challenge to the above-stated hypothesis pertains to a subgroup analysis of the SHARP trial patients with hepatitis C–related HCC.[60] Patients with hepatitis C–related HCC treated with sorafenib ($n = 93$) had a median survival advantage of 14 months compared to the whole sorafenib treated group of 10.7 months, suggesting a possible advantage for patients with hepatitis C–related HCC, which may be related to the virus core protein HCV-1 of hepatitis C induction of a high basal activity of Raf-1, one of the targets of sorafenib.[36] The placebo-controlled hepatitis C group did not have any added survival advantage to the placebo population of the study, thus proving the lack of any survival advantage for HCC patients with hepatitis C compared to other etiologies. A similar observation was noted in a retrospective analysis of the phase II trial evaluating sorafenib in patients with advanced HCC.[60] It was noted that patients who were infected with hepatitis C solely ($n = 13$) had a longer time to progression of 6.5 months compared to 4 months ($p = 0.05$) for the patients infected with hepatitis B ($n = 33$).[61] A similar trend for a survival advantage ($p = 0.29$) for the hepatitis C (12.4 months) versus hepatitis B patients (7.3 months) was also noted. With a predominant hepatitis B (73%) population accrued on the Asia-Pacific study versus only 18% of patients on the SHARP trial, this may offer another explanation for this difference in the median survival magnitude noted between the two studies. The outcome of the 18% of patients with hepatitis B in the SHARP trial was reported recently as 9.7 months.[62] This hepatitis B versus C observation does not however undermine the key efficacy of sorafenib. Thus, sorafenib remains a standard option for all patients with unresectable HCC with a reasonable Child–Pugh's score irrespective of the etiology of their cancer.

Patients with unresectable HCC and Child–Pugh A who are eligible for sorafenib based on the SHARP trial comprise approximately 70% of the patients seen by medical oncologists.[53] The safety and efficacy of sorafenib in patients with Child–Pugh B or C cirrhosis remains a subject of discussion. In a phase II study evaluating sorafenib in HCC, 28% of patients were Child–Pugh B cirrhosis.[63] The pharmacokinetic profiles including AUC and Cmax were comparable between Child–Pugh A and B patients, despite the anticipation that Child–Pugh B patients may metabolize sorafenib at a slower rate. Nonetheless, Child–Pugh B patients were noted to have more frequent worsening of their liver function, including elevated total serum bilirubin, worsening ascites, and encephalopathy.[60] Considering the lack of a control arm, it remains unclear if this observed worsening in liver function is part of the expected natural history of Child–Pugh B patients, due to sorafenib, or both. The elevated total bilirubin may also be due to sorafenib inhibitory effect of UGT1A1 and decreased bilirubin glucuronidation, which again cannot be proven considering that only total bilirubin was measured during the study. Median TTP for Child–Pugh A was 21 weeks (95% CI: 16–25 weeks) and Child–Pugh B 13 weeks (95% CI: 9–18 weeks), and median overall survival were 41 weeks (95% CI: 36.6–63.6 weeks) and 14 weeks (95% CI: 11.6–25.7 weeks), respectively. A Japanese phase I study evaluating two different doses of sorafenib in Japanese patients with advanced HCC did not show a similar phenomenon.[64] Geometric means of AUC_{0-12} and Cmax were slightly lower in patients with Child–Pugh B cirrhosis compared with Child–Pugh A, with no substantial differences in the incidence of adverse events between the two groups. One additional study evaluating sorafenib in 150 patients with different types of tumors in cohorts with differing levels of liver dysfunction raised concern about the safety of sorafenib in patients with liver dysfunction.[65] Among all the cohorts with higher than normal total bilirubin, the most commonly reported drug-limiting toxicity was further elevation of bilirubin. Even though the study accrued patients with different malignancies and was not limited to patients with HCC, it provides some guidance on the use of sorafenib in patients with HCC and advanced cirrhosis. Based on this study and the authors' opinion, sorafenib can be given at 400 mg PO twice per day for bilirubin up to 1.5 × upper limit of normal (ULN) and 200 mg PO twice per day (or 400 mg PO daily) for bilirubin 1.5–3 × ULN. Sorafenib should be avoided in patients with bilirubin above 3 × ULN, until more data are available regarding the safety and efficacy of sorafenib in patients with HCC and Child–Pugh B or C. An answer to the safety and efficacy of sorafenib in patients with advanced cirrhosis would require a randomized study to assess the natural history of the disease and ways of evaluating worsening cirrhosis in noninvasive ways that may be more accurate and sensitive than changes in bilirubin.

Bevacizumab, a potent anti-VEGF, has been studied extensively in patients with advanced HCC. Bevacizumab was evaluated as a single agent in 46 patients with advanced HCC at different doses of 5 and 10 mg/kg.[56] Median progression-free survival and overall survival were was 6.9 and 12.4 months, respectively. Grade 3–5 hemorrhage occurred in 11% of patients, including one death secondary to bleeding esophageal varices. In the initial phase of this study, of 18 patients accrued, 4 had to discontinue therapy because of serious adverse events, including 1 transient ischemic attack and 3 serious esophageal bleeding events. The study was thus modified to identify and treat esophageal varices before enrollment.[66] Another study evaluating single-agent bevacizumab in HCC yielded similar results.[67] Among 24 patients evaluable for response, 3 had a partial response and 13 had stable disease.

Sunitinib, a multitargeted RTK inhibitor and a potent antiangiogenic, was evaluated as a single agent in patients with advanced HCC in two separate phase II studies at two different dose levels. In a US study, 34 patients treated with sunitinib at 37.5 mg daily dose, 50% of patients had stable disease, with a median progression-free survival of 3.9 months and median overall survival was of 9.8 months.[68] Most common grade 3 and 4 adverse events included hematologic toxicities, fatigue, and transaminase elevation. Two deaths were noted and attributed to worsening disease and liver failure. The second, a European study, evaluated sunitinib at a higher dose of 50 mg/d in 37 patients with advanced HCC. This trial did not move to a planned second stage in view of a low response rate of 2.7% in the first stage of the study.[69] There were four deaths that were explained as possibly drug related. These included events of hepatic encephalopathy, hematologic toxicities, and a variceal bleed. Surprisingly and despite the lack of any observed advantage over sorafenib both in efficacy and safety, a phase III clinical trial randomizing patients with advanced HCC to sunitinib versus sorafenib and looking for superiority of the experimental arm was launched. The study accrued a total of 1073 patients and was stopped early for futility and safety concerns. Median OS was 8 months for the sunitinib arm versus 10 months for the sorafenib arm (HR 1.31 [95% CI: 1.13 -1.52], P=0.0019).[69] Another trial testing sunitinib combined with capecitabine is ongoing (www.clinicaltrials.gov, NCT00787787).

Brivanib, a dual inhibitor of VEGF and fibroblast growth factor (FGF), has been studied in HCC. In a study evaluating brivanib as first- and second-line therapy in 96 patients with advanced HCC, there were limited responses, the median overall survival was 10 months (95% CI: 6.8, 15.2) in the treatment naïve cohort and was not reached in the second-line cohort.[70] Although the median overall survival compared favorably to sorafenib, the historical control, progression-free survival was only 2.7 months in the treatment naïve group, and median TTP was only 2 months in the second-line group. The drug was well tolerated in the second-line setting.[71] Responses defined by modified RECIST criteria assessing both tumor size and viability correlated well with time to progression and overall survival.[72] A randomized phase III clinical trial comparing brivanib to sorafenib, that accrued 1155 patients, failed to meet its primary endpoint (Median OS = 9.9, sorafenib versus 9.5 months, brivanib) (HR (95% CI) 1.06 (0.93–1.22), p=0.3730).[73]

TABLE 21-1: Current Ongoing Phase III Clinical Trials in Hepatocellular Carcinoma

Latest Phase III Studies	
Single agent	**Versus**
ABT869	Sorafenib
Brivanib	Sorafenib
Sunitinib	Sorafenib
Combination	**Versus**
Doxorubicin plus sorafenib	Sorafenib
Erlotinib plus sorafenib[a]	Sorafenib

[a]Randomized phase II study.

ABT-869, a VEGF and PDGF inhibitor was studied as part of a phase II study of 44 patients of whom 38 had Child–Pugh A and 6 had Child–Pugh B cirrhosis.[74] The objective response rate for the entire cohort was 6.8%, all occurring in the Child–Pugh A group. The Child–Pugh A patients' outcome was equivalent to historical controls, with median TTP and Overall survival of 5.4 and 10.4 months, respectively. One fatal adverse event, an intracranial hemorrhage, possibly related to ABT-869 was reported. A large randomized phase III trial of ABT-869 versus sorafenib discontinued to the lack of evidence of improvement in survival: 9.1 months (95% CI: 8.1, 10.2) for linifanib versus 9.8 months (95% CI: 8.3, 11.0) for sorafenib (Hazard ratio (HR) 1.046 (95% CI: 0.896, 1.221).[75]

Combination Therapy Studies with Antiangiogenics

Several combinations of antiangiogenic agents plus biologic or chemotherapy agents have been studied in HCC, some serendipitously and others based on clear preclinical concepts that favor such combinations.

Bevacizumab remains the most studied antiangiogenic agent in combination therapy in HCC. Several phase II studies have evaluated bevacizumab in combination with chemotherapy. A combination of bevacizumab plus gemcitabine and oxaliplatin was examined in a phase II trial in 30 previously treated HCC patients.[76] The objective response rate was 20%, and 27% of patients had stable disease. Median progression-free survival and overall survival were 5.3 and 9.6 months, respectively. The addition of the chemotherapy agents added expected grade 3–4 toxicities, including leucopenia and neutropenia, in addition to elevation of transaminase liver enzymes, hypertension, and fatigue. Another phase II study evaluated oxaliplatin, and capecitabine in combination with bevacizumab was conducted.[77] In this phase II study of 30 patients with advanced HCC, a partial response rate of 13.3%, and stable disease of 76.7% were noted. Median progression-free survival and overall survival were 4.5 and 10.6 months, respectively. Nontrivial and expected toxicity included 33% rate of grade 2/3 peripheral neuropathy and 11% of grade 2/3 hand-foot syndrome. Three bleeding events were reported on the study. Bevacizumab plus capecitabine only was also studied in 25 patients with advanced HCC and yielded almost similar results.[78] Disease control rate (response plus stable disease) was 60% with median progression-free survival of 4.1 months and median overall survival of 10.7 months. The most common treatment-related grade 3 toxicity was hand-foot syndrome. One gastric ulcer hemorrhage was reported on the study.

The combination of bevacizumab with erlotinib, a RTK inhibitor, has carried the most promise. The combination was evaluated in a phase II study of 40 patients with HCC and Child–Pugh A or B and ECOG performance status of 0–2. Bevacizumab was administered at a dose of 10 mg/kg every two weeks and erlotinib was prescribed for daily oral dose of 150 mg.[8] The primary endpoint of progression-free survival after 16 weeks of therapy was met at a rate of 62.5%. Median progression-free survival and overall survival were 39 and 68 weeks, respectively. A high response rate of 25% was reported. Most common grades 3–4 drug-related toxicities included fatigue (20%), hypertension (15%), diarrhea (10%), elevated transaminases (10%), and gastrointestinal hemorrhage (12.5%). Although this remains a single institution study with possibly highly selected patients, its outcome compares favorably to single agent sorafenib. A randomized phase II study of bevacizumab plus erlotinib versus sorafenib is currently underway (www.clinicaltrials.gov, NCT00881751).

Sorafenib has been evaluated incombination with biologic therapy and chemotherapy. A phase I study has assessed the combination of sorafenib and erlotinib in patients with varying solid tumors.[61] This study included one patient with HCC. A randomized phase III study evaluating sorafenib plus crlotinib versus sorafenib alone in patients with advanced HCC recently showed a median overall survival of 9.5 months for the combination versus 8.5 months for single agent sorafenib (HR 0.929, 95% CI: 0.781-1.1.06, p=0.204 1-sided).[80]

A randomized phase II study evaluated sorafenib in combination with doxorubicin versus doxorubicin plus placebo in 96 patients with advanced HCC and Child–Pugh A.[63] Median TTP was nine months for the doxorubicin and sorafenib arm and 5 months for the doxorubicin and placebo arm. An exploratory comparison of overall survival between the two arms showed a significant difference of 13.7 months in favor of doxorubicin and sorafenib versus 6.5 months for doxorubicin and placebo ($p = 0.0049$, HR = 0.45). Grade 3–4 toxicities included fatigue (15%) and neutropenia (50%) in both arms. Expected sorafenib-related toxicities of grade 3–4 diarrhea (11%) and hand-foot syndrome (9%) were reported in the experimental arm. A concerning observation was a 19% rate of left ventricular dysfunction in the doxorubicin and sorafenib arm, most of which were subclinical and detected on MUltiple Gated Acquisition test (MUGA) scans or echocardiography evaluation with only 2% deemed to be clinically relevant (grade 3–4). This observation adds to the potential synergistic effect between doxorubicin and sorafenib that may explain the improved outcome compared to historical controls. Anthracyclines (e.g., doxorubicin) depend on ASK-1 in exerting their apoptotic effect. In cancer cells, a bFGF-mediated activation of Raf-1 may promote a complex between Raf-1 and ASK-1 at the mitochondria level, leading to the inhibition of ASK-1 kinase activity and prevention of stress-mediated apoptosis of anthracyclines. Inhibiting Raf-1 activity with sorafenib may help dissolve the ASK-1 Raf-1 dimer and release ASK-1 out of the mitochondria to restore the apoptotic activity of doxorubicin (Figure 21-3).[81] This potential synergy is currently being investigated in a randomized phase III trial by the US cooperative groups, evaluating the combination of sorafenib and doxorubicin versus sorafenib alone (www.clinicaltrial.gov, NCT01015833).

Second-Line Therapies

With the advent of sorafenib as a first line agent for the treatment of HCC, efforts looking at second-line treatments are underway. Brivanib showed evidence of

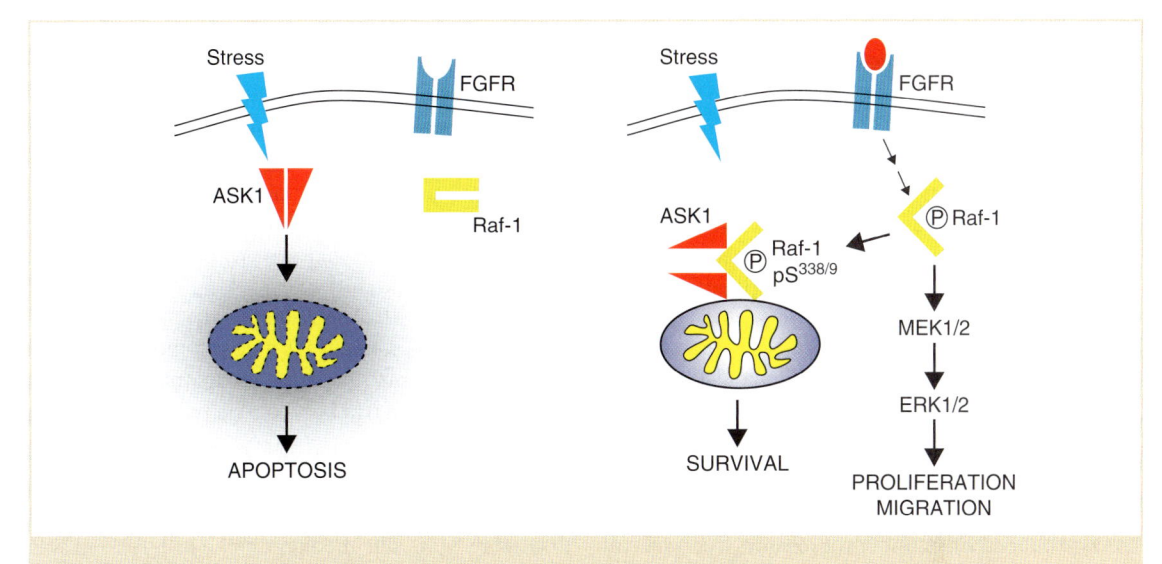

Figure 21-3: A model depicting the role of Raf-1 in regulation of ASK1-mediated apoptosis. bFGF-mediated activation of Raf-1 promotes a complex between Raf-1 and ASK1 at the mitochondria, leading to inhibition of ASK1 kinase activity and prevention of stress-mediated apoptosis.[79]

disease stabilizing activity in a second-line setting.[71] A Phase III study of brivanib versus placebo showed endpoint of median OS (9.4 versus 8.2 months, p=0.3307).[02] Other agents awaiting or undergoing investigation as second-line therapies post sorafenib include bevacizumab and erlotinib (www.clinicaltrials.gov, NCT01180959), lenalidomide (www.clinicaltrials.gov, NCT00717756), the IGF-1R inhibitor OSI 906 (www.clinicaltrials.gov, NCT01101906), and the anti-VEGFR2 antibody ramucirumab (www.clinicaltrials.gov, NCT01140347) and ADI-PEG 20 (www.clinicaltrials.gov, NCT01287585).

Adjuvant Therapy

There have been limited attempts thus far to evaluate biologic therapies in the adjuvant setting in HCC. Sorafenib is currently being evaluated in the adjuvant setting after potentially curative resection or ablation and following TACE in those with unresectable disease. Its safety is also being assessed post liver transplantation. (www.clinicaltrials.gov, NCT00618384, NCT00844168). Given the positive outcome, sorafenib demonstrated in the metastatic setting has led to developing sorafenib as part of adjuvant therapy.[54] This is however also supported by the well-described angiogenic drive that occurs after tumors are resected, which may be inhibited by the use of sorafenib. This approach should however be avoided out of a clinical trial setting until data are available and to ensure safety of patients. Brivanib is also undergoing evaluation in a phase III placebo-controlled study as adjuvant therapy following TACE (www.clinicaltrials.gov).

Biliary Tumors and Biologic Agents

As with HCC, the introduction of targeted agents into the therapeutic arsenal for biliary tract cancer is occurring in tandem with new insights into the molecular pathogenesis of these tumors. Differences in the gene expression profiles among gallbladder carcinoma, intrahepatic and extrahepatic cholangiocarcinomas are being recognized.[83] For example, β-catenin mutations have been documented more frequently in gallbladder carcinomas than in cholangiocarcinomas,[84] and KRAS mutations appear to occur more frequently in ICCs compared to gallbladder and extrahepatic cholangiocarcinomas.[85–91]

Activating mutations of the KRAS/MAPK and EGFR pathways appear to have a role in the pathogenesis of biliary tract tumors. Among ICCs, the frequency of KRAS mutations is 40%–50%.[85,87] BRAF, a downstream effector of the KRAS/MAPK pathway, is also mutated in approximately 20% of ICCs.[86] EGFR mutations have been found in approximately 13%–15% of biliary tract carcinomas, and EGFR amplifications occur in approximately 6% of cases.[92–94] EGFR overexpression occurs in approximately 15% of gallbladder carcinomas compared to 5% and 0% of extrahepatic cholangiocarcinomas and ICCs, respectively.[94,95]

Anti-EGFR therapies have been evaluated in clinical trials. A phase II study of erlotinib monotherapy in 42 patients with advanced biliary carcinoma produced a 6-month progression-free survival rate of 17% and 3 (7%) partial responses lasting 4 to 14 months. The median time to progression and overall survival times were 2.6 and 7.5 months, respectively. Notably, all three responding patients developed a grade 1/2 skin rash and two demonstrated HER1/EGFR tumor overexpression.[7] The randomized phase II BINGO study assessed gemcitabine and oxaliplatin with or without cetuximab. An interim analysis of 36 of 101 enrolled patients revealed a promising 4-month progression-free survival rate of 61% with combination therapy compared to 44% for chemotherapy alone.[96] Anti-EGFR therapies continue to be evaluated in clinical trials. A phase II study of erlotinib monotherapy in patients with unresectable HCC or biliary tract carcinoma has been completed (www.clinicaltrials.gov, NCT00033462). Erlotinib combined with gemcitabine and oxaliplatin is being studied in a phase I (www.clinicaltrials.gov, NCT0098776) and randomized phase III study (www.clinicaltrials.gov, NCT01149122). A phase I trial of this erlotinib, gemcitabine, and oxaliplatin with radiation in patients with advanced disease is also ongoing (www.clinicaltrials.gov, NCT00266097). Cetuximab in combination with gemcitabine (www.clinicaltrials.gov, NCT00747097) and in combination with both gemcitabine and oxaliplatin is being further assessed (www.clinicaltrials.gov, NCT00552149).

The VEGF pathway has also been implicated in the pathogenesis of biliary tract cancers. Upregulation of this pathway has been found in 53%–59% of cholangiocarcinomas and is a poor prognosticator associated with more aggressive disease biology.[97–99] Two phase II trials have evaluated sorafenib monotherapy in advanced biliary carcinoma with modest results. The SWOG 0514 study enrolled 36 patients and reported partial responses in 6% and stable disease in 29% of patients. The median progression-free survival and overall survival times were two and six months, respectively.[100] The second trial reported similar outcomes with partial response and stable disease rates of 2% and 30.6%, respectively.[101] Performance status correlated significantly with progression-free survival and overall survival times that were 2.3 and 4.4 months, respectively. A phase II study of bevacizumab plus erlotinib produced partial responses in 12% of patients and stable disease in 51%. The median time to progression was 4.4 months, and median survival was 9.9 months.[102] Another phase II study tested the combination of bevacizumab with gemcitabine and oxaliplatin.[103] A 40% partial response rate was observed, along with a 6-month progression-free survival rate of 63%, and median progression-free survival and overall survival times of 7 and 12.7 months, respectively. Overall survival was 14.7 months among the subset of patients with ICC. Current trials targeting the VEGF pathway include two phase II trials of bevacizumab with erlotinib, one of which was recently completed (www.clinicaltrials.gov, NCT00356889, NCT00350753). Bevacizumab and modified FOLFOX6 are also being studied in another phase II trial (www.clinicaltrials.gov, NCT00881504). The combination of sorafenib plus erlotinib is also being studied (www.clinicaltrials.gov, NCT01093222). Several phase II studies combining sorafenib with gemcitabine-based chemotherapy are currently underway. One phase I/II trial is testing sorafenib with gemcitabine and oxaliplatin (www.clinicaltrials.gov, NCT00955721). A randomized phase II trial is comparing gemcitabine with or without sorafenib (www.clinicaltrials.gov, NCT00661830). Another phase II trial is combining sorafenib with gemcitabine and cisplatin (www.clinicaltrials.gov, NCT00919061).

The PI3K/Akt/mTOR pathway has been shown to be upregulated in biliary tract cancers. In addition, the IGF-1R, which is a component of this pathway, is expressed in primary and metastatic gallbladder tumors.[104–106] In vitro studies show that IGF-1R inhibition results in antitumor activity and is synergistic with gemcitabine. Sirolimus had disease stabilizing activity in 33% of cholangiocarcinoma patients in a single-arm study, with a median survival time of seven months.[46] An ongoing phase II study of RAD001 monotherapy in patients who have progressed on first-line chemotherapy has reported a disease control rate of 55.5% lasting six to nine months.[108]

Other biologic agents that exhibit activity in biliary cancers are MEK1/2 inhibitors such as AZD684. A phase II trial of 29 patients reported a partial response rate of 14%, stable disease in 64% of patients, and median progression-free survival and overall survival times of 7 and 8.2 months, respectively.[109] Correlative biomarker studies showed that positive staining for pERK was present in 90% of patients with disease control and 0% of patients who progressed. A study evaluating MEK162 in combination with gemcitabine plus cisplatin is underway (www.clinicaltrials.gov, NCT01828034).

The current standard of care for the front-line management of biliary tract carcinomas was recently established in the ABC-02 trial.[110] In this pivotal phase III study, 410 patients with advanced biliary tract carcinomas or ampullary carcinoma were randomized to gemcitabine with or without cisplatin. Two hundred and four patients received combination chemotherapy, and 206 received gemcitabine alone. Treatment arms were well balanced for baseline characteristics; 36.9% and 35.8% had gallbladder carcinoma, and 57.8% and 59.8% had bile duct carcinomas. The addition of cisplatin significantly improved tumor control rates, as well as progression-free survival and overall survival. Bile duct and gallbladder tumors did not display differential responses to therapy.

Thus far, no biologic agent alone, or combined with chemotherapy or another biologic agent, has produced outcomes exceeding those of gemcitabine and cisplatin. An important consideration in evaluating the studies that have been conducted is that the study populations were very heterogeneous, including gallbladder, intrahepatic and extrahepatic cholangiocarcinomas, as well as previously treated and treatment naïve patients and that outcomes were not stratified for these variables. Emerging data suggest that tumors arising from the different sites along the biliary tract may be separate disease entities. Although biliary tract tumors are still treated uniformly, these discoveries are expected to provide further guidance on how to best integrate biologic therapy into the management of these diseases.

Summary

Novel therapeutics, such as sorafenib, are now established as part of the standard treatment of HCC. More importantly, this effort has led to others evaluating other novel therapeutics of similar or different mechanisms of action both as single agents and in combination.

Regardless of their specific targeting, novel therapeutics carry the risk of adverse events, some of which while rare, can be quite serious. Further efforts remain badly needed for evaluating biologic therapies in biliary tumors.

References

1. Abou-Alfa GK, Venook AP. The impact of new data in the treatment of advanced hepatocellular carcinoma. *Curr Oncol Rep.* 2008;10(3):199–205.
2. Huitzil-Melendez FD, Abou-Alfa GK, Morse MA. Novel therapies targeted at signal transduction in liver tumors. In: Clavien PA, ed. *Malignant Liver Tumors: Current And Emerging Therapies*. 3rd ed. Sudbury, MA: Jones and Bartlett; 2009:382.
3. Huether A, Hopfner M, Varadari V, et al. EGFR blockade by cetuximab alone or as combination therapy for growth control of hepatocellular carcinoma. *Biochem Pharmacol.* 2005;70:1568–1578.
4. Harada K. Shiota G. Kawasaki H. Transforming growth factor-alpha and epidermal growth factor receptor in chronic liver disease and hepatocellular carcinoma. *Liver.* August 1999;19(4):318–325.
5. Kira S, Nakanishi T, Suemori S, et al. Expression of transforming growth factor alpha and epidermal growth factor receptor in human hepatocellular carcinoma. *Liver.* 1997;17(4):177–182.
6. Kiss A, Wang NJ, Xie JP, Thorgeirsson SS. Analysis of transforming growth factor (TGF)-alpha/epidermal growth factor receptor, hepatocyte growth factor/c-met,TGF-beta receptor type II, and p53

expression in human hepatocellular carcinomas. *Clinical Cancer Research*. 1997;3(7):1059–1066.

7. Philip PA, Mahoney MR, Allmer C, et al. Phase II study of Erlotinib (OSI-774) in patients with advanced hepatocellular cancer. *J Clini Oncolo*. 2005;23:6657–6663.

8. Thomas MB, Morris JS, Chadha R, et al. Phase II trial of the combination of bevacizumab and erlotinib in patients who have advanced hepatocellular carcinoma. *J Clin Oncol*. 2009; 27(6):843–850. Epub 2009 January 12. Erratum in: *J Clin Oncol*. 2009;27(19):3263. Lin, Elinor [corrected to Lin, E].

9. Huether A, Höpfner M, Baradari V, Schuppan D, Scherübl H. EGFR blockade by cetuximab alone or as combination therapy for growth control of hepatocellular cancer. *Biochem Pharmacol*. 2005 Nov 25;70(11):1568–78. Epub 2005 Oct 13.

10. Hsu C, Huang CL, Hsu HC, et al. HER-2/neu overexpression is rare in hepatocellular carcinoma and not predictive of anti-HER-2/neu regulation of cell growth and chemosensitivity. *Cancer*. 2002;94(2):415–420.

11. Ramanathan RK, Belani CP, Singh DA, et al. A Phase II study of lapatinib in patients with advanced biliary tree and hepatocellular cancer. *Cancer Chemother Pharmacol*. 2009;64(4):777–783.

12. Huitzil FD, Sun MY, Capanu M, et al. Expression of the c-met and HGF in resected hepatocellular carcinoma (rHCC): correlation with clinicopathological features (CP) and overall survival (Overall survival). *J Clin Oncol*. 2008;26(suppl; abstr 4599).

13. Wang R, Ferrell LD, Faouzi S, et al. Activation of the Met receptor by cell attachment induces and sustains hepatocellular carcinomas in transgenic mice. *J Cell Biol*. 2001;153(5):1023–1034.

14. Johnson GL, Lapadat R. Mitogen-activated protein kinase pathways mediated by ERK, JNK, and p38 protein kinases. *Science*. 2002;298(5600): 1911–1912.

15. Garcia A, Rosen L, Cunningham CC, et al. Phase 1 study of ARQ 197, a selective inhibitor of the c-Met RTK in patients with metastatic solid tumors reaches recommended phase 2 dose. *J Clin Oncol*. 2007;25(18S suppl):3525; ASCO Annual Meeting Proceedings Part I.

16. Santoro A, Rimassa L, Borbath I, Daniele B, Salvagni S, Van Laethem JL, et al. Tivantinib for second-line treatment of advanced hepatocellular carcinoma: a randomised, placebo-controlled phase 2 study. *Lancet Oncol*. 2013 Jan;14(1):55–63.

17. Verslype C, Cohn AL, Kelley RK, Yang T-S, Su W-C, Ramies DA, et al. Activity of cabozantinib (XL184) in hepatocellular carcinoma: results from a randomized phase II discontinuation study. *J Clin Oncol* 30, 2012 (suppl; abstr 4007).

18. Salvi A, Arici B, Portolani N, et al. In vitro c-met inhibition by antisense RNA and plasmid-based RNAi down-modulates migration and invasion of hepatocellular carcinoma cells. *Int J Oncol*. 2007;31(2):451–460.

19. Heideman DA, Overmeer RM, van Beusechem VW, et al. Inhibition of angiogenesis and HGF-cMET-elicited malignant processes in human hepatocellular carcinoma cells using adenoviral vector-mediated NK4 gene therapy. *Cancer Gene Ther*. 2005;12(12): 954–962.

20. Salvi A, Sabelli C, Moncini S, et al. MicroRNA-23b mediates urokinase and c-met down-modulation and a decreased migration of human hepatocellular carcinoma cells. *FEBS J*. 2009;276(11):2966–2982. Epub 2009 April 16.

21. Wang SY, Chen B, Zhan YQ, et al. SU5416 is a potent inhibitor of hepatocyte growth factor receptor (c-met) and blocks HGF-induced invasiveness of human HepG2 hepatoma cells. *J Hepatol*. 2004;41(2):267–273.

22. Aleem E, Elshayeb A. Elhabachi N, et al: *Oncol Lett* 2012 March 3(3):704–712. Epub Dec 30 2011.

23. Desbois-Mouthon C, Baron A, Blivet-Van Eggelpoël MJ, et al. Insulin-like growth factor-1 receptor inhibition induces a resistance mechanism via the epidermal growth factor receptor/HER3/AKT signaling pathway: rational basis for cotargeting insulin-like growth factor-1 receptor and epidermal growth factor receptor in hepatocellular carcinoma. *Clin Cancer Res*. 2009;15(17): 5445–5456. Epub 2009 August 25.

24. Abou-Alfa GK, Gansukh B, Chou JF, et al: Phase II study of cixutumumab (IMC-A12, NSC742460; C) in hepatocellular carcinoma (HCC). *J Clin Oncol*. 29: 2011 (suppl; abstr 4043).

25. Hewish M, Chau I, Cunningham D. Insulin like growth-factor 1 receptor targeted therapeutics: novel compounds and novel treatment strategies for cancer medicine. *Recent Pat Anticancer Drug Discov*. 2009;4(1):54–72.

26. Bos JL. Ras oncogenes in human cancer: a review. *Cancer Res*. 1989;49(17):4682–4689.

27. Tada M, Omata M, Ohto M. Analysis of ras gene mutations in human hepatic malignant tumors by polymerase chain reaction and direct sequencing. *Cancer Research.* 1990;50(4):1121–1124.

28. Weihrauch M, Benicke M, Lehnert G, et al. Frequent k-ras-2 mutations and p16^{INK4A} methylation in hepatocellular carcinomas in workers exposed to vinyl chloride. *Br J Cancer.* 2001;84(7):982–989.

29. Weihrauch M, Benick M, Lehner G, et al. High prevalence of K-ras-2 mutations in hepatocellular carcinomas in workers exposed to vinyl chloride. *Int Arch Occup Environ Health.* 2001;74(6):405–410.

30. Kato K, Cox AD, Hisaka MM, et al. Isoprenoid addition to Ras protein is the critical modification for its membrane association and transforming activity. *Proc Natl Acad Sci USA.* 1992;89(14):6403–6407.

31. Carloni V, Vizzutti F, Pantaleo P. Farnesyl transferase inhibitor, ABT-100, is a potent liver cancer chemopreventive agent. *Clin Cancer Res.* 2005;11(11):4266–4274.

32. Mazume H, Nakata K, Hida D, et al. Effect of simvastatin, a 3-hydroxy-3-methylglutaryl coenzyme A reductase inhibitor, on alpha-fetoprotein gene expression through interaction with the ras-mediated pathway. *J Hepatol.* 1999;30(5):904–910.

33. Kawata S, Nagase T, Yamasaki E, et al. Modulation of the mevalonate pathway and cell growth by pravastatin and d-limonene in a human hepatoma cell line (Hep G2). *Br J Cancer.* 1994;69(6):1015–1020.

34. Kawata S, Yamasaki E, Nagase T, et al. Effect of pravastatin on survival in patients with advanced hepatocellular carcinoma. A randomized controlled trial. *Br J Cancer.* 2001;84(7):886–891.

35. Huynh H, Nguyen TT, Chow KH, et al. Over-expression of the mitogen-activated protein kinase (MAPK) kinase (MEK)-MAPK in hepatocellular carcinoma: its role in tumor progression and apoptosis. *BMC Gastroenterology.* 2003;3(1):19.

36. Giambartolomei S, Covone F, Levrero M, Balsano C. Sustained activation of the Raf/MEK/Erk pathway in response to EGF in stable cell lines expressing the Hepatitis C Virus (HCV) core protein. *Oncogene.* 2001;20(20):2606–2610.

37. Wilhelm SM, Carter C, Tang L, et al. BAY 43-9006 exhibits broad spectrum oral antitumor activity and targets the RAF/MEK/ERK pathway and receptor tyrosine kinases involved in tumor progression and angiogenesis. *Cancer Res.* 2004;64(19):7099–7109.

38. Stambolic V, Suzuk A, de la Pompa JL, et al. Negative regulation of PKB/Akt-dependent cell survival by the tumor suppressor PTEN. *Cell.* 1998;95:29–39.

39. Shiojima I, Walsh K. Role of Akt signaling in vascular homeostasis and angiogenesis. *Circ Res.* 2002;90:1243–1250.

40. Schmelzle T, Hall MN. Tor: a central controller of cell growth. *Cell.* 2000;103:253–262.

41. Villanueva A, Chiang DY, Newell P, et al. Pivotal role of mTOR signaling in hepatocellular carcinoma. *Gastroenterology.* 2008;135(6):1972–1983.

42. Toso S, Merani S, Bigam DL, et al. Sirolimus-based immunosuppression is associated with increased survival after liver transplantation for hepatocellular carcinoma. *Hepatology.* 2010;51(4):127–1243.

43. Zimmerman MA, Trotter JF, Wachs M, et al. Sirolimus-based immunosuppression following liver transplantation for hepatocellular carcinoma. *Liver Transpl.* 2008;14:633–638.

44. Chen YB, Sun YA, Gong JP. Effects of rapamycin in liver transplantation. *Hepatobiliary Pancreas Dis Int.* 2008;7:25–28.

45. Zhou J, Fan J, Wang Z, et al. Conversion to sirolimus immunosuppression in liver transplantation recipients with hepatocellular carcinoma: report of an initial experience. *World J Gastroenterol.* 2006;12:3114–3118.

46. Rizell M, Andersson M, Cahlin C, et al. Effects of the mTOR inhibitor sirolimus in patients with hepatocellular and cholangiocellular cancer. *Int J Clin Oncol.* 2008;13:66–70.

47. Treiber G. mTOR inhibitors for hepatocellular cancer: a forward-moving target. *Expert Rev Anticancer Ther.* 2009;9(2):247–261.

48. Yoshiji H, Kuriyama S, Yoshii J, et al. Halting the interaction between vascular endothelial growth factor and its receptors attenuates liver carcinogenesis in mice. *Hepatology.* 2004;39:1517–1524.

49. Zhang T, Sun HC, Xu Y, et al. Overexpression of platelet-derived growth factor receptor alpha in endothelial cells of hepatocellular carcinoma associated with high metastatic potential. *Clin Cancer Res.* 2005;11:8557–8563.

50. Abou-Alfa GK, Schwartz L, Ricci S, et al. Phase II study of sorafenib in patients with advanced hepatocellular carcinoma. *J Clin Oncol.* 2006;24(26):4293–300. Epub 2006 Aug 14.

51. Yeo W, Mok TS, Zee B, et al. A randomized phase III study of doxorubicin versus cisplatin/interferon alpha-2b/doxorubicin/fluorouracil (PIAF) combination chemotherapy for unresectable hepatocellular carcinoma. *J Natl Cancer Inst*. 19, 2005;97(20):1532–1538.

52. Zhao B, Schwartz LH, Jiang L, et al. Shape-constraint region-growing for delineation of hepatic metastases on contrast-enhanced CT scans. *Invest Radiol*. 2006;41(10):753–762.

53. Abou-Alfa GK, Zhao B, Capanu M, et al. *Necrosis as a Correlate for Response in Subgroup of Patients with Advanced Hepatocellular Carcinoma (HCC) Treated with Sorafenib*. ESMO 2008, Stockholm, Sweden.

54. Llovet JM, Ricci S, Mazzaferro V, et al. Investigators study group. Sorafenib in advanced hepatocellular carcinoma. *N Engl J Med*. 2008;359(4):378–390.

55. Huitzil Melendez FD, Capanu M, O'Reilly EM, et al. Advanced Hepatocellular Carcinoma: which Staging Systems Best Predict Prognosis? *J Clin Oncol*. 2010;28(17):2889–2895. Epub 2010 May 10.

56. Siegel AB, Cohen EI, Ocean A, et al. Phase II trial evaluating the clinical and biologic effects of bevacizumab in unresectable hepatocellular carcinoma. *J Clin Oncol*. 2008;26(18):2992–2998.

57. Faivre S, Raymond E, Boucher E, et al. Safety and efficacy of sunitinib in patients with advanced hepatocellular carcinoma: an open-label, multicentre, phase II study. *Lancet Oncol*. 2009;10(8):794–800.

58. Cheng AL, Kang YK, Chen Z, et al. Efficacy and safety of sorafenib in patients in the Asia-Pacific region with advanced hepatocellular carcinoma: a phase III randomised, double-blind, placebo-controlled trial. *Lancet Oncol*. 2009;10(1):25–34.

59. Abou-Alfa GK. Selection of patients with hepatocellular carcinoma for sorafenib. *J Natl Compr Canc Netw*. 2009;7(4):397–403.

60. Abou-Alfa, GK; Johnson, P; Knox, JK; Capanu, M; Davidenko, I; Lacava, J; Leung, T; Gansukh, B; Saltz, LB. Phase II randomized, double-blind study of doxorubicin plus sorafenib and doxorubicin plus placebo in patients with advanced hepatocellular carcinoma. *JAMA*. 2012;304(19):2154–2160.

61. Huitzil FD, Saltz LS, Song J, et al. Retrospective analysis of outcome in hepatocellular carcinoma (HCC) patients (pts) with Hepatitis C (C+) versus B (B+) treated with Sorafenib (S). Program and abstracts of the 2007 Gastrointestinal Cancers Symposium; January 19–21, 2008; Orlando, Florida. Abstract.

62. Bruix J, Raoul JL, Sherman M, Mazzaferro V, Bolondi L, Craxi A, et al. Efficacy and safety of sorafenib in patients with advanced hepatocellular carcinoma: subanalyses of a phase III trial. *J epatol*. 2012 Oct;57(4):821–9.

63. Abou-Alfa GK, Amadori D, Santoro A, Figer A, et al. Safety and efficacy of sorafenib in patients with hepatocellular carcinoma (hcc) and Child-Pugh A versus B cirrhosis. *Gastrointest Cancer Res*. 2011 Mar;4(2):40–4.

64. Furuse J, Ishii H, Nakachi K, et al. Phase I study of sorafenib in Japanese patients with hepatocellular carcinoma. *Cancer Sci*. 2008;99(1):159–165.

65. Miller AA, Murry DJ, Owzar K, Hollis DR, Kennedy EB, Abou-Alfa G, Desai A, Hwang J, Villalona-Calero MA, Dees EC, Lewis LD, Fakih MG, Edelman MJ, Millard F, Frank RC, Hohl RJ, Ratain MJ. Phase I and Pharmacokinetic Study of Sorafenib in Patients With Hepatic or Renal Dysfunction: CALGB 60301. *J Clin Oncol*. 2009 Apr 10;27(11):1800–5.

66. Schwartz JD, Schwartz M, Goldman J, et al: Bevacizumab in hepatocellular carcinoma (HCC) for patients without metastasis and without invasion of the portal vein. 2005 Gastrointestinal Cancer Symposium, #134.

67. Malka D, Dromain C, Farace F, et al. Bevacizumab in patients (pts) with advanced hepatocellular carcinoma (HCC): preliminary results of a phase II study with circulating endothelial cell (CEC) monitoring. *J Clin Oncol*. 2007; 25(18S, suppl):457; ASCO Annual Meeting Proceedings Part I.

68. Zhu AX, Sahani DV, Duda DG, et al. Efficacy, safety, and potential biomarkers of sunitinib monotherapy in advanced hepatocellular carcinoma: a phase II study. *J Clin Oncol*. 2009;27(18):3027–3035.

69. Cheng AL, Kang Y, Lin D, Park, J, Kudo M, Qin S, et al. Phase III study of sunitinib versus sorafenib in advanced hepatocellular carcinoma. *J Clin Oncol* 29: 2011 (suppl; abstr 4000).

70. Raoul JL, Finn RS, Kang YJ, et al. An open-label phase II study of first- and second-line treatment with brivanib in patients with hepatocellular carcinoma (HCC). *J Clin Oncol*. 2009;27(suppl):(15s) (abstr 4577).

71. Finn RS, Kang YK, Mulcahy M, Polite BN, Lim HY, Walters I, Baudelet C, Manekas D, Park JW. Phase II, open-label study of brivanib as second-line therapy in patients with advanced hepatocellular carcinoma. *Clin Cancer Res*. 2012 Apr 1;18(7):2090–8.

doi: 10.1158/1078-0432.CCR-11-1991. Epub 2012 Jan 11.

72. Finn RS, Raoul J, Manekas D, et al. Optimal assessment of treatment benefit with targeted agents for hepatocellular carcinoma (HCC): an analysis of brivanib phase II data. 2010 ASCO Annual Meeting. *J Clin Oncol* 28:15s, 2010 (suppl; abstr 4096).

73. Johnson P, Qin S, Park JW, et al. Brivanib versus sorafenib as first-line therapy in patients with unresectable advanced hepatocellular harcinoma (HCC): Results from the phase 3 BRISK-FL Study. Volume 56, Issue Supplement S1, LB-6, October 2012.

74. Toh H, Chen P, Carr BI, et al. Linifanib phase II trial in patients with advanced hepatocellular carcinoma (HCC). *J Clin Oncol.* 2010;28(suppl):15s (abstr 4038).

75. Cainap C, Qin S, Huang W-T, Chung I-J, Pan H, Cheng Y, et al. Phase III trial of linifanib versus sorafenib in patients with advanced hepatocellular carcinoma (HCC). *J Clin Oncol.* 30: 2012 (suppl 34; abstr 249).

76. Zhu AX, Blaskowsky LS, Ryan DP, et al. Phase II study of gemcitabine and oxaliplatin in combination with bevacizumab in patients with advanced hepatocellular carcinoma. *J Clin Oncol.* 2006;24:1898–1903.

77. Sun W, Haller DG, Mykulowycz K, et al. Combination of capecitabine, oxaliplatin with bevacizumab in treatment of advanced hepatocellular carcinoma (HCC): a phase II study. *J Clin Oncol.* 2007;25(18S, suppl):4574; 2007 ASCO Annual Meeting Proceedings Part I.

78. Hsu C, Yang T, Hsu C, Toh H, et al. Modified-dose capecitabine + bevaci-zumab for the treatment of advanced/metastatic hepatocellular carcinoma (HCC): a phase II, single-arm study. *J Clin Oncol.* 2007;25(18S, suppl):15190; 2007 ASCO Annual Meeting Proceedings Part I.

79. Duran I, Hotté SJ, Hirte H, et al. Phase I targeted combination trial of sorafenib and erlotinib in patients with advanced solid tumors. *Clin Cancer Res.* 2007;13(16):4849–4857.

80. Zhu AX, Rosmorduc O, Evans J, Ross P, Santoro A, Carrilho FJ, et al. SEARCH: A phase III, randomized, double-blind, placebo-controlled trial of sorafenib plus erlotinib in patients with hepatocellular carcinoma (HCC). *Ann Oncol* (2012) 23 (suppl 9): LBA2.

81. Alavi AS, Acevedo L, Min W, Cheresh DA. Chemoresistance of endothelial cells induced by basic fibroblast growth factor depends on Raf-1-mediated inhibition of the proapoptotic kinase, ASK1. *Cancer Res.* 2007;67(6):2766–2772.

82. Llovet JM, Decaens T, Raoul J-L, Boucher E, Kudo M, Chang C, et al. Brivanib versus placebo in patients with advanced hepatocellular carcinoma (HCC) who failed or were intolearent to sorafenib: Results from the phase 3 BRISK-PS study. *Journal of Hepatology* 2012; Vol. 56 Supplement 2, Page S549.

83. Hezel AF, Deshpande V, Zhu AX. Genetics of biliary tract cancers and emerging targeted therapies. *J Clin Oncol.* 2010;28(21):3531–3540.

84. Rashid A, Gao YT, Bhakta S, et al. Beta-catenin mutations in biliary tract cancers: a population-based study in China. *Cancer Res.* 2001;61:3406–3409.

85. Tannapfel A, Benicke M, Katalinic A, et al. Frequency of p16(INK4A) alterations and K-ras mutations in intrahepatic cholangiocarcinoma of the liver. *Gut.* 2000;47:721–727.

86. Tannapfel A, Sommerer F, Benicke M, et al. Mutations of the BRAF gene in cholangiocarcinoma but not in hepatocellular carcinoma. *Gut.* 2003;52:706–712.

87. Ohashi K, Nakajima Y, Kanehiro H, et al. Ki-ras mutations and p53 protein expressions in intrahepatic cholangiocarcinomas: relation to gross tumor morphology. *Gastroenterology.* 1995; 109:1612–1617.

88. Suto T, Habano W, Sugai T, et al. Aberrations of the K-ras, p53, and APC genes in extrahepatic bile duct cancer. *J Surg Oncol.* 2000;73: 158–163.

89. Hanada K, Tsuchida A, Iwao T, et al. Gene mutations of K-ras in gallbladder mucosae and gallbladder carcinoma with an anomalous junction of the pancreaticobiliary duct. *Am J Gastroenterol.* 1999;94:1638–1642.

90. Watanabe H, Date K, Itoi T, et al. Histological and genetic changes in malignant transformation of gallbladder adenoma. *Ann Oncol.* 1999;10(suppl 4):136–139.

91. Rashid A, Ueki T, Gao YT, et al. K-ras mutation, p53 overexpression, and microsatellite instability in biliary tract cancers: a population-based study in China. *Clin Cancer Res.* 2002; 8:3156–3316.

92. Leone F, Cavalloni G, Pignochino Y, et al. Somatic mutations of epidermal growth factor receptor in bile duct and gallbladder carcinoma. *Clin Cancer Res.* 2006;12:1680–1685.

93. Gwak GY, Yoon JH, Shin CM, et al. Detection of response-predicting mutations in the kinase domain of the epidermal growth factor receptor gene in cholangiocarcinomas. *J Cancer Res Clin Oncol.* 2005;131:649–652.
94. Nakazawa K, Dobashi Y, Suzuki S, et al. Amplification and overexpression of c-erbB-2, epidermal growth factor receptor, and c-met in biliary tract cancers. *J Pathol.* 2005;206:356–365.
95. Kiguchi K, Carbajal S, Chan K, et al. Constitutive expression of ErbB-2 in gallbladder epithelium results in development of adenocarcinoma. *Cancer Res.* 2001;61:6971–6976.
96. Malka D, Trarbach T, Fartoux L, et al. A multicenter, randomized phase II trial of gemcitabine and oxaliplatin (GEMOX) alone or in combination with biweekly cetuximab in the first-line treatment of advanced biliary cancer: interim analysis of the BINGO trial. *J Clin Oncol.* 2009;27(suppl):15s (abstr 4520).
97. Yoshikawa D, Ojima H, Iwasaki M, et al. Clinicopathological and prognostic significance of EGFR, VEGF, and HER2 expression in cholangiocarcinoma. *Br J Cancer.* 2008;98:418–425.
98. Park BK, Paik YH, Park JY, et al. The clinicopathologic significance of the expression of vascular endothelial growth factor-C in intrahepatic cholangiocarcinoma. *Am J Clin Oncol.* 2006;29:138–142.
99. Hida Y, Morita T, Fujita M, et al. Vascular endothelial growth factor expression is an independent negative predictor in extrahepatic biliary tract carcinomas. *Anticancer Res.* 1999;19:2257–2260.
100. El-Khoueiry AB, Rankin C, Lenz HJ, et al. SWOG 0514: a phase II study of sorafenib (BAY 43-9006) as single agent in patients (pts) with unresectable or metastatic gallbladder cancer or cholangiocarcinomas. *J Clin Oncol.* 2007;25(18S, suppl):4639; 2007 ASCO Annual Meeting Proceedings Part I.
101. Bengala C, Bertolini F, Malavasi N, et al. Sorafenib in patients with advanced biliary tract carcinoma: a phase II trial. *Br J Cancer.* 2010;102(1):68–72.
102. Lubner SJ, Mahoney MR, Kolesar JL, et al. Report of a multicenter phase II trial testing a combination of biweekly bevacizumab and daily erlotinib in patients with unresectable biliary cancer: a phase II Consortium study. *J Clin Oncol.* 2010;28(21):3491–3497.
103. Zhu AX, Meyerhardt JA, Blaszkowsky LS, et al. Efficacy and safety of gemcitabine, oxaliplatin, and bevacizumab in advanced biliary-tract cancers and correlation of changes in 18-fluorodeoxyglucose PET with clinical outcome: a phase 2 study. *Lancet Oncol.* 2010;11(1):48–54.
104. Hansel DE, Rahman A, Hidalgo M, et al. Identification of novel cellular targets in biliary tract cancers using global gene expression technology. *Am J Pathol.* 2003;163:217–229.
105. Kornprat P, Rehak P, Ruschoff J, Langner C. Expression of IGF-I, IGF-II, and IGF-IR in gallbladder carcinoma: a systematic analysis including primary and corresponding metastatic tumours. *J Clin Pathol.* 2006;59:202–206.
106. Alvaro D, Barbaro B, Franchitto A, et al. Estrogens and insulin-like growth factor 1 modulate neoplastic cell growth in human cholangiocarcinoma. *Am J Pathol.* 2006;169:877–888.
107. Wolf S, Lorenz J, Mössner J, et al. (2010) Treatment of biliary tract cancer with NVP-AEW541: Mechanisms of action and resistance. *World J Gastroenterol* 16:156–166.
108. Buzzoni R, Pusceddu S, Platania M, et al. Efficacy and safety of RAD001 in advanced biliary tract cancer (BTC) patients (pts) progressing after first-line chemotherapy: a phase II study. *J Clin Oncol.* 2010;28(suppl; abstr e14500).
109. Bekaii-Saab TMP, Xiaobai L, Saji M, et al. A multi-institutional study of AZD6244 (ARRY-142886) in patients with advanced biliary cancers 100th Annual Meeting of the American Association for Cancer Research, Denver, CO, April 18–22, 2009, abstr LB-129.
110. Valle J, Wasan H, Palmer DH, et al. Cisplatin plus gemcitabine versus gemcitabine for biliary tract cancer. *NEJM.* 2010;362:1273–1281.

CHAPTER 22

Immunotherapies for Liver Tumors

Tetsuya Nakatsura & Yusuke Nakamura

Introduction

Primary liver cancer, which consists predominantly of hepatocellular carcinoma (HCC), is the fifth most common cancer and the third leading cause of cancer-related death worldwide.[1] The incidence and mortality associated with HCC have been increasing steadily[2] as a consequence of epidemics of hepatitis C virus (HCV) and hepatitis B virus (HBV).

Although local ablative therapies as well as surgery have been shown to be very effective for the treatment of HCC, these therapies are limited by the size of tumor, the level of reserved hepatic function, and the presence or absence of intrahepatic metastases. The recurrence rates of liver cancer are still high[3] due to a high risk of metastasis and development of de novo HCC in a cirrhotic liver. Therefore, effective adjuvant therapy such as immunotherapy not only to effectively prevent the development of tumor metastasis but also to avoid the development of de novo tumors in patients with liver cirrhosis has been eagerly awaited.[4]

For the majority of patients with an advanced disease, the treatments with curative intent are no longer available. The patients can be treated by transarterial chemoembolization, Sorafenib, or systemic chemotherapy. Alternative treatments such as immunotherapy are currently being evaluated in patients with advanced HCC.

On the other hand, for the numerous patients infected with HCV and HBV, the establishment of an effective preventive method, such as cancer vaccine to prevent occurrence of HCC, is also required.

The liver is an immunologically privileged organ

Figure 22-1 shows the scheme how the various cells in the liver cause escape from the immune response. Abe and Thomson described that the liver immunoprivilege properties are likely due to its unique repertoire of antigen-presenting cell (APC) populations, consisting of Kupffer cells (KCs), liver sinusoidal endothelial cells (LSECs), and dendritic cells (DCs).[5] KCs and LSECs constitutively express anti-inflammatory cytokines like IL-10 and transforming growth factor beta (TGF-β) that affect T-cell differentiation and inhibit APC maturation in the liver.[6] As a consequence, the number of DCs, which are the most potent to elicit immune responses, is less than in spleen.[7]

In addition, hepatic stellate cells, called as Ito cells, were shown to be involved in liver immunological processes only in case of chronic liver injury. They are induced to transdifferentiate into myofibroblasts and secrete a number of cytokines and chemokines, such as TGF-β.[8,9] In fact, activated hepatic stellate cells have been shown to closely interact with lymphocytes[10] and have potent antigen-presenting properties.[11] Furthermore, stellate cells from hepatitis patients have been indicated to be more highly activated by lymphocyte proximity, especially by CD8+ cells, and to phagocyte CD45+ cells.[12] Those facts suggest that stellate cells are likely to downregulate the immune response in HCV/HBV-derived cirrhosis as well as in HCC.

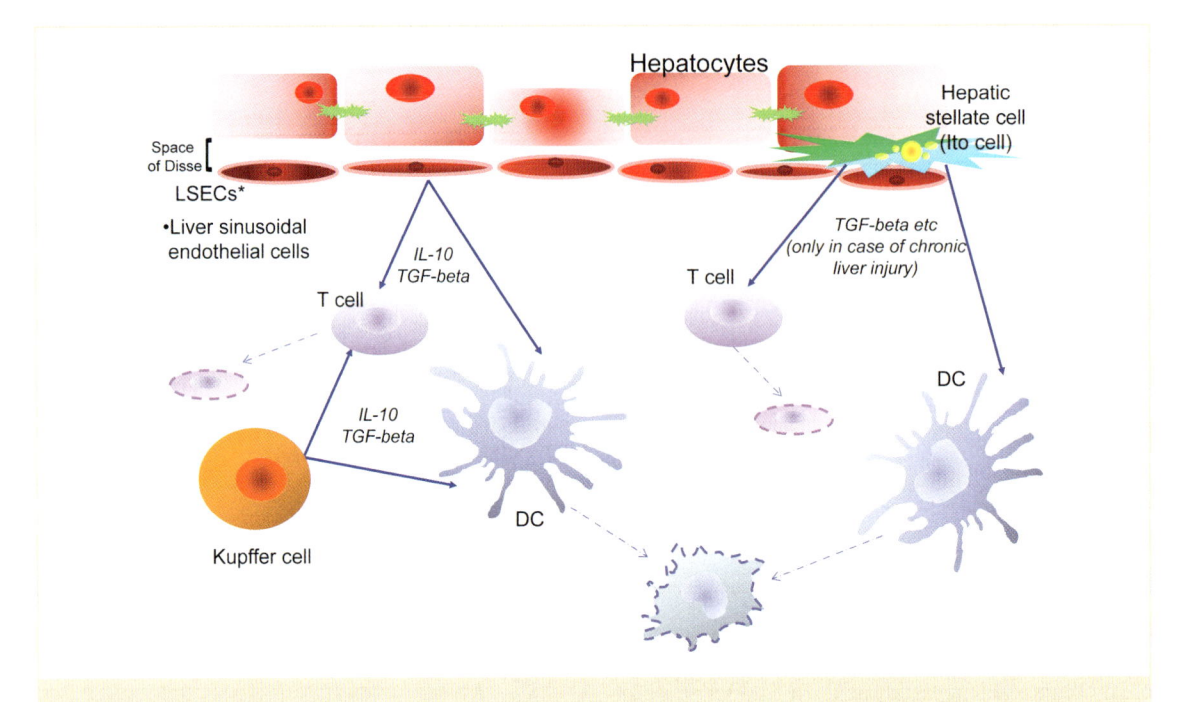

Figure 22-1: The liver is an immunological privileged organ. Liver immunoprivilege properties are due to its unique repertoire of antigen-presenting cell (APC) populations, consisting of Kupffer cells (KCs), liver sinusoidal endothelial cells (LSECs), and dendritic cells (DCs). Due to the fact that KCs and LSECs constitutively express IL-10 and transforming growth factor beta (TGF-β) anti-inflammatory cytokines, T-cell differentiation is affected and APC maturation inhibited in the liver. In addition, hepatic stellate cells, called as Ito cells, were shown to be involved in liver immunological processes only in case of chronic liver injury. They are induced to transdifferentiate into myofibroblasts and to secrete a number of cytokines and chemokines, such as TGF-β.

These findings open new therapeutic opportunities aimed to specifically target hepatic stellate cells in advanced cirrhosis and HCC.

Finally, when HCC is developed in HBV/HCV-derived cirrhosis, these viruses would likely exert direct and indirect effects on further downregulation of the immune response although the mechanisms are not well understood. They might influence the activity of hepatic stellate cells as well as that of resident or recruited immune cells, such as DCs, through direct viral and host protein interaction.[13–16] As reviewed by Liu et al.[17] in chronic B/C-viral hepatitis, a reduction in the myeloid and plasmacytoid DC populations in liver, downregulation of IL-12 and IFN-g levels, upregulation of IL-10, and impairment in DC capacity to prime naïve T cells may account for the insufficient immune response. Similarly, reduction of the number in circulating DC was found in the peripheral blood of patients with either chronic B hepatitis[18] or chronic C hepatitis.[19,20] HBV/HCV would likely contribute to the DC impairment of allostimulatory effect and IL-12 production capacities observed in patients with HCC,[21] although this remains to be elucidated.

Liver tumors have many kinds of mechanism of escape from the immune response

The various mechanisms of liver cancer cells to cause escape from the immune system are shown in Figure 22-2. As it was excellently reviewed by Matar

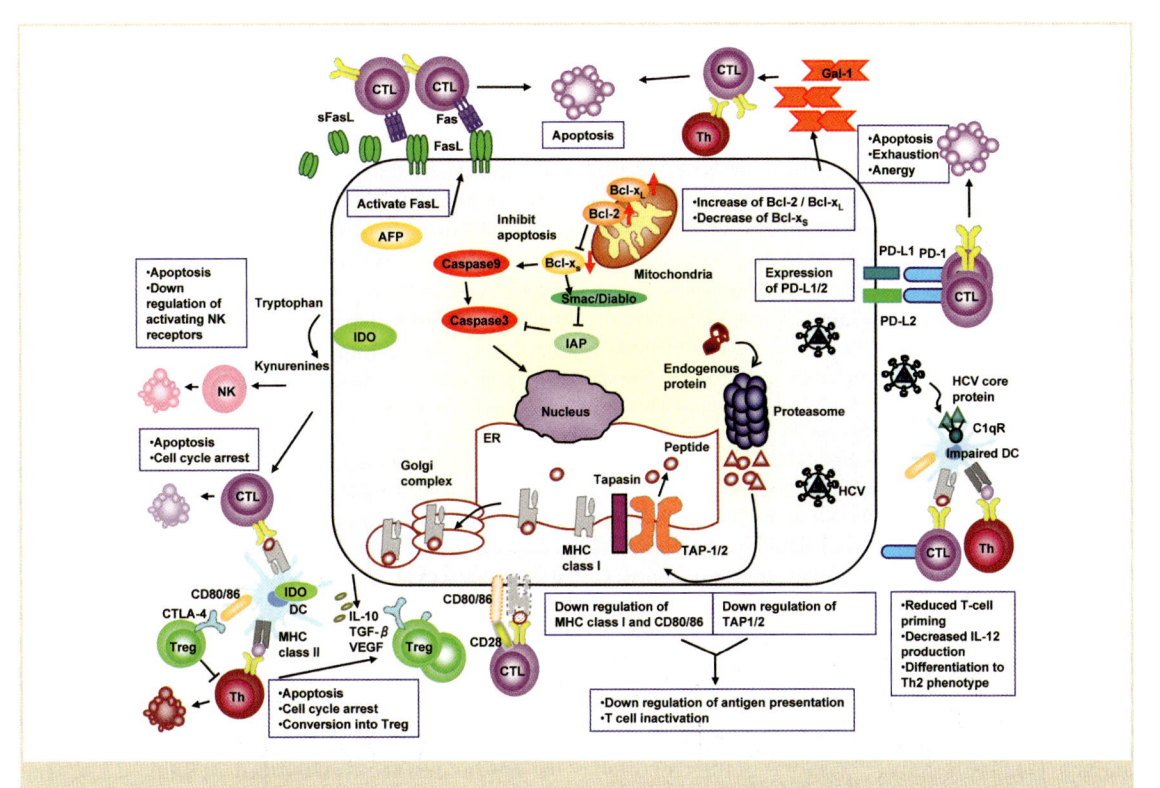

Figure 22-2: Liver tumors have many kinds of mechanism of escape from the immune response. Fas ligand (FasL) is a type II transmembrane protein reported to induce apoptosis of Fas expressing cells. The interaction of FasL or its secreted isoform produced by tumor cells, with their specific Fas receptor, expressed on T lymphocytes, was implicated in tumor cell evasion from immune surveillance. The α-fetoprotein (AFP), an oncofetal protein overexpressed in some hepatocellular carcinoma (HCC), was shown to induce FasL and tumor necrosis factor (TNF)-related apoptosis expression in HCC cells, as well as TRAIL receptor and Fas in lymphocytes. Another pathway developed to attack immune cells involves the interaction of PD-1 (programmed death-1) with its ligands PD-L1 and PD-L2. One further mechanism might implicate Galectin-1 (Gal-1)—a β-galactoside–binding protein with immunoregulatory properties, which is known to play a role in cytotoxic immune cells elimination. It is likely that Gal-1 contributes to tumor immune escape by killing activated T cells. Regulatory T-cell (Treg)–mediated immunosuppression is one of the central tumor immune-evasion mechanisms and may be the main obstacle of successful tumor immunotherapy. CD4+ CD25+ Treg mediates peripheral tolerance by suppressing self-antigen–reactive T cells. Tumor environmental factors such as vascular endothelial growth factor (VEGF), IL-10, and transforming growth factor-β (TGF-β), which all is elevated in HCC, might induce Treg. Another mechanism frequently used by tumors is the downregulation of major histocompatibility complex (MHC) class I, B7-1/B7-2 costimulatory molecules, or transporter associated with antigen processing (TAP)1/2 molecules in human HCC. In addition, HCC cells might escape from cytotoxic T lymphocyte (CTL)-induced apoptosis by increasing Bcl-2 and decreasing Bcl-xs expression and/or raising the surviving level, an important member of the inhibitor of apoptosis (IAP) family. Indoleamine 2,3 dioxygenase (IDO) catalyzes the degradation of the essential amino acid tryptophan and synthesizes immunosuppressive metabolites (sFasL, soluble Fas ligand).

et al., hepatic tumor cells escape from the immune response.[22] Fas ligand (FasL) is a type II transmembrane protein reported to induce apoptosis of Fas-expressing cells.[23] The interaction of FasL or its secreted isoform produced by tumor cells with their specific Fas receptor expressed on T lymphocytes was implicated as a possible mechanism of tumor cell evasion from immune surveillance.[24] The a-fetoprotein (AFP), an oncofetal protein overexpressed in the majority of HCCs, was shown to induce FasL and tumor necrosis factor (TNF) expression in HCC cells, as well as TRAIL receptor and Fas in lymphocytes.[25,26] Another pathway developed to attack immune cells involves the interaction of PD-1 (programmed death-1) with its ligands PD-L1 and PD-L2.[27] Another possible mechanism might implicate Galectin-1 (Gal-1)—a b-galactoside–binding protein with immunoregulatory properties, which is known to play a role in elimination of cytotoxic immune cells. It is likely that Gal-1 contributes to tumor immune escape by killing activated T cells.[28,29] In fact, the expression of Gal-1 was shown to be induced in HCC cell lines, HLF, HuH7, and HepG2.[30]

Regulatory T-cell–mediated immunosuppression is one of the central tumor immune-evasion mechanisms and may be the main obstacle of successful tumor immunotherapy.[31] CD4+ CD25+ regulatory T cells mediate peripheral tolerance of the immune attack to cancer cells by suppressing self-antigen–reactive T cells.[32,33] Several groups reported an increase in proportion of CD4+ CD25+ regulatory T cells in tumors as well as in malignant ascites and tumors from patients with HCC.[34–36]

Tumor environmental factors such as vascular endothelial growth factor (VEGF), IL-10, and TGF-β, all of which are elevated in HCC,[37–39] might induce regulatory T cells (Treg). It has also been suggested that impaired function of DCs might be an important factor in the escape of the tumor from the immune control in patients with cancer.[40] Several studies have shown that the number of DCs is significantly reduced in peripheral blood of patients with cancer.[41,42] Furthermore, several groups have shown that DCs from patients with cancer are often immature and cannot stimulate T cells.[43–45] The abnormal differentiation of DCs, which results in a decrease in the number, and the immature phenotype of DCs are proposed to be affected by tumor-derived factors, such as VEGF,[46] macrophage colony-stimulating factor, IL-6,[47] and IL-10.[48] Finally, AFP has also been identified as a possible inhibitor of DC function.[49] In addition, the downregulation of human leukocyte antigen (HLA) class I,[50] B7-1/B7-2 costimulatory molecules,[51] or transporter associated with antigen processing 1/2 molecules in human HCC is a well-known mechanisms to escape from the immune system.[52] HCC cells might also escape from cytotoxic T lymphocyte (CTL)-induced apoptosis by activation of Bcl-2 and surviving expression, and reduction of Bcl-xs expression.[53–55] Indoleamine 2,3 dioxygenase (IDO) catalyzes the degradation of the essential amino acid tryptophan and synthesizes immunosuppressive metabolites.[56] IDO constitutes an important mediator of peripheral immune tolerance in chronic HCV infection.[57] Understanding of the immune-escape mechanisms should help us to design immunotherapy protocols to increase the probability of therapeutic success.

Cytokine therapy and immunostimulating monoclonal antibodies

Cytokine therapy and immunostimulating monoclonal antibodies are summarized in Table 22-1. One of the most explored cytokines is interferon alpha (IFN-α).[58] The mechanisms of IFN-α antitumor action include direct effect on tumor cells, induction of lymphocyte and macrophage cytotoxic activities, and antiangiogenesis.[59] IL-2, an immunostimulatory cytokine, has been administered alone or in combination with other treatments against liver tumors. Systemic IL-2 treatment was able to produce objective responses against HCC when given alone[60] or with lymphokine-activated killer (LAK) cells.[61]

The immunostimulating monoclonal antibodies are defined as a new family of drugs aiming to augment immune responses. They consist in either agonistic or antagonistic mAbs that are aimed to bind key immune system receptors, thereby enhancing antigen presentation, providing costimulation or counteracting immune regulation.[62] Antibodies against CD28 are known to potentiate antitumor immunity in combination with bispecific antibodies that bind to both the tumor antigen and the T cell receptor (TCR)–CD3 complex.[63] Some anti-CD28 antibodies, termed *superagonist* antibodies, can activate T cells without concomitant TCR engagement. Unfortunately, reports of severe toxicity in a phase I dose-escalation trial with an

TABLE 22-1: Cytokine Therapy and Immunostimulating Monoclonal Antibodies

	Mechanisms of Action
IFN-α	Enhances cytotoxicity, tumor antigen presentation, and antiangiogenesis
IL-2	Enhances NK cell and CD8+ T-cell function; increases vascular permeability
Anti-CD28 mAbs	Activate T cells without concomitant TCR engagement
Anti-CD137 (4-1BB) mAbs	Promote survival of T cells and prevent activation-induced cell death
Anti-OX-40 mAbs	Ensure T-cell long-term survival
Anti-CTLA-4 mAbs	Generate inhibitory signals mediating reduction in T-cell proliferation and in IL-2 secretion
Anti-PD-1 and PD-L1 mAbs	Produce CTL-mediated antitumor effects

Abbreviations: Cytotoxic T-lymphocyte antigen 4.

anti-CD28 mAb caused the serious concerns to this approach.[64] Another costimulatory molecule, CD137 (also known as 4-1BB), is a member of the TNF-receptor superfamily, expressed in antigen-activated T cells (CD4+, CD8+, Treg, and natural killer [NK] cells), DCs, cytokine-activated NK cells, eosinophils, mast cells, and, intriguingly, endothelial cells of some metastatic tumors.[65] The natural ligand for CD137 (CD137 ligand) is constitutively produced by activated APCs. Agonistic anti-CD137 Abs strongly promote survival of T cells by preventing cell death.[66] OX40 (also known as CD134 and TNR4) is another member of the TNF-receptor family, specifically expressed in activated CD4+ and CD8+ T lymphocyte, B cells, DCs, and eosinophils.[67] OX40 ligand (OX40L) is expressed in activated APCs and can also be found in activated T cells and endothelial cells.[68] OX40 seems to be particularly important to ensure long-term survival of T cells, probably through upregulation of the antiapoptotic proteins Bcl-xL and Bcl-2.[69] Phase I clinical trials, using a murine antihuman OX40 mAb, have been initiated in patients with advanced cancer originated from multiple tissues; however, it cannot be administered in several repeated doses because of its xenogeneic nature, which is likely to trigger immune responses against murine sequences.[70] The cytotoxic T-lymphocyte–associated protein 4 (CTLA-4, also known as CD152) is an inhibitory receptor with a structural homology to the costimulatory receptor CD28.[71] Under antigenic stimulation, ligand binding to CTLA-4 generates inhibitory signals mediating reduction in T-cell proliferation and in IL-2 secretion. Administration of antagonistic anti-CTLA-4 mAbs demonstrated antitumor effects in different murine tumor models including colon, prostate, and renal carcinomas, as well as fibrosarcoma and lymphoma.[72,73] As mentioned earlier, PD-1 and its ligands PD-L1 and PD-L2[74] deliver inhibitory signals to T cells. Administration of anti-PD-1 or anti-PD-L1 mAbs induced CTL-mediated antitumor effects in mice.[75]

Tumor antigens in primary liver cancer

There are many types of antigen-specific immunotherapy such as the use of autologous and allogeneic tumor cells (engineered to secrete cytokines), peptides, proteins, and DNAs as well as tumor-specific antibodies. The use of whole tumor cells has the advantage that they express all potential tumor antigens while peptide vaccines cover one or a few antigen epitopes. Whole tumor cells can activate CD4+ T helper cell responses as well as CD8+ T cells and were shown that induction of tumor-specific CD4+ T cells might be crucial not only to activate CD8+ T cells but also to mediate antitumor effector functions.[76]

However, most immunotherapeutic approaches have been based on the generation of tumor-specific CD8+ T cells, which recognize 8–11 amino acid peptides derived from intracellular proteins called as tumor antigens and presented on HLA class I complexes. Although it is also possible to adoptively transfer antigen-specific T cells into patients, most cancer vaccines rely on the generation of antigen-specific T cells in vivo.

The identification of tumor antigens represents an important step for the development of potent cancer vaccines. These antigens can be tumor-specific proteins, which are expressed exclusively in tumor tissue, tumor-associated or cancer-testis antigens, which are overexpressed in tumors but are also detected in placenta and/or testis, or differentiation antigens, which are overexpressed in tumors and are also expressed in corresponding normal tissues. Table 22-2 summarizes results from numerous studies analyzing the expression of different tumor antigens in HCC. AFP, which is expressed in up to 80% of HCC tumors but not in normal adult tissue, represents a classical tumor antigen for HCC. AFP has been a target for immunotherapy of HCC in several studies. Different HLA class I and II restricted epitopes from AFP have been identified.[77-81]

TABLE 22-2: Tumor Antigens and Cytotoxic T-lymphocyte Epitopes in HCC

Antigen	Expression in HCC (%)	CTL Epitope Sequence	HLA Restriction	Position	References
MAGE-A1	19–80	EADPTGHSY	A1	161–169	114–122
MAGE-A2	30–34	YLQLVFGIEV	A2	157–166	119, 121, 123
MAGE-A3	24–70	FLWGPRALV	A2	271–279	114, 115, 117–120, 122, 124, 125
MAGE-A10	19–37	GLYDGMEHL	A2	254–262	114, 120, 126
SSX-2	10–47	KASEKIFYV	A2	41–49	114, 117, 123, 126–128
NY-ESO-1	13–51	MLMAQEALAFL	A2	1–11	83–85, 114, 123, 126, 127
		SLLMWITQC	A2	157–165	
		SLLMWITQA	A2	157–165	
MAGE-C2	68	LLFGLALIEV	A2	191–200	114, 123
		ALKDVEERV	A2	336–344	
HCA587	56–70	TLDEKVAELV	A2	140–149	116, 129–131
		KVAELVEFL	A2	144–152	
		VIWEVLNAV	A2	248–256	
		FLAKLNNTV	A2	317–325	
HTERT	80–90	AYQVCGPPL	A24	167–175	87, 132
		VYAETKHFL	A24	324–332	
		VYGFVRACL	A24	461–469	
		DYVVGARTF	A24	637–645	
		CYGDMENKL	A24	845–853	
		TYVPLLGSL	A24	1088–1096	
CEA	93–100	YLSGANLNL	A2	571–579	133–135
WT1	95	RMFPNAPYL	A2	126–134	135, 136
MRP3	55	LYAWEPSFL	A24	503–511	137
		AYVPQQAWI	A24	692–700	
		VYSDADIFL	A24	765–773	

p53	68	STPPPGTRV	A2	149–157	138, 139
		LLGRNSFEV	A2	264–272	
AFP	70–85	PLFQVPEPV	A2	137–145	80, 96, 105, 140
		FMNKFIYEI	A2	158–166	
		GLSPNLRFL	A2	325–334	
		GVALQTMKQ	A2	542–550	
		EYSRRHPQL	A24	357–365	
		KYIQESQAL	A24	403–411	
		RSCGLFQKL	A24	414–422	
		EYYLQNAFL	A24	424–432	
		AYTKKAPQL	A24	434–442	
Glypican-3	72–81	FVGEFFTDV	A2	144–152	90, 141–143
		EYILSLEEL	A24	298–306	

Abbreviations: AFP, α-fetoprotein; CTL, cytotoxic T lymphocyte; HCC, hepatocellular carcinoma; HLA, human leukocyte antigen.

Most of the other HCC-specific antigens were derived mainly from different types of tumor such as melanoma. Cancer-testis antigens are exclusively found in tumors with the exception of testis and therefore do not encompass the risk of autoimmune reactions during immunotherapy.[82] Best-characterized cancer-testis antigens in HCC are the melanoma-associated antigen (MAGE) antigens. NY-ESO-1, one of cancer-testis antigens, was identified by serological analysis of recombinant cDNA expression libraries (SEREX) using tumor mRNA and autologous serum from a patient with esophageal squamous cell carcinoma.[83] Several groups have shown that NY-ESO-1 is expressed in up to 50% of HCC.[84,85] The catalytic telomerase subunit (hTERT) expressed in >85% of human cancers is considered to be an attractive tumor antigen for a variety of tumors[86] and is an interesting candidate tumor antigen for HCC.[87]

The authors previously reported that Glypican-3 (GPC3) was uniquely overexpressed in human HCC[88] and an ideal tumor antigen for immunotherapy in mouse models.[89] They also identified both HLA-A24(A*2402) and H-2K^d-restricted GPC3$_{298-306}$ (EYILSLEEL) as well as HLA-A2(A*0201)-restricted GPC3$_{144-152}$ (FVGEFFTDV), both of which can induce GPC3-reactive cytotoxic T cells (CTLs).[90] When BALB/c mice were intradermally vaccinated at the base of the tail with K^d-restricted GPC3$_{298-306}$ peptide mixed with incomplete Freund's adjuvant (IFA), the peptide-specific CTLs were induced. However, the peptide without IFA could not induce peptide-specific CD8$^+$ T cells. Furthermore, proteomic analyses showed that IFA protected the peptide against degradation in the human serum. Peptide-reactive CTLs were induced by peptide vaccine in a dose-dependent manner. Similarly, induction of an Ag-specific immune response by HLA-A2 GPC3$_{144-152}$ depended on the dose administered. Our results suggested that IFA is one of indispensable adjuvants for peptide based immunotherapy and that the immunological effect of peptide vaccines depends on the dose of peptide injected.[91]

The authors recently identified a target antigen of cholangiocarcinoma, Forkhead box M1 (FOXM1) for immunotherapy.[92,93] The level of FOXM1 mRNA was more than four times higher in cancer cells in comparison to adjacent normal epithelial cells, in all of 24 cholangiocarcinoma tissues. An immunohistochemical analysis also detected FOXM1 protein in the cancer cells but not in the normal cells. FOXM1(362–370) (YLVPIQFPV), FOXM1 (373–382) (SLVLQPSVKV), and FOXM1(640–649) (GLMDLSTTPL) peptides primed HLA-A2-restricted CTLs in the HLA-A2 transgenic mice. Human CTL lines reactive to these three peptides could also be established from HLA-A2-positive healthy donors and patients with cancer. Natural processing of the three epitopes from FOXM1 protein was confirmed by specific killing of HLA-A2-positive FOXM1 transfectants by peptide-induced CTLs. FOXM1 is expressed in various types of cancer, and it is also functionally involved in the oncogenic transformation and the survival of cancer cells. Therefore, FOXM1 may be a suitable target for immunotherapy against various cancers including cholangiocarcinoma.

Human clinical trials

Many immunotherapeutic clinical trials have been evaluated in patients with HCC and are summarized in Table 22-3. Most of these trials are nonrandomized phase I or II studies in which <30 patients were enrolled. Therefore, these studies mainly demonstrate feasibility and safety, but still lack definite proof of the efficacy of immunotherapy for HCC.

Only one randomized clinical trials demonstrated efficacy of adoptive T-cell transfer. Takayama et al.[94] reported benefits of adoptive transfer with an adjuvant setting for HCC after surgical resection of the primary tumor. In this study, autologous peripheral blood T cells were precultured in medium supplemented with CD3-specific antibody and IL-2, and cell infusion was shown to reduce the risk of cancer recurrence by 41% when compared to a control group receiving only surgery. However, this trial remains unconfirmed, and the mechanism involved in the antitumoral effect remains unclear.

Several studies have shown the potential for DC-based immunotherapy for patients with HCC. However, it should be noted that a DC-based therapeutic approach is a very complex process depending on several factors: type and quality of DCs, manner of antigen loading, and dose and route of vaccination. In addition, DCs have to be prepared for every individual patient making this approach only feasible for a selected patient group. It has been shown that DCs from patients with HCC can be transduced using an AFP-expressing adenovirus in order to stimulate

TABLE 22-3: Immunotherapeutic Clinical Trials in HCC

Author Year References	Country	Indication	Immunotherapy	n	Clinical Result
Onishi (1989)[144]	Japan	Advanced HCC	LAK + IL-2	10	RR: 2/10 (20%), DCR: 10/10 (100%)
					MST: NA
Yoshida (1990)[145]	Japan	Advanced HCC	IFN-γ	14	RR: 0/14 (0%), DCR: 9/14 (64%)
					MST: NA
The GI Tumor Study Group (1990)[146]	USA	Advanced HCC	IFN-α2b	28	RR: 2/28 (7%), DCR: NA
					MST: 5.5 mo
Takayama (1991)[147]	Japan	Advanced HCC	Tumor-infiltrating lymphocyte	3 (1 HCC)	PR (tumor reduction rate: 55%)
					Survival time: NA
Lai (1993)[148]	Hong Kong	Advanced HCC	RCT: IFN-α vs. no treatment	35 vs. 36	RR: 11/35 (31%), DCR: 23/35 (66%)
					MST: 3.6 mo
					Significantly longer survival after IFN-α therapy ($P = 0.0471$)
Colleoni (1993)[149]	Italy	Advanced HCC	Mitoxantrone + IFN-β	40	RR: 9/40 (23%), DCR: 21/40 (53%)
					MST: 8 mo
Kardinal (1993)[150]	USA	Advanced HCC	Doxorubicin + IFN-α	31	RR: 1/31 (3%), DCR 13/31 (42%)
					MST: 10 mo
Aldeghi (1994)[151]	Switzerland	Advanced HCC	Melatonin + IL-2	14	RR: 5/14 (36%), DCR: 11/14 (79%)
					MST: NA
Lotz (1994)[152]	France	Advanced HCC	Doxorubicin + IFN-α2b	21	RR: 3/21 (14%), DCR: 4/21 (19%)
					MST: 4 mo
Feun (1994)[153]	USA	Advanced HCC	Doxorubicin + IFN-γ	22	RR: 3/22 (14%), DCR: 4/22 (18%)
					MST: NA

Lygidakis (1995)[154]	Greece	Adjuvant (resection)	RCT: pre- and postoperative targeting loco regional chemo-immunotherapy vs. no treatment	20 and 20	Significantly lower recurrence rate after adjuvant therapy
Lygidakis (1995)[155]	Greece	Advanced HCC	IL-2 + IFN-γ + lipiodol	20	RR: 11/20 (55%), DCR 18/20 (90%) MST: NA
Kawata (1995)[156]	Japan	Adjuvant (resection)	RCT: doxorubicin + IL-2 + LAK vs. doxorubicin alone	12 and 12	No significant difference in overall and recurrence-free survival
Kountouras (1995)[157]	Greece	Advanced HCC	Doxorubicin + IFNα + tamoxifen + desferrioxamine + ascorbic acid	7	RR: 2/7 (29%), DCR: 6/7 (86%) MST: 10.7 mo
Bokemeyer (1995)[158]	Germany	Advanced HCC	Epirubicin + IFN-α2b	31	RR: 1/31 (3%), DCR: 12/31 (39%) MST: 9.5 mo
Stuart (1996)[159]	USA	Advanced HCC	5-FU + IFN-α	10	RR: 0/10 (0%), DCR: 2/10 (2%) MST: 10 mo
Haruta (1996)[160]	Japan	Advanced HCC	RCT: LAK vs. CTL	8 and 18	LAK group; RR: 0/8 (0%), DCR: 6/8 (75%), MST: 4 mo CTL group; RR: 5/18 (28%), DCR: 18/18 (100%), MST: 21 mo Significantly longer survival after CTL therapy ($P < 0.01$)
Ji (1996)[161]	Korea	Advanced HCC	Non-RCT (retrospective): Cisplatin + IFN-α vs. no treatment	30 and 26	RR: 4/30 (13%), DCR: 19/30 (63%) MST: 8.3 mo Significantly longer survival after chemo-immunotherapy ($P = 0.0001$)
Wang (1997)[162]	China	Adjuvant (resection)	TIL	12 (11 HCC)	Comparison with historic control shows lower recurrence rate
Stefanini (1998)[163]	Italy	Advanced HCC	TACE + α-1-thymosin	12	Comparison with historic control shows survival benefit ($P < 0.05$)
Takayama (2000)[94]	Japan	Adjuvant (resection)	RCT: activated autologous lymphocyte vs. no treatment	76 and 74	Significantly longer recurrence-free survival after transfer of activated lymphocytes ($P = 0.008$)
Llovet (2000)[164]	Spain	Advanced HCC	RCT: IFN-α2b vs. no treatment	30 and 28	RR: 2/30 (7%), DCR: NA No significant difference in RR and survival
Ikeda (2000)[165]	Japan	Adjuvant (resection or ethanol injection)	RCT: IFN-β vs. no treatment	10 and 10	Significantly longer recurrence-free survival after IFN-β therapy ($P = 0.0004$)

(Continued)

TABLE 22-3: Immunotherapeutic Clinical Trials in HCC (Continued)

Author Year References	Country	Indication	Immunotherapy	n	Clinical Result
Kubo (2001)[166]	Japan	Adjuvant (resection)	RCT: IFN-α vs. no treatment	15 and 15	Significantly longer recurrence-free survival after IFN-α therapy ($P = 0.037$)
Reinisch (2002)[167]	Austria	Advanced HCC	GM-CSF + IFN-γ	15	RR: 1/15 (7%), DCR: 10/15 (67%)
					MST: 5.5 mo
Palmieri (2002)[60]	Italy	Advanced HCC	Low-dose IL-2	18	RR: 3/18 (17%), DCR: 16/18 (89%)
					MST: 24.5 mo
Ladhams (2002)[168]	Australia	Advanced HCC	Dendritic cell pulsed with autologous tumor	2	Slowing in the rate of tumor growth in one of two patients
Sakon (2002)[169]	Japan	Advanced HCC	5-FU + IFN-α	11	RR: 8/11 (73%), DCR: 9/11 (82%)
					MST: NA
Iwashita (2003)[102]	Japan	Advanced HCC	Dendritic cell pulsed with autologous tumor	10 (8 HCC)	RR: 0/8 (0%), DCR 6/8 (75%)
					MST: NA
Patt (2003)[170]	USA	Advanced HCC	5-FU + IFN-α2b	43	RR: 9/36 (25%), DCR 22/36 (61%)
					MST: 19.5 mo
Stift (2003)[171]	Austria	Advanced HCC	Dendritic cell pulsed with autologous tumor	20 (2 HCC)	RR: NA, DCR: NA
					MST: 10.5 mo
					Constant remaining of AFP over a period of 6 mo in one of two patients
Feun (2003)[172]	USA	Advanced HCC	Doxorubicin + 5-FU + IFN-α2b	30	RR: 2/30 (7%), DCR: 3/30 (10%)
					MST: 3 mo
Komorizono (2003)[173]	Japan	Advanced HCC	Cisplatin + 5-FU + IFN-α	6	RR: 2/6 (33%), DCR 3/6 (50%)
					MST: NA
Butterfield (2003)[105]	USA	Advanced HCC	AFP peptide vaccination	6	RR: 0/6 (0%), DCR 0/6 (0%)
					MST: 8 mo
Shiratori (2003)[174]	Japan	adjuvant (ethanol injection)	RCT: IFN-α vs. no treatment	49 and 25	Longer recurrence-free and overall survival after IFN-α therapy (P value not shown)
Kuang (2004)[104]	China	Adjuvant	RCT: autologous formalin-fixed tumor vaccine vs. no treatment	18 and 21	Significantly longer recurrence-free survival after vaccination ($P = 0.003$)
Shi (2004)[175]	China	Advanced and early HCC	Cytokine-induced killer cell	13	RR: NA, DCR: NA
					MST: NA
Sangro (2004)[176]	Spain	Advanced HCC	Intratumoral adenovirus encoding IL-12 genes	21 (8 HCC)	RR: 1/8 (13%), DCR 7/8 (88%)
					MST: NA

Lee (2005)[103]	Taiwan	Advanced HCC	Dendritic cell pulsed with autologous tumor	31	RR: 4/31 (13%), DCR 21/31 (68%) MST: NA
Kumagai (2005)[99]	Japan	Advanced HCC	Intratumoral dendritic cell injection after ethanol injection	4	Feasibility study
Yin (2005)[177]	China	Advanced HCC	Cisplatin + doxorubicin + 5-FU + IFN-2α	26	RR: 4/26 (15%), DCR 13/26 (50%) MST: 6 mo
Chi (2005)[100]	Taiwan	Advanced HCC	Local radiation + intratumoral DC injection	14	RR: 2/14 (14%), DCR 9/14 (64%) MST: 5.6 mo
Mazzolini (2005)[178]	Spain	Advanced HCC	Dendritic cell transfected with adenovirus encoding IL-12 gene	17 (8 HCC)	RR: 0/0 (0%), DCR: 2/8 (25%) MST: NA
Butterfield (2006)[96]	USA	Advanced HCC	Dendritic cell pulsed with AFP peptide	10	RR: 0/10 (0%), DCR 0/10 (0%) MST: 7.5 mo
Nakamoto (2007)[179]	Japan	Advanced and early HCC	Non-RCT: TACE + dendritic cell vs. TACE alone	10 and 11	No significant difference in survival
Vitale (2007)[180]	Italy	Advanced HCC	5-FU + IFN-α2b	9	RR: 3/9 (33%), DCR 4/9 (44%) MST: 11.5 mo
Weng (2000)[181]	China	Adjuvant (TACE and RFA)	RCT: cytokine-induced killer cell vs. no treatment	45 and 40	Significantly longer recurrence-free survival after immunotherapy ($P = 0.01$)
Hui (2009)[182]	China	Adjuvant (resection)	RCT: cytokine-induced killer cell 3 courses vs. 6 courses vs. no treatment	41, 43, and 43	Significantly longer recurrence-free survival after immunotherapy ($P = 0.001$ and 0.004)
Palmer (2009)[183]	UK	Advanced HCC	Dendritic cell pulsed with liver tumor cell line lysate (HepG2)	35	RR: 1/25 (4%), DCR 7/25 (28%) MST: 5.6 mo
Olioso (2009)[184]	Italy	Advanced HCC	Cytokine-induced killer cell + IFN-α	12 (1 HCC)	Complete response Survival time: 33 mo (alive)
Hao (2010)[185]	China	Advanced HCC	Non-RCT: TACE + cytokine-induced killer cell vs. TACE alone	72 and 74	Significantly longer survival after combination therapy ($P < 0.001$)

Abbreviations: AFP, α-fetoprotein; CTL, cytotoxic T lymphocyte; DCR, disease control rate; GM-CSF, granulocyte macrophage colony-stimulating factor; HCC, hepatocellular carcinoma; IFN, interferon; IL, interleukin; LAK, lymphokine-activated killer cell; MST, median survival time; NA, not assessed; RCT, randomized control trial; RFA, radiofrequency ablation therapy; RR, response rate; TACE, transcatheter arterial chemoembolization; TIL; tumor-infiltrating lymphocyte.

AFP-specific immune responses.[95] Results from the first phase I/II clinical trial using AFP peptide-pulsed DCs were recently reported. Significant levels of AFP-specific T-cell responses were detected in six patients who received the vaccination.[96]

In addition, DCs loaded with RNAs from HepG2 tumor cells were also able to generate anti-HCC T cells.[97] Loading of DCs with Hsp70-peptide complexes derived from human HCC cells resulted in maturation of DCs, which in turn stimulated proliferation of autologous HCC-specific CTLs.[98]

Two small pilot studies have performed intratumoral injection of DCs in patients with HCC. Intratumoral injection of DCs relies on the ability of DCs to capture antigens from the tumor cells and transport them to draining lymph nodes, where the tumor antigen is presented to T cells. This approach has the advantage that neither autologous tumor material is needed nor the vaccine is restricted to a single antigen.[99,100] In addition, trials using DCs pulsed with autologous HCC tumors or tumor cell lines have just been initiated.[101] One phase I study showed the safety and feasibility of autologous DC in 10 patients with HCC.[102] Another study has also used DC pulsed with tumor lysate and demonstrated that about 10% of the patients with HCC showed a partial response confirming the feasibility and safety of the DC vaccination in these patients.[103]

Results from a randomized phase II trial using a mixture of GM-CSF (granulocyte macrophage colony-stimulating factor), IL-2, formalin-fixed autologous tumor material indicated that the vaccine was well tolerated and no major side effect was induced. More than 85% of all patients were HBV-positive and approximately 50% of the patients had liver cirrhosis. Progression-free survival and overall survival were significantly improved in the vaccinated group with an overall survival of 18/19 in the vaccinated group and 13/21 in the control group after 24 months.[104]

Antigen-specific vaccinations in patients with HCC have been tested using four immunodominant AFP peptides emulsified in Montanide ISA-51 in a phase I clinical trial including six patients with advanced HCC.[105] Although, no clinical responses or the decrease of AFP serum level were detected in these patients, detailed immunomonitoring clearly demonstrated induction of AFP-specific CD8+ T cells in the majority of the patients. In contrast to DC-based therapies, antigen-specific vaccines do not have to be prepared for every individual patient if shared tumor antigens are used, which makes production of the vaccine much less complex and expensive.

The authors analyzed the safety and efficacy of GPC3 peptide vaccination for patients with advanced HCC in the nonrandomized, open-label, phase I clinical trial.[106] Thirty-three advanced patients with HCC were given GPC3 vaccination intradermally (injections on days 1, 15, and 29 with dose escalation). The primary endpoint was the safety of GPC3 vaccination. The secondary endpoints were immune response, as measured by an enzyme-linked immunospot assay, and clinical outcomes, as measured by tumor response, time to tumor progression, and overall survival. GPC3 vaccination was well tolerated. One patient showed a partial response, and 19 patients showed stable disease 2 months after initiation of treatment. The levels of the tumor markers AFP and des-g-carboxy prothrombin temporarily decreased in nine patients. GPC3 peptide vaccine could induce the GPC3-specific CTL response in 30 patients, and the GPC3-specific CTL frequency after vaccination correlated with overall survival. Overall survival was significantly more prolonged in patients with high frequency of GPC3-specific CTLs ($N = 15$) ($P = 0.033$) than in those with a low frequency ($N = 18$). GPC3-derived peptide vaccination was well tolerated, and measurable immune responses and antitumor efficacy were noted. The authors show that GPC3-specific CTL frequency can be a predictive marker for overall survival in patients receiving peptide vaccination.

The potential of synergistic effect of combined therapy

A recent study analyzing T-cell–specific immune responses in 20 patients with HCC undergoing RFA demonstrated an increase in the frequency of tumor-reactive circulating T cells.[107] In this study, IFN-γ secretion by CD8+ T cells was tested before and four weeks after treatment, upon stimulation with autologous tumor lysate. Ablation therapy increased not only the number of tumor-specific T cells circulating in peripheral blood but also the frequency of T cells specific for recall antigens. No correlation between T-cell responses and protection from tumor relapse was found. Although this study was not primarily designed to show an effect of RFA on T-cell responses, results from this study suggest that RFA can activate nonspecific immune responses of T lymphocytes. Some chemotherapeutical agents were shown to induce upregulation of some tumor-associated antigen expression or to reduce tumor cell resistance to specific CTLs. Some of these combinations have been found to produce synergistic rather than additive effects.

The immune-inhibitory mechanisms developed by tumor cells, such as overproduction of immunosuppressive cytokines (TGF-β and IL-10) or induction of Treg cells, are important obstacles that a successful cancer immunotherapy strategy has to face. Inhibition of one or more of these mechanisms appears to be a good strategy to induce antitumor immunity.[108] Elimination or inhibition of Treg activity by low-dose cyclophosphamide[109] or antibodies against CD25 or CTLA-4 may modify tumor immunosuppressive microenvironment, thereby increasing the efficacy of immunotherapy. Adoptive transfer efficacy can also be enhanced by alternative immunotherapies such as cytokine administration[110] and in some cases by standard cytotoxic chemotherapy and radiotherapy.[111,112]

Preclinical models support the rationale for combining cancer vaccines with conventional therapies, such as radiation, chemotherapy, surgery, hormone therapy, as well as other immunotherapies. One of the most promising results was obtained from clinical trials combining antibodies against CTLA-4 with other immunotherapies such as application of GM-CSF-transduced tumor-cell vaccines. This treatment resulted in the alteration of the intratumor balance of Tregs–T effector cells and in tumor rejection.[113] Further research is required to optimize the combination of different immunotherapies to obtain maximal clinical benefits. The combination of well-designed clinical trials with innovative immunotherapeutic approaches will lead to the development of efficient new therapies for the treatment of HCC.

Acknowledgments

The authors thank Drs Noriko Sakemura, Munehide Nakatsugawa, Shiro Suzuki, Daisuke Nobuoka, Kazutaka Horie, Toshiaki Yoshikawa, Yumi Saito, and Manami Shimomura (Division of Cancer Immunotherapy, Research Center for Innovative Oncology, National Cancer Center Hospital East) for assistance.

References

1. Parkin DM, Bray F, Ferlay J, Pisani P. Global cancer statistics, 2002. *CA Cancer J Clin.* 2005; 55: 74–108.
2. El-Serag HB, Mason AC. Rising incidence of hepatocellular carcinoma in the United States. *N Engl J Med.* 1999;340:745–750.
3. Kumada T, Nakano S, Takeda I, et al. Patterns of recurrence after initial treatment in patients with small hepatocellular carcinoma. *Hepatology.* 1997;25:87–92.
4. Colombo M, Donato MF. Prevention of hepatocellular carcinoma. *Semin Liver Dis.* 2005; 25:155–161.
5. Abe M, Thomson AW. Antigen processing and presentation in the liver. In: *Liver Immunology Principles and Practice.* Gershwin M Eric, Vierling John M, Manns Michael P. (Eds.) Humana Press Inc. (New York); 2007:49–59.
6. Crispe IN. Hepatic T cells and liver tolerance. *Nat Rev Immunol.* 2003;3:51–62.
7. Pillarisetty VG, Shah AB, Miller G, et al. Liver dendritic cells are less immunogenic than spleen dendritic cells because of differences in subtype composition. *J Immunol.* 2004; 172:1009–1017.
8. De Minicis S, Seki E, Uchinami H, et al. Gene expression profiles during hepatic stellate cell activation in culture and in vivo. *Gastroenterology.* 2007;132:1937–1946.
9. Friedman SL. Liver fibrosis—from bench to bedside. *J Hepatol.* 2003;38:S38–S53.
10. Muhanna N, Horani A, Doron S, Safadi R. Lymphocyte-hepatic stellate cell proximity suggests a direct interaction. *Clin Exp Immunol.* 2007;148:338–347.
11. Vinas O, Bataller R, Sancho-Bru P, et al. Human hepatic stellate cells show features of antigen-presenting cells and stimulate lymphocyte proliferation. *Hepatology.* 2003;38:919–929.
12. Muhanna N, Doron S, Wald O, et al. Activation of hepatic stellate cells after phagocytosis of lymphocytes: a novel pathway of fibrogenesis. *Hepatology.* 2008;48:963–977.
13. Bain C, Fatmi A, Zoulim F, et al. Impaired allostimulatory function of dendritic cells in chronic hepatitis C infection. *Gastroenterology.* 2001;120:512–524.

14. Sarobe P, Lasarte JJ, Zabaleta A, et al. Hepatitis C virus structural proteins impair dendritic cell maturation and inhibit in vivo induction of cellular immune responses. *J Virol.* 2003;77:10862–10871.
15. Waggoner SN, Hall CH, Hahn YS. HCV core protein interaction with gC1q receptor inhibits Th1 differentiation of CD4+ T cells via suppression of dendritic cell IL-12 production. *J Leukoc Biol.* 2007;82:1407–1419.
16. Zimmermann M, Flechsig C, La Monica N, et al. Hepatitis C virus core protein impairs in vitro priming of specific T cell responses by dendritic cells and hepatocytes. *J Hepatol.* 2008;48:51–60.
17. Liu B, Woltman AM, Janssen HL, Boonstra A. Modulation of dendritic cell function by persistent viruses. *J Leukoc Biol.* 2009;85:205–214.
18. Duan XZ, Zhuang H, Wang M, et al. Decreased numbers and impaired function of circulating dendritic cell subsets in patients with chronic hepatitis B infection (R2). *J Gastroenterol Hepatol.* 2005;20:234–242.
19. Kanto T, Inoue M, Miyatake H, et al. Reduced numbers and impaired ability of myeloid and plasmacytoid dendritic cells to polarize T helper cells in chronic hepatitis C virus infection. *J Infect Dis.* 2004;190:1919–1926.
20. Wertheimer AM, Bakke A, Rosen HR. Direct enumeration and functional assessment of circulating dendritic cells in patients with liver disease. *Hepatology.* 2004;40:335–345.
21. Ninomiya T, Akbar SM, Masumoto T, et al. Dendritic cells with immature phenotype and defective function in the peripheral blood from patients with hepatocellular carcinoma. *J Hepatol.* 1999;31:323–331.
22. Matar P, Alaniz L, Rozados V, et al. Immunotherapy for liver tumors: present status and future prospects. *J Biomed Sci.* 2009;16:30.
23. Curtin JF, Cotter TG. Live and let die: regulatory mechanisms in Fas-mediated apoptosis. *Cell Signal.* 2003;15:983–992.
24. Song E, Chen J, Ouyang N, et al. Soluble Fas ligand released by colon adenocarcinoma cells induces host lymphocyte apoptosis: an active mode of immune evasion in colon cancer. *Br J Cancer.* 2001;85:1047–1054.
25. Li M, Liu X, Zhou S, et al. Effects of alpha fetoprotein on escape of Bel 7402 cells from attack of lymphocytes. *BMC Cancer.* 2005;5:96.
26. Li MS, Ma QL, Chen Q, et al. Alpha-fetoprotein triggers hepatoma cells escaping from immune surveillance through altering the expression of Fas/FasL and tumor necrosis factor related apoptosis-inducing ligand and its receptor of lymphocytes and liver cancer cells. *World J Gastroenterol.* 2005;11:2564–2569.
27. He YF, Zhang GM, Wang XH, et al. Blocking programmed death-1 ligand-PD-1 interactions by local gene therapy results in enhancement of antitumor effect of secondary lymphoid tissue chemokine. *J Immunol.* 2004;173:4919–4928.
28. Rubinstein N, Alvarez M, Zwirner NW, et al. Targeted inhibition of galectin-1 gene expression in tumor cells results in heightened T cell-mediated rejection; A potential mechanism of tumor-immune privilege. *Cancer Cell.* 2004;5:241–251.
29. Rabinovich GA, Rubinstein N, Matar P, et al. The antimetastatic effect of a single low dose of cyclophosphamide involves modulation of galectin-1 and Bcl-2 expression. *Cancer Immunol Immunother.* 2002;50:597–603.
30. Kondoh N, Hada A, Ryo A, et al. Activation of Galectin-1 gene in human hepatocellular carcinoma involves methylation-sensitive complex formations at the transcriptional upstream and downstream elements. *Int J Oncol.* 2003;23:1575–1583.
31. Zou W. Regulatory T cells, tumour immunity and immunotherapy. *Nat Rev Immunol.* 2006;6:295–307.
32. Shevach EM. CD4+ CD25+ suppressor T cells: more questions than answers. *Nat Rev Immunol.* 2002;2:389–400.
33. Zou W. Immunosuppressive networks in the tumour environment and their therapeutic relevance. *Nat Rev Cancer.* 2005;5:263–274.
34. Ormandy LA, Hillemann T, Wedemeyer H, et al. Increased populations of regulatory T cells in peripheral blood of patients with hepatocellular carcinoma. *Cancer Res.* 2005;65:2457–2464.
35. Unitt E, Rushbrook SM, Marshall A, et al. Compromised lymphocytes infiltrate hepatocellular carcinoma: the role of T-regulatory cells. *Hepatology.* 2005;41:722–730.
36. Yang XH, Yamagiwa S, Ichida T, et al. Increase of CD4+ CD25+ regulatory T-cells in the liver of patients with hepatocellular carcinoma. *J Hepatol.* 2006;45:254–262.
37. Yamaguchi R, Yano H, Iemura A, et al. Expression of vascular endothelial growth factor in human hepatocellular carcinoma. *Hepatology.* 1998;28:68–77.
38. Beckebaum S, Zhang X, Chen X, et al. Increased levels of interleukin-10 in serum from patients with hepatocellular carcinoma correlate with profound numerical deficiencies and immature phenotype of circulating dendritic cell subsets. *Clin Cancer Res.* 2004;10:7260–7269.

39. Giannelli G, Fransvea E, Marinosci F, et al. Transforming growth factor-beta1 triggers hepatocellular carcinoma invasiveness via alpha3beta1 integrin. *Am J Pathol.* 2002;161:183–193.
40. Gabrilovich D. Mechanisms and functional significance of tumour-induced dendritic-cell defects. *Nat Rev Immunol.* 2004;4:941–952.
41. Hoffmann TK, Muller-Berghaus J, Ferris RL, et al. Alterations in the frequency of dendritic cell subsets in the peripheral circulation of patients with squamous cell carcinomas of the head and neck. *Clin Cancer Res.* 2002;8:1787–1793.
42. Della Bella S, Gennaro M, Vaccari M, et al. Altered maturation of peripheral blood dendritic cells in patients with breast cancer. *Br J Cancer.* 2003;89:1463–1472.
43. Gabrilovich DI, Corak J, Ciernik IF, et al. Decreased antigen presentation by dendritic cells in patients with breast cancer. *Clin Cancer Res.* 1997;3:483–490.
44. Ishida T, Oyama T, Carbone DP, Gabrilovich DI. Defective function of Langerhans cells in tumor-bearing animals is the result of defective maturation from hemopoietic progenitors. *J Immunol.* 1998;161:4842–4851.
45. Ormandy LA, Farber A, Cantz T, et al. Direct ex vivo analysis of dendritic cells in patients with hepatocellular carcinoma. *World J Gastroenterol.* 2006;12:3275–3282.
46. Gabrilovich DI, Ishida T, Nadaf S, et al. Antibodies to vascular endothelial growth factor enhance the efficacy of cancer immunotherapy by improving endogenous dendritic cell function. *Clin Cancer Res.* 1999;5:2963–2970.
47. Park SJ, Nakagawa T, Kitamura H, et al. IL-6 regulates in vivo dendritic cell differentiation through STAT3 activation. *J Immunol.* 2004;173:3844–3854.
48. Yang AS, Lattime EC. Tumor-induced interleukin 10 suppresses the ability of splenic dendritic cells to stimulate CD4 and CD8 T-cell responses. *Cancer Res.* 2003;63:2150–2157.
49. Um SH, Mulhall C, Alisa A, et al. Alpha-fetoprotein impairs APC function and induces their apoptosis. *J Immunol.* 2004;173:1772–1778.
50. Kurokohchi K, Carrington M, Mann DL, et al. Expression of HLA class I molecules and the transporter associated with antigen processing in hepatocellular carcinoma. *Hepatology.* 1996;23:1181–1188.
51. Fujiwara K, Higashi T, Nouso K, et al. Decreased expression of B7 costimulatory molecules and major histocompatibility complex class-I in human hepatocellular carcinoma. *J Gastroenterol Hepatol.* 2004;19:1121–1127.
52. Matsui M, Machida S, Itani-Yohda T, Akatsuka T. Downregulation of the proteasome subunits, transporter, and antigen presentation in hepatocellular carcinoma, and their restoration by interferon-gamma. *J Gastroenterol Hepatol.* 2002;17:897–907.
53. Chiu CT, Yeh TS, Hsu JC, Chen MF. Expression of Bcl-2 family modulated through p53-dependent pathway in human hepatocellular carcinoma. *Dig Dis Sci.* 2003;48:670–676.
54. Fields AC, Cotsonis G, Sexton D, et al. Survivin expression in hepatocellular carcinoma: correlation with proliferation, prognostic parameters, and outcome. *Mod Pathol.* 2004;17:1378–1385.
55. Kannangai R, Wang J, Liu QZ, et al. Survivin overexpression in hepatocellular carcinoma is associated with p53 dysregulation. *Int J Gastrointest Cancer.* 2005;35:53–60.
56. Munn DH. Indoleamine 2,3-dioxygenase, tumor-induced tolerance and counter-regulation. *Curr Opin Immunol.* 2006;18:220–225.
57. Larrea E, Riezu-Boj JI, Gil-Guerrero L, et al. Upregulation of indoleamine 2,3-dioxygenase in hepatitis C virus infection. *J Virol.* 2007;81:3662–3666.
58. Kirkwood J. Cancer immunotherapy: the interferon-alpha experience. *Semin Oncol.* 2002;29:18–26.
59. Belardelli F, Ferrantini M, Proietti E, Kirkwood JM. Interferon-alpha in tumor immunity and immunotherapy. *Cytokine Growth Factor Rev.* 2002;13:119–134.
60. Palmieri G, Montella L, Milo M, et al. Ultra-low-dose interleukin-2 in unresectable hepatocellular carcinoma. *Am J Clin Oncol.* 2002;25:224–226.
61. Ishikawa T, Imawari M, Moriyama T, et al. Immunotherapy of hepatocellular carcinoma with autologous lymphokine-activated killer cells and/or recombinant interleukin-2. *J Cancer Res Clin Oncol.* 1988;114:283–290.
62. Zhu Y, Chen L. Cancer therapeutic monoclonal antibodies targeting lymphocyte co-stimulatory pathways. *Curr Opin Investig Drugs.* 2003;4:691–695.
63. Chen L, Ashe S, Brady WA, et al. Costimulation of antitumor immunity by the B7 counterreceptor for the T lymphocyte molecules CD28 and CTLA-4. *Cell.* 1992;71:1093–1102.
64. Suntharalingam G, Perry MR, Ward S, et al. Cytokine storm in a phase 1 trial of the anti-CD28

monoclonal antibody TGN1412. *N Engl J Med.* 2006;355:1018–1028.

65. Myers LM, Vella AT. Interfacing T-cell effector and regulatory function through CD137 (4-1BB) co-stimulation. *Trends Immunol.* 2005;26:440–446.

66. Shuford WW, Klussman K, Tritchler DD, et al. 4-1BB costimulatory signals preferentially induce CD8+ T cell proliferation and lead to the amplification in vivo of cytotoxic T cell responses. *J Exp Med.* 1997;186:47–55.

67. Croft M. Costimulation of T cells by OX40, 4-1BB, and CD27. *Cytokine Growth Factor Rev.* 2003;14:265–273.

68. Watts TH. TNF/TNFR family members in costimulation of T cell responses. *Annu Rev Immunol.* 2005;23:23–68.

69. Rogers PR, Song J, Gramaglia I, et al. OX40 promotes Bcl-xL and Bcl-2 expression and is essential for long-term survival of CD4 T cells. *Immunity.* 2001;15:445–455.

70. Melero I, Hervas-Stubbs S, Glennie M, et al. Immunostimulatory monoclonal antibodies for cancer therapy. *Nat Rev Cancer.* 2007;7:95–106.

71. Teft WA, Kirchhof MG, Madrenas J. A molecular perspective of CTLA-4 function. *Annu Rev Immunol.* 2006;24:65–97.

72. Leach DR, Krummel MF, Allison JP. Enhancement of antitumor immunity by CTLA-4 blockade. *Science.* 1996;271:1734–1736.

73. Chambers CA, Kuhns MS, Egen JG, Allison JP. CTLA-4-mediated inhi-bition in regulation of T cell responses: mechanisms and manipulation in tumor immunotherapy. *Annu Rev Immunol.* 2001;19:565–594.

74. Chen L. Co-inhibitory molecules of the B7-CD28 family in the control of T-cell immunity. *Nat Rev Immunol.* 2004;4:336–347.

75. Hirano F, Kaneko K, Tamura H, et al. Blockade of B7-H1 and PD-1 by monoclonal antibodies potentiates cancer therapeutic immunity. *Cancer Res.* 2005;65:1089–1096.

76. Hung K, Hayashi R, Lafond-Walker A, et al. The central role of CD4(+) T cells in the antitumor immune response. *J Exp Med.* 1998;188:2357–2368.

77. Butterfield LH, Koh A, Meng W, et al. Generation of human T-cell responses to an HLA-A2.1-restricted peptide epitope derived from alpha-fetoprotein. *Cancer Res.* 1999;59:3134–3142.

78. Butterfield LH, Meng WS, Koh A, et al. T cell responses to HLA-A*0201-restricted peptides derived from human alpha fetoprotein. *J Immunol.* 2001;166:5300–5308.

79. Meng WS, Butterfield LH, Ribas A, et al. Fine specificity analysis of an HLA-A2.1-restricted immunodominant T cell epitope derived from human alpha-fetoprotein. *Mol Immunol.* 2000;37: 943–950.

80. Mizukoshi E, Nakamoto Y, Tsuji H, et al. Identification of alpha-fetoprotein-derived peptides recognized by cytotoxic T lymphocytes in HLA-A24+ patients with hepatocellular carcinoma. *Int J Cancer.* 2006;118:1194–1204.

81. Alisa A, Ives A, Pathan AA, et al. Analysis of CD4+ T-cell responses to a novel alpha-fetoprotein-derived epitope in hepatocellular carcinoma patients. *Clin Cancer Res.* 2005;11:6686–6694.

82. Scanlan MJ, Gure AO, Jungbluth AA, et al. Cancer/testis antigens: an expanding family of targets for cancer immunotherapy. *Immunol Rev.* 2002;188:22–32.

83. Chen YT, Scanlan MJ, Sahin U, et al. A testicular antigen aberrantly expressed in human cancers detected by autologous antibody screening. *Proc Natl Acad Sci U S A.* 1997; 94:1914–1918.

84. Korangy F, Ormandy LA, Bleck JS, et al. Spontaneous tumor-specific humoral and cellular immune responses to NY-ESO-1 in hepatocellular carcinoma. *Clin Cancer Res.* 2004;10:4332–4341.

85. Shang XY, Chen HS, Zhang HG, et al. The spontaneous CD8+ T-cell response to HLA-A2-restricted NY-ESO-1b peptide in hepatocellular carcinoma patients. *Clin Cancer Res.* 2004; 10:6946–6955.

86. Vonderheide RH, Hahn WC, Schultze JL, Nadler LM. The telomerase catalytic subunit is a widely expressed tumor-associated antigen recognized by cytotoxic T lymphocytes. *Immunity.* 1999;10:673–679.

87. Mizukoshi E, Nakamoto Y, Marukawa Y, et al. Cytotoxic T cell responses to human telomerase reverse transcriptase in patients with hepatocellular carcinoma. *Hepatology.* 2006; 43:1284–1294.

88. Nakatsura T, Yoshitake Y, Senju S, et al. Glypican-3, overexpressed specifically in human hepatocellular carcinoma, is a novel tumor marker. *Biochem Biophys Res Commun.* 2003;306:16–25.

89. Nakatsura T, Komori H, Kubo T, et al. Mouse homologue of a novel human oncofetal antigen, glypican-3, evokes T-cell-mediated tumor rejection without autoimmune reactions in mice. *Clin Cancer Res.* 2004;10:8630–8640.

90. Komori H, Nakatsura T, Senju S, et al. Identification of HLA-A2- or HLA-A24-restricted CTL epitopes possibly useful for glypican-3-specific immunotherapy of hepatocellular carcinoma. *Clin Cancer Res.* 2006;12:2689–2697.

91. Motomura Y, Ikuta Y, Kuronuma T, et al. HLA-A2 and -A24-restricted glypican-3-derived peptide vaccine induces specific CTLs: preclinical study using mice. *Int J Oncol.* 2008;32:985–990.

92. Obama K, Ura K, Li M, et al. Genome-wide analysis of gene expression in human intrahepatic cholangiocarcinoma. *Hepatology.* 2005;41:1339–1348.

93. Yokomine K, Senju S, Nakatsura T, et al. The forkhead box M1 transcription factor as a candidate of target for anti-cancer immunotherapy. *Int J Cancer.* 2010,126.2153–2163.

94. Takayama T, Sekine T, Makuuchi M, et al. Adoptive immunotherapy to lower postsurgical recurrence rates of hepatocellular carcinoma: a randomised trial. *Lancet.* 2000;356.802–807.

95. Gonzalez-Carmona MA, Marten A, Hoffmann P, et al. Patient-derived dendritic cells transduced with an a-fetoprotein-encoding adenovirus and co-cultured with autologous cytokine-induced lymphocytes induce a specific and strong immune response against hepatocellular carcinoma cells. *Liver Int.* 2006;26:369 379.

96. Butterfield LH, Ribas A, Dissette VB, et al. A phase I/II trial testing immunization of hepatocellular carcinoma patients with dendritic cells pulsed with four alpha-fetoprotein peptides. *Clin Cancer Res.* 2006;12:2817–2825.

97. Zhang L, Zhang H, Liu W, et al. Specific antihepatocellular carcinoma T cells generated by dendritic cells pulsed with hepatocellular carcinoma cell line HepG2 total RNA. *Cell Immunol.* 2005;238:61–66.

98. Wang XH, Qin Y, Hu MH, Xie Y. Dendritic cells pulsed with hsp70-peptide complexes derived from human hepatocellular carcinoma induce specific anti-tumor immune responses. *World J Gastroenterol.* 2005;11:5614–5620.

99. Kumagi T, Akbar SM, Horiike N, et al. Administration of dendritic cells in cancer nodules in hepatocellular carcinoma. *Oncol Rep.* 2005;14:969–973.

100. Chi KH, Liu SJ, Li CP, et al. Combination of conformal radiotherapy and intratumoral injection of adoptive dendritic cell immunotherapy in refractory hepatoma. *J Immunother.* 2005;28:129–135.

101. Palmer DH, Hussain SA, Johnson PJ. Gene- and immunotherapy for hepatocellular carcinoma. *Expert Opin Biol Ther.* 2005;5:507–523.

102. Iwashita Y, Tahara K, Goto S, et al. A phase I study of autologous dendritic cell-based immunotherapy for patients with unresectable primary liver cancer. *Cancer Immunol Immunother.* 2003;52:155–161.

103. Lee WC, Wang HC, Hung CF, et al. Vaccination of advanced hepatocellular carcinoma patients with tumor lysate-pulsed dendritic cells: a clinical trial. *J Immunother.* 2005;28:496–504.

104. Kuang M, Peng BG, Lu MD, et al. Phase II randomized trial of autologous formalin-fixed tumor vaccine for postsurgical recurrence of hepatocellular carcinoma. *Clin Cancer Res.* 2004;10:1574–1579.

105. Butterfield LH, Ribas A, Meng WS, et al. T-cell responses to HLA-A*0201 immunodominant peptides derived from alpha-fetoprotein in patients with hepatocellular cancer. *Clin Cancer Res.* 2003;9:5902–5908.

106. Sawada Y, Yoshikawa T, Nobuoka D, et al. Phase I Trial of a Glypican-3-Derived Peptide Vaccine for Advanced Hepatocellular Carcinoma: Immunologic Evidence and Potential for Improving Overall Survival. Clin Cancer Res. 2012;18:3686–3696.

107. Zerbini A, Pilli M, Penna A, et al. Radiofrequency thermal ablation of hepatocellular carcinoma liver nodules can activate and enhance tumor-specific T-cell responses. *Cancer Res.* 2006;66:1139–1146.

108. Curiel TJ. Tregs and rethinking cancer immunotherapy. *J Clin Invest.* 2007;117:1167–1174.

109. Rico M, Matar P, Zacarías Fluck M, et al. Low dose Cyclophosphmide (Cy) treatment induces a decrease in the percentage of regulatory T cells in lymphoma-bearing rats. *Proc Am Assoc Cancer Res.* 2007;48:233.

110. Cheever MA, Greenberg PD, Fefer A, Gillis S. Augmentation of the anti-tumor therapeutic efficacy of long-term cultured T lymphocytes by in vivo administration of purified interleukin 2. *J Exp Med.* 1982;155:968–980.

111. Ganss R, Ryschich E, Klar E, et al. Combination of T-cell therapy and trigger of inflammation induces remodeling of the vasculature and tumor eradication. *Cancer Res.* 2002;62:1462–1470.

112. Chakraborty M, Abrams SI, Camphausen K, et al. Irradiation of tumor cells up-regulates Fas and enhances CTL lytic activity and CTL adoptive immunotherapy. *J Immunol.* 2003;170:6338–6347.

113. Quezada SA, Peggs KS, Curran MA, Allison JP. CTLA4 blockade and GM-CSF combination immunotherapy alters the intratumor balance of effector and regulatory T cells. *J Clin Invest.* 2006;116:1935–1945.

114. Peng JR, Chen HS, Mou DC, et al. Expression of cancer/testis (CT) antigens in Chinese hepatocellular carcinoma and its correlation with clinical parameters. *Cancer Lett.* 2005;219:223–232.

115. Zerbini A, Pilli M, Soliani P, et al. Ex vivo characterization of tumor-derived melanoma antigen encoding gene-specific CD8+ cells in patients with hepatocellular carcinoma. *J Hepatol.* 2004;40:102–109.

116. Zhao L, Mou DC, Leng XS, et al. Expression of cancer-testis antigens in hepatocellular carcinoma. *World J Gastroenterol.* 2004;10:2034–2038.

117. Luo G, Huang S, Xie X, et al. Expression of cancer-testis genes in human hepatocellular carcinomas. *Cancer Immun.* 2002;2:11.

118. Kobayashi Y, Higashi T, Nouso K, et al. Expression of MAGE, GAGE and BAGE genes in human liver diseases: utility as molecular markers for hepatocellular carcinoma. *J Hepatol.* 2000;32:612–617.

119. Chen CH, Huang GT, Lee HS, et al. High frequency of expression of MAGE genes in human hepatocellular carcinoma. *Liver.* 1999;19:110–114.

120. Tahara K, Mori M, Sadanaga N, et al. Expression of the MAGE gene family in human hepatocellular carcinoma. *Cancer.* 1999;85:1234–1240.

121. Yamashita N, Ishibashi H, Hayashida K, et al. High frequency of the MAGE-1 gene expression in hepatocellular carcinoma. *Hepatology.* 1996;24:1437–1440.

122. Kariyama K, Higashi T, Kobayashi Y, et al. Expression of MAGE-1 and -3 genes and gene products in human hepatocellular carcinoma. *Br J Cancer.* 1999;81:1080–1087.

123. Gehring AJ, Ho ZZ, Tan AT, et al. Profile of tumor antigen-specific CD8 T cells in patients with hepatitis B virus-related hepatocellular carcinoma. *Gastroenterology.* 2009;137:682–690.

124. Zhang HG, Chen HS, Peng JR, et al. Specific CD8(+) T cell responses to HLA-A2 restricted MAGE-A3 p271-279 peptide in hepatocellular carcinoma patients without vaccination. *Cancer Immunol Immunother.* 2007;56:1945–1954.

125. Zhou M, Peng JR, Zhang HG, et al. Identification of two naturally presented MAGE antigenic peptides from a patient with hepatocellular carcinoma by mass spectrometry. *Immunol Lett.* 2005;99:113–121.

126. Bricard G, Bouzourene H, Martinet O, et al. Naturally acquired MAGE-A10- and SSX-2-specific CD8+ T cell responses in patients with hepatocellular carcinoma. *J Immunol.* 2005;174:1709–1716.

127. Chen CH, Chen GJ, Lee HS, et al. Expressions of cancer-testis antigens in human hepatocellular carcinomas. *Cancer Lett.* 2001;164:189–195.

128. Wu LQ, Lu Y, Wang XF, et al. Expression of cancer-testis antigen (CTA) in tumor tissues and peripheral blood of Chinese patients with hepatocellular carcinoma. *Life Sci.* 2006;79:744–748.

129. Wang Y, Han KJ, Pang XW, et al. Large scale identification of human hepatocellular carcinoma-associated antigens by autoantibodies. *J Immunol.* 2002;169:1102–1109.

130. Xing Q, Pang XW, Peng JR, et al. Identification of new cytotoxic T-lymphocyte epitopes from cancer testis antigen HCA587. *Biochem Biophys Res Commun.* 2008;372:331–335.

131. Li B, Wang Y, Chen J, et al. Identification of a new HLA-A*0201-restricted CD8+ T cell epitope from hepatocellular carcinoma-associated antigen HCA587. *Clin Exp Immunol.* 2005;140:310–319.

132. Liu YC, Chen CJ, Wu HS, et al. Telomerase and c-myc expression in hepatocellular carcinomas. *Eur J Surg Oncol.* 2004;30:384–390.

133. Morrison C, Marsh W Jr, Frankel WL. A comparison of CD10 to pCEA, MOC-31, and hepatocyte for the distinction of malignant tumors in the liver. *Mod Pathol.* 2002;15:1279–1287.

134. Lau SK, Prakash S, Geller SA, Alsabeh R. Comparative immunohistochemical profile of hepatocellular carcinoma, cholangiocarcinoma, and metastatic adenocarcinoma. *Hum Pathol.* 2002;33:1175–1181.

135. Koido S, Homma S, Hara E, et al. In vitro generation of cytotoxic and regulatory T cells by fusions of human dendritic cells and hepatocellular carcinoma cells. *J Transl Med.* 2008;6:51.

136. Sera T, Hiasa Y, Mashiba T, et al. Wilms' tumour 1 gene expression is increased in hepatocellular carcinoma and associated with poor prognosis. *Eur J Cancer.* 2008;44:600–608.

137. Mizukoshi E, Honda M, Arai K, et al. Expression of multidrug resistance-associated protein 3 and cytotoxic T cell responses in patients with hepatocellular carcinoma. *J Hepatol.* 2008;49:946–954.

138. Stroescu C, Dragnea A, Ivanov B, et al. Expression of p53, Bcl-2, VEGF, Ki67 and PCNA

and prognostic significance in hepatocellular carcinoma. *J Gastrointestin Liver Dis.* 2008;17: 411–417.
139. Cicinnati VR, Zhang X, Yu Z, et al. Increased frequencies of CD8⁺ T lymphocytes recognizing wild-type p53-derived epitopes in peripheral blood correlate with presence of epitope loss tumor variants in patients with hepatocellular carcinoma. *Int J Cancer.* 2006;119: 2851–2860.
140. Mizejewski GJ. Biological role of alpha-fetoprotein in cancer: prospects for anticancer therapy. *Expert Rev Anticancer Ther.* 2002;2:709–735.
141. Capurro M, Wanless IR, Sherman M, et al. Glypican-3: a novel serum and histochemical marker for hepatocellular carcinoma. *Gastroenterology.* 2003;125:89–97.
142. Shirakawa H, Suzuki H, Shimomura M, et al. Glypican-3 expression is correlated with poor prognosis in hepatocellular carcinoma. *Cancer Sci.* 2009;100:1403–1407.
143. Shirakawa H, Kuronuma T, Nishimura Y, et al. Glypican-3 is a useful diagnostic marker for a component of hepatocellular carcinoma in human liver cancer. *Int J Oncol.* 2009;34:649–656.
144. Onishi S, Saibara T, Fujikawa M, et al. Adoptive immunotherapy with lymphokine-activated killer cells plus recombinant interleukin 2 in patients with unresectable hepatocellular carcinoma. *Hepatology.* 1989;10:349–353.
145. Yoshida T, Okazaki N, Yoshino M, et al. Phase II trial of high dose recombinant gamma-interferon in advanced hepatocellular carcinoma. *Eur J Cancer.* 1990;26:545–546.
146. The Gastrointestinal Tumor Study Group. A prospective trial of recombinant human interferon alpha 2B in previously untreated patients with hepatocellular carcinoma. *Cancer.* 1990;66:135–139.
147. Takayama T, Makuuchi M, Sekine T, et al. Distribution and therapeutic effect of intraarterially transferred tumor-infiltrating lymphocytes in hepatic malignancies. A preliminary report. *Cancer.* 1991;68:2391–2396.
148. Lai CL, Lau JY, Wu PC, et al. Recombinant interferon-alpha in inoperable hepatocellular carcinoma: a randomized controlled trial. *Hepatology.* 1993;17:389–394.
149. Colleoni M, Buzzoni R, Bajetta E, et al. A phase II study of mitoxantrone combined with beta-interferon in unresectable hepatocellular carcinoma. *Cancer.* 1993;72:3196–3201.
150. Kardinal CG, Moertel CG, Wieand HS, et al. Combined doxorubicin and alpha-interferon therapy of advanced hepatocellular carcinoma. *Cancer.* 1993;71:2187–2190.
151. Aldeghi R, Lissoni P, Barni S, et al. Low-dose interleukin-2 subcutaneous immunotherapy in association with the pineal hormone melatonin as a first-line therapy in locally advanced or metastatic hepatocellular carcinoma. *Eur J Cancer.* 1994;30A:167–170.
152. Lotz JP, Grange JD, Hannoun L, et al. Treatment of unresectable hepatocellular carcinoma with a combination of human recombinant alpha-2b interferon and doxorubicin: results of a pilot study. *Eur J Cancer.* 1994;30A:1319–1325.
153. Feun LG, Savaraj N, Hung S, et al. A phase II trial of recombinant leukocyte interferon plus doxorubicin in patients with hepatocellular carcinoma. *Am J Clin Oncol.* 1994;17:393–395.
154. Lygidakis NJ, Pothoulakis J, Konstantinidou AE, Spanos H. Hepatocellular carcinoma: surgical resection versus surgical resection combined with pre- and post-operative locoregional immunotherapy-chemotherapy. A prospective randomized study. *Anticancer Res.* 1995;15:543–550.
155. Lygidakis NJ, Kosmidis P, Ziras N, et al. Combined transarterial targeting locoregional immunotherapy-chemotherapy for patients with unresectable hepatocellular carcinoma: a new alternative for an old problem. *J Interferon Cytokine Res.* 1995;15:467–472.
156. Kawata A, Une Y, Hosokawa M, et al. Adjuvant chemoimmunotherapy for hepatocellular carcinoma patients. Adriamycin, interleukin-2, and lymphokine-activated killer cells versus adriamycin alone. *Am J Clin Oncol.* 1995;18:257–262.
157. Kountouras J, Boura P, Karolides A, et al. Recombinant a2 interferon (a-IFN) with chemohormonal therapy in patients with hepatocellular carcinoma (HCC). *Hepatogastroenterology.* 1995;42:31–36.
158. Bokemeyer C, Kynast B, Harstrick A, et al. No synergistic activity of epirubicin and interferon-alpha 2b in the treatment of hepatocellular carcinoma. *Cancer Chemother Pharmacol.* 1995;35:334–338.
159. Stuart K, Tessitore J, Huberman M. 5-Fluorouracil and alpha-interferon in hepatocellular carcinoma. *Am J Clin Oncol.* 1996;19:136–139.
160. Haruta I, Yamauchi K, Aruga A, et al. Analytical study of the clinical response to two distinct adoptive immunotherapies for advanced hepatocellular

carcinoma: comparison between LAK cell and CTL therapy. *J Immunother Emphasis Tumor Immunol* 1996;19:218–223.
161. Ji SK, Park NH, Choi HM, et al. Combined cisplatinum and alpha interferon therapy of advanced hepatocellular carcinoma. *Korean J Intern Med.* 1996;11:58–68.
162. Wang Y, Chen H, Wu M, et al. Postoperative immunotherapy for patients with hepatocarcinoma using tumor-infiltrating lymphocytes. *Chin Med J (Engl).* 1997;110:114–117.
163. Stefanini GF, Foschi FG, Castelli E, et al. Alpha-1-thymosin and transcatheter arterial chemoembolization in hepatocellular carcinoma patients: a preliminary experience. *Hepatogastroenterology.* 1998;45:209–215.
164. Llovet JM, Sala M, Castells L, et al. Randomized controlled trial of interferon treatment for advanced hepatocellular carcinoma. *Hepatology.* 2000;31:54–58.
165. Ikeda K, Arase Y, Saitoh S, et al. Interferon beta prevents recurrence of hepatocellular carcinoma after complete resection or ablation of the primary tumor-A prospective randomized study of hepatitis C virus-related liver cancer. *Hepatology.* 2000;32:228–232.
166. Kubo S, Nishiguchi S, Hirohashi K, et al. Effects of long-term postoperative interferon-alpha therapy on intrahepatic recurrence after resection of hepatitis C virus-related hepatocellular carcinoma. A randomized, controlled trial. *Ann Intern Med.* 2001;134:963–967.
167. Reinisch W, Holub M, Katz A, et al. Prospective pilot study of recombinant granulocyte-macrophage colony-stimulating factor and interferon-gamma in patients with inoperable hepatocellular carcinoma. *J Immunother.* 2002;25:489–499.
168. Ladhams A, Schmidt C, Sing G, et al. Treatment of non-resectable hepatocellular carcinoma with autologous tumor-pulsed dendritic cells. *J Gastroenterol Hepatol.* 2002;17:889–896.
169. Sakon M, Nagano H, Dono K, et al. Combined intraarterial 5-fluorouracil and subcutaneous interferon-alpha therapy for advanced hepatocellular carcinoma with tumor thrombi in the major portal branches. *Cancer.* 2002;94:435–442.
170. Patt YZ, Hassan MM, Lozano RD, et al. Phase II trial of systemic continuous fluorouracil and subcutaneous recombinant interferon Alfa-2b for treatment of hepatocellular carcinoma. *J Clin Oncol.* 2003;21:421–427.
171. Stift A, Friedl J, Dubsky P, et al. Dendritic cell-based vaccination in solid cancer. *J Clin Oncol.* 2003;21:135–142.
172. Feun LG, O'Brien C, Molina E, et al. Recombinant leukocyte interferon, doxorubicin, and 5FUDR in patients with hepatocellular carcinoma-A phase II trial. *J Cancer Res Clin Oncol.* 2003;129:17–20.
173. Komorizono Y, Kohara K, Oketani M, et al. Systemic combined chemotherapy with low dose of 5-fluorouracil, cisplatin, and interferon-alpha for advanced hepatocellular carcinoma: a pilot study. *Dig Dis Sci.* 2003;48:877–881.
174. Shiratori Y, Shiina S, Teratani T, et al. Interferon therapy after tumor ablation improves prognosis in patients with hepatocellular carcinoma associated with hepatitis C virus. *Ann Intern Med.* 2003;138:299–306.
175. Shi M, Zhang B, Tang ZR, et al. Autologous cytokine-induced killer cell therapy in clinical trial phase I is safe in patients with primary hepatocellular carcinoma. *World J Gastroenterol.* 2004;10:1146–1151.
176. Sangro B, Mazzolini G, Ruiz J, et al. Phase I trial of intratumoral injection of an adenovirus encoding interleukin-12 for advanced digestive tumors. *J Clin Oncol.* 2004;22:1389–1397.
177. Yin XY, Lu MD, Liang LJ, et al. Systemic chemo-immunotherapy for advanced-stage hepatocellular carcinoma. *World J Gastroenterol.* 2005;11:2526–2529.
178. Mazzolini G, Alfaro C, Sangro B, et al. Intratumoral injection of dendritic cells engineered to secrete interleukin-12 by recombinant adenovirus in patients with metastatic gastrointestinal carcinomas. *J Clin Oncol.* 2005;23:999–1010.
179. Nakamoto Y, Mizukoshi E, Tsuji H, et al. Combined therapy of transcatheter hepatic arterial embolization with intratumoral dendritic cell infusion for hepatocellular carcinoma: clinical safety. *Clin Exp Immunol.* 2007;147:296–305.
180. Vitale FV, Romeo P, Vasta F, et al. Hepatic intra-arterial interferon alpha 2b-based immunotherapy combined with 5-fluorouracil (5-FU)-based systemic chemotherapy for patients with hepatocellular carcinoma (HCC) not responsive and/or not eligible for conventional treatments: a pilot study. *Anticancer Res.* 2007;27:4077–4081.
181. Weng DS, Zhou J, Zhou QM, et al. Minimally invasive treatment combined with cytokine-induced killer cells therapy lower the short-term recurrence

rates of hepatocellular carcinomas. *J Immunother.* 2008;31:63–71.

182. Hui D, Qiang L, Jian W, et al. A randomized, controlled trial of postoperative adjuvant cytokine-induced killer cells immunotherapy after radical resection of hepatocellular carcinoma. *Dig Liver Dis.* 2009;41:36–41.

183. Palmer DH, Midgley RS, Mirza N, et al. A phase II study of adoptive immunotherapy using dendritic cells pulsed with tumor lysate in patients with hepatocellular carcinoma. *Hepatology.* 2009;49:124–132.

184. Olioso P, Giancola R, Di Riti M, et al. Immunotherapy with cytokine induced killer cells in solid and hematopoietic tumours: a pilot clinical trial. *Hematol Oncol.* 2009;27:130–139.

185. Hao MZ, Lin HL, Chen Q, et al. Efficacy of transcatheter arterial chemoembolization combined with cytokine-induced killer cell therapy on hepatocellular carcinoma: a comparative study. *Chin J Cancer.* 2010;29:172–177.

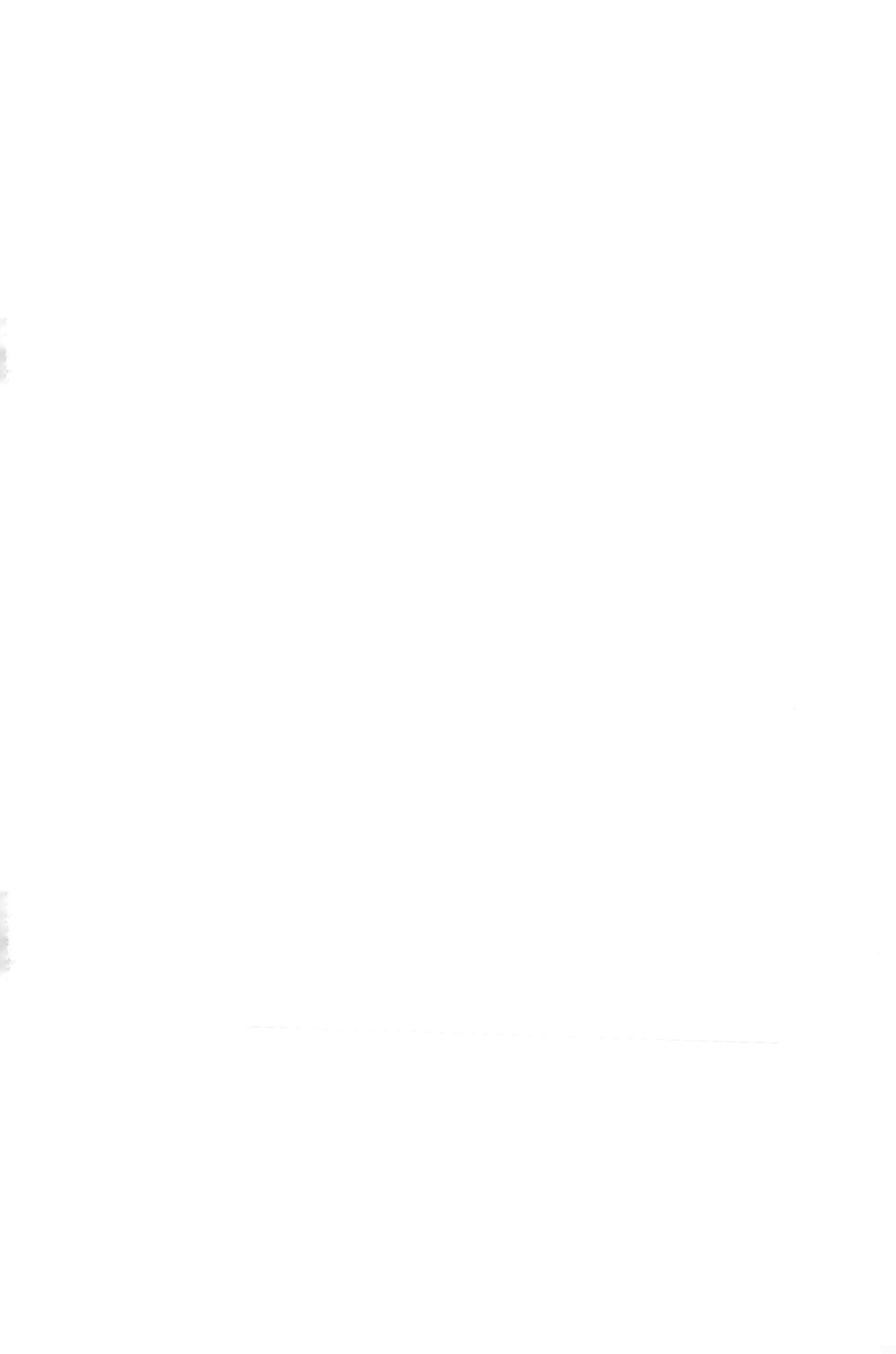

SECTION VII

Complementary Therapies and Supportive Care

Gary E. Deng

CHAPTER 23

Integrative Oncology: Complementary Therapies in Cancer Care

Gary E. Deng & Barrie Cassileth

Introduction

Integrative oncology refers to the use and study of complementary modalities that are used as adjuncts to mainstream medicine to control symptoms associated with cancer and cancer treatment. Unfortunately, the term was paired with "alternative medicine" to form the acronym CAM (for Complementary and Alternative Medicine), thus blurring critical distinctions between the two.

"Alternative medicine" refers to the use of unproven methods, most of which lack data to support purported benefits and safety. These alternatives are often promoted for use instead of mainstream cancer care as viable cancer treatments, but they are typically fraudulent, deliver misleading pseudoscientific information with a heavy commercial bias,[1] endorse unproven, potentially harmful therapies,[2] and discourage conventional therapies such as surgery, chemotherapy, and radiotherapy, which are referred to as "cutting, poisoning, and burning." Many so-called "alternative" cancer treatments are especially harmful to patients with cancer who postpone needed and proper treatment, thus diminishing the possibility of remission and cure.[3]

"Complementary therapies," conversely, are rational, evidence-based techniques that alleviate physical and emotional symptoms, improve quality of life (QoL), and may improve adherence to oncology treatment regimens. "Integrative medicine" and "integrative oncology" are now widely accepted as the appropriate terms that describe the adjunctive role played by complementary therapies as part of multidisciplinary mainstream cancer care.[4,5]

The application and insistence of rigorous evidence within the field of integrative oncology is well established with the 2009 Society for Integrative Oncology Practice Guidelines, which are the only comprehensive evidence-based recommendations for incorporating complementary therapies into conventional clinical oncology practice.[6] As complementary therapies are proven to be safe and effective, they are subsequently integrated in a supporting role to standard of care.

Recommended complementary therapies include massage and other touch modalities, acupuncture, nutritional guidance, and mind–body approaches such as meditation, yoga, music therapy, and fitness. Multiple fitness programs are available for patients at all levels of clinical status and include gentle or chair aerobics, qigong, tai chi, strength and balance training, and more. These are safe, evidence-based approaches that optimally should be provided by licensed practitioners who are also trained to work with patients with cancer.[7] These adjunctive therapies are pleasant and noninvasive, offering patients the opportunity to select therapies that appeal to them, thus enabling them to play a role in their own care and providing a means of control over what patients often feel to be an uncontrollable disease.

This chapter presents the issues associated with usage prevalence of complementary and alternative therapies among patients with cancer, along with recommendations on how to navigate the conversation with patients, and subsequently focuses on those complementary therapies that are safe, effective, and appropriate in the practice of integrative oncology.

Complementary and Alternative Therapies: Usage Prevalence and Patient Considerations

CAM is widely used by the American public and complementary modalities that are offered at many hospitals. A 2010 US survey indicates that such services are driven both by consumer interest and evolving attitudes. Among 714 survey respondents, patient demand (85%) and clinical effectiveness (70%) were the leading reasons that hospitals offer complementary therapies, whereas insurance coverage (4%) was the last consideration.[8]

In the 2007 National Health Interview Survey, overall prevalence of CAM usage was estimated at 4 in 10 adults (38.3%; 83 million) and 1 in 9 children (11.8%; 8.5 million under age 18 years).[9,10] In patients with cancer, the usage prevalence varies from 10% to >60%, depending on the definitions of CAM which were applied.[11-20] When stratified by cancer diagnoses, prevalence of use was the highest in patients with lung cancer (53%) according to a nationwide survey in Japan.[21] A European survey reports greater complementary therapy use among those diagnosed with pancreatic, liver, bone/spinal, and brain cancers.[22] A more recent survey found that up to 40% of patients with cancer in the United States use complementary modalities during the survivorship period following acute cancer therapies.[23]

In all surveys, patients who seek these modalities tend to be younger, more educated, and more affluent, representing a health-conscious segment of the population that is more proactive in finding health information, takes initiative in their health care, and can afford to pay for typically uncovered services.

Patients may also seek out these therapies because of a poor prognosis even if receiving standard of care, a fear of adverse effects from conventional treatment, a lack of a sense of control in the complicated health care system, a cultural and social affinity to therapies of natural origin, and the belief that unfamiliar therapies may yet hold surprising benefit.[24-28] Those concerns are even more prominent in patients with hepatobiliary cancer, given the nature of their disease and the limited treatment options. A Canadian survey of 357 patients conducted from 2002 to 2005 at the outpatient clinics of three participating subspecialist hepatobiliary/surgical oncologists and general surgeons showed that 58% of all patients surveyed used herbs and supplements. It also found that the three most commonly cited reasons for using adjunctive therapies were to "boost immunity" (41%), "enhance energy" (33%), and "fight cancer" (19%). Furthermore, significantly more patients with malignant than benign disease reported such use to fight cancer (27% vs. 9%) or to not specify any reason at all (44% vs. 5%).[29]

In a sense, these attempts to do something more speak of the unmet psychological and physical needs of these patients, which, if not evaluated and addressed, will not resolve on their own. In addition, there is the risk of potential side effects or interference with concurrent conventional treatment. Complications related to hepatobiliary surgery can include bleeding, infection, and liver function impairment,[29] and the use of natural products such as herbs and dietary supplements may contribute to such complications. In the context of a hepatobiliary and surgical oncology practice, this has led some institutions to routinely provide preoperative instructions to stop using all herbs and supplements one week before any surgery.[29] In the larger context of integrative oncology, it requires careful and consistent review and management of patient participation in such therapies.

Complementary Therapies: the Physician–Patient Discussion

Healthcare professionals should communicate openly and clearly with patients about the use of complementary therapies regarding benefits, risks, and realistic expectations. Furthermore, it may be particularly useful to initiate the conversation, as studies reveal that 38% to 60% of patients with cancer take complementary medicines without informing their healthcare team,[15,16] and most patients with cancer rely on friends, family members, the media, and the Internet rather than healthcare professionals for knowledge on the subject,[21,22] potentially undermining the efficacy and safety of a mainstream regimen that a patient may undergo.

Reasons for not broaching the discussion of complementary therapies during clinical encounters are bidirectional and manifold. Patients may not think it is important, may fear being ridiculed, or may feel that healthcare professionals do not know enough about the myriad therapies available to render a trustworthy opinion. Healthcare professionals may also choose to avoid the topic, which tends to initiate a time-consuming discussion, the proverbial "opening a can of worms."[15,16] In addition, there may be an underlying lack of confidence on the part of the healthcare professional to successfully address the specifics of patients' queries to their satisfaction, due to unfamiliarity with a given therapy. Furthermore, a healthcare professional may not believe that any particular complementary therapy is of any value to the patient.

These issues underscore the important role that healthcare professionals play in soliciting information from patients about their use of adjunctive therapies and in maintaining an open and receptive demeanor when patients disclose their use. Not asking could put patients at risk from adverse interactions or prevent them from undergoing effective therapies due to erroneous advice they receive from unconventional sources.[30] Open communication will help patients make informed treatment decisions. A dismissive attitude hinders a healthcare professional's ability to deliver optimal clinical care and to meet the ethical and legal obligations to their patients.

The value or lack thereof for any given complementary therapy must be evaluated individually to determine whether it does in fact support a patient's treatment program and should be part of the integrative oncology arsenal. Although many therapies are unproven or have been disproved, some therapies have demonstrated safety and potential benefits to patients. Blanket advice such as "don't use it, it is useless" will not be very effective, because the underlying needs of the patient have not been addressed. In this case, a patient should be referred to a qualified healthcare professional trained and skilled in discussing the use of complementary therapies as an integrated part of their overall care. Today, most major cancer centers and many community hospitals have established integrative medicine programs to study and combine helpful complementary therapies with mainstream oncology care.[31] They also teach patients with cancer to avoid therapies that lack safety or efficacy data, to avoid potentially harmful therapies, and to be aware of possible supplement–drug interactions. The health professionals in these programs are valuable resources for busy oncologists who lack the time or knowledge for in-depth discussions with patients about complementary therapies.

The ever-growing number of adjunctive modalities available has precluded many healthcare professionals from being familiar with those therapies or products that interest many patients. Additionally, the likelihood that a new therapy "may go viral" on the Internet almost ensures that it will become a subsequent consideration to patients. Until recently, medical degree courses rarely included a review of common complementary therapies, and many physicians who provide cancer care may be unable to discuss these approaches in an informed, open, patient-centered fashion. An increasing number of medical schools now integrate current information on complementary modalities within the context of their standard curriculum, establishing the proper application of these therapies within the clinical setting.[32,33] An Academic Consortium for Complementary and Alternative Health Care (http://accahc.org/) was formed to create and sustain a network of national CAM educational organizations and agencies that promote mutual understanding, collaborative activities, and interdisciplinary healthcare education. For practicing healthcare professionals, educational resources including review articles, books,[31,34,35] continuing medical education courses, and reliable websites and databases are available (Table 23-1).

Patients can also be directed to these credible sites, but the best approach is direct dialog within the clinical setting and to vet any adjunctive therapies that may be contraindicated with surgery or standard of care.

TABLE 23-1: Recommended Websites for Evidence-Based Cam Resources and Legal Issues

Organization/Website	Address/URL
National Cancer Institute Office of Cancer Complementary and Alternative Medicine (OCCAM)	http://www.cancer.gov/cancertopics/pdq/cam
PubMed	http://nccam.nih.gov/research/camonpubmed/
Memorial Sloan-Kettering Cancer Center	http://www.mskcc.org/mskcc/html/44.cfm
University of Texas M. D. Anderson Cancer Center Complementary/Integrative Medicine Education Resources	http://www.mdanderson.org/CIMER
The Cochrane Review Organization Complementary Medicine Database	http://www2.cochrane.org/reviews/en/topics/22.html http://www2.cochrane.org/reviews/en/subtopics/22.html
Natural Standard	http://www.naturalstandard.com/
Natural Medicines Comprehensive Database	http://www.naturaldatabase.com/
American Botanical Council	http://www.herbalgram.org

Evidence-Based Complementary Therapies in Integrative Oncology

Massage and other touch modalities

Massage therapy involves applying pressure to muscle and connective tissue to reduce tension and pain, improve circulation, and encourage relaxation. Massage techniques most commonly used in oncology include Swedish massage, aromatherapy massage, reflexology, and acupressure. All involve manual manipulation of soft tissues of the body by the therapist. However, the methods of applying touch, degree of educational preparation, regulatory requirements, and underlying theoretical frameworks vary widely among these modalities.

Massage therapy helps relieve symptoms commonly experienced by patients with cancer. It reduces anxiety and pain[36-40] as well as fatigue and distress.[36] A randomized controlled trial (RCT) of 380 patients with advanced cancer showed that both a series of six 30-minute massage sessions and simple-touch sessions over two weeks reduced pain and improved mood. Massage was significantly superior for both immediate pain and mood, but not for sustained pain, worst pain, QoL, symptom distress, or analgesic medication use.[41]

Sometimes patients are exposed to aroma during a massage session for additional therapeutic benefit. In a large study, aromatherapy massage did not appear to confer benefit for anxiety and/or depression in the long term but was associated with clinically important benefits up to two weeks after the intervention.[42] One type of massage known as manual lymph drainage uses precise light rhythmic motions to reduce edema. Several studies have evaluated this for patients with edema of the arm following mastectomy, and today, it is generally accepted as part of physical therapy standard of care in combination with compression bandaging.

Reflexology is a unique form of bodywork in that it may be preferable for some patients who are frail, nonambulatory, or uncomfortable with body massage. It has been found to relieve anxiety and pain when administered either by trained therapist or properly tutored caregiver.[43]

Reiki, a practice from Japan, promotes the healing of physical and emotional ailments through gentle touch and may also be helpful in the postoperative and nonambulatory setting, although limited study has been conducted with respect to its effects on pain management.[44]

Massage therapy is generally safe when given by credentialed practitioners. Serious adverse events are rare and associated with exotic types of massage or untrained or inexperienced practitioners.[45,46] In work with patients with cancer, the application of deep or intense pressure should be avoided, especially near lesions or enlarged lymph nodes or other anatomic distortions such as postoperative changes or on or near medical devices to prevent dislodging the device or increasing discomfort and potential infection. Patients with bleeding tendencies should receive only gentle, light-touch massage.

Acupuncture

Acupuncture, is integral to traditional Chinese medicine (TCM) and involves the placement of needles at selected points on the body, followed by manipulation with physical forces, heat, or electrical stimuli (Figure 23-1). Acupuncture has been used traditionally for many ailments, but few such applications are supported by rigorous clinical studies, although there is an abundance of preclinical and clinical data. Recent scientific research suggests that its effects are likely mediated by the nervous system. Release of neurotransmitters and change of brain-functional magnetic resonance imaging (MRI) signals have been observed during acupuncture.[47,48]

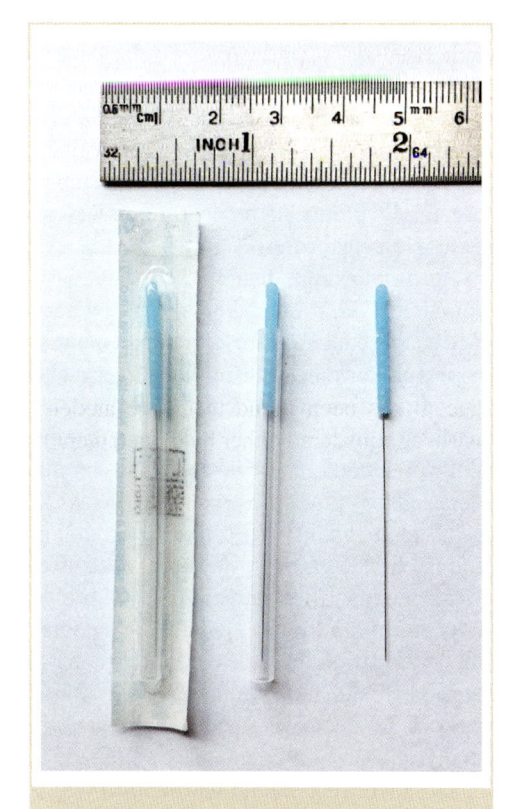

Figure 23-1: Acupuncture needles.

Clinical trial data support the use of acupuncture in treating some common symptoms experienced by patients with cancer, such as pain, nausea, and vomiting. Acupuncture has been shown to reduce many forms of pain including adult postoperative pain and osteoarthritis of the knee.[49,50] It also appears to be effective against cancer-related pain. A randomized placebo-controlled trial tested auricular (outer ear) acupuncture in 90 patients with cancer with pain despite stable medication. Pain intensity decreased by 36% at two months from baseline in the treatment group, a statistically significant difference compared with the two control groups (no acupuncture or pressure at nonacupuncture points) for whom little pain reduction was seen.[51] Skin penetration per se showed no significant analgesic effect. In this study, most of the patients had neuropathic pain, which rarely responds to conventional treatment. Acupuncture was also evaluated in a pilot study of 21 enrolled patients with breast cancer experiencing aromatase-inhibitor-induced arthralgia. The worst pain scores, pain severity, and pain-related functional interference were all significantly reduced by acupuncture treatment.[52]

Acupuncture and acupressure can help lessen chemotherapy-induced nausea and vomiting.[50,53,54] Electroacupuncture (EA, application of electrical pulses to acupuncture needles) significantly reduced the number of total emetic episodes from a median of 15 to 5 when compared with pharmacotherapy only in an RCT of 104 patients receiving myeloablative chemotherapy.[55] The combination of acupuncture and serotonin receptor antagonist antiemetics showed mixed results.[56,57]

A number of reviews continue to strongly recommend acupuncture for acute chemotherapy-induced nausea and vomiting, and positive clinical trials also support this claim.[58,59] The general consensus suggests that EA is more effective than manual acupuncture, which is more effective than acupressure (without needles).[59] For delayed chemotherapy-induced nausea and vomiting, however, more studies on EA, acupuncture, and acupressure are necessary.

Several recent papers on the benefits of acupuncture in the perioperative setting have also been published. A systematic review of 15 RCTs comparing acupuncture with sham control found that perioperative acupuncture may be a useful adjunct in the management of acute postoperative pain.[60]

A common complication after upper abdominal surgery in patients with primary liver cancer is postoperative gastroparesis syndrome. In a recent RCT at a hepatobiliary surgical hospital in China, 63 patients experiencing postoperative gastroparesis syndrome were randomized to acupuncture applied to acupoint ST 36 and other acupoints once daily, or metoclopramide (20 mg IM tid). The study suggests that acupuncture is a good treatment option for patients with postoperative gastroparesis syndrome, reporting significant differences in both gastric drainage volume ($F = 2.132$, $P < 0.05$) and cure rate (90.6% vs. 32.3% for metoclopramide, $P < 0.01$), with fewer required treatments.[61]

EA has been found to have an antipruritic effect in the animal studies,[62] but there is a lack of evidence-based clinical data in humans. This could become an area of further interest, however, as pruritus is a common symptom for patients with hepatobiliary disease[63] and can often require combined pharmacologic interventions and in some instances remain therapy resistant.[64,65]

When used for the prevention of postoperative nausea and vomiting, EA or ondansetron was more effective than placebo with a greater degree of patient satisfaction, but EA seems to be more effective in controlling nausea compared with ondansetron.[66]

Acupuncture needles are regulated as a medical device in the United States. They are filiform, sterile, single-use, and very thin (28 to 40 gauge). Insertion of acupuncture needles causes minimal or no pain and less tissue injury than phlebotomy or parenteral injection. Acupuncture performed by experienced, well-trained practitioners is safe, and serious adverse events are extremely rare. The most common minor adverse events included local bleeding and needling pain, both in <5% of patients.[67] It is prudent to use acupuncture with caution at the site of tumor or metastasis, in limbs with lymphedema, in areas with considerable anatomic distortion from surgery, and in patients with severe thrombocytopenia, coagulopathy, or neutropenia. Patients should receive treatment only from acupuncturists trained and experienced in treating patients with malignant diseases.

Nutritional Guidance and Issues Concerning Natural Products

Providing nutritional guidance to help patients improve their health and manage both weight gain and loss, as well as possible changes in appetite and taste has become increasingly important in the oncology setting. Most hospitals are staffed with certified dieticians and nutrition counselors to assess patients' current dietary habits and make appropriate recommendations.

Of particular concern, however, are natural products that are available in the United States as dietary supplements and are popular among patients with cancer.[21,22,68] These include vitamins, minerals, amino acids, herbal extracts, complex botanical formulations, and other substances of animal origin. Most users expect the supplements to help cancer treatment or reduce side effects, but such expectations are often unrealistic and unmet.[22] Furthermore, quality control and adulteration of dietary supplements are also issues, as product inconsistency and contamination have been reported.[69,70]

In general, any benefit ascribed to a therapeutic agent, such as anticancer activity, is usually supported by preclinical studies. Natural products such as botanicals are a valuable resource for the development of these therapeutic agents when they are carefully studied for safety and efficacy. About one-quarter of all prescription drugs contain active ingredients that are plant-derived, including several chemotherapeutic agents (paclitaxel, docetaxel), camptothecins (irinotecan, topotecan), and vinca alkaloids (vincristine, vinblastine, vinorelbine).

Contrastingly, the natural products available as dietary supplements have not been proven efficacious and are rarely produced at pharmaceutical grade. Some supplements cause significant side effects, such as gastrointestinal distress, hepatotoxicity, and nephrotoxicity.[71] Detrimental herb–drug interactions may occur and concurrent use of supplements such as complex botanical agents during surgery, chemotherapy, or radiation therapy can be problematic.[72–74]

Garlic has been used to treat many conditions including infections, heart disease, and circulatory disorders and may also have protective effects against stomach,[75] colorectal,[76,77] prostate,[78] hematologic,[79] and endometrial cancers.[80] However, excessive use of garlic is the identified cause in cases of prolonged bleeding time with spinal epidural hematoma and platelet dysfunction,[81] and renal hematoma after extracorporeal shock-wave lithotripsy.[82] Garlic is also known to decrease platelet aggregation and potentially elevate international normalized ratio values and, therefore, should not be used with anticoagulants or in patients with platelet dysfunction.[83]

Milk thistle, used to treat various liver ailments, may result in increased levels of medications metabolized by the cytochrome p4503A4 pathway.[84] It also modulates uridine 5′-diphospho-glucuronosyltransferase enzymes in vitro and can increase the side effects of drugs metabolized by them.[85] Sweating, nausea, vomiting, and weakness are also reported side effects. In one case, these events were accompanied by diarrhea, abdominal pain, and collapse.[86] A severe case of epistaxis was suggested to have been caused by a patient's self-medication with aspirin, garlic, and milk thistle.[87] At high dosage, silibinin, the major active constituent of the flavonolignan silymarin in milk thistle, can elevate bilirubin and liver enzymes.[88]

Many herbs such as St. John's wort interfere with cytochrome p450 enzymes. Reduced plasma levels of SN38, an active metabolite of irinotecan, have been reported following simultaneous use.[89] Such metabolic interactions preclude St. John's wort for patients on medications metabolized by cytochrome p4503A4.[90] Other supplements such as vitamin E, fish oil, gingko biloba, feverfew, and ginger may have adverse effects in perioperative use such as increased bleeding tendency.

In the demographic of hepatobiliary and surgical patients, supplement use is particularly concerning. The survey conducted by Schieman et al. found that 56 patients reported using one or more herbs or supplements perioperatively and that 27 reported using specific herbal ingredients, 10 of which have known associations with excessive bleeding and or hepatotoxicity.[29]

Although many herbs have documented benefits, caution is warranted in the surgical oncology setting. These issues should be discussed with patients to discourage self-treatment with natural products while reviewing their use of dietary supplements. Patients interested in taking natural products which show a health benefit in preliminary studies should do so under close medical monitoring and after a thorough evaluation of the risks. Presurgical screening should revisit this discussion.

Natural products under investigation

Research on specific natural products that merit further study is ongoing at most oncology research facilities, and there are many considerations regarding which substances should actually be studied in clinical trials.[91]

There has been recent interest in *sho-saiko-to*, a Chinese herbal medicine used in Asia for many years to treat liver disease, as it may slow the growth of tumor cells and stimulate the immune system. A phase II study found that sho-saiko-to improves liver pathology caused by chronic hepatitis C in patients who are not candidates for interferon-based therapy.[92]

Mind–Body Modalities

The mind–body connection is an important aspect of cancer care. The Institute of Medicine (IOM) issued a report "Cancer Care for the Whole Patient" in 2007, which stated that "cancer care today often provides state-of-the-science biomedical treatment, but fails to address the psychological and social (psychosocial) problems associated with the illness. These problems—including anxiety, depression, or other emotional problems—cause additional suffering, weaken adherence to prescribed treatments, and threaten patients' return to health."[93] Extensive research has documented that mind–body interventions address many of the issues mentioned in the Institute of Medicine report.

The role of the mind, emotions, and behaviors in health and well-being is central to many traditional medicine systems. Some techniques in mind–body modalities, including meditation, yoga, hypnosis, relaxation techniques, cognitive-behavioral therapy, biofeedback, and guided imagery, are quickly becoming part of mainstream care. A meta-analysis of 116 studies found that mind–body therapies reduced anxiety, depression, and mood disturbance in patients with cancer and assisted them in their coping skills.[94] These types of therapy can transform the meaning of cancer and lessen the stress of having a cancer diagnosis. They reduce both psychological vulnerability to stress and associated physiological consequences. Each time a patient feels the benefit of a technique they are using, they reinforce a sense of control over their own lives and counter feelings of hopelessness and helplessness.[95] Mind–body techniques must be practiced regularly to produce beneficial effects, so estimation of compliance needs to be a component when evaluating their use.[96]

Meditation is derived from the Latin word *meditari*, which means "to think, contemplate, devise, ponder." The practice trains attention and awareness in order to bring mental processes under greater voluntary control. There are two general types of meditation. Concentrative meditation focuses attention on increasing mental awareness and clearing the mind. Mindfulness meditation opens attention to whatever goes through the mind and to the flow of sensations experienced from moment to moment. The most extensively studied form of meditation in oncology is a multicomponent program called mindfulness-based stress reduction that includes mindfulness meditation, yoga stretching, and group dynamics.[97,98] In a randomized wait-list control study of 109 patients with cancer, participation in a seven-week mindfulness-based stress reduction program was associated with significant improvement in mood disturbance and stress symptoms.[99] Importantly, the effect was maintained six months after the program ended.[100] mindfulness-based stress reduction has been associated with improved mood, aspects of QoL, and decreased cortisol levels, as well as a decrease in inflammatory cytokines (IFN-γ, TNF, and IL-4), and these improvements continued for 6 to 12 months after the training.[101–103] The limitation of this research is that most of the studies were single-arm trials.[96,97,104,105] More recent research suggests that mindfulness-based stress reduction can be a useful clinical intervention in patients who have received transplants or have failed back surgery syndrome.[106,107]

Yoga, a physical, mental, and spiritual practice originating in ancient India, combines components of physical movement, breath control, and meditation. In clinical research, yoga was found to reduce hot flashes, joint pain, fatigue, sleep disturbance, and related symptoms in postmenopausal breast cancer survivors.[108] Practicing a form of Tibetan yoga that incorporates controlled breathing and visualization significantly decreased sleep disturbance in lymphoma patients.[109] A yoga intervention based on Hatha Yoga techniques improved overall QoL, social and emotional well-being, and spirituality in women treated for breast cancer,[110] and an RCT comparing the effects of a yoga program with supportive therapy and exercise rehabilitation on postoperative outcomes and wound healing suggest possible benefits.[111] The limitation of yoga research is that most studies were conducted with a "wait-list" control group in which patients did not receive interventions other than usual care.

Hypnosis is an artificially induced state of consciousness in which a person is made highly receptive to suggestions. A trancelike state similar to deep daydreaming can be achieved by first inducing relaxation and then directing attention to specific thoughts or objects. For best results, the patient and therapist must have good rapport with a strong level of trust; the environment must be comfortable and free from distractions; and the patient must be willing to undergo the process and wish to be hypnotized.

Research shows that hypnosis is beneficial in reducing pain and anxiety,[112–115] as well as anticipatory and postoperative nausea and vomiting.[113,116,117] Hypnosis was also found to reduce presurgical distress in 90 patients who underwent biopsy with significantly reduced scores for emotional upset, depressed mood, and anxiety, along with increased level of relaxation before surgery.[118] Some oncology centers provide hypnotherapy services and instructional CDs to help patients prepare for surgery using self-hypnosis techniques. A small percentage of patients may experience dizziness, nausea, or headache, symptoms that usually result from being brought out of a trance by an inexperienced hypnotherapist.

Relaxation techniques can significantly ameliorate anxiety and distress. An NIH consensus panel concluded that behavioral techniques, particularly relaxation and biofeedback, produce improvements in some aspects of sleep, but improvement in sleep onset and time did not achieve clinical significance.[115] It compares favorably with alprazolam in decreasing anxiety and depression, although the effect of alprazolam was slightly quicker for anxiety and stronger for depressive symptoms.[119] Generally, brief use of relaxation techniques has only short-term effects, whereas ongoing practice throughout and beyond the course of conventional treatment is likely to produce more lasting benefits.[120–122]

Music therapy includes listening to music, actively creating music with instruments, talking about music, and lyric writing, among others. Music can produce profound psychological, physiological, and social effects in people. The use of music in the oncology setting has become more common in recent years. Reviews of music therapy literature reveal extensive descriptive research, but a limited number of RCTs.[123–126] Several quantitative studies have established the impact of music on pain reduction, anxiety, and nausea. Music therapy has also been successful in mitigating mood and side effects of treatment, and RCTs support similar findings. Evidence shows that listening to specially selected music reduces anxiety.[127,128] Music therapy can be particularly helpful in palliative care. In terminally ill patients, music therapy reduced anxiety as well as pain, tiredness, and drowsiness.[129] QoL increased as a result of music therapy sessions, whereas life quality decreased in the control group.[130] Patients undergoing radiation experienced less anxiety and treatment-related distress than controls.[131] Limitations to research of music therapy include small samples and nonrandomized designs. Many interventions also had the participants listen to music from a predetermined selection. It is not clear, therefore, what role, if any, a music therapist played in the process.

Fitness

Exercise regimens such as *gentle or chair aerobics, qigong, tai chi*, or *strength and balance training* can help patients with cancer recover from treatment and improve their functional status. Most research has focused on supportive care endpoints in breast cancer survivors, such as QoL, physical functioning, emotional well-being, and fatigue, and included health-related endpoints such as cardiovascular fitness, muscular strength, body composition, and objective physical functioning. McNeely et al. conducted a systematic review and meta-analysis of 14 RCTs involving exercise interventions in 717 breast cancer survivors 35 to 72 years of age.[132] Pooled data from these trials showed significant positive effects of exercise on QoL, cardiorespiratory fitness, and cardiovascular fitness. The pooled data also demonstrated a statistically significant impact on fatigue reduction, but only during the survivorship phase.

Large epidemiologic studies have suggested an association between post-diagnosis physical activity levels and survival in patients with cancer. In the Nurses Health Study, women with regular exercise enjoyed a 50% lower risk of breast cancer-specific mortality compared with women reporting less than an hour of walking per week. Similar risk reductions were observed for breast cancer recurrence and all-cause mortality.[133] These observations were supported by subsequent research.[134–136]

Tai Chi, also spelled "Tai-ji," is a form of physical exercise originating from martial arts. It emphasizes fluid movement, situation awareness, and flexibility. It appears to lead to favorable changes in biomarkers for bone formation in breast cancer survivors when compared with standard exercise control.[137] Tai chi was also found to be associated with increased aerobic capacity, muscular strength and flexibility, and improved health-related QoL and self-esteem in women with breast cancer when compared with a psychosocial support therapy control group.[138,139]

Summary

Patients with cancer are very much interested in exploring therapies that have not been part of conventional mainstream medicine. Hospitals and other research institutions recognize the added value that complementary therapies can bring by supporting standard of care, and the critical role that evidence-based research plays in selecting proper therapies for inclusion. In the context of surgical oncology, this can present specific and critical issues with respect to the optimal delivery of needed mainstream treatment. Recommended and noninvasive therapies with favorable benefit–risk profiles specific to integrative cancer care can help navigate the terrain with patients interested in pursuing supportive modalities. At the same time, educating the patient to the dangers of self-treatment using natural products and close monitoring by healthcare professionals of the self-treatment activities of patients receiving mainstream therapy can ensure optimal integrity in overall disease management. This dual approach to complementary modalities can help alleviate the underlying psychological and physical symptoms that many patients with cancer experience, whereas supporting, as opposed to hindering, standard of care.

References

1. Schmidt K. CAM and the desperate call for cancer cures and alleviation what can websites offer cancer patients? *Complement Ther Med*. 2002;10(3):179–180.
2. Schmidt K, Ernst E. Assessing websites on complementary and alternative medicine for cancer. *Ann Oncol*. 2004;15(5):733–742.

3. Cassileth BR, Deng G. Complementary and alternative therapies for cancer. *Oncologist*. 2004;9(1):80–89.
4. Cassileth B, Deng G, Vickers A, Yeung KS. *PDQ Integrative Oncology*. Hamilton, Canada: BC Decker; 2005.
5. Remen RN. Practicing a medicine of the whole person: an opportunity for healing. *Hematol Oncol Clin North Am*. 2008;22(4):767–773.
6. Deng GE, Frenkel M, Cohen L, et al. Evidence-based clinical practice guidelines for integrative oncology: complementary therapies and botanicals. *J Soc Integr Oncol*. Summer 2009;7(3):85–120.
7. Center MS-KC. Online Workshops & Educational Programs. 2011; http:// www.mskcc.org/mskcc/html/ 97377.cfm.
8. Ananth S, Institute S. *2010 Complementary and Alternative Medicine Survey of Hospitals*. 2011. http://www.siib.org/news/2468-SIIB/version/default/part/AttachmentData/data/CAM%20Survey%20FINAL.pdf. Accessed September 21, 2011.
9. Barnes PM, Bloom B, Nahin RL. *Complementary and Alternative Medicine Use among Adults and Children: United States, 2007*. Hyattsville, MD: National Center for Health Statistics; 2008.
10. Nahin RL, Barnes PM, Stussman BJ, Bloom B. *Costs of Complementary and Alternative Medicine (CAM) and Frequency of Visits to CAM Practitioners: United States, 2007*. Hyattsville, MD: National Center for Health Statistics; 2009.
11. Adams J, Sibbritt DW, Easthope G, Young AF. The profile of women who consult alternative health practitioners in Australia. *Med J Aust*. 15, 2003;179(6):297–300.
12. Chrystal K, Allan S, Forgeson G, Isaacs R. The use of complementary/alternative medicine by cancer patients in a New Zealand regional cancer treatment centre. *N Z Med J*. 24, 2003;116(1168):U296.
13. Lee MM, Chang JS, Jacobs B, Wrensch MR. Complementary and alternative medicine use among men with prostate cancer in 4 ethnic populations. *Am J Public Health*. 2002;92(10):1606–1609.
14. Weiger WA, Smith M, Boon H, et al. Advising patients who seek complementary and alternative medical therapies for cancer. *Ann Intern Med*. 3, 2002;137(11):889–903.
15. Navo MA, Phan J, Vaughan C, et al. An assessment of the utilization of complementary and alternative medication in women with gynecologic or breast malignancies. *J Clin Oncol*. 15, 2004;22(4):671–677.
16. Richardson MA, Sanders T, Palmer JL, et al. Complementary/alternative medicine use in a comprehensive cancer center and the implications for oncology. *J Clin Oncol*. 2000;18(13):2505–2514.
17. Amin M, Glynn F, Rowley S, et al. Complementary medicine use in patients with head and neck cancer in Ireland. *Eur Arch Otorhinolaryngol*. 2010;267(8):1291–1297.
18. Davis SR, Lijovic M, Fradkin P, et al. Use of complementary and alternative therapy by women in the first 2 years after diagnosis and treatment of invasive breast cancer. *Menopause (New York, NY)*. 2010;17(5):1004–1009.
19. Habermann TM, Thompson CA, LaPlant BR, et al. Complementary and alternative medicine use among long-term lymphoma survivors: a pilot study. *Am J Hematol*. 2009;84(12):795–798.
20. Vapiwala N, Mick R, Hampshire MK, et al. Patient initiation of complementary and alternative medical therapies (CAM) following cancer diagnosis. *Cancer J*. 2006;12(6):467–474.
21. Hyodo I, Amano N, Eguchi K, et al. Nationwide survey on complementary and alternative medicine in cancer patients in Japan. *J Clin Oncol*. 20, 2005;23(12):2645–2654.
22. Molassiotis A, Fernadez-Ortega P, Pud D, et al. Use of complementary and alternative medicine in cancer patients: a European survey. *Ann Oncol*. 2005;16(4):655–663.
23. Gansler T, Kaw C, Crammer C, Smith T. A population-based study of prevalence of complementary methods use by cancer survivors: a report from the American Cancer Society's studies of cancer survivors. *Cancer*. 2008;113(5):1048–1057.
24. White MA, Verhoef MJ. Decision-making control: why men decline treatment for prostate cancer. *Integr Cancer Ther*. 2003;2(3):217–224.
25. Shumay DM, Maskarinec G, Kakai H, Gotay CC. Why some cancer patients choose complementary and alternative medicine instead of conventional treatment. *J Fam Pract*. 2001;50(12):1067.
26. Montbriand MJ. Abandoning biomedicine for alternate therapies: oncology patients' stories. *Cancer Nurs*. 1998;21(1):36–45.
27. Verhoef MJ, Balneaves LG, Boon HS, Vroegindewey A. Reasons for and characteristics associated with complementary and alternative medicine use among adult cancer patients: a systematic review. *Integr Cancer Ther*. 2005;4(4):274–286.

28. Druss BG, Rosenheck RA. Association between use of unconventional therapies and conventional medical services. *JAMA*. 18, 1999;282(7):651–656.
29. Schieman C, Rudmik LR, Dixon E, et al. Complementary and alternative medicine use among general surgery, hepatobiliary surgery and surgical oncology patients. *Can J Surg*. 2009;52(5):422–426.
30. Ernst E. Complementary medicine: its hidden risks. *Diabetes Care*. 2001;24(8):1486–1488.
31. Cohen L, Markman M, eds. *Integrative Oncology: Incorporating Complementary Medicine into Conventional Cancer Care*. Hamilton, Canada: Humana Press; 2008.
32. Lee MY, Benn R, Wimsatt L, et al. Integrating complementary and alternative medicine instruction into health professions education: organizational and instructional strategies. *Acad Med*. 2007;82(10):939–945.
33. Brokaw JJ, Tunnicliff G, Raess BU, Saxon DW. The teaching of complementary and alternative medicine in U.S. medical schools: a survey of course directors. *Acad Med*. 2002;77(9):876–881.
34. Abrams D, Weil A, eds. *Integrative Oncology*. USA: Oxford University Press; 2009.
35. Mumber MP, ed. *Integrative Oncology: Principles and Practice*. Hamilton, Canada: Informa HealthCare; 2005.
36. Ahles TA, Tope DM, Pinkson B, et al. Massage therapy for patients undergoing autologous bone marrow transplantation. *J Pain Symptom Manage*. 1999;18(3):157–163.
37. Stephenson NL, Weinrich SP, Tavakoli AS. The effects of foot reflexology on anxiety and pain in patients with breast and lung cancer. *Oncol Nurs Forum*. 2000;27(1):67–72.
38. Grealish L, Lomasney A, Whiteman B. Foot massage. A nursing intervention to modify the distressing symptoms of pain and nausea in patients hospitalized with cancer. *Cancer Nurs*. 2000;23(3):237–243.
39. Wilkinson S, Aldridge J, Salmon I, et al. An evaluation of aromatherapy massage in palliative care. *Palliat Med*. 1999;13(5):409–417.
40. Cassileth BR, Vickers AJ. Massage therapy for symptom control: outcome study at a major cancer center. *J Pain Symptom Manage*. 2004;28(3):244–249.
41. Kutner JS, Smith MC, Corbin L, et al. Massage therapy versus simple touch to improve pain and mood in patients with advanced cancer: a randomized trial. *Ann Intern Med*. 16, 2008;149(6):369–379.
42. Wilkinson SM, Love SB, Westcombe AM, et al. Effectiveness of aromatherapy massage in the management of anxiety and depression in patients with cancer: a multicenter randomized controlled trial. *J Clin Oncol*. 10, 2007;25(5):532–539.
43. Stephenson NL, Swanson M, Dalton J, et al. Partner-delivered reflexology: effects on cancer pain and anxiety. *Oncol Nurs Forum*. 2007;34(1):127–132.
44. Olson K, Hanson J, Michaud M. A phase II trial of Reiki for the management of pain in advanced cancer patients. *J Pain Symptom Manage*. 2003;26(5):990–997.
45. Ernst E. The safety of massage therapy. *Rheumatology (Oxford)*. 2003;42(9):1101–1106.
46. Cambron JA, Dexheimer J, Coe P, Swenson R. Side-effects of massage therapy: a cross-sectional study of 100 clients. *J Altern Complement Med*. 2007;13(8):793–796.
47. Han JS. Acupuncture: neuropeptide release produced by electrical stimulation of different frequencies. *Trends Neurosci*. 2003;26(1):17–22.
48. Wu MT, Hsieh JC, Xiong J, et al. Central nervous pathway for acupuncture stimulation: localization of processing with functional MR imaging of the brain-preliminary experience. *Radiology*. 1999;212(1):133–141.
49. Berman BM, Lao L, Langenberg P, et al. Effectiveness of acupuncture as adjunctive therapy in osteoarthritis of the knee: a randomized, controlled trial. *Ann Intern Med*. 2004;141(12):901–910.
50. NIH Consensus Conference. Acupuncture. *JAMA*. 1998;280(17):1518–1524.
51. Alimi D, Rubino C, Pichard-Leandri E, et al. Analgesic effect of auricular acupuncture for cancer pain: a randomized, blinded, controlled trial. *J Clin Oncol*. 2003;21(22):4120–4126.
52. Crew KD, Capodice JL, Greenlee H, et al. Pilot study of acupuncture for the treatment of joint symptoms related to adjuvant aromatase inhibitor therapy in postmenopausal breast cancer patients. *J Cancer Surviv*. 2007;1(4):283–291.
53. Ezzo JM, Richardson MA, Vickers A, et al. Acupuncture-point stimulation for chemotherapy-induced nausea or vomiting. *Cochrane Database Syst Rev*. 2006(2):CD002285.
54. Lee A, Done ML. Stimulation of the wrist acupuncture point P6 for preventing postoperative nausea and vomiting. *Cochrane Database Syst Rev*. 2004(3):CD003281.

55. Shen J, Wenger N, Glaspy J, et al. Electroacupuncture for control of myeloablative chemotherapy-induced emesis: a randomized controlled trial. *JAMA*. 2000;284(21):2755–2761.
56. Josefson A, Kreuter M. Acupuncture to reduce nausea during chemotherapy treatment of rheumatic diseases. *Rheumatology (Oxford)*. 2003;42(10):1149–1154.
57. Streitberger K, Friedrich-Rust M, Bardenheuer H, et al. Effect of acupuncture compared with placebo-acupuncture at P6 as additional antiemetic prophylaxis in high-dose chemotherapy and autologous peripheral blood stem cell transplantation: a randomized controlled single-blind trial. *Clin Cancer Res*. 2003;9(7):2538–2544.
58. Ernst E. Acupuncture: what does the most reliable evidence tell us? *J Pain Symptom Manage*. 2009;37(4):709–714.
59. Naeim A, Dy SM, Lorenz KA, et al. Evidence-based recommendations for cancer nausea and vomiting. *J Clin Oncol*. 10, 2008;26(23):3903–3910.
60. Sun Y, Gan TJ, Dubose JW, Habib AS. Acupuncture and related techniques for postoperative pain: a systematic review of randomized controlled trials. *Br J Anaesth*. 2008;101(2):151–160.
61. Sun BM, Luo M, Wu SB, et al. Acupuncture versus metoclopramide in treatment of postoperative gastroparesis syndrome in abdominal surgical patients: a randomized controlled trial. *Zhong Xi Yi Jie He Xue Bao*. 2010;8(7):641–644.
62. Han JB, Kim CW, Sun B, et al. The antipruritic effect of acupuncture on serotonin-evoked itch in rats. *Acupunct Electrother Res*. 2008;33(3–4):145–156.
63. Kremer AE, Oude Elferink RP, Beuers U. Pathophysiology and current management of pruritus in liver disease. *Clin Res Hepatol Gastroenterol*. 2011;35(2):89–97.
64. Bergasa NV. Pruritus in chronic liver disease: mechanisms and treatment. *Curr Gastroenterol Rep*. 2004;6(1):10–16.
65. Talwalkar JA, Souto E, Jorgensen RA, Lindor KD. Natural history of pruritus in primary biliary cirrhosis. *Clin Gastroenterol Hepatol*. 2003;1(4):297–302.
66. Gan TJ, Jiao KR, Zenn M, Georgiade G. A randomized controlled comparison of electro-acupoint stimulation or ondansetron versus placebo for the prevention of postoperative nausea and vomiting. *Anesth Analg*. 2004;99(4):1070–1075, table of contents.
67. Melchart D, Weidenhammer W, Streng A, et al. Prospective investigation of adverse effects of acupuncture in 97 733 patients. *Arch Intern Med*. 12, 2004;164(1):104–105.
68. Kumar NB, Hopkins K, Allen K, et al. Use of complementary/integrative nutritional therapies during cancer treatment: implications in clinical practice. *Cancer Control*. 2002;9(3):236–243.
69. Cassileth B, Lucarelli C. *Herb-drug Interactions in Oncology*. Hamilton, Canada: BC Decker; 2003.
70. Ko RJ. A U.S. perspective on the adverse reactions from traditional Chinese medicines. *J Chin Med Assoc*. 2004;67(3):109–116.
71. Kumar NB, Allen K, Bell H. Perioperative herbal supplement use in cancer patients: potential implications and recommendations for presurgical screening. *Cancer Control*. 2005;12(3):149–157.
72. Labriola D, Livingston R. Possible interactions between dietary antioxidants and chemotherapy. *Oncology (Williston Park)*. 1999;13(7):1003–1008; discussion 1008, 1011–1002.
73. Seifried HE, McDonald SS, Anderson DE, et al. The antioxidant conundrum in cancer. *Cancer Res*. 1, 2003;63(15):4295–4298.
74. Cassileth BR, Heitzer M, Wesa K. The public health impact of herbs and nutritional supplements. *Pharm Biol*. 1, 2009;47(8):761–767.
75. Fleischauer AT, Poole C, Arab L. Garlic consumption and cancer prevention: meta-analyses of colorectal and stomach cancers. *Am J Clin Nutr*. 2000;72(4):1047–1052.
76. Ngo SN, Williams DB, Cobiac L, Head RJ. Does garlic reduce risk of colorectal cancer? A systematic review. *J Nutr*. 2007;137(10):2264–2269.
77. Tanaka S, Haruma K, Yoshihara M, et al. Aged garlic extract has potential suppressive effect on colorectal adenomas in humans. *J Nutr*. 2006;136(3 suppl):821S–826S.
78. Hsing AW, Chokkalingam AP, Gao YT, et al. Allium vegetables and risk of prostate cancer: a population-based study. *J Natl Cancer Inst*. 6, 2002;94(21):1648–1651.
79. Walter RB, Brasky TM, Milano F, White E. Vitamin, mineral, and specialty supplements and risk of hematologic malignancies in the prospective VITamins and lifestyle (VITAL) study. *Cancer Epidemiol Biomarkers Prev*. 23, 2011;20(10):2298–308.
80. Galeone C, Pelucchi C, Dal Maso L, et al. Allium vegetables intake and endometrial cancer risk. *Public Health Nutr*. 2009;12(9):1576–1579.
81. Rose KD, Croissant PD, Parliament CF, Levin MB. Spontaneous spinal epidural hematoma

81. with associated platelet dysfunction from excessive garlic ingestion: a case report. *Neurosurgery.* 1990;26(5):880–882.
82. Gravas S, Tzortzis V, Rountas C, Melekos MD. Extracorporeal shock-wave lithotripsy and garlic consumption: a lesson to learn. *Urol Res.* 2010;38(1):61–63.
83. Ang-Lee MK, Moss J, Yuan CS. Herbal medicines and perioperative care. *JAMA.* 11, 2001;286(2):208–216.
84. Venkataramanan R, Ramachandran V, Komoroski BJ, et al. Milk thistle, a herbal supplement, decreases the activity of CYP3A4 and uridine diphosphoglucuronosyl transferase in human hepatocyte cultures. *Drug Metab Dispos.* 2000;28(11):1270–1273.
85. Mohamed ME, Frye RF. Effects of herbal supplements on drug glucuronidation. Review of clinical, animal, and in vitro studies. *Planta medica.* 2011;77(4):311–321.
86. An adverse reaction to the herbal medication milk thistle (Silybum marianum). Adverse drug reactions advisory committee. *Med J Aust.* 1, 1999;170(5):218–219.
87. Shakeel M, Trinidade A, McCluney N, Clive B. Complementary and alternative medicine in epistaxis: a point worth considering during the patient's history. *Eur J Emerg Med.* 2010;17(1):17–19.
88. Flaig TW, Gustafson DL, Su LJ, et al. A phase I and pharmacokinetic study of silybin phytosome in prostate cancer patients. *Invest New Drugs.* 2007;25(2):139–146.
89. Mathijssen RH, Verweij J, de Bruijn P, et al. Effects of St. John's wort on irinotecan metabolism. *J Natl Cancer Inst.* 21, 2002;94(16):1247–1249.
90. Markowitz JS, Donovan JL, DeVane CL, et al. Effect of St John's wort on drug metabolism by induction of cytochrome P450 3A4 enzyme. *JAMA.* 17, 2003;290(11):1500–1504.
91. Vickers AJ. Which botanicals or other unconventional anticancer agents should we take to clinical trial?. *J Soc Integr Oncol.* Summer 2007;5(3):125–129.
92. Deng G, Kurtz RC, Vickers A, et al. A single arm phase II study of a Far-Eastern traditional herbal formulation (sho-sai-ko-to or xiao-chai-hu-tang) in chronic hepatitis C patients. *J Ethnopharmacol.* 14, 2011;136(1):83–87.
93. Holland J, Weiss T. The new standard of quality cancer care: integrating the psychosocial aspects in routine cancer from diagnosis through survivorship. *Cancer J.* 2008;14(6):425–428.
94. Devine EC, Westlake SK. The effects of psychoeducational care provided to adults with cancer: meta-analysis of 116 studies. *Oncol Nurs Forum.* 1995;22(9):1369–1381.
95. Gordon JS. Mind-body medicine and cancer. *Hematol Oncol Clin North Am.* 2008;22(4):683–708, ix.
96. Shapiro SL, Bootzin RR, Figueredo AJ, et al. The efficacy of mindfulness-based stress reduction in the treatment of sleep disturbance in women with breast cancer: an exploratory study. *J Psychosom Res.* 2003;54(1):85–91.
97. Ott MJ, Norris RL, Bauer-Wu SM. Mindfulness meditation for oncology patients: a discussion and critical review. *Integr Cancer Ther.* 2006;5(2):98–108.
98. Smith JE, Richardson J, Hoffman C, Pilkington K. Mindfulness-Based Stress Reduction as supportive therapy in cancer care: systematic review. *J Adv Nurs.* 2005;52(3):315–327.
99. Speca M, Carlson LE, Goodey E, Angen M. A randomized, wait-list controlled clinical trial: the effect of a mindfulness meditation-based stress reduction program on mood and symptoms of stress in cancer outpatients. *Psychosom Med.* 2000;62(5):613–622.
100. Carlson LE, Ursuliak Z, Goodey E, et al. The effects of a mindfulness meditation-based stress reduction program on mood and symptoms of stress in cancer outpatients: 6-month follow-up. *Support Care Cancer.* 2001;9(2):112–123.
101. Carlson LE, Speca M, Faris P, Patel KD. One year pre-post intervention follow-up of psychological, immune, endocrine and blood pressure outcomes of mindfulness-based stress reduction (MBSR) in breast and prostate cancer outpatients. *Brain Behav Immun.* 2007;21(8):1038–1049.
102. Carlson LE, Speca M, Patel KD, Goodey E. Mindfulness-based stress reduction in relation to quality of life, mood, symptoms of stress and levels of cortisol, dehydroepiandrosterone sulfate (DHEAS) and melatonin in breast and prostate cancer outpatients. *Psychoneuroendocrinology.* 2004;29(4):448–474.
103. Witek-Janusek L, Albuquerque K, Chroniak KR, et al. Effect of mindfulness based stress reduction on immune function, quality of life and coping in women newly diagnosed with early stage breast cancer. *Brain Behav Immun.* 2008;22(6):969–981.
104. Carlson LE, Garland SN. Impact of mindfulness-based stress reduction (MBSR) on sleep, mood, stress and fatigue symptoms in cancer outpatients. *Int J Behav Med.* 2005;12(4):278–285.
105. Carlson LE, Speca M, Patel KD, Goodey E. Mindfulness-based stress reduction in relation to quality of life, mood, symptoms of stress, and immune parameters in breast and prostate cancer outpatients. *Psychosom Med.* 2003;65(4):571–581.

106. Gross CR, Kreitzer MJ, Thomas W, et al. Mindfulness-based stress reduction for solid organ transplant recipients: a randomized controlled trial. *Altern Ther Health Med*. 2010;16(5):30 38.

107. Esmer G, Blum J, Rulf J, Pier J. Mindfulness-based stress reduction for failed back surgery syndrome: a randomized controlled trial. *J Am Osteopath Assoc*. 2010;110(11):646–652.

108. Carson JW, Carson KM, Porter LS, et al. Yoga of Awareness program for menopausal symptoms in breast cancer survivors: results from a randomized trial. *Support Care Cancer*. 2009;17(10):1301–1309.

109. Cohen L, Warneke C, Fouladi RT, et al. Psychological adjustment and sleep quality in a randomized trial of the effects of a Tibetan yoga intervention in patients with lymphoma. *Cancer*. 2004;100(10):2253–2260.

110. Moadel AB, Shah C, Wylie-Rosett J, et al. Randomized controlled trial of yoga among a multiethnic sample of breast cancer patients: effects on quality of life. *J Clin Oncol*. 2007;25(28):4387–4395.

111. Rao RM, Nagendra HR, Raghuram N, et al. Influence of yoga on postoperative outcomes and wound healing in early operable breast cancer patients undergoing surgery. *Int J Yoga*. 2008;1(1):33–41.

112. Montgomery GH, Weltz CR, Seltz M, Bovbjerg DH. Brief presurgery hypnosis reduces distress and pain in excisional breast biopsy patients. *Int J Clin Exp Hypn*. 2002;50(1):17–32.

113. Faymonville ME, Mambourg PH, Joris J, et al. Psychological approaches during conscious sedation. Hypnosis versus stress reducing strategies: a prospective randomized study. *Pain*. 1997;73(3):361–367.

114. Flory N, Lang E. Practical hypnotic interventions during invasive cancer diagnosis and treatment. *Hematol Oncol Clin North Am*. 2008;22(4):709–725, ix.

115. Integration of behavioral and relaxation approaches into the treatment of chronic pain and insomnia. NIH technology assessment panel on integration of behavioral and relaxation approaches into the treatment of chronic pain and insomnia. *JAMA*. 24–31, 1996;276(4):313–318.

116. Zeltzer LK, Dolgin MJ, LeBaron S, LeBaron C. A randomized, controlled study of behavioral intervention for chemotherapy distress in children with cancer. *Pediatrics*. 1991;88(1):34–42.

117. Morrow GR, Morrell C. Behavioral treatment for the anticipatory nausea and vomiting induced by cancer chemotherapy. *N Engl J Med*. 9, 1982;307(24):1476–1480.

118. Schnur JB, Bovbjerg DH, David D, et al. Hypnosis decreases presurgical distress in excisional breast biopsy patients. *Anesth Analg*. 2008;106(2):440–444, table of contents.

119. Holland JC, Morrow GR, Schmale A, et al. A randomized clinical trial of alprazolam versus progressive muscle relaxation in cancer patients with anxiety and depressive symptoms. *J Clin Oncol*. 1991;9(6):1004–1011.

120. Krischer MM, Xu P, Meade CD, Jacobsen PB. Self-administered stress management training in patients undergoing radiotherapy. *J Clin Oncol*. 2007;25(29):4657–4662.

121. Campos de Carvalho E, Martins FT, dos Santos CB. A pilot study of a relaxation technique for management of nausea and vomiting in patients receiving cancer chemotherapy. *Cancer Nurs*. 2007;30(2):163–167.

122. Anderson KO, Cohen MZ, Mendoza TR, et al. Brief cognitive-behavioral audiotape interventions for cancer-related pain: immediate but not long-term effectiveness. *Cancer*. 2006;107(1):207–214.

123. Hanser SB. Music therapy research in adult oncology. *J Soc Integrative Oncol*. 2006;4:62–66.

124. Hilliard RE. Music therapy in pediatric oncology: a review of the literature. *J Soc Integrative Oncol*. 2006;4:75–79.

125. Hilliard RE. Music therapy in hospice and palliative care: a review of the empirical data. *Evid Based Complement Alternat Med*. 2005;2(2):173–178.

126. Rykov M, Salmon D. Bibliography for music therapy in palliative care, 1963–1997. *Am J Hosp Palliat Care*. 1998;15(3):174–180.

127. Frank JM. The effects of music therapy and guided visual imagery on chemotherapy induced nausea and vomiting. *Oncol Nurs Forum*. 1985;12(5):47–52.

128. Sabo CE, Michael SR. The influence of personal message with music on anxiety and side effects associated with chemotherapy. *Cancer Nurs*. 1996;19(4):283–289.

129. Horne-Thompson A, Grocke D. The effect of music therapy on anxiety in patients who are terminally ill. *J Palliat Med*. 11(4):582–590.

130. Hilliard RE. The effects of music therapy on the quality and length of life of people diagnosed

with terminal cancer. *J Music Ther*. Summer 2003;40(2):113–137.
131. Clark M, Isaacks-Downton G, Wells N, et al. Use of preferred music to reduce emotional distress and symptom activity during radiation therapy. *J Music Ther*. Fall 2006;43(3):247–265.
132. McNeely ML, Campbell KL, Rowe BH, et al. Effects of exercise on breast cancer patients and survivors: a systematic review and meta-analysis. *CMAJ*. 2006;175(1):34–41.
133. Holmes MD, Chen WY, Feskanich D, et al. Physical activity and survival after breast cancer diagnosis. *JAMA*. 2005;293(20):2479–2486.
134. Holick CN, Newcomb PA, Trentham-Dietz A, et al. Physical activity and survival after diagnosis of invasive breast cancer. *Cancer Epidemiol Biomarkers Prev*. 2008;17(2).379–386.
135. Meyerhardt JA, Giovannucci EL, Holmes MD, et al. Physical activity and survival after colorectal cancer diagnosis. *J Clin Oncol*. 2006;24(22):3527–3534.
136. Meyerhardt JA, Heseltine D, Niedzwiecki D, et al. Impact of physical activity on cancer recurrence and survival in patients with stage III colon cancer: findings from CALGB 89803. *J Clin Oncol*. 2006;24(22):3535–3541.
137. Peppone LJ, Mustian KM, Janelsins MC, et al. Effects of a structured weight-bearing exercise program on bone metabolism among breast cancer survivors: a feasibility trial. *Clin Breast Cancer*. 2010;10(3):224–229.
138. Mustian KM, Katula JA, Zhao H. A pilot study to assess the influence of tai chi chuan on functional capacity among breast cancer survivors. *J Support Oncol*. 2006;4(3):139–145.
139. Mustian KM, Katula JA, Gill DL, et al. Tai Chi Chuan, health-related quality of life and self-esteem: a randomized trial with breast cancer survivors. *Support Care Cancer*. 2004;12(12):871–876.

CHAPTER 24

Natural Medicine and Complementary and Alternative Therapy in Primary Liver Cancer: Scientific Research and Clinical Applications

Hao Chen & Zhiqiang Meng

The ancient literature about liver cancer mainly came from East Asia, especially in the books of Traditional Chinese Medicine (TCM).[1] For example, in a chapter entitled "Miraculous Pivot Water Expansion," the phrase "Ganmai weiji wei feiqi, zai xiexia, ru fubei" appears. This means that the *feiqi* disease in liver is induced by the accumulation of *ganqi* in the right upper abdomen: The patient has a mass in the liver, and it appears like an upside-down cup on the surface of body. Also appears the phrase "Fuliang, zai xinxia, shangxia xing, shi tuoxue," which means that the patient feels a movable bulge under the diaphragm and has symptoms of hematemesis occasionally. In a chapter entitled "Miraculous Pivot • Xieqi Zangfu Bingxing," "Xiben, zai you xiexia, fu da ru bei" means patients are short of breath, with a lump in the right upper abdomen, resembling a large cup. There was no special term for liver cancer in ancient times, but the symptoms described in the literature are similar to clinical findings in patients with liver cancer.[2]

Although having little efficacy, Sorafenib (marketed as Nexavar by Bayer) is still the only drug approved by the Food and Drug Administration for the treatment of liver cancer. Thus, there are many reports on complementary and alternative therapy for liver cancer all over the world. In China, the treatment of liver cancer is mainly focused on the prescription of herbal combinations for alleviating symptoms (such as fever, pain, poor appetite, and abdominal distension) while producing minimal side effects, maintaining quality of life, lowering levels of α-fetoprotein (AFP) in some patients, reducing tumor size, or prolonging survival. But from other countries, such as India, Japan, Korea, and Egypt, reports were mainly on the use of single natural product as complementary therapy for advanced liver cancer to improve appetite, relieve pain, and reduce chemotherapy-induced nausea. Experimental data have demonstrated that some extracts, such as ingredients from ginseng and turmeric, have some antitumor effects. These effects still need clinical validation. In addition to herbs, other complementary therapies, such as acupuncture and yoga, have shown positive effects in relieving pain in patients with advanced liver cancer.

Treatments with Single Herbs or Extracts from a Single Herb

Cinobufotalin (Huachansu) extracted from dried toad venom taken from the skin glands of *Bufo gargarizans* or *Bufo melanostictus* is a widely used drug for treatment of liver cancer in China. Many studies confirm its antitumor effect in liver cancer.[3–7] The results of phase I clinical trials for Cinobufotalin carried out in China showed that 6 of 15 patients with advanced cancer (11 with primary liver cancer) were stable after treatment, with a reduction of tumor size in one patient by 20%. The median survival time was 7.6 months, quality of life was improved, and there was no dose-related toxicity. A phase II clinical trial is currently under way.[8]

Kanglaite (KLT Injection) is a drug extracted from the natural herb Semen Coicis. A multicenter study investigating the therapeutic effect of KLT in primary liver cancer showed an effective rate of 11.42%, which is not significantly different than that of chemotherapy (cisplatin + 5-fluorouracil + adriamycin plan) which has an effective rate of 9.8%. KLT can attenuate symptoms and improve quality of life and immune function in patients without bone marrow suppression and damage to the liver or kidney function. The only side effects were mild nausea or fever, which resolved without further intervention after discontinuation of the drug.[9] A randomized phase III trial investigating the effect of KLT combined with interventional therapy included 198 patients with primary liver cancer. The efficacy rate complete response (CR) and partial response (PR) of a combination of KLT and transcatheter arterial chemoembolization (TACE) was 69.23% (90 of 130 patients), compared with only 38.23% (36 of 68 patients) in the group treated with TACE alone. In the group with combined treatment of KLT and TACE, symptom relief, quality of life score, weight ratings, and improvement of immune function were all significantly better than the TACE alone group.[10]

Arsenic trioxide (As_2O_3) is an antitumor drug extracted from arsenicum sublimatum, a traditional Chinese medicine. It has been used in the treatment of acute promyelocytic leukemia via its induction of apoptosis in tumor cells. It has also shown an antitumor effect in liver cancer. In a phase I clinical trial, 28 patients with primary liver cancer were treated with AS_2O_3. Among them, 3 had PR, 21 had SD, and 4 had PD. The improvement rate was 10.7%.[11]

Cannabis sativa is often used as adjunctive therapy for the treatment of advanced liver cancer in both ancient and modern times. *Cannabis* is widespread throughout the world, including Kyrgyzstan, Afghanistan, parts of China, Hungary, Poland, Bulgaria, India, and Nepal. Historically the use of cannabis is best known in ancient India. Cannabis is called *ganjika* in Sanskrit and *ganja* in modern Hindi. It can increase appetite, relieve pain, and attenuate side effects such as nausea and other symptoms after chemotherapy.[12]

Panax ginseng belongs to the Araliaceae family of flowering plants and mainly grows in East Asia, especially in cold climates. It has been used to promote longevity and prevent cancer for thousands of years in the Orient. It is widely distributed and used in China, Russia, Japan, South Korea, and North America. A study from Korea has confirmed that *Radix ginseng rubra* had a positive effect in the prevention of liver cancer.

A survey conducted in 1987 in the Seoul National Cancer Hospital of Korea suggested that appropriate use of ginseng may prevent cancer. The Odds ratios (ORs) for liver cancer was 0.48 in people taking ginseng.[13–15] Subsequently, a prospective cohort study of 4634 people conducted in Korea since 1987 found that the occurrence rate of tumors in people taking ginseng was significantly lower than those who did not (relative risk: 0.31; 95% confidence interval [CI]: 0.13–0.74).[16,17] Mechanistic studies in an animal model of liver cancer support the anticancer effect of ginseng.[18]

Viscum album, also known as European mistletoe, is a widely used anticancer drug in Egypt and has been proven to have clinical effects in a variety of tumors. Mabed et al. conducted a phase II clinical trial in Egypt for the effect of viscum fraxini-2, a sprig extract of *Viscum album*, combined with systemic chemotherapy in the treatment of advanced liver cancer. The results showed that 3 of 23 patients who participated achieved a complete response, 2 had partial responses, and 9 had progressive disease. The median overall survival was five months, and median progression-free survival was two months.

No significant hematologic toxicity was observed in this study; 34.8% patients had 3°–4° drug-related fever, 13.1% had erythema at the injection site, 17.4% experienced local pain at the injection site, and no drug-related deaths occured.[19] A meta-analysis summarizing 23 studies showed that *Viscum album* could significantly improve the survival time of patients, suppress the tumor growth, and improve quality of life.[20] *Viscum album* has continued to be used in Egypt and many other places.

Cirsium has been used for many centuries as a liver protectant. The earliest record could be found in classic Greek and Roman literature from the first-century AD. The extract from Cirsium or *Silybum marianum*, commonly known as milk thistle is a very commonly used hepatoprotective medicine. In addition to its hepatoprotective effect shown in clinical trials, Cirsium also appears to have activity against liver cancer in laboratory studies, as summarized in this chapter.[21]

Treatment with Combination Natural Medicine

In China, natural medicines used in liver cancer treatment are mainly in the form of compound formulations. Many clinical studies showed that natural medicine when combined with modern treatments especially TACE could improve the efficacy, reduce the side effects of treatment, improve quality of life, and increase the long-term survival rate.

Liver cancer is not sensitive to radiation therapy, but one study has shown that whole liver moving split fields radiotherapy combined with a TCM formulation (*Astragalus*, Radix codonopsis, *Wolfiporia cocos*, Fructus Akebiae, etc.) could increase the efficiency of radiotherapy in the treatment of large hepatocellular carcinoma. In one study of 157 patients who completed more than four courses of radiotherapy, it was demonstrated that those treated with combination of radiotherapy and TCM had a five-year survival rate of 42.97% ± 11.98% and median survival of 53.4 months. Those treated with radiotherapy alone had a survival rate of 14.48% ± 7.19% and median survival of 11.1 months.[22]

The *PingXiao capsule* (*Curcuma aromatica* Salisb, Fructus Aurantii, Faeces Trogopterori, aluminum potassium sulfate dodecahydrate, Semen Strychni, etc.) has also been studied in combination with TACE for the treatment of liver cancer. Compared with the control group, the tumor size in the combined treatment group was markedly reduced ($P < 0.05$). The median survival of the combined group was 24.50 ± 17.08 months, whereas it was 12.18 ± 9.71 months in the control group ($P < 0.01$). The average time of continuous decline in AFP level in the combined group was 11.2 ± 5.5 months, longer than that of control group (5.3 ± 3.8 months). These data suggested that taking the PingXiao capsule during TACE could improve the long-term therapeutic effect for patients.[23]

Combined with TACE, *Qianggan pills* (Ingredients: *Astragalus*, Radix Codonopsis, *Salvia miltiorrhiza*, *Angelica sinensis*, White Peony Root, Radix Rehmanniae, *Curcuma aromatica* Salisb, *Polygonatum sibiricum*) also showed positive effects in a study of 80 patients with liver cancer. One group of patients who had undergone repeated TACE administrations (more than three times) was compared with another group of patients who took the Qianggan pills and received TACE one time. The group treated with the combined therapy had better liver function and longer survival rate ($P < 0.01$). One-, two-, and three-year survival rates of the group receiving repeated TACE were lower than the single-TACE plus TCM group (confirmed by follow-up). Three-year survival rates of the two groups were as follows: 19.23% in repeated-TACE group and 26.25% in single-TACE plus TCM. The difference in survival rates was significant ($P < 0.05$). These results confirmed that receiving TACE in combination with TCM could protect liver function and improve survival rates of patients with liver cancer.[24]

Ren Huaping reported that the side effects of TACE (nausea and vomiting, leukopenia, thrombocytopenia) were attenuated in patients who started taking Jianpiliqi formulation (Ingredients: Radix Codonopsis, *Wolfiporia cocos*, Rhizoma Atractylodis Macrocephalae, Pinellia Tuber, Fructus Aurantii, Fructus Amomi) one week before TACE administration, compared with the patients undergoing TACE administration without TCM ($P < 0.05$).[25] Liu Chenlin evaluated Qinggan Jidu Sanjie Tang (Ingredients: Bupleurum chinense DC, Radix Paeoniae Rubra, Carapax Trionycis, *Salvia miltiorrhiza*, *Wolfiporia cocos*) as a supplementary therapy for TACE in liver cancer. The incidence of liver dysfunction in the combination group was lower than that of the TACE alone group ($P < 0.05$). The incidence and aggravation rates of cirrhosis were 35% and 50%, respectively, in the combination group, which are significantly lower than the TACE group ($P < 0.05$).[26] Several other studies also have similar results.[27,28] This indicates that TCM could be an effective supplementary strategy for TACE in the treatment of liver cancer.

A meta-analysis of the literature, consisting of 2653 cases drawn from 37 clinical trials, compared the therapeutic effect and damage to liver function of patients who underwent TACE administration with and without TCM. The results showed that patients with advanced liver cancer received more beneficial treatment from TACE combined with TCM than from TACE alone.[29] For this meta-analysis, we searched the Cochrane Library, MEDLINE, CENTRAL, EMBASE, CBMdisc, and CNKI as well as manual searches. Meta-analysis was performed on the results of homogeneous studies. Analyses subdivided by study design were also performed.

Laboratory Studies of Natural Medicine

Natural medicines have been used in the treatment of cancer for thousands of years, but the efficacy of natural medicine is not consistent because of the variations in origin, storage, transportation, processing, and other conditions. With the increasing need for drug research and development in recent years, a strategy has emerged in which a drug is developed not from chemical synthesis but via extraction from natural medicine followed by resynthesis of extracts. Renewed efforts have been carried out to study commonly used natural medicine with antitumor properties. The research has produced encouraging results.

One study compared the inhibitory effects of Sorafenib, arsenic trioxide (As_2O_3), or the combination of these two drugs on hepatocellular carcinoma, xenograft, and angiogenesis. Results showed that tumor volume and weight were significantly reduced in all three groups when compared with the no-intervention control. Moreover, the combination of As_2O_3 and Sorafenib exerts synergistic inhibition on cancer cell growth and angiogenesis.[30]

Oxymatrine, extracted from *Sophora flavescens Alt.*, can suppress transformation of live cancer cells and reduce cytotoxicity to the cells, probably due to its inhibition of the metabolic activation of hepatotoxin. Oxymatrine can attenuate chemical liver damage, as estimated by the pathological results.[31] This review shows that for cells without oxymatrine pretreatment, cell injury was implicated as indicated by the decrease in cell viability. Ku Shen showed protective effects on cells from the dimethyl sulfoxide-induced toxicity. The results show that oxymatrine can inhibit the G(2) and M phase of H4IIE. The findings suggest that antiinflammatory constituents such as oxymatrine could mediate cell division of cancer cells and reduce cell cytotoxicity likely due to its capacity to inhibit the metabolic activation of hepatotoxin, a critical factor in the pathogenesis of chemical-induced liver injury.

Cinnamomum cassia, commonly known as Chinese cinnamon, is a traditional flavor or spice used as a natural medicine in ancient times. Gamal-Eldeen et al. recently found five new compounds in *Cinnamomum cassia*: 7-acetonyl-5-hydroxy-2-methylchromone, 7-(propan-2'-ol-l'-yl)-5-hydroxy-2-methylchromone, 5-methyl-3-(propan-2'-on-1'-yl) benzoic acid, 5-(methoxymethyl)-3-(propan-2'-ol-1'-yl) benzoic acid, and glyceryl-1-tetracosanoate.

Among these five compounds, glyceryl-1-tetracosanoate showed high levels of activity in suppressing liver cancer, inducing proliferation of T cells and macrophages, and acting as an antiinflammatory agent.[32]

Abdel-Hameed et al. found three components in the extracts of Tribulus plants: (22S, 25S)-16β,22, 26-trihydroxy-cholest-4-en-3-one-16-*O*-β-D-glucopyranosyl-(1→3)-β-D-xylopyranoside, (22S,25S)-16β,22,26-trihydroxy-cholest-4-en-3-one-16-*O*-β-D-glucopyranosyl-(1→3)-β-D-glucopyranoside, and 3β-hydroxy-5a-pregn-16(17)en-20-one-3-*O*-β-D-xylopyranosyl-(1→2)-[β-D-xylopyranosyl-(1→3)]-β-D-glucopyranosyl-(1→4)-[α-L-rhamnopyranosyl-(1→2)]-β-D-galactopyranoside.

The IC50 of these three components in HepG2 cell line were 2.4, 2.2, and 1.1 mg/mL. They showed the high potential of these three components in suppressing liver cancer in vitro. So the author suggested that these components merited further investigation.[33]

In 2006, Marzouk et al. detected the antitumor activity of a variety of new compounds that they found in *Tecoma stans* (*yellow trumpetbush*).[34]

By using the 1,1-diphenyl-2-picrylhydrazyl (DPPH) assay, they found that 4-OE-caffeoyl-α-L-rhamno-pyranosyl-(1'→ 3)-α/β E/Z-acetoside had strong antioxidant activity, and cytotoxic and growth suppressive activity against the HepG2 cell line.[34]

In 2002, Lin et al. found that *Coptis groenlandica Salisb* (*Ranunculaceae*) had a strong antitumor effect on five cell lines This discovery was made by comparing the cytotoxicity of 15 herbs commonly used in Canada for liver cancer on 5 hepatoma cell lines in vitro: HepG2/C3A, SK-HEP-1, HA22T/VGH, Hep3B, and PLC/PRF/5.[35]

Zingiber officinale, commonly known as ginger, is widely used as both food and drug throughout the world. Its antitumor effect has been confirmed in in vitro experiments. Vijaya Padma from India reported that the IC_{50} of *Zingiber officinale* on the HepG2 cell line was 900 μg/mL. When the dose reached 250 μg/mL, the cancer cells would undergo morphological changes, including cell shrinkage and nuclear deformation. Using the gas chromatograph/mass spectrometer (GC-MS) screening, they confirmed that the active constituents in the extract were clavatol, geraniol, and pinostrobin. This study also demonstrated ginger's potential as an anticancer agent.[36]

The rhizome *Curcuma longa*, commonly known as *turmeric*, is a spice from India often used in the treatment of cancer, diabetes, heart disease, and skin diseases. Recently, it was found to contain methyl and hydroxyl compounds.[37] In 2005, Adams et al. found that 2,6 bis-piperidone in *Curcuma longa* was active in antiangiogenesis and in inducing cell cycle arrest and apoptosis in cancer cells. The study also found that the activity of metabolites of the rhizome *Curcumae longae* was greater than that of the rhizome itself.[38] Ning et al. found that Rhizoma Curcumae Longae could inhibit cell growth of liver cancer cell lines HEP3B, SK-Hep-1, and SNU449 by down-regulating the notch intracellular domain pathway.[39]

Silybum marianum, commonly known as milk thistle, is an herb predominantly or commonly used for the liver and gallbladder diseases. In recent years, it has been used in the treatment of liver disease, chemotherapy-induced liver damage, and liver cancer.[40] In 2009, García-Maceira and Mateo found that *Silybum marianum* could suppress the increase of vascular endothelial growth factor induced by hypoxemia in Hep3B cell lines. This phenomenon might be attributed to the inhibitory effect of *Silybum marianum* on the PI3K/Akt pathway through LY294002. Milk thistle has a strong inhibitory effect on H1F1, thereby inhibiting tumor cells.[41]

In another study, García-Maceira and Mateo found that silibinin, a compound extracted from *Silybum marianum*, could inhibit the growth of human hepatocellular carcinoma cell lines through inhibition of Hypoxia-inducible factor-1α and the mammalian target of rapamycin/p70S6K/4E-BP1 signal transduction pathway.[41] Recently, researchers investigated the effect of silibinin on a mice model of urethane-induced liver cancer. The results showed that the incidence rate of large tumor and formation of nutritive blood vessels for the tumor in the silibinin-treated group were all lower than those of the control group.[42]

BM-ANF1 is an extract from the skin of Indian hoptoad. It can inhibit proliferation of U937, K562, and HepG2 cell lines in a dose-dependent manner. In the HepG2 cell line, BM-ANF1 can arrest the cell cycle at the G1 phase by up-regulating the expression of p53 and modulating the expression of p21 and p27, which might be the main mechanism of BM-ANF1–induced inhibition in cancer cells. Therefore, BM-ANF1 can significantly inhibit human liver cancer cells.[43]

In North America, *black cohosh*, a perennial herb, is frequently used as an alternative to hormone replacement therapy. In recent years, the liver-protective and antitumor activities of black cohosh have been discovered. To investigate the effect of one of its major constituent, actein, Einbond et al. treated Sprague-Dawley rats bearing HepG2 xenografts with 35.7 mg/kg of actein for 6 and 24 hours. The results demonstrated that the 24-hour treatment could significantly inhibit the growth of the HepG2 cell, which might be induced by inhibition of HMGCS1, HMGCR, HSD17B7, NQO1, S100A9 and up-regulation of BZRP and CYP7A1.[44]

Coptis chinensis Franch has been a commonly used herb in China for more than 2000 years. It can purge "heart fire" and protect the liver. It has been used as a new antibiotic and antiviral drug in clinical practice in recent years. *Coptis chinensis* Franch was mainly used in the treatment of chronic liver disease, liver fibrosis, cirrhosis, and liver cancer.[45] Wu et al. studied the effects of berberine (a constituent of *Coptis chinensis*) on the Hep3B cancer cell line and found that it could restrain growth of cancer cells in a dose-dependent manner.[46] The mechanism of cytotoxicity may be related to caspase3-induced apoptosis. *Coptis chinensis* Franch is the major component of Sanhuang

Xiexin Tang, which showed an inhibitory effect on the HepG2 cell line. To clarify the mechanism of the inhibition from molecular and genetic level, Cheng et al.[47] investigated the effects of roots of *Coptis* on HepG2 cells. The results showed that roots of *Coptis* could repress HepG2 cell proliferation by activating the *P53* gene.

Geranylgeranoic acid (GGA) is found in many herbs (e.g., *Rubia cordifolia, Schisandra chinensis* (Turcz.) Baill, *Epimedium brevicornum*, and *Radix glycyrrhizae*). Shidoji and Ogawa from Japan found that GGA could induce apoptosis in human hepatoma cell lines HuH-7 and PLC/PRF-5 and mouse hepatoma cell line MLE-10. They further confirmed that the GGA extract from *Schisandra* exerted effects similar to synthetic GGA after hydrogenation and methylation. It has been confirmed that GGA can be extracted from 24 natural medicines.[48]

Antrodia camphorata is a fungus widely used for the treatment of liver cancer in Taiwan. Recently, Li et al.[49] from Taiwan demonstrated that the synthetic drug acetone-chloroform extracted from *Cinnamomum* showed good activity against the human HepG2 cell line. It can down-regulate MDR-1, up-regulate PARP-1, and induce apoptosis by down-regulating COX-2 and p-AKT.

Other Complementary and Alternative Therapies

In addition to natural medicine, many other remedies of complementary medicine are used throughout the world for the prevention and treatment of liver cancer, including diet, acupuncture, and massage therapy. Many have shown effects in alleviation of symptoms or the prevention and treatment of liver cancer.

One Japanese study in 2005 demonstrated the relationship between soy and liver cancer. The authors investigated the effects of eating traditional Japanese miso soup and tofu in hepatitis B or hepatitis C carriers, patients at high risk of developing liver cancer. The study, conducted from 1964 to 1988, included 176 biopsy-proven liver cancer patients and 560 hepatitis B or hepatitis C carriers who died of diseases other than liver cancer. The authors compared the dietary habits of these patients two years before death or cancer diagnosis. The results showed the ORs of liver cancer incidence were 0.5 (95% CI: 0.29–0.95) in hepatitis B carriers and 0.5 (95% CI: 0.20–0.99) in hepatitis C carriers, in favor of patients eating traditional Japanese miso soup and tofu over the long term versus those who did not.[50] A similar study was also done in Haimen, China in which the authors found that a high-protein diet can reduce the rate of liver cancer in patients carrying hepatitis B or hepatitis C virus (OR: 0.32; 95% CI: 0.12–0.86).[51]

A study of 40 patients in Taiwan was conducted to investigate the effect of massage therapy in liver cancer patients. Patients were randomly assigned into two groups: the intervention group received massage therapy primarily focused on the back before undergoing TACE and the control group did not. The tension indices of patients in the intervention group were significantly lower than those of the control group at the time before TACE and at two, four, six, and seven days after TACE.[52]

In one study in China, Sun and Yu (2000) compared the analgesic effect of combined therapy of acupuncture and sustained-release morphine tablets with morphine tablets alone. The intervention group (80 patients) received acupuncture (triple needling and needle retention in Ashi point) and morphine tablets, whereas the control group (40 patients) received only morphine tablets. The total rate of effectiveness was 96.2% in the combined therapy group and 68.3% in the control group. This suggests that the analgesic effect of acupuncture significantly increases pain relief as compared to the control group who did not receive acupuncture.[53]

Alimi et al.[54] from the Gustave Roussy Centre in France had 90 patients with cancer-related pain randomly assigned into three groups: an ear-point acupuncture group, a non-ear-point acupuncture control group, and a seeds-pressure control group. As measured by Visual Analogue Scale (VAS), the pain of patients in the ear-point acupuncture group was relieved by 36%, compared with only 2% in the control group. Therefore, the authors suggested that a combination of pain medication and ear-point acupuncture could significantly relieve pain in cancer patients ($P < 0.05$).

In another study, Zhou et al. treated cancer patients suffering moderate and severe pain with wrist–ankle acupuncture, MS-Contin (sustained-release morphine sulfate), or both. The rate of pain relief in patients suffering moderate pain treated with wrist–ankle acupuncture was 83.3% and in patients suffering severe pain was 63.0%. After combined wrist–ankle acupuncture with morphine sulfate, the relief rate increased to 85.0% in patients suffering severe pain. These results indicate that the combination of wrist–ankle acupuncture and morphine sulfate was better than treatment with either approach alone and could reduce the incidence rate of adverse effects.[55]

In the study of Chen and Liu in 2006, 60 patients with hiccup due to liver cancer were randomly assigned in 2:1 ratio to an acupuncture treatment group of 40 patients and a control group of 20 patients receiving metoclopramide intramuscular injections. The acupuncture group was given treatments at the PE6, REN17, ST36, and UB2 acupuncture points and other points. After 10 days of treatment, the total effective rate was 82.5% in the acupuncture group, much better than the 55% in the metoclopramide group ($P < 0.05$). The results showed that the acupuncture treatment has positive effects on cancer-related hiccup.[56]

Summary and Outlook

The prognosis for patients with liver cancer is still poor. Most patients are diagnosed with liver cancer in the middle or late stage of the disease. Few treatment options are available to them. Even diagnosed at an early stage, patients face the problem of a high recurrence rate after surgery. Thus, complementary and alternative therapies are a valuable addition in the treatment of liver cancer, especially in Asian countries. Although complementary and alternative therapies, especially natural medicine, have shown therapeutic or adjuvant effects in many clinical studies, many problems and shortcomings remain. Most studies reflect simple single-center clinical observations. In the absence of standardized, well-designed, multicenter clinical trials, reliable and convincing conclusions cannot be drawn, hindering the application of complementary and alternative therapies to clinical practice.

In recent years, great interest has developed worldwide for seeking more new drugs from natural plants, particularly from Chinese herbal medicine, that are safe, nontoxic or minimally toxic, fast acting, and easy to administrate. Modern science and technology have helped to accelerate the process of modernization of traditional natural medicine. We anticipate the development of more effective antitumor drugs in the future. But before transitioning to the next level, complementary and alternative therapy must first fit into the current environment of global scientific and technological exchange and competition, while trying to maintain and develop its own unique characteristics. Standardized clinical trials are the only way to verify the therapeutic effect of natural medicines. Thus, it is imperative that good clinical trials are designed and performed when complementary and alternative medicine is studied in the treatment of liver cancer.

References

1. Yu EX. *The Status and Consideration of the Role of Traditional Chinese Medicine in the Treatment of Tumors. Domestic and Foreign Progress in Scientific Technology of Traditional Chinese Medicine*. Shanghai Science and Technology Literature Press Shanghai, China; 1992:55.
2. Yu EX. 38 years of exploration for the role of traditional Chinese medicine in the treatment of cancer. *China Oncol*. 1994;4:153–155.
3. Ma YJ, Ma YP. Cinobufacini injection treatment of advanced primary liver cancer clinical observation. *J Liaoning Univ TCM*. 2010;12(1):123–124.
4. Sun ZJ, Pan CE, Wang GJ. Clinical observation in the therapeutic effect of combination of Huachansu and TACE. *Cancer Res Prev Treat*. 2002;29:67–68.
5. Su YH, Yin XC, Xie JM, et al. Inhibition effects of three kinds of bufotoxinson human SMMC-7721 and BEL-7402 hepatoma cells line. *Acad JSec Mil Med Univ*. 2004;24(4):393–395.
6. Liu YQ, Yu ZH, Shao ZH, et al. Clinical observation oncombination of Huachansu injection and TACE inliver cancer. *Chinese RuralHealth Serv Admin*. 2010;30(5):402–404.
7. Zuo XD, Cui YA, Qin SK, et al. Progress of clinical research in the anti-tumor effect of Huachansu. *Chinese Clin Oncol*. 2003;8(3):232–235.
8. Meng Z, Yang P, Shen Y, et al. Pilot study of huachansu in patients with hepatocellular carcinoma, nonsmall-cell lung cancer, or pancreatic cancer. *Cancer*. 2009;115(22):5309–5318.
9. Li DP. The clinical application of KLT injection. *Chinese J Clin Oncol*. 2001;28(4):300–302.

10. Qian MS. *The Study of Kanglaite Injection Against Tumor*. Hangzhou: Zhejiang University Press; 1998:214–229.
11. Qin SK. Progress in the study of arsenic trioxide for hepatocellular and gallbladder carcinoma. *J Oncol*. 2001;7(2):115–118.
12. Izzo AA, Borrelli F, Capasso R, et al. Non-psychotropic plant cannabinoids: new therapeutic opportunities from an ancient herb. *Trends Pharmacol Sci*. 2009;30(10):515–527.
13. Yun TK, Choi SY. A case-control study of ginseng intake and cancer. *Int J Epidemiol*. 1990;19:871–876.
14. Yun TK, Choi SY. Preventive effect of ginseng intake against various human cancers: a case-control study on 1987 pairs. *Cancer Epidemiol Biomarkers Prev*. 1995;4(4):401–408.
15. Yun TK, Choi SY, Yun HY. Epidemiological study on cancer prevention by ginseng: are all kinds of cancers preventable by ginseng? *J Korean Med Sci*. 2001;16:S19–S27.
16. Yun TK, Choi SY. Non-organ specific cancer prevention of ginseng: a prospective study in Korea. *Int J Epidemiol*. 1998;27:359–364.
17. Yun TK. Panax ginseng—a non-organ-specific cancer preventive? *Lancet Oncol*. 2001;2(1):49–55.
18. Wu XG, Zhu DH. Influence of ginseng upon the development of liver cancer induced by diethylnitrosamine in rats. *J Tongji Med Univ China*. 1990;10:141–145.
19. Mabed M, El-Helw L, Shamaa S. Phase II study of viscum fraxini-2 in patients with advanced hepatocellular carcinoma. *British J Cancer*. 2004;90(1):65–69.
20. Kienle GS, Berrino F, Bussing A, et al. Mistletoe in cancer—a systematic review on controlled clinical trials. *Eur J Med Res*. 2003;8(3):109–119.
21. Kroll DJ, Shaw HS, Oberlies NH. Milk thistle nomenclature: why it matters in cancer research and pharmacokinetic studies. *Integr Cancer Ther*. 2007;6(2):110–119.
22. Yu EX, Liu LM, Song MZ, et al. Clinical trials for the therapeutic effect of combination of whole liver moving split fields radiotherapy and traditional Chinese medicine in large liver cancer. *Chinese J Oncol*. 1992;14(1):57–59.
23. Wu WY, Guo WJ, Lin JH. The therapeutic effect of TACE in combination with Pingxiao capsule in primary liver cancer. *Chin J Integr Tradit Western Med Liver Dis*. 2001;11(1):50–51.
24. Song AY, Cheng YP, Liu SJ, et al. Comparison of therapeutic effect between combination of one time TACE with TCM and multi-course TACE. *Acta Chin Med Pharmacol*. 2000;(2):8.
25. Ren HP, Song MZ, Cheng L. Observation of therapeutic effect of "spleen nourishing and qi-regulating prescription" on negative effects after TACE in patient with Hepatocarcinoma. *Shanghai J Tradit Chin Med*. 2000;(3):24–25.
26. Zhang SF, Chen Z, Li B. Progresson on research and application of traditional Chinese medicine in intervention treatment of primary liver carcinoma. *Chin J Integr Tradit Western Med*. 2006;26(8):759–761.
27. Li HL, Li X, Guo CY, et al. Clinical study on combined treatment of TCM with post hepatocellular carcinoma LP-TAE. *Chin J Integr Tradit Western Med Dig*. 2001;9(2):97–98.
28. Qiang Y, Zhang T. The therapeutic effect of combination of Jianpi Liqi method and TACE in pixu subtype of primary liver cancer: 31 cases report. *J Nanjing TCM Univ (Nat Sci)*. 2000;16(2):86–87.
29. Meng MB, Cui YL, Guan YS, et al. Traditional Chinese medicine plus transcatheter arterial chemoembolization for unresectable hepatocellular carcinoma. *J Altern Complem Med*. 2008;14(8):1027–1042.
30. Zhang H, Luo RC, Wu J. Sorafenib combined with arsenic trioxide inhibiting hepatocellular carcinoma xenografts and angiogenesis in nude mice. *Chinese J Cancer Prev Treat*. 2009;16(8):578–582.
31. Ho JW, Ngan Hon PL, Chim WO. Effects of oxymatrine from Ku Shen on cancer cells. *Anticancer Agents Med Chem*. 2009;9(8):823–826.
32. Gamal-Eldeen AM, Djemgou PC, Tchuendem M, et al. Anti-cancer and immunostimulatory activity of chromones and other constituents from Cassia petersiana. *Z Naturforsch C. A Journal of Biosciences* 2007;62(5–6):331–338.
33. Abdel-Hameed el-SS, El-Nahas HA, El-Wakil EA, et al. Cytotoxic cholestane and pregnane glycosides from *Tribulus macropterus*. *Z Naturforsch C. A Journal of Biosciences* 2007;62(5–6):319–325.
34. Marzouk M, Gamal-Eldeen A, Mohamed M, El-Sayed M. Anti-proliferative and antioxidant constituents from *Tecoma stans*. *Z Naturforsch C. A Journal of Biosciences* 2006;61(11–12):783–791.
35. Lin LT, Liu LT, Chiang LC, Lin CC. In vitro anti-hepatoma activity of fifteen natural medicines from Canada. *Phytother Res*. 2002;16(5):440–444.
36. Vijaya Padma V, Arul Diana Christie S, Ramkuma KM. Induction of apoptosis by ginger in HEp-2 cell line is mediated by reactive oxygen species. *Basic Clin Pharmacol Toxicol*. 2007;100(5):302–307.

37. Anand P, Thomas SG, Kunnumakkara AB, et al. Biological activities of curcumin and its analogues (Congeners) made by man and mother nature. *Biochem Pharmacol.* 2008;76(11):1590–1611.
38. Adams BK, Cai J, Armstrong J, et al. EF24, a novel synthetic curcumin analog, induces apoptosis in cancer cells via a redox-dependent mechanism. *Anticancer Drugs.* 2005;16:263–275.
39. Ning L, Wentworth L, Chen H, Weber SM. Downregulation of Notch1 signaling inhibits tumor growth in human hepatocellular carcinoma. *Am J Transl Res.* 2009;1(4):358–366.
40. Greenlee H, Abascal K, Yarnell E, Ladas E. Clinical applications of *Silybum marianum* in oncology. *Integr Cancer Ther.* 2007;6(2):158–165.
41. García-Maceira P, Mateo J. Silibinin inhibits hypoxia-inducible factor-1alpha and mTOR/p70S6K/4E-BP1 signalling pathway in human cervical and hepatoma cancer cells: implications for anticancer therapy. *Oncogene.* 2009;28(3):313–324.
42. Kroll DJ, Shaw HS, Oberlies NH. Milk thistle nomenclature: why it matters in cancer research and pharmacokinetic studies. *Integr Cancer Ther.* 2007;6(2):110–119.
43. Gomes A, Giri B, Kole L, et al. A crystalline compound (BM-ANF1) from the Indian toad (Bufo melanostictus, Schneider) skin extract, induced antiproliferation and apoptosis in leukemic and hepatoma cell line involving cell cycle proteins. *Toxicon.* 2007;50(6):835–849.
44. Einbond LS, Soffritti M, Esposti DD, et al. Actein activates stress- and statin-associated responses and is bioavailable in Sprague-Dawley rats. *Fundam Clin Pharmacol.* 2009;23:311–321.
45. Feng YB, Luo WQ, Zhu SQ. Explore new clinical application of Huanglian and corresponding compound prescriptions from their traditional use. *Zhongguo Zhong Yao Za Zhi.* 2008;33(10):1221–1225.
46. Wu G, Liu ZS, Qian Q, Jiang C. Effect of Berberine on the growth of hepatocellular carcinoma cell lines. *Med J Wuhan Univ.* 2008;29(1):102–105.
47. Cheng WY, Wu SL, Hsiang CY, et al. Relationship between San-Huang-Xie-Xin-Tang and its herbal components on the gene expression profiles in HepG2 cells. *Am J Chin Med.* 2008;36(4):783–797.
48. Shidoji Y, Ogawa H. Natural occurrence of cancer-preventive geranylgeranoic acid in medicinal herbs. *J Lipid Res.* 2004;45(6):1092–1103.
49. Li SL, Huang ZN, Hsieh HH, et al. The augmented anti-tumor effects of Antrodia camphorata co-fermented with Chinese medicinal herb in human hepatoma cells. *Am J Chin Med.* 2009;37(4):771–783.
50. Sharp GB, Lagarde F, Mizuno T, et al. Relationship of hepatocellular carcinoma to soya food consumption: a cohort-based, case-control study in Japan. *Int J Cancer.* 2005;115(2):290–295.
51. Yu SZ, Huang XE, Koide T, et al. Hepatitis B and C viruses infection, lifestyle and genetic polymorphisms as risk factors for hepatocellular carcinoma in Haimen, China. *Jpn J Cancer Res.* 2002;93(12):1287–1292.
52. Lin ML, Tsang YM, Hwang SL. Efficacy of a stress management program for patients with hepatocellular carcinoma receiving transcatheter arterial embolization. *J Formos Med Assoc.* 1998;97(2):113–117.
53. Sun YL, Yu LR. The therapeutic effect of triple needling and needle retention in liver cancer related pain: 80 cases report. *Chin Acupunct Moxibust.* 2000;20(4):211–212.
54. Alimi D, Rubino C, Pichard-Léandri E, et al. Analgesic effect of auricular acupuncture for cancer pain: a randomized, blinded, controlled trial. *J Clin Oncol.* 2003;21(22):4120–4126.
55. Zhou QH, Hu X, Gu W, et al. Clinical observation on efficacy of wrist-ankle acupuncture in relieving moderate and severe pain of patients with liver cancer. *J Zhejiang College of Tradit Chin Med.* 2005;29(11):53–56.
56. Chen HT, Liu B. Clinical observation on the effect of acupuncture in hiccup due to liver cancer. *J Clin Acupunct Moxi.* 2006;22(5):18–19.

INDEX

Note: Page numbers followed by f, or t indicate material in figures, or tables, respectively.

A

Ablation process, 371
Ablation therapy, 464
Ablative technologies, 146
Ablative therapies
    cryoablation, 167
    ethanol ablation, 167
    microwave ablation, 167
    radiofrequency ablation, 166–167
Abscesses, hepatic pyogenic, 258–259
Academic Consortium for Complementary and Alternative Health Care, 479
ACR guidelines. *See* American College of Radiology (ACR) guidelines
Acupuncture, 481–482, 481f
Adenocarcinomas, 3
Adenoma, 91–94, 93t, 95t
    hepatic, 258, 260
    imaging studies, 92–93
    incidence and characteristics, 91–92
    indications for surgery, 93–94
    laboratory testing, 92–93
    MRI for diagnosing, 259f
    physical exam, 92–93
Adenomyomatosis, 63, 251
Adjuvant HAI posthepatic resection, 432–433, 433t
Adjuvant systemic chemotherapy, 147–149, 148f
Adjuvant therapy
    biliary tumors and biologic agents, 445–447
    for hepatocellular carcinoma, 419
    role of, 44
Adoptive transfer efficacy, 465
α-fetoprotein (AFP), 114, 255, 455f, 456, 493
    as biomarker of response to chemotherapy, 419
    serum level of, 125
Aflatoxins, 113
Age-adjusted mortality rates, for extrahepatic cholangiocarcinoma, 4, 4f
AJCC. *See* American Joint Committee on Cancer (AJCC)
Albendazole, 100
Alcohol, 113
Alcoholic liver cirrhosis, 439
Alpha interferon (αIFN), 169
Alternative therapies
    cancer treatments, 477
    prevalence and patient considerations, 478

Amebic cysts, 99
American Association for the Study of Liver Disease (AASLD), 117
American College of Radiology (ACR) guidelines, 223
American Joint Committee on Cancer (AJCC), 8, 9, 68, 69, 69t, 320
Anatomical tumor staging, 320
Angiogenesis, 169
Angiographic embolization, 93
Angiographic methods, 355
Angiography, 98, 400, 401, 401f
    GBC, 66
    selective, 363f
Angiomyolipoma, 233
Anomalous pancreaticobiliary ductal junction, 63
Antagonistic anti-CTLA-4 mAbs, 457
Anthracendione, 415
Anthracycline, 413, 415
Antiangiogenic agents, combination of, 418
Antiangiogenics, combination therapy studies with, 443–444
Antibiotic prophylaxis, 168
Anticancer drugs, development of, 420
Anti-EGFR therapies, 446
Antigen presenting cell (APC), 453, 454f
Antigen-specific immunotherapy, 417
Antihelminth therapy, 100
Antitumor effect in liver cancer, 494
Anti-viral therapy, reactivation reduction by, 420
Antrodia camphorata, 498
APC. *See* Antigen-presenting cell (APC)
Arsenic trioxide (As_2O_3), 494, 496
Arsenicum sublimatum, 494
Arteriography, 427
Ascitic fluid cytology, 67
ASK-1 kinase activity, 444
ASK1-mediated apoptosis, 445f
Aspartate aminotransferase (AST), 428
Asymptomatic gallstones, prophylactic cholecystectomy for, 82
Atrophy-hypertrophy complex, 5
Auto-phosphorylation, 437
Axial computed tomography, 6f

B

Barcelona Clinic Liver Cancer (BCLC), 118, 320, 321
BCA. *See* Biliary cystadenomas (BCA)
BCLC. *See* Barcelona Clinic Liver Cancer (BCLC)

BCLM. *See* Breast cancer liver metastases (BCLM)
Benign biliary tumors
    BCA, 100–101
    bile duct adenoma, 101
    biliary microhamartoma, 101
    biliary papillomatosis, 101
    treatment of, 102
Benign lesions
    angiomyolipoma, 233
    biliary cystadenoma, 233
    biliary hamartoma, 232–233
    cysts, 227–228
    fatty infiltration, 227
    focal nodular hyperplasia, 229–230, 231f
    hemangioma, 228–229, 229f
    hepatic adenoma, 230–232
    hepatic solid lesions, 260–261
Benign periablational enhancement, 346
Best-characterized cancer-testis antigens in HCC, 459
Bevacizumab, 441, 442, 446
    with erlotinib, 444
    with gemcitabine and oxaliplatin, 443
Bile duct, 428
    adenoma, 101
    in GBC, 70
Biliary cystadenocarcinoma, 101, 242
Biliary cystadenomas (BCA), 100–101, 101f, 233
Biliary disease, clinical presentation of, 247–248
Biliary hamartoma, 232–233
Biliary infiltration, 79
Biliary microhamartoma, 101
Biliary obstruction, 79
Biliary papillomatosis, 101
Biliary tract carcinomas, 447
Biliary tree, direct imaging of, 7
Biliary tumors, 445–447
Bilirubin, 414, 442
BINGO study, 446
Biologic agents, 445–447
Bipolar electrodes, 327
Bismuth–Corlette classification, 304
    of hilar cholangiocarcinoma, 8, 9f
Black cohosh, 497
Bland embolization, 356–357, 358f, 365f
Body surface area method, 403, 409
Bortezomib, 418
β-particle, 391, 405–406
Brachytherapy, 14
    for GBC, 81
    ovarian cancer liver metastases, 197
Breast cancer, 211–212
    hepatic metastasectomy outcomes, 178–179, 179t
    outcomes of additional liver-directed therapeutic modalities, 180–182, 181t
    predictive risk factors assessment, 213t
Breast cancer liver metastases (BCLM), 178–182, 179t, 181t, 198, 212f, 213f
Breathing motion
    control technique, 377
    management of, 381–382
Bremsstrahlung imaging, 403, 404f
Bremsstrahlung radiation, 403
Brivanib, 443–445
Bufo gargarizans, 494
Bufo melanostictus, 494

C

CA 19-9. *See* Carbohydrate antigen (CA) 19-9
Cabozantinib, 438–439
CAM. *See* Complementary and Alternative Medicine (CAM)
Cancer-testis antigens, 459
Cannabis sativa, 494
Capecitabine, 81, 443
Carbohydrate antigen (CA) 19-9, 5, 100
Carbon ion radiotherapy, for liver cancer, 385
Carcinoembryonic antigen (CEA), 5, 26, 100, 253, 392
Carcinoid, 158
    heart disease, 312
    vs. pancreatic NE, 163f
Cardiotoxicity, 413–414
CASH. *See* Chemotherapy-associated hepatic steatohepatitis (CASH)
Catheter, 403
Catheter-based therapies, 319, 321, 342, 347
Catheter-related complications, HAI, 428, 428t
Caudate lobe bile ducts, 11
Cavernous hemangioma, 96
Cavitation of HIFU, 370, 370f
CBD. *See* Common bile duct (CBD)
CCA. *See* Cholangiocarcinoma (CCA)
CD134. *See* OX40
CD152, 457
CD137 ligand, 457
CEA. *See* Carcinoembryonic antigen (CEA)
Cell membrane
    Ras processing and anchoring to, 439
    receptors, 439
Cervical cancers, 213
Cetuximab, 438
CgA. *See* Chromogranin A (CgA)
CHD. *See* Common hepatic duct (CHD)
Chemical ablation techniques of HCC
    PAI, 324–325
    PEI, 321–324, 322f

Chemical carcinogens, GBC, 62–63
Chemoembolization, 374
    conventional transarterial, 356–357
    for metastatic NETs, 168
Chemotherapeutical agents, 465
Chemotherapeutic regimens, 137, 141
Chemotherapy, 169
    AFP as biomarker of response to, 419
    vs. chemotherapy plus SIRT, 393
    in combination with novel targeted agents, 418–419
    GBC, 81–82
    HBV reactivation in, 420
    for hepatocellular carcinoma, 413–417, 414t
Chemotherapy-associated hepatic steatohepatitis (CASH), 148
Chest X-ray, 65
Child-Pugh A cirrhosis, 441
Child-Pugh A patients, 443
Child-Pugh B patients, 442
Chinese cinnamon. *See Cinnamomum cassia*
Cholangioadenoma, 101
Cholangiocarcinoma (CCA), 239–241, 239f, 240f. *See also* Hilar cholangiocarcinoma
    biliary tree distribution frequency of, 304, 305f
    definition, 3
    description, 304
    epidemiology and risk factors, 3–4
    intrahepatic, 260
    jaundice, 249
    MELD-based allocation, 305–306
    MRCP for, 262
    neoadjuvant therapy, 306
    patient selection, 304–305
    PCC. *See* Peripheral cholangiocarcinoma (PCC)
    preoperative evaluation, 5–8
    recurrence and survival, OLT, 306–308, 307t, 308f, 309f
    resection *vs.* transplantation, 308–310
    treatment of, 293
Cholangiography, 66, 262
Cholangitis, 5
Cholecystectomy, gallbladder polyps, 63
Cholecystocoeliac pathway, 70
Cholecystoenteric fistula, 63
Cholecysto-mesenteric pathway, 70
Cholecysto-retropancreatic pathway, 70
Choledochal cysts, 4
Cholesterol polyps, 251
Choloroquin, 99
Chromogranin A (CgA), 159
Cinnamomum cassia, 496
Cinobufotalin, 494
Cirrhosis, 305, 319, 321, 325
Cirrhotic liver, Child-Pugh grading scale for, 380
Cirsium, 495

Cisplatin, 15, 44, 124, 125, 300, 417, 447
Classic radiation-induced liver disease, 380
Clinical outcome, determination of, 217
Clinical risk score (CRS), 142–143, 142t, 143t, 146, 147
Coagulation necrosis, 325
Collins formula, 425–426
Color-Doppler analysis, 323
Color Doppler ultrasound image, 322f
Colorectal cancer (CRC), 392
    diagnostic imaging of patients with, 253–254
    liver metastases
        adjuvant systemic chemotherapy, 147–149, 148f
        chemotherapeutic regimens, 137
        clinical risk score, 142–143, 142t, 143t
        epidemiology, 137
        Foster's multi-institutional review, 138
        history of, 137–138
        long-term results, 138, 140
        metachronous lesions, 141
        operative considerations, 145–147, 146t
        patient selection, 144–145
        perioperative morbidity and mortality, 147
        prognostic variables, 140–142
        recurrence and re-resection, 140, 141t
        resectable liver disease, 138
        resection, results of, 138
    treatment, 254–255
Combination chemotherapy, for hepatocellular carcinoma, 415t, 417–418
Combination therapy
    of HCC, 342–344
    studies with antiangiogenics, 443–444
Common bile duct (CBD), 66, 74
Common hepatic artery (CHA), 360
Common hepatic duct (CHD), 66
Compartmental macrodosimetry method, 403, 410
Complementary and Alternative Medicine (CAM), 477, 478
Complementary therapies, 477
    acupuncture, 481–482, 481f
    fitness, 485
    integrative oncology, 480–481
    mind-body modalities. *See* Mind-body modalities
    physician-patient communication, 478–479, 480t
    prevalence and patient considerations, 478
Complete margin-negative (R_0) resection, 160
Complete response (CR), 345
Computed tomography (CT), 100, 116, 144–145, 223–225, 271, 392
    angiomyolipoma, 233
    biliary cystadenoma, 233
    biliary hamartoma, 232
    CCA, 305
    characteristics of, 6, 32, 32t
    cholangiocarcinoma, 240, 240f

Computed tomography (CT) (*continued*)
  classic appearance of hemangioma on, 258f
  contrast-enhanced, 346
  cryoablation, 338–339
  cysts, 227
  diagnosis
    of CRC, 253
    of HA, 92
  in excretory phase demonstrating an echinococcal cyst, 99f
  fatty infiltration, 227
  fibrolamellar carcinoma, 238
  fibronodular hyperplasia lesion, 259f
  focal nodular hyperplasia, 98, 229
  gallbladder carcinoma, 241
  guidance, 328
  HCC, 358f
  HCC before RT, 378f
  hemangioma, 228
  hepatic adenoma, 231
  hepatic epithelioid hemangioendothelioma and hepatic angiosarcoma, 242
  hepatic metastasis, 234, 234f
  hepatocellular carcinoma, 235–236, 236f
  intraprocedural, 361
  laser ablation, 340–341
  lymphoma, 242
  mass-forming PCC, 34, 35f
  MCT, 335–336, 336f
  nonhepatic collateral supply identified, 360
  RFA, 328–329, 331f–333f
  triphasic, 116
  unenhanced, 345
Contrast enhanced computed tomography, 65
Conventional angiography, 66
Conventional transarterial chemoembolization, 356–357
Cool-tip system, 329
Coptis chinensis, 497–498
Coptis groenlandica Salisb, 497
Correlative biomarker studies, 447
CR. *See* Complete response (CR)
CRC. *See* Colorectal cancer (CRC)
Cross-sectional imaging, 5–7, 65
  of liver, 428
Cross-sectional radiologic evaluation of tumor, 399–400
CRS. *See* Clinical risk score (CRS)
Cryoablation, 167, 264, 338–340
  basic principles, 338
  complications and contraindications, 340
  results, 339–340
  TACE and, 343–344
  technique, 338–339
CTL. *See* Cytotoxic T lymphocyte (CTL)
Curcuma longa, 497

Cutaneous malignant melanoma, 182–183
Cyclin-dependent kinase inhibitors, 438
Cystadenocarcinomas, 249, 257
Cystic hepatic disease, 98–99
  amebic cysts, 99
  hepatic cysts, 100
  hydatid cysts, 99–100
Cystic lesions, 249
Cysts, 227–228, 228f
Cytokine therapy, 456–457, 457t
Cytoplasmic downstream targets, 439–440
Cytoreduction, 160, 164
Cytotoxic T cells, 459
Cytotoxic T lymphocyte (CTL)
  epitopes in HCC, 458t–459t
  induced apoptosis, 455f, 456

D

DC-based therapeutic approach, 460
DCE MRI. *See* dynamic contrast-enhanced (DCE) MRI
DCs. *See* Dendritic cells (DCs)
DEB. *See* Drug-eluting beads (DEB)
Deep vein thromboses, 146
Defibrillator, 335
Dendritic cells (DCs), 453, 454f
DFI. *See* Disease-free interval (DFI)
DFS. *See* Disease-free survival (DFS)
Diarrhea, 441
Diffusion weighting, MR technique, 364
Dihydropyrimidine dehydrogenase (DPD), 416
Diloxanide, 99
1,1-Diphenyl-2-picrylhydrazyl (DPPH) assay, 496
Direct cholangiography, 7–8
Direct cholangioscopy, 7–8
Disease-free interval (DFI), 179
Disease-free survival (DFS), 178
DNs. *See* Dysplastic nodules (DNs)
Doppler imaging, 5
Doppler ultrasound, GBC, 66
Dosimetry, treatment planning and Y-90 microsphere, 402–403
Doxorubicin, 124, 356, 413, 416, 444
  pegylation of, 414–415
  toxicity for, 414
DPD. *See* Dihydropyrimidine dehydrogenase (DPD)
Drug-eluting beads (DEB), 356, 357, 359
Ductal dilatation. *See* Intrahepatic ductal dilatation
Duodenal infiltration, 66
Duplex imaging, 5
Dynamic contrast-enhanced (DCE) MRI, 224
  scanning phases of, 226
Dysplastic nodules (DNs), 115

E

EA. *See* Electroacupuncture (EA)
EBRT. *See* External beam radiation therapy (EBRT)
EC. *See* Extended cholecystectomy (EC)
Echinococcal cysts, 99, 256
EFLV. *See* Essential functional liver volume (EFLV)
EGFR. *See* Epidermal growth factor receptor
18-Fluorodeoxyglucose positron emission tomography (FDG-PET), 32–33, 254f, 392
    applicability of, 225
    follow-up studies, 403
    functional imaging, 400
    hepatic metastasis, 234–235, 234f
    lymphoma, 242
    preoperative, 142
    scans, 144–145
    usefulness of, 7
Electroacupuncture (EA), 481
Electrocautery, 288
Elevated carcinoembryonic antigen (CEA), 141
Embolization, 168, 356
Emetine, 99
Endocrine tumors, 102
Endoscopic retrograde cholangiopancreatography (ERCP), 6, 247, 250, 262
    direct cholangiography with, 7
Endoscopic stenting (ES), 79
Endoscopic ultrasound (EUS), 250, 262
    GBC, 66
Entamoeba histolytica, 99
Epidemiology, 137
Epidermal growth factor receptor (EGFR), 437–439
Epirubicin, 415
Epithelial ovarian cancer, 213
Equivalent uniform dose, 383
ERCP. *See* Endoscopic retrograde cholangiopancreatography (ERCP)
Erlotinib, 438
Erlotinib monotherapy, 446
ES. *See* Endoscopic stenting (ES)
Essential functional liver volume (EFLV), 120
Ethanol ablation, 167
EUS. *See* Endoscopic ultrasound (EUS)
Everolimus, 440
Extended cholecystectomy (EC), 63, 67, 73
    for T2 disease, 77
External beam radiation therapy (EBRT), 48
Extrahepatic biliary tree, 12f
    cholangiocarcinoma lesions arise in, 3
Extrahepatic cholangiocarcinoma, age-adjusted incidence of, 3, 4
Extrahepatic collateral supply, 362f
Extrahepatic ductal dilatation
    intrahepatic and, 250–251
    treatment of patient with, 251f
Extrahepatic metastases, 141

F

Fas-expressing cells, 455, 455f
Fas ligand (FasL), 455–456, 455f
Fatty infiltration, 227
FDG-PET. *See* 18-Fluorodeoxyglucose positron emission tomography (FDG-PET)
Fibrolamellar carcinoma (FLCs), 238
Fibronodular hyperplasia (FNH), 258, 259f, 261f
    resection of, 263
Fine needle aspiration cytology (FNAC), 67
5 Fluoro-2-deoxyuridine (FUDR), 426
5-Fluorouracil (5-FU), 14, 15, 416
    based adjuvant chemotherapy, 147, 148
5-FU, leucovorin, capecitabine (CAPOX), 254
5-FU, leucovorin, irinotecan (FOLFIRI), 254
5-FU, leucovorin, oxaliplatin (FOLFOX), 256
FLCs. *See* Fibrolamellar carcinoma (FLCs)
Floxuridine (FUDR), 148
FLR. *See* Future liver remnant (FLR)
Fluorocarbon liquid, 427
Fluoroscopic guidance, 8
FNAC. *See* Fine needle aspiration cytology (FNAC)
Focal nodular hyperplasia (FNH), 91, 229, 225f–30, 231f, 255, 256
    imaging studies, 97–98
    incidence and characteristics, 97
    laboratory testing, 97–98
    physical examination, 97–98
FOLFOX 4, 393
Foregut carcinoid, 159t
Forkhead box M1 (FOXM1), 459
4-dimensional (4-D) radiotherapy, 382
FOXM1. *See* Forkhead box M1 (FOXM1)
Fraction size of radiation dose, 380–381
FUDR. *See* 5 Fluoro-2-deoxyuridine (FUDR); Floxuridine (FUDR)
Functional imaging, pretreatment evaluation, 400, 400f
Functional volume, liver function evaluation, 399
Future liver remnant (FLR), 8, 145, 391

G

Gadolinium, 96
Gadolinium-enhanced MR, 364
Gal-1. *See* Galectin-1 (Gal-1)
Galectin-1 (Gal-1), 455f, 456
Gallbladder cancer (GBC)
    clinical features, 63–65
    description, 61

Gallbladder cancer (GBC) (*continued*)
   diagnosis
      angiography, 66
      ascitic fluid cytology, 67
      chest X-ray, 65
      cholangiography, 66
      contrast enhanced CT, 65
      differential, 67–68
      Doppler ultrasound, 66
      endoscopic ultrasound, 66
      fifth to sixth edition changes, 69–70
      laparoscopic ultrasound, 67
      laparoscopy, 67
      MRI, 65–66
      PET, 66
      staging systems, 68, 69t
      thick-walled, 68
      timing of, 64–65
      tissue, 67
      tumor markers, 67
      ultrasound, 65
      upper gastrointestinal endoscopy, 66
   epidemiology, 61–62
   incidental, 75–76
   laparoscopic surgery, 76
   management, 71, 72f
      incidental, 75–76
      laparoscopic surgery, 76
      noncurative simple cholecystectomy, 76
      palliation, 79–81, 80f
      port site metastases, 76–77
      radiotherapy and chemotherapy, 81–82
      surgery and prognosis, 77–79, 77t–80t
      suspected, 71, 73–74, 73f
      unsuspected, 74–75, 75f
   noncurative simple cholecystectomy, 76
   palliation, 79–81, 80f
   pathology, 69–70
   port site metastases, 76–77
   prevention, 82
   radiotherapy and chemotherapy, 81–82
   resections in, 78t
   risk factors, 62–63
   spreads, 70–71, 71t
   surgery and prognosis, 77–79, 77t–80t
   surgical implications, 70–71, 71t
   suspected, 71, 72f, 73–74, 73f
   unsuspected, 74–75, 75f
Gallbladder carcinoma, 241, 241f
Gallbladder polyps, 63, 251, 252f
   diagnostic imaging of patients, 252, 252f
   treatment of patients with, 252–253
Gallstones, 62
   jaundice without, 248–251, 248f

Gas chromatograph/mass spectrometer (GC-MS) screening, 497
Gastric cancer, 190, 215, 215t
Gastroduodenal artery, 400, 401
Gastroenteropancreatic NE tumors (GEP NETs), 157
   clinical and biochemical features, 159t
   drugs and targets, 169
Gastrointestinal (GI) branches, 400
Gastrointestinal (GI) complications, 428
Gastrointestinal NE tumors (GI-NETs), 157
Gastrointestinal stromal tumors (GISTs), 186, 188–189, 190t, 198, 215–216, 216t
Gastrointestinal tumors, 189–193, 191t, 192t, 198–199
Gastrojejunostomy, 80–81
Gd-BOPTA, 226, 256, 260
Gd-EOB-DTPA, 226, 231f, 232f
Gefitinib, 439
Gemcitabine, 81–82, 417, 443, 446, 447
Gemcitabine-based chemotherapy, 15, 446
Gemcitabine-induced thrombocytopenia, 417
Gene expression profiles, 445
General anesthesia, 371
Genetic abnormalities, 438
Genitourinary tumors, 193–196, 195t, 196t, 199
GEP NETs. *See* Gastroenteropancreatic NE tumors
Geranylgeranoic acid (GGA), 498
German Cooperative group study, 429
GGA. *See* Geranylgeranoic acid (GGA)
GI-NETs. *See* Gastrointestinal NE tumors
Ginger. *See* Zingiber officinale
GISTs. *See* Gastrointestinal stromal tumors (GISTs)
Glass microspheres, 391–392
Glutamine synthetase (GS), 116
Glyceryl-1-tetra-cosanoate, 496
Glypican-3 (GPC3), 116, 459
   peptide vaccination for patients, 464
Granular cell myoblastomas, 102
GS. *See* Glutamine synthetase (GS)
Gynecological tumors, 196–198, 197t, 199, 212–214

H

HA. *See* Hepatic adenoma (HA)
HAE. *See* Hepatic arterial embolization (HAE)
HAIC. *See* Hepatic arterial infusion chemotherapy (HAIC)
HAI therapy. *See* Hepatic arterial infusion (HAI) therapy
Hand-foot syndrome, 441
Hanging maneuver, 289–290, 290f
HBV. *See* Hepatitis B virus (HBV)
HCC. *See* Hepatocellular carcinoma (HCC)

Index

HCV. *See* Hepatitis C virus (HCV)
HCV-1. *See* Hepatitis C virus 1
HDL. *See* Hepato-duodenal ligament (HDL)
Heat deposition in tissue, limitations of, 326–327
Heat shock protein 70 (HSP70), 116
Hemangioma, 93t, 223
    hepatic solid masses, 257–258, 258f
    imaging images, 96, 96f
    incidence and characteristics, 94–96, 95t
    indications for surgery, 96–97
    laboratory testing, 96
    MRI, 228–229, 229f
    physical examination, 96
Hemihepatectomy, 11–13f
    left. *See* Left hemihepatectomy
    right. *See* Right hemihepatectomy
Hepatectomy, 7
Hepatic adenoma (HA), 91–94, 95f, 230–232, 258
Hepatic angiosarcoma, 242
Hepatic arterial embolization (HAE), 356, 357
Hepatic arterial infusion chemotherapy (HAIC)
    breast cancer, 180
    gastrointestinal tumors, 191–193
    genitourinary tumors, 195–198
    melanoma, 183–185
    soft-tissue sarcoma, 187, 188
Hepatic arterial infusion (HAI) therapy
    catheter-related complications, 428, 428t
    catheter, technique for insertion, 427–428
    in combination with systemic chemotherapy, 431–432, 431t
    conversion to resectability, 432
    5 fluoro-2-deoxyuridine (FUDR), 426
    ideal drug properties for, 425t
    implantable pump for, 427f
    infusion pump, 426–427
    meta-analyses of, 430t
    with nonfluoropyrimidine chemotherapy agents, 430–431
    with nonfluoropyrimidine drugs, 426
    pharmacological principles for drug selection in, 425–426
    posthepatic resection, 432–433, 433t
    preoperative evaluation, 427
    for primary liver cancer, 433–434
    randomized trials of, 429, 429t
    toxicity of, 428
    unresectable colorectal hepatic metastases, 428–430
Hepatic artery infusion, 148
Hepatic cirrhosis, 377–379
Hepatic colorectal metastases, 426
    clinical data for, 392–396
    recurrence after resection of, 141t

Hepatic cystic lesions, 256
    diagnostic imaging of patients with, 257
    treatment of patients with, 257
Hepatic cysts, aspiration of, 100
Hepatic epithelioid hemangioendothelioma, 242
Hepatic extraction ratio, 425
Hepatic hemangiomas, 96
Hepatic injury, 404–405
Hepatic metastasectomy
    breast cancer, 178–179, 179t
    gastrointestinal tumors, 190–191, 191t
    genitourinary tumors, 194, 195t, 199
    GISTs, 188–189
    gynecological malignancies, 196–197, 197t
    melanoma, 183, 183t
    soft-tissue sarcoma, 186–187, 187t
Hepatic metastases, 144t, 233–235, 234f
Hepatic resection, 160–161, 164–165
    anatomy, 269, 270f
    left hemihepatectomy. *See* Left hemihepatectomy
    left lateral sectionectomy. *See* Left lateral sectionectomy
    left trisectionectomy, 283, 285
    morbidity of, 145–146
    operative preparation, 272
    operative strategies
        anterior approach and hanging maneuver, 288–290, 290f
        laparoscopic partial hepatectomy, 287–288, 288f, 289f
        nonanatomic resections, 287
        two-stage hepatectomy, 286
    preoperative considerations
        chemotherapy-associated hepatotoxicity, 270–271
        cirrhosis, 270
        PVE, 271–272, 271f
    results, 140t
    right hemihepatectomy. *See* Right hemihepatectomy
    right trisectionectomy, 283
    segmentectomy I, 285–286, 285f–287f
    survival rate achieved by, 161f, 163f
    use of, 11
Hepatic scintigraphy, Tc-99m MAA, 402
Hepatic shunting, detection and quantitation of, 401, 402f
Hepatic solid masses
    abscesses, 258–259
    adenoma, 258
    cholangiocarcinoma, 260
    fibronodular hyperplasia, 258
    hemangioma, 257–258
    hepatocellular carcinoma, 259–260
    metastases with unknown primary, 260–264
Hepatic stellate cells, 453
Hepatic transplantation, 167, 168t

Hepatic tumors, resection of, 211
Hepatitis B virus (HBV), 30, 112
  reactivation in chemotherapy, 420
Hepatitis C virus 1(HCV-1), 439
Hepatitis C virus (HCV), 30, 112–113
Hepatoblastoma
  diagnosis, 125
  epidemiology, 124–125
  pathology, 125
  treatment, 125
Hepatocellular carcinoma (HCC), 119, 235–238, 259–260, 293, 369, 373, 433
  adjuvant systemic therapy for, 419
  AFP as biomarker of response to chemotherapy, 419
  antiangiogenic drug in, 440
  chemical ablation techniques. *See* chemical ablation techniques
  chemotherapy for, 413–417
  clinical data for, 396, 397–398
  combination in, 437
    chemotherapy for, 415t, 417–418
  CT image of patient with, 378f
  cytotoxic drugs for, 420
  definition, 413
  description, 294, 294f
  diagnosis of, 116–117, 117f, 261–262, 322f
  epidemiology, 111
  etiology
    aflatoxin, 113
    alcohol, 113
    HBV, 112
    HCV, 112–113
    risk factors, 113–114
  fractionation and total doses of RT, 383
  HBV reactivation in chemotherapy, 420
  HIFU for, 373
  hypervascular, 362f
  International Consensus Conference on, 299t
  intrahepatic spread of, 382
  in vitro and in vivo models of, 440
  LDLT, 302
  listing criteria, 298, 300
  local ablation therapies for, 321
  malignant lesions, 235–238
  massive, 365f
  MELD, 297–298, 300f
  neoplasia in form of, 91
  pathology, 114–116
  patient selection, 295–297, 295f–298f
  patients' risk factors for, 441
  phase III clinical trials in, 433t
  potential targets for, 438f
  progressive imaging changes in treated, 359f
  radiologic criteria, 297, 299t
  radiosensitivity of, 377
  radiotherapy, 381
  recurrent, 363f
  resection *vs.* transplantation, 302–304, 303f, 304f
  single-agent chemotherapy in, 414t
  specific antigens, 459
  staging systems, 117–118, 118t
  surveillance, 114
  thermal ablation techniques. *See* thermal ablation techniques of HCC
  transplantation for, 440
  treatment
    algorithms for, 319
    liver resection, 119–121
    liver transplantation, 122, 123t
    local ablative therapy, 122–123
    locoregional treatments, 123–124
    options for, 264
    single-agent therapy, 124
    sorafenib, 124
    tamoxifen, 124
  tumor
    necrosis in, 440f
    staging, 319–321
  wait list management, 300–302, 301f
Hepatocyte growth factor (HGF), 438
Hepatocytes, 439
Hepato-duodenal ligament (HDL), 70
HepG2 cell line, 496–498
HepG2 tumor cells, 464
HER1/EGFR tumor overexpression, 446
HGF. *See* Hepatocyte growth factor (HGF)
Hiccup due to liver cancer, 499
HIFU. *See* High-intensity focused ultrasound (HIFU)
High bile duct obstruction, 249
High-intensity focused ultrasound (HIFU), 369–373
  applications for liver cancer, 373–375, 374f
  cavitation effect of, 370f
  initial development of, 373
  mechanical effect, 370
  thermal effect of, 370
  three-dimensional therapeutic planning of, 372f
  tumor response to, 374
Hilar cholangiocarcinoma, 12f.
    See also Cholangiocarcinoma
  adjuvant therapy for, 15–16
  Bismuth–Corlette classification of, 8, 9f
  classification and staging of, 8–10
  CT characteristics of, 6
  in jaundiced patient, 5
  palliative therapy for, 16–18
  surgery for, 10–15, 14t

Index   511

Hilar tumors, 3
Hilus of liver, 13f
Hindgut carcinoid, 159t
Hong Kong, HCC clinical data from, 396, 397
Hormone receptor, 178
HSP70. See Heat shock protein 70 (HSP70)
Huachansu, 494
Human clinical trials, 460, 460t–463t, 464
Hydatid cysts, 99–100, 103
Hypervascular liver mass, MR characteristics of, 257t
Hypervascular mass, 250
Hypervascular metastases, 253
Hypovascular liver lesions, 225, 235

I

ICC. See Intrahepatic cholangiocarcinoma (ICC)
Ideal drug properties for HAI, 425t
IDO catalyzes. See Indoleamine 2,3 dioxygenase (IDO) catalyzes
IFA. See Incomplete Freund's adjuvant (IFA)
IFN-α. See Interferon alpha (IFN-α)
IGF. See Insulin growth factors (IGF)
IGF-1R. See IGF-1 receptor (IGF-1R)
IGFBP-3. See Insulin growth factor binding protein-3 (IGFBP-3)
IHP. See Isolated hepatic perfusion (IHP)
IL-10, 455f, 456
Image-guided ablation therapy for HCC, 321
Image-guided RT, 377, 381
  clinical experience, 382–383
Immune-inhibitory mechanisms, 465
Immunostimulating monoclonal antibodies, 456–457, 457t
Immunotherapeutic approaches, 457
Immunotherapeutic clinical trials in HCC, 460t–463t
Implantable pump for HAI, 427f
Incidental gallbladder cancer, 64, 75–76
Incomplete Freund's adjuvant (IFA), 459
Indocyanine green (ICG), 381
Indoleamine 2,3 dioxygenase (IDO) catalyzes, 455f, 456
Inferior vena cava, 289, 290f
Infusion pump, HAI, 426–427
Institute of Medicine (IOM), 483
Insulin growth factor binding protein-3 (IGFBP-3), 439
Insulin receptor (IR), 439
Intensity-modulated conformal RT, clinical experience, 382–385
Intensity-modulated RT, 377
Interferon alpha (IFN-α), 456
International Consensus Conference on liver transplantation for HCC, 299t
International Union Against Cancer (UICC), staging systems, 68, 69t
International Working Party (IWP), 115

Intraarterial chemotherapy for liver tumors, HAI therapy. See Hepatic arterial infusion (HAI) therapy
Intra-arterial doxorubicin, 356
Intra-arterial therapy, 357
Intrahepatic biliary dilation, 5
Intrahepatic cholangiocarcinoma (ICC), 5, 262, 433, 437
Intrahepatic ductal dilatation
  and extrahepatic ductal dilatation, 250–251
  and jaundice, 249f
  patients with
    diagnostic imaging of, 249–250
    treatment of, 251f
Intraoperative ultrasound (IOUS), 146, 148, 253, 263
Intratumoral injection of DCs, 464
IOM. See Institute of Medicine (IOM)
Ionic agitation, 326
IOUS. See Intraoperative ultrasound (IOUS)
IR. See Insulin receptor (IR)
Irinotecan, 393, 426
Isolated hepatic perfusion (IHP), 185, 186
Ito cells, 453
IWP. See International Working Party (IWP)

J

Jarnagin–Blumgart T-stage criteria, 9t
Jaundice
  intrahepatic ductal dilatation and, 249f
  prehepatic and hepatic causes of, 248
  without gallstones, 248–251, 248f
JC HIFU system, 371, 372f
Joule–Thompson (J–T) effect, 338

K

Kanglaite, 494
Kasabach–Merritt syndrome, 96, 97, 263
KCs. See Kupffer cells (KCs)
Klatskin tumors, 3, 249, 250
KLT Injection. See Kanglaite
KRAS mutations, 445
Kupffer cells (KCs), 226, 227, 453, 454f

L

Lactate dehydrogenase (LDH) level, 183, 184, 186
Lanreotide, 169
Laparoscopic approaches, 340
Laparoscopic cholecystectomy (LC), 76
Laparoscopic excision, 100
Laparoscopic hepatic resection, 103
Laparoscopic intervention, 100
Laparoscopic liver resections, 103, 105t
Laparoscopic mobilization, 289f
Laparoscopic partial hepatectomy, 287–288, 288f, 289f

Index

Laparoscopic surgery, 99, 103, 105t, 263
   GBC, 76
Laparoscopic ultrasonography, 287
Laparoscopic ultrasound, GBC, 67
Laparoscopy, 145
   GBC, 67
Laser ablation therapy, 340–342
   basic principles, 340
   complications and contraindications, 342
   real-time monitoring of, 345
   results, 341–342
   TACE and, 344
   technique, 340–341
Laser interstitial tumor therapy (LITT), 340–342
LC. *See* Laparoscopic cholecystectomy (LC)
LDH level. *See* Lactate dehydrogenase (LDH) level
LDLT. *See* Living donor liver transplant (LDLT)
Left hemihepatectomy
   incision and exploration, 280
   inflow control, 280–282f
   liver mobilization, 280, 280f
   outflow control, 281, 282f
   parenchymal transection, 281
Left lateral sectionectomy
   incision, 282
   inflow control, 282–283, 283f, 284f
   outflow control, 283
   parenchymal transection, 283, 285f
Left trisectionectomy, 283, 285
Left ventricular ejection fraction (LVEF), 416
Lenalidomide, 445
Lesions
   biopsies of, 98
   hepatic and biliary, 92f
LFTs. *See* Liver function tests (LFTs)
Ligamentum teres, 11
Ligation, 427
Lipiodol, 363–364
Liquefactant necrosis, 99
LITT. *See* Laser interstitial tumor therapy (LITT)
Liver
   hepatoblastoma. *See* Hepatoblastoma
   hepatocellular carcinoma. *See* Hepatocellular carcinoma
   hilus of, 13f
   immunologically privileged organ, 453–454, 454f
   NET, metastatic. *See* Neuroendocrine tumors (NETs), metastatic
   resection *vs.* transplantation
      CCA, 308–310
      HCC, 302–304, 303f, 304f
   transplantation, role of, 49–50, 49t
   in tumor metastases, 177
Liver cancer, 498
   antitumor effect in, 494
   conformal radiotherapy for, 384t
   hiccup due to, 499
   natural medicines used in, 495–496
   SBRT for, 383–385
   soy and, 498
   tumor antigens in, 457–459, 458t–459t
Liver-directed therapeutic modalities
   breast cancer, 180–182, 181t
   gastrointestinal tumors, 191–193, 192t
   genitourinary tumors, 195, 196t, 197–198
   GISTs, 189, 190t
   melanoma, 183–185, 184t
   soft-tissue sarcoma, 187–188
Liver-directed therapies, metastatic NET
   ablation therapies, 165–166
      cryoablation, 166–167
      ethanol ablation, 167
      microwave ablation, 167
      radiofrequency ablation, 166–167
   chemoembolization/radioembolization, 168
   hepatic resection, 160–161, 164–165
   hepatic transplantation, 167, 168t
Liver disease, clinical presentation of, 247–248
Liver failure, 147, 334
   patients with, 319, 320
Liver function, evaluation, 399
Liver function tests (LFTs), 33, 147
Liver irradiation tolerance in predicting RILD, 380
Liver lesions, 91
   imaging characteristics of, 95t
   management workup of, 94f
Liver mass
   colorectal cancer metastases, 253–255
   malignancy, 255–256
      workup of patients with history of, 253, 254f
   MR characteristics of hypervascular, 257t
   neuroendocrine metastases, 255
Liver metastases (LM), 177
   BCLM, 178–182, 179t, 181t
   breast cancer, 212f, 213f
   GISTs, 188–189, 190t
   melanoma, 182–186, 183t, 184t, 198
   ovarian tumors, 196–198, 197t
   pancreatic acinar cell carcinoma, 214f
   pre-RT CT image of, 379f
   SBRT for, 379
   STS, 186–188, 187t, 198
Liver regeneration, 379
Liver resection, 73–74, 119–121, 138, 145
   complications of, 139t
   morbidity and mortality of, 138
   postoperative care, 147
   safety limits for, Chinese consensus for, 120–121, 121f
Liver sinusoidal endothelial cells (LSECs), 453, 454f

Liver transaction, devices for, 104t
Liver transplantation, 122
    for CCA
        biliary tree distribution frequency of, 304, 305f
        description, 304
        MELD-based allocation, 305–306
        neoadjuvant therapy, 306
        patient selection, 304–305
        recurrence and survival, OLT, 306–308, 307t, 308f, 309f
        resection *vs.* transplantation, 308–310
    description, 293–294
    frequencies distribution of, 293, 293f
    for HCC
        description, 294, 294f
        International Consensus Conference on, 299t
        LDLT, 302
        listing criteria, 298, 300
        MELD, 297–298, 300f
        patient selection, 295–297, 295f–298f
        radiologic criteria, 297, 299t
        resection *vs.* transplantation, 302–304, 303f, 304f
        wait list management, 300–302, 301f
    for NETs
        description, 310
        MELD-based allocation, 312
        patient selection, 310–312, 310f, 311f, 311t
        recurrence and survival, OLT, 312–313, 313f, 313t
Liver tumors
    description, 453
    escape mechanisms, immune system, 454–456, 455f
Living donor liver transplant (LDLT), 302
LM. *See* Liver metastases (LM)
LN. *See* Lymph nodes (LN)
Local ablative therapy, 122–123, 321
Locoregional therapies, 319–321
    thermal ablation, 325, 342, 346
Loco-regional therapies, 15–16
LSECs. *See* Liver sinusoidal endothelial cells (LSECs)
LVEF. *See* Left ventricular ejection fraction (LVEF)
Lyman model in predicting RILD, 380
Lymph flow in gallbladder, 70
Lymph nodes (LN), 70–71, 71t, 78–79, 79t
    dissection, 74
Lymphoma, 242

M

MAA. *See* Macroaggregate albumin (MAA)
Macroaggregate albumin (MAA), 401–402
Magnetic resonance cholangiopancreatography (MRCP), 225, 249, 250f
    for cholangiocarcinoma, 262
    hilar cholangiocarcinoma, 6–7

Magnetic resonance–guided thermotherapy, 181–182
Magnetic resonance imaging (MRI), 144–145, 223, 225–227, 345, 373
    acupuncture, 481
    angiomyolipoma, 233
    biliary cystadenoma, 233
    biliary hamartoma, 232–233
    characteristics, 32, 32t
    cholangiocarcinoma, 239f, 240–241
    classic appearance of hemangioma on, 258f
    contrast-enhanced, 346
    cryoablation, 338–339
    cysts, 227, 228f
    diagnosis for adenoma, 259f
    encapsulated hepatocellular carcinoma, 117f
    fatty infiltration, 227
    fibrolamellar carcinoma, 238
    fibronodular hyperplasia lesion, 261f
    focal nodular hyperplasia, 230
    gallbladder carcinoma, 241, 241f
    GBC, 65–66
    guidance, use of, 341
    guided HIFU, 372
    hemangioma, 228–229
    hepatic adenoma, 92, 231–232
    hepatic epithelioid hemangioendothelioma and hepatic angiosarcoma, 242
    hepatic metastasis, 235
    hepatocellular carcinoma, 236–238, 237f
    hilar cholangiocarcinoma, 6–7
    laser ablation, 340, 341
    lymphoma, 242
    mass-forming PCC, 34, 36f
Malignancy
    diagnostic imaging of patients with no history, 255–256
    workup of patients
        with history, 253
        with no history of, 255, 256f
Malignant ascites, 68
Malignant lesions
    biliary cystadenocarcinoma, 242
    cholangiocarcinoma, 239–241
    fibrolamellar carcinoma, 238
    gallbladder carcinoma, 241, 241f
    hepatic angiosarcoma, 242
    hepatic epithelioid hemangioendothelioma, 242
    hepatic metastasis, 233–235
    hepatocellular carcinoma, 235–238
    lymphoma, 242
Malignant liver tumors, 211
Malignant solid lesions, diagnostic imaging of patients with, 261–262
Malignant tumors, 356

514　Index

Mammalian target of rapamycin (mTOR), 439
    inhibition, 440
    inhibitors, 169
    pathway, 446
MAP Kinase signaling, 418
Margin-negative resection, 14
Massage therapy, 480–481
    in liver cancer patients, 498
Mayo protocol, 307
MCT. *See* Microwave coagulation therapy (MCT)
MDCT protocols. *See* multidetector CT (MDCT) protocols
Mebendazole, 100
Medical internal radiation dosimetry
    compartmental macrodosimetry method, 410
    noncompartmental macrodosimetry method, 409–410
MEK1/2 inhibitors, 447
Melanoma, 182–186, 183t, 184t, 198
MELD. *See* Model for end-stage liver disease (MELD)
Melphalan-based isolated hepatic perfusion, 185
Memorial Sloan Kettering Cancer Center (MSKCC), 8, 16, 138, 142, 146, 147
Meta-analyses of HAI therapy, 430t
Metastases
    colorectal cancer, 253–255
    neuroendocrine, 255
    with unknown primary, 260–264
Metastatic cancers, clinical data for, 398
Metastatic liver cancers, 386
Metastatic neuroendocrine tumors
    multicenter studies, liver transplantation for, 311t
    OLT criteria, 313t
Metronidazole, 99
Microsphere therapy, 406t
Microwave ablation (MWA), 167, 335
Microwave coagulation therapy (MCT), 335–338
    basic principles, 335
    complications and contraindications, 337–338
    devices, 336
    results, 337
    vs. RFA, 337
    TACE and, 343, 344f
    technique, 335–336, 336f
Midgut carcinoid, 159t
Milan criteria, 295, 300f, 303
Milk thistle, 483
Mind-body modalities
    meditation, 483–484
    music therapy, 484–485
    relaxation techniques, 484
    yoga and hypnosis, 484
Mirizzi's syndrome, 62
Mitomycin C (MMC), 180
Mitoxantrone, 415
MMC. *See* Mitomycin C (MMC)

Mn-DPDP, 226
Model for end-stage liver disease (MELD), 297–298, 300f
    CCA, 305–306
    NETs, 312
Modern RT technology, 377
Modification of RECIST (mRECIST), 364
Morbidity rates of liver resection, 138
Mortality rates of liver resection, 138
MPR. *See* Multiplanar reformations (MPR)
MRCP. *See* Magnetic resonance cholangiopancreatography (MRCP)
MRI. *See* Magnetic resonance imaging (MRI)
MR-thermometry imaging, use of, 341
MSKCC. *See* Memorial Sloan Kettering Cancer Center (MSKCC)
mTOR. *See* Mammalian target of rapamycin (mTOR)
MUGA scans. *See* Multiple Gated Acquisition test (MUGA) scans
Multidetector CT (MDCT) protocols, 224–225
Multiplanar reformations (MPR), 224
Multiple Gated Acquisition test (MUGA) scans, 444
Multiple phase I-II studies, 440
Multiple therapeutic agents, 426
Multipronged needles, use of, 321–322
Multitined devices, use of, 329
Multivariate analyses of clinical factors, 142
MWA. *See* Microwave ablation (MWA)
Myelosuppression, 414

N

National Medicare Database, 140
Natural medicine
    laboratory studies of, 496–498
    treatment with combination, 495–496
Natural products, 482–483
NCNN metastases. *See* Noncolorectal, nonneuroendocrine (NCNN) metastases
NCRGI metastases. *See* Noncolorectal gastrointestinal (NCRGI) metastases
NCRLM. *See* Noncolorectal liver metastases (NCRLM)
NE cells. *See* Neuroendocrine (NE) cells
Neoadjuvant chemotherapy, 148, 254
Neoadjuvant therapy, CCA, 306
Neoplastic cysts, 100
Neoplastic disease, 91
NETs. *See* Neuroendocrine tumors (NETs)
Neuroendocrine cancers. *See* Colorectal cancer (CRC)
Neuroendocrine (NE) cells, 101, 157, 167
Neuroendocrine metastases, 255
    to liver, clinical data for, 398, 399f
Neuroendocrine tumors (NETs), 294, 355, 360, 364, 398
    description, 310
    MELD-based allocation, 312

Index   515

patient selection, 310–312, 310f, 311f, 311t
recurrence and survival, OLT, 312–313, 313f, 313t
Neuroendocrine tumors (NETs), metastatic, 157
   ablative therapies, 165–166
     cryoablation, 167
     ethanol ablation, 167
     microwave ablation, 167
     radiofrequency ablation, 166–167
   chemoembolization/radioembolization, 168
   chemotherapy, 169
   classification, 157–158
   cytoreduction in, 160, 164
   diagnosis and staging of, 158–160
   epidemiology, 158
   hepatic resection, 160–161, 164–165
   hepatic transplantation, 167, 168t
   management algorithm for, 170f
   management options, 158
   natural history and prognosis, 158
   new drugs and targets, 169–170
   somatostatin analogs, 168–169
   survival rate by hepatic resection, 161f
Nevin Stage Grouping, 68
New Zealand, CRC retrospective data from, 392
Nolatrexed, 416
Nonalcoholic fatty liver disease, 114
Nonanatomic resections, 287
Nonclassic radiation-induced liver disease, 380
Noncolorectal gastrointestinal (NCRGI) metastases, 189–190
Noncolorectal liver metastases (NCRLM), 177
Noncolorectal, nonneuroendocrine (NCNN) metastases, 177
   gastrointestinal tumors, 190–193
   genitourinary tumors, 194
Noncompartmental macrodosimetry method, medical internal radiation dosimetry, 409–410
Noncurative simple cholecystectomy, 76
Nondoxorubicin-based chemotherapy, 417
Nonfluoropyrimidine chemotherapy agents, HAI with, 430–431
Nonfluoropyrimidine drugs, HAI with, 426
Nonhepatic arteries, embolization of, 361
Nonobstructive jaundice, 248
Nonoperative biliary drainage, 264
Nonoperative palliation, 17–18
Nonseminomatous germ cell tumors (NSGCTs), 194, 196
Non-surgical treatment of HCC, 324
Nontarget embolization, 361
Normalized total dose (NTD), 380
Normal-tissue complication probability (NTCP), 380, 381
North American Neuroendocrine Society, 157

"No touch" technique, 12, 14
Novel therapeutics for liver tumors
   adjuvant therapy, biliary tumors and biologic agents, 445–447
   therapeutic biologic pathways
     combination therapy studies with antiangiogenics, 443–444
     cytoplasmic downstream targets, 439–440
     EGFR, 437–439
     inhibitors of proangiogenic pathway, 440–443
     second-line therapies, 444–445
NSGCTs. *See* Nonseminomatous germ cell tumors (NSGCTs)
Nutritional guidance, 482–483

O

Obstructive jaundice, 248
Obvious gallbladder cancer, 64
OCPs. *See* Oral contraceptive pills (OCPs)
Octreotide, 168, 169
Ocular melanoma, 182
Odds ratios (ORs) for liver cancer, 494
OLT. *See* Orthotopic liver transplantation (OLT)
Open surgical approaches, 340
Oral contraceptive pills (OCPs), 91, 97, 98, 258
   cessation of, 92–94
Organ Procurement and Transplantation Network criteria, 305–306
Orthotopic liver transplantation (OLT), 14, 15, 94, 293–294, 325
   CCA
     recurrence and survival, 306–308, 307t, 308f
     treatment algorithm of, 309f
   HCC, 298f, 303–304f
   metastatic NET, treatment of, 167
   recurrence and survival, NETs, 312–313, 313f, 313t
Ovarian cancer, 213
Ovarian tumors, 196–198, 197t
OX40, 457
Oxaliplatin, 443, 446
   phase I/II dose-escalation study, 392–393
Oxaliplatin-induced neurotoxicity, 417
Oxymatrine, 496

P

Pacemakers, 335
PAI therapy. *See* Percutaneous acetic acid injection (PAI) therapy
Pakistan, GBC in, 61–62
Palliation, GBC, 79–81, 80f
Palliative efficacy of radiotherapy, 14

Palliative therapy
    for hilar cholangiocarcinoma, 16–18
    palliative chemotherapy, 44, 45t
    palliative radiation therapy, 48–49, 48t
    regional intra-arterial chemotherapy, 44, 46t, 47, 47t, 48
Panax ginseng, 494
Pancreatic acinar cell carcinoma, liver metastases, 214f
Pancreatic cancer, 214–215
Pancreatic neuroendocrine tumors (PNET), 157, 158
Pancreatico-duodenectomy (PD), 74
Parenchymal transection, 288, 289
Partial response (PR), 346
Particle therapy, clinical experience of, 385
Partition method, 410
Pathologic analysis of liver metastases, 142
Patient selection, 360
Patients with intrahepatic ductal dilatation, 249–251, 249f
PCC. *See* Peripheral cholangiocarcinoma (PCC)
PD. *See* Pancreatico-duodenectomy (PD); Progressive disease (PD)
PD-L1. *See* Programmed death-1 (PD-L1)
PDT. *See* Photodynamic therapy (PDT)
PEI therapy. *See* Percutaneous ethanol injection (PEI) therapy
Pennes' bioheat equation, 326
Peptide-reactive CTLs, 459
Peptide receptor radionuclide therapy, 170
Percutaneous acetic acid injection (PAI) therapy, 324–325
Percutaneous biopsy, 262
Percutaneous cryoablation, 338, 339
Percutaneous endovascular embolization, 97
Percutaneous ethanol injection (PEI) therapy, 122, 165, 302
    basic principles, 321–322
    complications and contraindications, 324
    results, 323
    TACE and, 342–343
    technique, 322–323
Percutaneous laser ablation, 340, 341
Percutaneous transhepatic cholangiography (PTC), 6, 247, 250, 262
    direct cholangiography with, 7
Percutaneous transhepatic drain (PTD), 12f
Perihilar cholangiocarcinoma, TNM system for, 10t
Perioperative morbidity, 147
Perioperative mortality, 147
Peripheral cholangiocarcinoma (PCC)
    adjuvant therapy, 44
    assessment, 34, 38
    clinical presentation and demographics, 31–32, 31t
    diagnosis
        biochemical investigations, 33
        imaging characteristics, 32, 32t
        percutaneous biopsy, role of, 34
        radiographic studies, 33–34, 35f–36f
        tumor markers, 33
    etiology
        chemical carcinogen exposure, 29
        fibropolycystic liver disease, 29
        genetic factors, 26, 29f
        hepatolithiasis, 26
        parasitic infection, 26
        PSC, 29
        risk factors, 26, 28t
        viral hepatitis, 30
    incidence of, 30–31
    location and pathology
        histologic classification, 24, 26t
        histopathological and immunohistochemical features, 25, 28t
        subtype, 24, 27t
    natural history, 30, 30t
    palliative therapy
        palliative chemotherapy, 44, 45t
        palliative radiation therapy, 48–49, 48t
        regional intra-arterial chemotherapy, 44, 46t, 47, 47t, 48
    recurrence, 50
    staging of, 34, 37t, 38t
    surgical embryology and anatomy, 23–24, 24t, 25f
    transplantation, role of, 49–50, 49t
    treatment
        CT and MRI, 39
        hepatectomy and aggressive resection, 41–42
        laparoscopy, 39
        LN metastases, 42
        noncurative resection (R1 and R2 resection), 41, 41t
        results, 43
        routine LN sampling/dissection, 42–43, 43f
        surgical margin status, 39, 40f
PES. *See* Postembolization syndrome (PES)
PET. *See* Positron emission tomography (PET)
Peutz-Jeghers syndrome, 251
Pharmacokinetic studies of HAI, 426
Pharmacological principles for drug selection, HAI therapy, 425–426
Phase I/II dose-escalation, combination with
    irinotecan, 393
    oxaliplatin, 392–393
Photodynamic therapy (PDT), 16
PI3K/Akt pathway, 439, 446
PingXiao capsule, 495
PNET. *See* Pancreatic neuroendocrine tumors (PNET)
Polycystic disease, 257
Polyvinyl alcohol (PVA), 357
Porcelain gallbladder, 63

Portal vein embolization (PVE), 8, 145, 148, 255, 271–272, 391
Portal vein tumor thrombus, 360
Port site metastases, management of, 76–77
Positron emission tomography (PET), 160
    CCA, 305
    diagnosis of CRC, 253
    GBC, 66
Postablation syndrome, 334
Postcholecystectomy jaundice, 68
Postembolization imaging, 363–364
Postembolization syndrome (PES), 403, 404
Posthepatic resection, adjuvant HAI, 432–433, 433t
Postoperative care, 147
PR. *See* Partial response (PR)
Pretreatment evaluation/patient selection, 399–403
    cross-sectional radiologic evaluation, tumor, 399–400
    functional imaging, 400
    liver function, 399
Primary cancers, clinical data for, 398
Primary hepatic malignancies
    epithelioid hemangioendothelioma, 126–127
    HCC. *See* Hepatocellular carcinoma (HCC)
    hepatoblastoma. *See* Hepatoblastoma
    mesenchymal origin, 125–126
    primary angiosarcoma, 126
    primary hepatic lymphoma, 127
Primary liver cancer, HAI for, 433–434
Primary sclerosing cholangitis (PSC), 3–4, 29, 31, 249, 305
Primary tumor, removal of, 71
Proangiogenic pathway, inhibitors of, 440–443
Prognosis, 141, 142
Prognostic scoring system, 217
Prognostic variables, 140–142
Programmed death-1 (PD-L1), 455f, 456
Progression-free survival, 438
Progressive disease (PD), 346
Proper hepatic (PH) arteries, 360, 361f
Prophylactic cholecystectomy for asymptomatic gallstones, 82
Proton radiotherapy for liver cancer, 385
Pruritus, GBC, 64
PSC. *See* Primary sclerosing cholangitis (PSC)
Pseudolesions, 227
PTC. *See* Percutaneous transhepatic cholangiography (PTC)
PTD. *See* Percutaneous transhepatic drain (PTD)
Pulmonary complications, 147
PVE. *See* Portal vein embolization (PVE)

Q

Qianggan pills, 495
Quality of life (QoL), 477

R

Radiation cholecystitis, 405
Radiation dose
    determination of, 381
    fraction size of, 380–381
Radiation-induced liver disease (RILD), 377, 379–380
    after 3-D conformal RT, 383
    predicting, liver irradiation tolerance and Lyman model in, 380
Radiation pneumonitis, 405
Radiation therapy (RT), 378f
    clinical experience, 382–385
    for HCC, 381
    for liver cancers, 377, 386
    pre-RT CT image of liver metastasis, 379f
    transcatheter arterial chemoembolization before, 382
Radioembolization (RAE), 168, 356
Radiofrequency ablation (RFA), 166–167, 325–335, 369, 374
    basic principles, 325–326
    breast cancer, 180
    complications and contraindications, 334–335
    devices, 329–330
    gastrointestinal tumors, 193
    genitourinary tumors, 197, 198
    HCC, 302
    heat deposition in tissue, 326–327
    of hepatic colorectal metastases, 146, 146t
    results, 330–334, 331f–333f
    soft-tissue sarcoma, 187
    TACE, 343
    technique, 328–329
Radiological test, 114
Radiomicrosphere therapy (RMT), 391
    clinical data for
        hepatic colorectal metastases, 392–396
        hepatocellular carcinoma, 396–398
        primary and metastatic cancers, 398
    clinical practice of
        pretreatment evaluation/patient selection, 399–403
        treatment and follow-up procedures, 403
    Y-90 microsphere therapy, complications of, 403–406
Radiosensitivity of hepatocellular carcinoma, 377
Radiotherapy
    clinical efficacy of, 48, 48t
    GBC, 81–82
    palliative efficacy of, 14
    role of, 16
    use of, 15
Radix ginseng rubra, 494
RAD001 monotherapy, 447
Raf/MEK/ERK signaling pathway, 439
Raf-1, role of, 445f

Index

Randomized controlled trial (RCT), 114, 480
Randomized phase II, chemo-SIRT trial, 393
Randomized trial
    of HAI therapy, 429, 429t
        systemic chemotherapy *vs.* RMT plus chemotherapy, 396, 397f
Ranunculaceae, 497
Ras mutations, 439
RCC. *See* Renal cell carcinoma (RCC)
RCT. *See* Randomized controlled trial (RCT)
Real-time ultrasound, guidance, 322–323
Receptor dimerization, 437
Receptor tyrosine kinase (RTK) inhibitors, 438, 439, 442, 444
RECIST. *See* Response Evaluation Criteria in Solid Tumors (RECIST)
Recurrence of colorectal cancer liver metastases, 140
Regional chemotherapy *vs.* RMT plus regional chemotherapy, randomized phase III, 393, 394, 396, 396f
Renal cell carcinoma (RCC), 193–196
RES. *See* Reticuloendothelial system (RES)
Resection margin status, 141
Resin microspheres, 391
    phase II clinical trial, 393
Response evaluation criteria in solid tumors (RECIST), 364, 365f, 393
    criteria, 443
Reticuloendothelial system (RES), 226
RFA. *See* Radiofrequency ablation (RFA)
RF energy, 103
Right hemihepatectomy
    exploration and intraoperative hepatic ultrasonography, 272
    incision, 272, 273f
    inflow control, 274, 274f
    liver mobilization, 272, 273f, 274
    outflow control, 274, 275, 277f
    parenchymal transection, 276, 277, 278f–279f
Right phrenic artery, embolization of, 364
Right trisectionectomy, 283
Right upper quadrant (RUQ) pain, 247–248
RILD. *See* Radiation-induced liver disease (RILD)
RMT. *See* Radiomicrosphere therapy (RMT)
RTK inhibitors. *See* Receptor tyrosine kinase (RTK) inhibitors
RUQ pain. *See* Right upper quadrant pain (RUQ)

S

Salmonella typhi, 62
Sanhuang Xiexin Tang, 497–498
Sarcoma, 216–217, 216f, 217f
Schisandra, 498

SD. *See* Stable disease (SD)
SEER database. *See* Surveillance Epidemiology and End Results (SEER) database
Segmental adenomyomatosis, 63
Segmentectomy I, 285–286, 285f–287f
Selective internal radiation therapy (SIRT), 48, 393
Sepsis failure, 334
Sequential therapy, TACE, 344
SEREX. *See* Serological analysis of recombinant cDNA expression libraries (SEREX)
Serial serum, α-fetal protein, 92
Serological analysis of recombinant cDNA expression libraries (SEREX), 459
Serological tests, 114
Sex GBC, risk factors, 62
SHARP trial, 441, 442
Silibinin, 483
Silybum marianum, 495, 497
Single-agent therapy, 124
Single-arm study, 447
Single herbs, treatments with, 494–495
Single Positron Emission Computed Tomography (SPECT), 401
Sirolimus, 440, 447
SIRT. *See* Selective internal radiation therapy (SIRT)
Small particles of iron oxide (SPIO), 226
Soft-tissue sarcoma (STS), 186–188, 187t, 198
Soft-tissue sarcoma liver metastases (STSLM), 186–188, 187t
Solid benign liver tumors, treatment for, 262–263, 263t
Solid hepatic masses
    adenoma, 91–94, 93t
        focal nodal hyperplasia, 93t, 97–98
        hemangioma, 93t, 94–97, 96f
Solid malignant liver tumors, treatment for, 263
Solid masses, hepatic. *See* Hepatic solid masses
Solitary liver metastasis, 145
Somatostatin analogs, in metastatic NET treatment, 168–169
Somatostatin receptors (SSTR), 160
    scintigraphy, 223
Sophora flavescens Alt., 496
Sorafenib, 124, 418, 439–442, 444–445, 493, 496
Soy cancer, 498
SPECT. *See* Single Positron Emission Computed Tomography (SPECT)
SSTR. *See* Somatostatin receptors (SSTR)
Stable disease (SD), 346
Staging laparoscopy, 67
Staging systems, GBC, 68, 69t
Standard lymph node dissection, 74
Staplers, 102–103
Stereotactic body radiation therapy (SBRT)
    characteristics of, 383
        for liver

cancer, 383–385
   metastases, 379
STS. *See* Soft-tissue sarcoma (STS)
STSLM. *See* Soft-tissue sarcoma liver metastases (STSLM)
Sunitinib, 441, 442
Surgical palliation, 16–17
Surgical resection, 138, 211
   of hilar cholangiocarcinoma, 10–15
   of liver metastases, 212, 213
   of pancreatic cancer, 214–215
   results of, 14t
Surgical techniques and respective outcomes
   laparoscopic surgery, 103, 105t
   "open" surgery, 102–103
Surveillance Epidemiology and End Results (SEER) database, 4, 158
Suspected gallbladder cancer, 64, 71, 72f, 73–74, 73f
Swiss review reports, 103
SWOG 0514 study, 446
Synergistic effect of combined therapy, potential of, 464–465
Synergistic therapies for HCC treatment, 347
Systemic chemotherapy, 15, 215
   HAI with, 431–432, 431t
   vs. RMT plus chemotherapy, randomized trial of, 396, 397f

T

TACE. *See* Transcatheter arterial chemoembolization (TACE)
TACI. *See* Transcatheter arterial chemoinfusion (TACI)
Tai Chi, 485
Tamoxifen, 124
T cells, 455f, 456
TCM. *See* Traditional Chinese medicine (TCM)
Technetium-99m macroaggregated albumin scanning (Tc-99m MAA), 401–402, 402f
Tecoma stans, 496
Temsirolimus, 440
Testicular cancers, 194
TGF-β. *See* Transforming growth factor-β (TGF-β)
Therapeutic biologic pathways
   combination therapy studies with antiangiogenics, 443–444
   cytoplasmic downstream targets, 439–440
   EGFR, 437–439
   inhibitors of proangiogenic pathway, 440–443
   second-line therapies, 444–445
Thermal ablation techniques of HCC, 321
   combination therapies, 342–344, 344f
   cryoablation, 338–340
   follow-up assessment, 345–346

future directions, 346–347
immediate imaging assessment, 345
laser ablation, 340–342
MCT, 335–338, 336f
overview, 325
posttreatment imaging assessment, 345–346
RFA. *See* Radiofrequency ablation (RFA)
Thermodynamics law, 338
3-dimensional (3-D) conformal RT, 377, 381, 382
   clinical experience, 382–385
   hypofractionation by, 386
Thrombocytopenia, 417
Time to symptomatic progression (TTSP), 441
Time-to-tumor progression (TTP), 440
Tissue heating *vs.* cell death, 326
Tissue vaporization, 326, 327
Tivantinib, 438
TLG. *See* Total Lesion Glycolysis (TLG)
TN. *See* Tumor necrosis (TN)
TNF. *See* Tumor necrosis factor (TNF)
TNM. *See* Tumor node metastasis (TNM)
Total Lesion Glycolysis (TLG), 393, 395f
Toxicity of HAI chemotherapy, 428
Traditional Chinese medicine (TCM), 481, 493
   for treatment of liver cancer, 495–496
Transabdominal ultrasound, 5
Transcatheter arterial chemoembolization (TACE), 44, 264, 333–334, 356, 373, 494
   breast cancer, 180–181
   conventional, 357
   cryoablation and, 343–344
   gastrointestinal tumors, 193
   genitourinary tumors, 195–197
   HCC, 300, 301, 301f
   laser ablation and, 344
   lipiodol used as carrier in, 363
   MCT and, 343, 344f
   melanoma, 185, 186
   PEI and, 342–343
   before radiation therapy, 382
   RFA and, 343
   RT combined with, 381, 382
   soft-tissue sarcoma, 187, 188
   for treatment of liver cancer, 495–496
   use of, 342
Transcatheter arterial chemoinfusion (TACI), 44
Transcatheter intra-arterial therapy, categories of, 356
Transcatheter therapy for liver tumors, 355
   anatomic considerations, 360–363
   bland embolization, 357
   conventional transarterial chemoembolization, 356–357
   drug-eluting beads, 357, 359
   evaluation of response to regional therapies, 365t

Transcatheter therapy for liver tumors (*continued*)
    patient selection, 360
    postembolization imaging, 363–364
Transforming growth factor-β (TGF-β), 455f, 456
Transgenic mouse models, 438
Transplantation for cholangiocarcinoma, 14–15
Trisectionectomy, 283, 285
T-stage classification, 8–9, 9t
TTP. *See* Time-to-tumor progression (TTP)
TTSP. *See* Time to symptomatic progression (TTSP)
Tubulin polymerization, 416
Tumor antigens in primary liver cancer, 457–459, 458t–459t
Tumor burden, 295–297, 295f–298f
Tumor necrosis (TN), 440
Tumor necrosis factor (TNF), 455f, 456
Tumor node metastasis (TNM), 8, 158
    for perihilar cholangiocarcinoma, 10t
Tumors
    ablation, 374
    environmental factors, 455f, 456
    gynecological, 212–214
    markers, GBC, 67
    staging, 319–321
Turmeric. *See Curcuma longa*
Two-stage hepatectomy, 286–287
Tyrosine residues, 437

U

UCSF. *See* University of California, San Francisco (UCSF)
UFT, 415–416
UGIE. *See* Upper gastro-intestinal endoscopy (UGIE)
UICC. *See* International Union Against Cancer (UICC)
ULN. *See* Upper limit of normal (ULN)
Ultrasonography (US), 144, 223, 224
    angiomyolipoma, 233
    biliary cystadenoma, 233
    biliary hamartoma, 232
    cholangiocarcinoma, 239–240
    cysts, 227, 228
    fatty infiltration, 227
    fibrolamellar carcinoma, 238
    focal nodular hyperplasia, 229
    gallbladder carcinoma, 241, 241f
    hemangioma, 228, 229f
    hepatic adenoma, 230–231
    hepatic epithelioid hemangioendothelioma and angiosarcoma, 242
    hepatic metastasis, 233–234
    hepatocellular carcinoma, 235
    lymphoma, 242
Ultrasound (US), 98, 99, 369
    characteristics, 32, 32t
    GBC, 65
UMLM. *See* Uveal melanoma liver metastases (UMLM)
United Network for Organ Sharing (UNOS), Milan criteria, 295, 300f
United States
    CRC retrospective data from, 392
    HCC clinical data from, 397–398
University of California, San Francisco (UCSF), tumor burden criteria, 296, 297f
Unresectable colorectal hepatic metastases, HAI therapy, 428–429
Unsuspected gallbladder cancer, 64, 74–75, 75f
Upper gastro-intestinal endoscopy (UGIE), 80
    GBC, 66
Upper limit of normal (ULN), 442
US. *See* Ultrasonography (US); Ultrasound (US)
Uterine cancers, 213
Uveal melanoma, 182
Uveal melanoma liver metastases (UMLM), 182–186

V

Valley Lab/Covidien device, 329
VAS. *See* Visual Analogue Scale (VAS)
Vascular encasement, 5
Vascular endothelial growth factor (VEGF), 455f, 456
    pathway, 446
Vascular endothelial growth factor receptor (VEGFR), 439
Vascular malformation, 97
Vascular resections, 74
VEGF. *See* Vascular endothelial growth factor (VEGF)
VEGFR. *See* Vascular endothelial growth factor receptor (VEGFR)
Vein resection, 12
"Veno-occlusive disease," 404
Viscum album, 494–495
Visual Analogue Scale (VAS), 498
Viverrini, 4
von Meyenburg's complex, 232

W

Wait list management for HCC, 300–302, 301f
Wedge resections, 142
Whole tumor cells, 457
World Health Organization (WHO), 157, 364
Wrist–ankle acupuncture, 498–499

X

Xanthogranulomatous cholecystitis, 63, 67

Y

Yellow trumpetbush. *See Tecoma stans*
Yttrium-90 (Y-90) microsphere therapy, 391, 392f
　adverse events/complications, 406t
　body surface area method, 403, 409
　clinical data for
　　hepatic colorectal metastases, 392–396
　　hepatocellular carcinoma, 396–398
　　neuroendocrine metastases, 398, 399f
　　primary and metastatic cancers, 398
　complications of, 403–405
　HCC data from, 396–398
　medical internal radiation dosimetry, compartmental macrodosimetry method, 403, 409–410
　products in clinical use, 391–392
　RMT, clinical practice of, 399–403
　therapy, complications of, 403–406
Yttrium-90 TheraSpheres®, 168

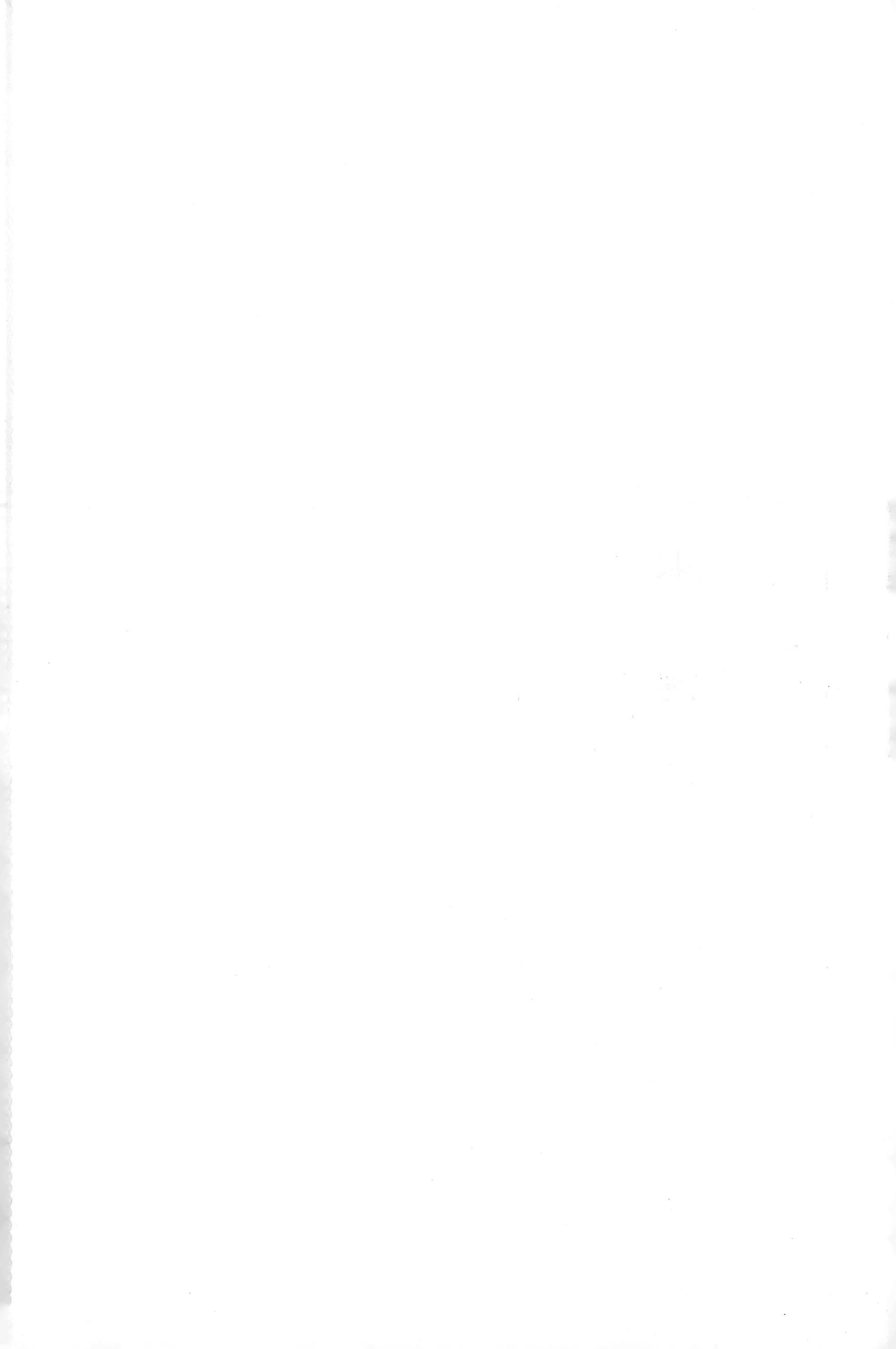